Cardiology
1996

WILLIAM C. ROBERTS, MD
Executive Director
Baylor Cardiovascular Institute
Dean, A. Webb Roberts Center for Continuing Education
Baylor University Medical Center
Dallas, Texas
Editor in Chief, The American Journal of Cardiology
Editor in Chief, The Baylor University Medical Center Proceedings

JAMES T. WILLERSON, MD
Edward Randall III Professor and Chairman
Department of Internal Medicine
University of Texas Medical School at Houston
Chief of Medical Service
Hermann Hospital
Medical Director and Director of
Cardiology Research
The Texas Heart Institute
Editor in Chief, Circulation

THOMAS P. GRAHAM, JR, MD
Director of Pediatric Cardiology
Vanderbilt University Medical Center
Nashville

WILLIAM W. PARMLEY, MD
Professor of Medicine
University of California
San Francisco, School of Medicine
Chief of Cardiology
Moffitt/Long Hospital, San Francisco
Editor in Chief, Journal of the
American College of Cardiology

CHARLES E. RACKLEY, MD
Professor of Medicine
Division of Cardiology
Department of Medicine
Georgetown University Medical Center
Washington, D.C.

DEAN T. MASON, MD
Physician in Chief, Western Heart Institute
Chairman, Department of
Cardiovascular Medicine
St. Mary's Medical Center
at Golden Gate Park, San Francisco
Editor in Chief, American Heart Journal

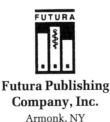

**Futura Publishing
Company, Inc.**
Armonk, NY

Copyright © 1996
Futura Publishing Company, Inc.

Published by
Future Publishing Company, Inc.
135 Bedford Road
Armonk, New York 10504

ISBN #: 0-87993-643-6
ISSN #: 0275-0066

Every effort has been made to ensure that the information in this book is as up to date and accurate as possible at the time of publication. However, due to the constant developments in medicine, neither the author, nor the editor, nor the publisher can accept any legal or any other responsibility for any errors or omissions that may occur.

Printed in the United States of America.

∞ Printed on acid-free paper.

Preface

Cardiology 1996 is the 16th book to be published in this series. In contains summaries of 784 articles, all published in 1995. A total of 20 medical journals (Table 1) were examined and at least 1 and usually many articles were summarized from each journal. The number of articles summarized by each of the 6 authors are listed in Table 2. All of Dr. Willerson's submissions were from *Circulation;* Dr. Parmley's from *The Journal of the American College of Cardiology;* and Dr. Mason's from *The American Heart Journal.* The contributions of Dr. Graham and myself were from a variety of medical journals. The summaries from each contributor were submitted to me, organized into the various sections in each of the 10 chapters, and edited.

A book of this type is made possible because of unselfish contributions from several individuals, none of whom is rewarded by authorship. I am enormously grateful to Anita Rawlinson for typing the summaries contributed by me; to Angie Esquivel, Leslie Flatt, Azora L. Irby, and Joy Phillips also for typing many summaries.

The present book will end my tenure as the "main man" on this project after 16 years in this role. Dr. James T. Willerson will take over beginning with *Cardiology 1997.* I have enjoyed the role for the last 16 years, but that is enough. Dr. Willerson has asked me to continue to provide summaries of the articles from *The American Journal of Cardiology* for *Cardiology 1997,* and of course, I am delighted to do so. Dr. Willerson, I am certain, will move this book forward and upward and I wish him the best. I would like to thank the publisher for their understanding and support, and also thank Ann Kerr for her excellent copy editing.

William C. Roberts, MD

Tables 1. Journals Containing Articles Summarized in *Cardiology 1996.*

1. *American Heart Journal*
2. *American Journal of Cardiology*
3. *American Journal of Medicine*
4. *American Journal of Surgery*
5. *Annals of Internal Medicine*
6. *Annals of Thoracic Surgery*
7. *Archives of Internal Medicine*
8. *Arteriosclerosis and Thrombosis*
9. *British Heart Journal*
10. *British Medical Journal*
11. *Chest*
12. *Circulation*
13. *Clinical Therapeutics*
14. *European Heart Journal*
15. *Journal of the American College of Cardiology*
16. *Journal of the American Medical Association*
17. *Journal of Thoracic and Cardiovascular Surgery*
18. *Lancet*
19. *Medicine*
20. *New England Journal of Medicine*

Table 2. Contributions of the Six Authors to CARDIOLOGY 1996

	Author	1	2	3	4	5	6	7	8	9	10	TOTALS	
1	WCR	70	48	26	21	20	16	10	2	9	30	252	(32.14%)
2	JTW	13	50	27	16	3	6	11	2	10	14	152	(19.39%)
3	TPG, Jr	0	0	0	0	0	0	1	118	0	4	123	(15.69%)
4	WWP	0	35	23	10	0	4	1	0	10	5	88	(11.22%)
5	CER	14	27	30	8	0	1	0	0	4	1	85	(10.84%)
6	DTM	0	34	11	24	0	4	1	1	3	6	84	(10.71%)
	TOTALS	97	194	117	79	23	31	24	123	36	60	784	(100.00%)
	Figures	12	34	30	5	4	5	0	1	1	11	103	
	Tables	5	16	16	7	5	0	0	1	0	0	50	

Contents

Preface iii

1. **Factors Causing, Accelerating, or Preventing Coronary Arterial Atherosclerosis**

Risk Factors—General and/or Multiple 1
Blood Lipids 5

    Determining Atherosclerotic Risk 5
    Low Values 9
    Lipoprotein(a) 11
    Apolipoprotein E 11
    High-Density Lipoprotein Subfractions 12
    Effects of Fasting 13
    Effects of Insulin Levels 13
    In Coronary Artery Disease 14
    In Stroke 15
    In Suicide, Parasuicide, and Trauma 15
    In Hairy-Cell Leukemia 16
    Frequency of Hypothyroidism 16
    Effect of Running 17
    Effect of Soy Protein Intake 18
    Effects of Naproxen and Nabumetone 18

Low-Fat and/or Low-Cholesterol Diet 19
Drug Therapy of Hyperlipidemia 22

    Lovastatin—Cost Effectiveness 22
    Pravastatin 23
    Fluvastatin 24
    Simvastatin vs. Gemfibrozil 24
    Colestipol 27
    Colestipol + Lovastatin 27
    Colestipol + Lovastatin vs. Colestipol + Niacin 28
    Colestipol + Psyllium Mucilloid 28
    Cholestyramine vs. Cholestyramine + Lovastatin vs. Lovastatin 29
    Niacin 29
    Antioxidant Vitamins 29
    Low-Density Lipoprotein Apheresis 30

Obesity, Body Fat, Body Weight, and Weight Change 31
Physical Activity and Fitness 34
Cigarette Smoking 36

    Prevalence in USA 36
    Nicotine Therapy 36
    Cessation and Weight Gain 38

Effects on Endothelial Function 38
Effect on Myocardial Blood Flow 39
Passive Smoking 40

Diabetes Mellitus 41
Endothelial-Cell Dysfunction 42
Estrogen and Estrogen Replacement Therapy 43
Homocysteine 46
Left Ventricular Hypertrophy 49
Miscellaneous Topics 50

Fetal and Infant Growth 50
Risk Factors in Black and White Men 50
French Paradox 51
Fibrinolytic Parameters 51
Dietary Fish and Mercury 51
Shift Work 52
Anti-Cardiolipid Antibodies 53
Mutation in Gene Coding or Coagulation Factor 53
Angiotensin-Converting–Enzyme Gene Polymorphism 54
Green Tea 55

2. Coronary Artery Disease

Miscellaneous Topics 61

Modifying Risk Factors After Events 61
Preoperative Assessment 61
American vs. Canadian Functional Status 62
Survival in Various Time Periods 62
Heart Rate Variability and Depression 63
Costs of Psychological Distress 63
Dilatation of Atherosclerotic Arteries 64
Myocardial Bridges 64
In Heterozygous Familial Hypercholesterolemia 65
Cocaine-Associated Myocardial Ischemia—Review 65
Waiting Times for Cardiovascular Procedures 65
Intravascular Ultrasound in Coronary Aneurysms 66
Energy Expenditure From Household Tasks 67

Detection 67

Costs of Diagnostic Tests 67
Coronary Calcium by Ultrafast Computed Tomography 69
Pharmacologic Stress Testing 71
Stress Echocardiography 72
Transesophageal Echocardiography 72
Intravascular Ultrasonography 73
Angiographic Predictors of New Narrowings 75
Angioscopy in "Normal" Coronary Arteries 75
Left Main "Equivalent" Disease 76

Prognosis 77

    Exercise Testing 77
    Heart Rate Response to Mental Stress 78
    Coronary Patency 78

Unstable Angina Pectoris 79

    Cardiologist vs. Internist Management 79
    Risk Stratification 79
    Angiographic Narrowing Compared with Other Coronary Subsets ...80
    Angiographic Progression 81
    Angiography in Octogenarians 82
    Intracoronary Angioscopy and/or Ultrasonography 83
    Acute Thrombotic Reactant Markers 84
    Early Morning Ischemic Threshold 84
    P-Selectin 85
    Diltiazem vs. Glyceryl Trinitrate 86
    Subcutaneous Heparin vs. Intravenous Heparin vs. Aspirin 86
    Hirulog Treatment 88

Stable Angina Pectoris 88

    Patient Preferences in Treatment 88
    Risk of Infarction or Sudden Death 89
    Narrowing Progression 89
    Percutaneous Coronary Angioscopy 90
    Circadian Variation in Coronary Tone 91
    Intensive Exercise and Low-Fat Diet 92

Silent Myocardial Ischemia 92

    With Mental Stress 92
    With Exercise Testing 93
    Magnitude of Myocardial Dysfunction 94
    Outcome 94

Variant, Spastic, or Microvascular Angina 95
Diet and Drugs for Myocardial Ischemia 98

    Aspirin 98
    Nitrates 99
    Diltiazem 102
    Metoprolol vs. Diltiazem 102
    Metoprolol vs. Nifedipine 103
    Metoprolol vs. Verapamil (on Platelet Aggregability) 103
    Nitroglycerin vs. Nitroprusside (on Platelet Aggregability) 104
    Amlodipine vs. Atenolol vs. Amlodipine + Atenolol 104
    Low–Molecular Weight Heparin vs. Regular Heparin or Aspirin 105
    Lovastatin 105
    Lovastatin + Cholestyramine vs. Lovastatin + Probucol 106
    Pravastatin 106
    Simvastatin 110

n-3 vs. n-6 Fatty Acids 110
Estrogen 112
Zatebradine 112

Coronary Angioplasty vs. Bypass..113
Percutaneous Transluminal Coronary Angioplasty 119

Transradial Approach 119
In Rest Angina Pectoris 119
For Saphenous Venous Graft Narrowing 120
In Men vs. Women 120
Sixty-Millimeter Balloon..121
Gender Bias? 121
In-Laboratory Closure 121
Platelet IIb/IIIa Inhibitor Therapy..123
Treatment with Bivalirudin (Hirulog) Afterwards 124
Novel Hemostatic Device..124
Intravascular Ultrasonic Findings Afterwards...............................125
In-Hospital Costs...125
*Relation Between Procedure Volume and Length of Hospital Stay
and Complications* 126
Quality of Life Afterwards..128
Long-term Follow-up...129
Influence of Diabetes on Outcome..130
Restenosis 131

Directional Coronary Atherectomy 136
Coronary Stenting 141
Coronary Artery Bypass Grafting...148

Review..148
Society of Thoracic Surgeons National Cardiac Database 148
Relation of Volume to Outcome 149
Regionalization of Bypass Surgery 150
Wait Before Bypass..150
In Octogenarians..151
In Chronic Obstructive Pulmonary Disease 152
After Successful Angioplasty 152
After Failed Angioplasty 153
After Failed Stenting 153
In Familial Hypercholesterolemia 154
With Peripheral Vascular Disease 154
*Concomitant Insertion of an Implantable Cardioverter
Defibrillator*..155
Concomitant Carotid Endarterectomy 155
Concomitant Abdominal Aortic Aneurysmal Surgery....................156
Body Size and Outcome 157
Predicting Atrial Fibrillation Afterwards 158
Left Ventricular Function Afterwards...158
Recurrence of Angina Afterwards...159
Risk Factors Afterwards 159

Deep Vein Thrombosis Afterwards..159
Rehabilitation Afterwards 160
Physical and Psychological Function Afterwards 161
Restenotomy for Bleeding..161
Blood Urea Nitrogen as Mortality Determinant.............................161
Thyroid Hormone Treatment Afterwards..163
Survival After Left Main Narrowing 163
Graft Patency by Computed Tomography...164
Venous Graft Angioplasty and Atherectomy 165
Late Survival 166
Minimal Access Bypass 166
Decline in Mortality...166
Without Cardiopulmonary Bypass...167

3. Acute Myocardial Infarction

General Topics 181

Variation in Use of Cardiac Procedures...181
Effect of Psychosocial Factors...186
Relation to Smoking 187
Relation to Gray Hair, Baldness, and Facial Wrinkling.................187
Effect of Previous Aspirin Therapy...188
Risk of Serum C3 Levels...189
Quality of Care of Medicare Patients 190
Characteristics When "Unrecognized"...190
Decreasing Mortality...194
Associated With Cocaine Use 195

Diagnosis and Early Testing..195

Creatine Kinase–MB Isoenzyme, Troponin T, Myoglobin, and
    Leukocyte Differential...195
Echocardiography..197
Heart Rate Variability...198
Predictors of Non–Q-Wave Infarction..198
Early vs. Late Responders 199
Relation of Pain Location and Infarct Site......................................200

Prognostic Indices 200

Ischemic Time..200
Blood Pressure 201
Previous Angina Pectoris...202
When in Young Adults 204
ST Segment Elevation on Holter Monitoring 204
Maximal Exercise Testing 204
Older Age 206
Sex 207
Depression...207
Neurohumoral Factors...208
Infarct Size 209

Signal-Averaged Electrocardiography 209
Pharmacological Echocardiography 210
Exercise Capacity 211

Complications 212

Angina Pectoris Afterwards 212
Right Ventricular Infarction 212
Congestive Heart Failure 212
Cardiogenic Shock 213
Cardiac Rupture 214

General Treatment 215

Regional Differences in Management 215
Aspirin 216
Oral Anticoagulant 218
β-Blocker 220
Aspirin, β-blocker, Angiotensin-Converting Enzyme Inhibitor,
  Calcium Antagonist, and Anticoagulant 220
Magnesium Sulfate 221
Antiarrhythmic Drug 221
Theophylline 222
Captopril 222
Captopril + Mononitrate + Magnesium Sulfate 223
Enalapril 226
Trandolapril 227
Zofenopril 228
Insulin-Glucose Infusion 229
L-Carnitine 230
Partial Ileal Bypass 230

Thrombolysis 230

Review 230
Variation in Use 230
In Men vs. Women 231
In Menstruating Women 236
In Smokers vs. Non Smokers 237
Effect of Previous Angina on Outcome 237
Tissue Plasminogen Activator 238
Tissue Plasminogen Activator vs. Streptokinase 242
Anistreplase 243
Reteplase vs. Streptokinase 243
Reteplase vs. Alteplase 244
Streptokinase + Hirulog + Heparin 245
Recombinant Staphylokinase vs. Alteplase 246
Recombinant Urokinase Type Plasminogen Activator (Saruplase).246
Patency Afterwards 246
Effect of Nitroglycerin 247
Elevated ST Segment Augmentation and Resolution 248
Biochemical Markers of Reperfusion 248

Q-Wave Regression Afterwards...249
Impaired Tissue Reperfusion...249
Recurrent Myocardial Ischemia or Infarction Afterwards.............250
Early and Late Mortality..251

Coronary Angioplasty 254

Coronary Bypass 256
Rehabilitation..257

4. Arrhythmias, Conduction Disturbances, Syncope, and Cardiac Arrest

Atrial Fibrillation/Flutter 269

Historical Development 269
Risk Factors for Development 269
Prevalence, Ages, and Gender 270
Natural History 270
Cerebral Infarction..271
Anticoagulant Therapy..273
Warfarin and Aspirin 275
Warfarin vs. Quinidine or Amiodarone..................................276
Diltiazem 276
Cardioversion 277
Radiofrequency Catheter Ablation.......................................278
Treatment of Resistant Type 279
Atrial Thrombi 280

Supraventricular Tachycardia with or without the Short P-R Interval
Syndrome 280

Review...280
Incidence of Associated Atrial Fibrillation 281
Propafenone 281
Sotalol...281

Ventricular Arrhythmias...282

Prognostic Predictors 282
Localizing the Arrhythmic Origin..285
Patterns of Coronary Narrowing 285
Amiodarone...286
Amiodarone vs. Bretylium..287
Sotalol vs. Procainamide..287
Radiofrequency Catheter Ablation.......................................288

Cardiac Arrest..288

Cardiopulmonary Resuscitation..288
In Morbid Obesity 290
Effect of Smoking Cessation..290
Effect of β-Blockers...291
Effect of n-3 Polyunsaturated Fatty Acids 291

Effect of Heart Rate Variability...292
Frequency of "Active" Coronary Lesions 292

Syncope 293

Importance of History for Delineation of Types 293
Provocation Maneuvers 293
In Athletes 295
Pindolol 295
Cardiac Pacing...296

Long Q-T Interval Syndrome..296

Review..296

Genetic Abnormality..296
Bundle Branch Block..299
Heart Block...300
Pacemakers...300
Cardioverters-Defibrillators 301
Miscellaneous..308

Palpitations 308
Ambulatory Electrocardiography...309
Amiodarone..309

5. Systemic Hypertension

General Topics 315

Drugs, Poisons, and Foods Increasing Blood Pressure.....................315
*Effects of Nonsteroidal Anti-inflammatory Drugs on Blood
Pressure*..315
Implications of Small Reductions...316
Relation of Blood Pressure and Mortality 316
Association of Midlife Pressure and Late-Life Cognition 317
Atrial Natriuretic Peptide..317
Endothelial Function 317

Treatment 319

Regular Exercise..319
Trends in Management..319
Risk of Myocardial Infarction from Antihypertensive Agents 320
Change of Treatment 321
Effects of Drugs on Serum Lipids 324
Effect on Proteinuria and Renal Function 325
Thiazides...326
Enalapril..326
Losartan...328
Losartan ± Captopril..331
Dexamethasone (for Alcohol-Induced Hypertension) 331

6. Valvular Heart Disease

Mitral Stenosis 335

    Massive Calcium in Left Atrial Wall.................................335
    Percutaneous Balloon Valvuloplasty.............................335

Mitral Regurgitation...337

    Quantification by Echocardiography.............................337
    Quantification by Magnetic Resonance Imaging 338
    Operative Valve Repair 338

Mitral Valve Prolapse 338
Aortic Valve Stenosis...339
Aortic Regurgitation..340
Infective Endocarditis 340
Valve Replacement...342

    St. Jude Medical Prosthesis...342
    Porcine Bioprostheses...343
    Tricuspid Valve Replacement..345
    Aortic Valve Replacement with Small Aortic "Root" 346
    Pericardial Aortic Valve...347
    Homovital Homografts for Aortic Valve Replacement 348
    Warfarin ± Dipyridamole..348
    Mechanical Valve Thrombosis.......................................349
    Mechanical Valve Strut Fracture...................................350
    Reoperations...351

7. Myocardial Heart Disease

Idiopathic Dilated Cardiomyopathy.....................................355

    Risk of Alcoholic Type by Gender..................................355
    With Ventricular Tachycardia 355
    Effect of Exercise Training 356
    Location of Gene in the Familial Variety.......................357
    Interleukin-2 Receptor Levels.......................................357

Hypertrophic Cardiomyopathy...357

    Prevalence 357
    Natural History 358
    Response to Isoproterenol 358
    Paced Electrogram Fractionation..................................359
    Genetic Studies 360
    Nonsurgical Reduction of Septum..................................361
    Operative Treatment...361
    Pseudoform After Tacrolimus Therapy...........................362

Association with a Condition Affecting Primarily a Noncardiac
  Structure(s)..362

    HIV Involvement 362

Myotonic Dystrophy...363
β-Thalassemia Major 364

Miscellaneous Topics 364

Right Ventricular Dysplasia 364
Idiopathic Restrictive Cardiomyopathy...365
Immunosuppression for Myocarditis...365
Hepatitis C Viral Infection 366

8. Congenital Heart Disease

Atrial Septal Defect..369
Atrioventricular Septal Defect...370
Ventricular Septal Defect...372
Pulmonic Valve Stenosis..374
Tetralogy of Fallot...374
Pulmonic Valve Atresia...378
Complete Transposition...380
Corrected Transposition 383
Truncus Arteriosus 384
Valvular Aortic Stenosis..384
Supravalvular Aortic Stenosis..385
Aortic Valve Atresia and Other Hypoplastic Left-Sided Cardiac
      Syndromes...385
Aortic Isthmic Coarctation 387
Anomalous Pulmonary Venous Connection 389
Coronary Arterial Anomaly...390
Mitral Valve Disease 392
Arrhythmias and Conduction Defects 393
Transhepatic Cardiac Catheterization...396
Intravascular Stents..397
Cavopulmonary Anastomotic Procedures 399
Homograft or Allograft..402
Fontan Procedure..403
Miscellaneous Topics 406

*Single-Stage Repair of Aortic Arch Obstruction and Associated
      Defects*..406
Systemic Obstruction in Univentricular Heart 407
Norwood Procedure for Nonhypoplastic Left-Sided Anomalies......408
Extracorporeal Membrane Oxygenation...408
*Neurological Status After Hypothermic Cardiac Arrest or
      Low-Flow Cardiopulmonary Bypass* 409
Modified Blalock-Taussig Shunt..409
Coronary Sinus Atresia 410
Thoracoscopic Surgery...410
Intra-aortic Spring Coll Loops..411
Renal Replacement Therapy After Operation..................................411
Right Ventricular Function 411
Associated Pulmonary Arteriovenous Malformation.......................412

Cardiac Isomerism 412
Prenatal Echocardiography in Left-Sided Obstruction....................413
Intravascular Ultrasonic Imaging 413
In-Hospital Mortality and Hospital-Case Volume 414
Fetal Cardiac Neoplasms 414
Tuberous Sclerosis and Cardiac Rhabdomyoma..............................414
Kawasaki Disease..415
Knowledge of Infective Endocarditis Prophylaxis 415
Superior Vena Caval Flow in Normal Children.............................416

9. Congestive Heart Failure

General Topics 425

Rate of Hospitalization...425
Preventing Readmission 425
Home Care...426
Survival While Awaiting Transplantation.................................426
Cheyne-Stokes Respirations 427
Sleep-Disordered Breathing..427
Right Ventricular Ejection Fraction as Prognostic Factor................428
Skeletal Muscle Oxygenation...428
Neurohumoral Variability 429
Signal-Averaged Electrocardiogram and Prolonged QRS 430
Endothelial-Cell Dysfunction 430
Tumor Necrosis Factor Soluble Receptors 431
Implantable Defibrillators 432

Treatment 432

ACE Inhibitors—Trials 432
Captopril vs. Digoxin..433
Enalapril..433
Losartin...434
Losartin vs. Enalapril...434
Fosinoprin 435
Digoxin + Diuretic + ACE Inhibitor 435
Ibopamine + Digoxin 436
Carvedilol 437
Metoprolol 438
Candoxatrilat 438
Nitrate + Hydralazine..438
Amiodarone...439
Thiamine 439
L-Arginine...440
Respiratory Muscle Training 440
Dual-Chamber Pacing..441
Left Ventricular Assist Device...441

10. Miscellaneous Topics

Cardiac and/or Pulmonary Transplantation.................................445

Pericardial Heart Disease...457
   Tamponade 457
   In AIDS..459

Venous Thrombosis and/or Pulmonary Embolism.............................459
Aortic Disease..461
   The Marfan Syndrome...461
   Protruding Plaque 463
   Abdominal Aortic Aneurysm 463
   Dissection 465

Peripheral Arterial Disease..466
   Carotid Arteries...466
   Leg Arteries 469

Odds and Ends...470
   Left Atrial Size and Stroke..470
   Diagnosing Left Atrial Thrombi 471
   Atrial Septal Aneurysm...471
   Energy of Heavy Snow Shoveling 473
   Carcinoid Heart Disease..473
   Primary Pulmonary Hypertension 474
   Raynaud's Disease 475
   Necropsy Findings in Octogenarians...475

Author Index 487
Subject Index...494

Cardiology
1996

Conversion of Units

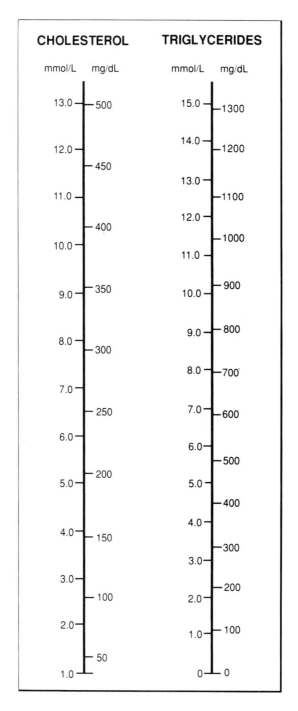

CHOLESTEROL

TRIGLYCERIDES

Cholesterol mg/dL = mmol/L x 38.6
Triglyceride mg/dL = mmol/L x 88.5

1

Factors Causing, Accelerating, or Preventing Coronary Arterial Atherosclerosis

Risk Factors—General and/or Multiple

A national program for detection and control of systemic hypertension was implemented in the 1970s, and a similar program for control of hypercholesterolemia has been implemented in recent years. Nieto and associates[1] from Baltimore, Maryland; Barcelona, Spain; Chapel Hill and Winston-Salem, North Carolina; Bethesda, Maryland; and Minneapolis, Minnesota, studied the levels of awareness, treatment, and control of these conditions in US population samples during a 3-year period (1987–1989) (Tables 1–1 and 1–2). The levels of awareness, treatment (by medication), and adequate control of hypertension (systolic BP, ≥140 mm Hg; diastolic BP, ≥90 mm Hg; or antihypertensive medication) and hypercholesterolemia (serum cholesterol level, ≥6.21 mmol/L [≥240 mg/dL], or lipid-lowering medication) were studied among participants in the baseline examination of the Atherosclerosis Risk in Communities Study, including 15 739 individuals aged 45 to 64 years. Eighty-four percent of the hypertensive subjects and 42% of the hypercholesterolemic subjects were aware of their conditions. Overall, 50% of the hypertensive subjects and only 4% of the hypercholesterolemic subjects had their conditions both treated and controlled. Rates of hypertension prevalence, awareness, and control remained stable during the 3-year study period. Hypercholesterolemia prevalence decreased from 30% in 1987 to 25% in 1989; its awareness increased from 31% to 50% during the same period. Hypertensive women were more likely than hypertensive men to be aware of their condition and obtain treatment, whereas hypercholesterolemia awareness was higher in men than in women. Hypertension awareness was highest in black women, but black hypertensive subjects were less likely than white patients to be treated and to have their hypertension controlled. Black hypercholesterolemic subjects were less likely to be either aware or treated. After the recent implementation of the National Cholesterol Education Program, the levels of awareness, treatment, and control of hypercholesterolemia are improving at a high rate, although they are still substantially lower than those for hypertension.

To examine the association between a variety of baseline lifestyle and biological factors in a middle-aged cohort of Japanese-American men and the 20-year incidence rates of total atherosclerotic end points and each of the initial clinical manifestations of this disease, including fatal and nonfatal CAD, angina pectoris, thromboembolic strokes, and aortic aneurysms, Goldberg and associ-

1

TABLE 1-1. Baseline Prevalence of Hypertension and Hypercholesterolemia by Sex, Race, Age, and Examination Year: The Atherosclerosis Risk in Communities Study, 1987 to 1989

	Hypertension*		Hypercholesterolemia†	
	No. (%)	P	No. (%)	P
All Subjects	**5494** (35)		**4202** (27)	
Sex				
M	2428 (35) ⎤	0.23	1693 (24) ⎤	<0.001
F	3066 (35) ⎦		2509 (29) ⎦	
Race				
W	3121 (27) ⎤	<0.001	3068 (27) ⎤	0.12
B	2373 (56) ⎦		1134 (28) ⎦	
Age, y				
45-54	2342 (28) ⎤	<0.001	1840 (23) ⎤	<0.001
55-64	3152 (43) ⎦		2362 (32) ⎦	
Year				
1987	1471 (35) ⎤	0.13‡	1226 (30) ⎤	<0.001‡
1988	1829 (34)		1481 (28)	
1989	2194 (36) ⎦		1495 (25) ⎦	

*Blood pressure of 140 mm Hg or more systolic or 90 mm Hg or more diastolic, or antihypertensive treatment.

†Total serum cholesterol level of 6.21 mmol/L (240 mg/dL) or more, or lipid-lowering treatment. Cholesterol levels are adjusted for laboratory drift (see the "Subjects and Methods" section).

‡Cochran's trend test.

Reproduced with permission from Nieto et al.[1]

ates[2] from Worcester, Massachusetts; Honolulu, Hawaii; Bethesda, Maryland; and Novato, California, studied 2710 Japanese-American men aged 55–64 years at the time of the initial clinical examination of the Honolulu Heart Program (1965–1968) and who were free from evidence of CAD, cerebrovascular disease, cancer, or aortic aneurysms (Table 1-3). Among the men studied, 602 atherosclerotic events developed during the 23-year period of follow-up (1965 through 1988). After adjustment for each of the baseline characteristics examined, significant positive associations between quartile cutoffs of body mass index (BMI), systolic BP, serum levels of cholesterol, triglycerides, glucose, and uric acid, as well as cigarette smoking, and the occurrence of any atherosclerotic end point were seen, whereas an inverse association with alcohol consumption was observed. Characteristics associated with the development of other fatal and nonfatal clinical events in this cohort, including coronary heart disease, thromboembolic stroke, and aortic aneurysms, are presented with accompanying relative and attributable risks. The results of this prospective epidemiological study provide insights to the long-term predictive utility of the commonly accepted risk factors for coronary heart disease in relation to the different clinical manifestations of atherosclerosis in a middle-aged male cohort followed up for approximately 20 years. These results provide additional support for risk factor modification in middle-aged men and for the encouragement of positive long-term lifestyle changes.

Individual studies have not clearly answered 2 questions: what is the relation, if any, between serum total cholesterol and stroke, and how does the strength of the relation between diastolic BP and stroke vary with age. The Prospective Studies Collaborators[3] investigated the associations of blood choles-

TABLE 1-2. Percentages Aware, Treated with Medication, and Controlled Among Hypertensive and Hypercholesterolemic Subjects, by Sex, Race, and Age: The Atherosclerosis Risk in Communities Study, 1987 to 1989

	% Aware Among Those With Condition	% Treated With Medication Among Those Aware	% Controlled Among Those Treated
Hypertension*			
Total (No.)	84	87	68
	(4582/5473)	(3994/4582)	(2714/3994)
Sex			
M	81	84	68
F	86†	90†	68
Race			
W	83	88	73
B	85‡	86‡	61†
Age, y			
<55	83	87	71
≥55	84	88	66†
Hypercholesterolemia§			
Total (No.)	42	27	35
	(1748/4202)	(446/1664)‖	(155/446)¶
Sex			
M	44	26	36
F	40‡	27	33
Race			
W	47	28	34
B	26†	20#	40
Age, y			
<55	38	26	34
≥55	44†	27	34

*Blood pressure of 140 mm Hg or more systolic or 90 mm Hg or more diastolic, or antihypertensive treatment.

†P <0.001.

‡P <0.05.

§Total serum cholesterol level of 6.21 mmol/L (240 mg/dL) or more, adjusted for laboratory drift, or lipid-lowering treatment.

‖The denominator for the proportion treated included those aware hypercholesterolemics who either were treated or fit the National Cholesterol Education Program criteria: low-density lipoprotein cholesterol level (LDL-C) of 4.91 mmol/L (190 mg/dL) or more, or LDL-C of 4.14 mmol/L (160 mg/dL) or more and two or more other risk factors, or LDL-C of 3.36 mmol/L (130 mg/dL) or more and prevalent coronary or other atherosclerotic disease.

¶Controlled were participants with lipid-lowering drug treatment who fit the National Cholesterol Education Program criteria: LDL-C less than 4.14 mmol/L (160 mg/dL) if less than two risk factors and no atherosclerotic disease, or LDL-C less then 3.36 mmol/L (130 mg/dL) if no atherosclerotic disease but two or more other risk factors, or LDL-C of 2.59 mmol/L (100 mg/dL) or less if prevalent coronary or other atherosclerotic disease.

#P <0.01.

Reproduced with permission from Nieto et al.[1]

terol and diastolic BP with subsequent stroke rates by review of 45 prospective observational cohorts involving 450 000 individuals with 5–30 years of follow-up (mean, 16 years; total, 7.3 million person-years of observation) during which 13 397 participants were reported as having a stroke. Most of these were fatal strokes in studies that recorded only mortality and not incidence, but about

TABLE 1-3. Age-Adjusted Means of Selected Biological and Lifestyle Characteristics According to the Development of Selected Atherosclerotic Events in Middle-aged Men: Honolulu Heart Program

Characteristic	No Atherosclerotic End Point (n = 2108)	Any Atherosclerotic End Point (n = 602)	Definite CHD* (n = 352)	Angina (n = 176)	Thromboembolic Stroke (n = 184)	Aortic Aneurysm (n = 119)
Ventricular rate, beats/min	77.1	77.0	76.5	76.2	78.5	76.9
Body mass index, kg/m²	23.3	24.1	24.2	24.3	24.0	23.9
Systolic blood pressure, mm Hg	134.8	143.8	144.9	142.2	144.4	146.0
Serum cholesterol, mmol/L (mg/dL)	5.54 (214.1)	5.85 (226.4)	5.98 (231.4)	5.98 (231.1)	5.73 (221.6)	5.94 (229.8)
Serum triglycerides, mmol/L (mg/dL)	2.37 (209.7)	2.81 (249.0)	2.88 (255.2)	2.89 (255.8)	2.64 (233.5)	2.79 (247.4)
Serum glucose, mmol/L (mg/dL)	9.09 (163.9)	10 (181.1)	10.4 (187.8)	9.5 (171.9)	10.1 (182.2)	8.9 (160.8)
Serum uric acid, µmol/L	345	357	357	369	351	375
Hematocrit	0.44	0.45	0.45	0.45	0.45	0.45
Current cigarette smoking, %	38.5	47.4	46.7	36.3	52.8	64.4
Alcohol consumption, mL/mo	396	336	261	255	465	405
Physical activity index	33.0	32.6	32.6	32.5	32.7	33.2
Forced expiratory volume, L/m²†	2.55	2.50	2.48	2.57	2.49	2.43

*CHD indicates coronary heart disease.

†In 1 s corrected for height.

Reproduced with permission from Goldberg et al.[2]

one quarter were from studies that recorded both fatal and nonfatal strokes. After standardization, there was no association between blood cholesterol and stroke except, perhaps, in those under 45 years of age when screened. This lack of association was not influenced by adjustment for sex, diastolic BP, history of CAD, or ethnicity (Asian or non-Asian). However, because the types of the strokes were not centrally available, the lack of any overall relation might conceal a positive association with ischemic stroke together with a negative association with hemorrhagic stroke. When the highest and the lowest of the six BP categories were compared, the difference in usual diastolic BP was 27 mm Hg (102 vs. 75 mm Hg), and there was a 5–fold difference in stroke risk. This 5–fold difference was seen both in those with a preexisting history of CAD and in those without it. The proportional difference in stroke risk, however, was more extreme in middle than in old age. Among those more than 45 years old (45–64, and 65+ when screened), the differences in the relative risks of stroke (between the highest diastolic BP category and a combination of the lowest two categories) were 10-fold, 5–fold, and 2–fold, respectively. However, because the absolute stroke risks are greater in old age, the absolute differences in the annual stroke rates showed an opposite pattern: 2, 5, and 8 per thousand, respectively.

Several reports have shown that migrants from Southeast Asia tend to have an increased risk of CAD when settling in their new country. Bhatnagar and associates[4] from Uxbridge and Manchester, UK; Chandrashekhar, India; and Charleston, South Carolina, compared coronary risk factors in a randomly selected group of 247 migrants from the Indian subcontinent of Punjabi origin living in West London and 117 of their siblings living in Punjab, India. The West London cohort had a greater BMI, systolic BP, serum cholesterol, apolipoprotein B, lower HDL cholesterol, and higher fasting blood glucose than their siblings in the Punjab. Insulin sensitivity, derived from the homeostatic assessment mathematical model, was lower in men in West London than in their counterparts in India. Indians in West London had lower β-cell function than those in the Punjab. Serum lipoprotein (a) concentrations were similar in both the West London and Punjab population, but were significantly higher than those of white European populations in the UK. Increases in serum cholesterol after migration from India led to increased coronary risk conferred by high serum lipoprotein (a) concentrations and greater insulin resistance.

Blood Lipids

Determining Atherosclerotic Risk

During 23 years of follow-up of 7049 middle-aged men of Japanese ancestry living on the island of Oahu, Hawaii, Iribarren and associates[5] from Los Angeles, Calif.; Honolulu, Hawaii; and Bethesda, Maryland, analyzed 1954 deaths among their study group: 38% from cancer, 25% from cardiovascular disease, and 37% from other causes. Men with low serum total cholesterol levels (<180 mg/dL) had several adverse health characteristics, including a high prevalence of current smoking, heavy alcohol drinking, and certain gastrointestinal conditions. Those in the lowest total cholesterol group (<180 mg/dL) were at significantly higher risk of mortality from hemorrhagic stroke (relative risk [RR], 2.41), cancer (RR, 1.41), and all causes (RR, 1.23). Adjustment for confounders in multivariant analysis (excluding cases with prevalent disease at baseline and deaths through year 5) did not explain the risk of fatal hemorrhagic stroke but reduced the risk of cancer mortality by 51% and reduced the excess risk of all-cause mortality by 56% in the low total cholesterol group. In addition, there were clear differences in patterns of risk when comparing men with and without risk factors (smoking, alcohol consumption, and untreated hypertension). The authors concluded that the excess mortality at low total cholesterol levels can be partially explained by confounding with other determinants of death and preexisting disease at baseline, and total cholesterol mortality associations are not homogeneous in the population. Total cholesterol level was not associated with increased cancer or all-cause mortality in the absence of smoking, high alcohol consumption, and untreated systemic hypertension.

To compare the relation between serum total cholesterol and long-term mortality from CAD and different cultures, Verschuren and associates[6] measured total cholesterol at baseline (1958–1964) and at 5- and 10-year follow-up in 12 467 men aged 40–59 years in 16 cohorts located in 7 countries: 5 European countries, the USA, and Japan. The age standardized CAD mortality in the 6 cohorts ranged from 3% to 20%. The RR values for the highest compared with the lowest cholesterol quartile ranged from 1.5 to 2.3, except for Japan's RR of 1.1. For a cholesterol level of around 5.45 mmol/L (210 mg/dL), CAD mortality rates varied from 4% to 5% in Japan and Mediterranean Southern Europe to about 15% in Northern Europe (Figure 1-1). However, the relative increase in CAD mortality caused by a given cholesterol increase was similar in all cultures except Japan. Using a linear approximation, a 0.50-mmol/L (20-mg/dL) increase in total cholesterol corresponded to an increase in CAD mortality risk of 12%, which became an increase in mortality risk of 17% when adjusted for regression dilution bias. Across cultures, cholesterol is linearly

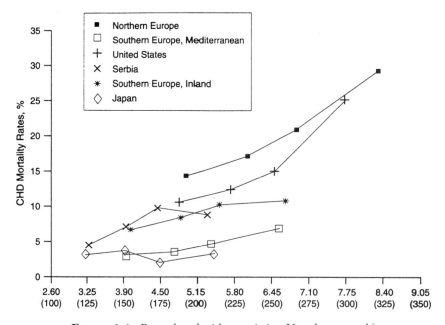

FIGURE 1-1. Reproduced with permission Verschuren et al.[6]

related to CAD mortality, and the relative increase in CAD mortality rates with a given cholesterol increase is the same. The large difference in absolute CAD mortality rates at a given cholesterol level, however, indicates that other factors, such as diet, that are typical for cultures with a low CAD risk are also important with respect to primary prevention.

Burchfiel and colleagues[7] determined whether a combination of a low level of HDL cholesterol and a high level of triglyceride is associated with an increased risk of cardiovascular disease and whether the risk varies across levels of total cholesterol. Combined effects of HDL, triglycerides, and total cholesterol on the incidence of atherosclerotic disease were examined prospectively in Japanese-American men from the Honolulu Heart Program. Among 1646 men aged 51 to 72 years and free of CAD, stroke, and cancer, and not taking lipid-lowering medications, 318 developed atherosclerotic events, including angina, myocardial ischemia, aortic aneurysm, definite CAD, or thromboembolic stroke, and 170 developed definite CAD between 1970 and 1988. Subjects were stratified by total cholesterol level, HDL cholesterol level, and triglyceride level. With Cox regression with HDL cholesterol and low triglycerides as references, age-adjusted relative risk of atherosclerotic events were increased in men with low HDL cholesterol and high triglycerides (Figure 1-2), but not in men with desirable triglyceride levels. Elevated risks of CAD were present independent of BP, obesity, fat distribution, diabetes, smoking, and alcohol. Results were not altered by exclusion of subjects with angina alone and triglyceride levels when total cholesterol was borderline high or high irrespective of other risk factors. These findings indicate that combined effects of HDL cholesterol and triglycerides may be important as risk factors for atherogenesis.

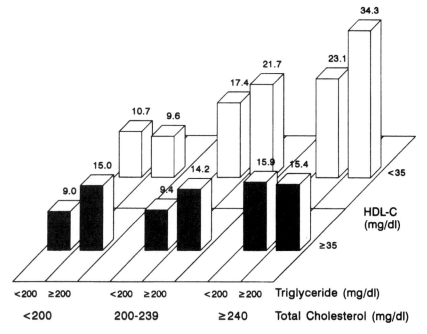

FIGURE 1-2. Age-adjusted incidence of atherosclerotic events per 1000 person-years by HDL cholesterol (HDL-C), triglyceride, and total cholesterol levels for Honolulu Heart Program, 1970 to 1988. Reproduced with permission from Burchfiel et al.[7]

To investigate the relation between total cholesterol concentration and mortality from CAD, cardiovascular diseases, noncardiovascular causes and all causes, Verschuren and Kromhout[8] from BA Bilthoven, the Netherlands, studied 23 000 men and 26 000 women aged 30–54 years who had been examined between 1974 and 1980. Mortality from CAD in men was five times higher than in women. A strong positive association between total serum cholesterol concentration and mortality from CAD and cardiovascular diseases was observed in both men and women (Figure 1-3). The RR values for the highest compared with the lowest fifth of the cholesterol distribution was for mortality from CAD in men and for mortality from cardiovascular disease in men and in women. No increase of noncardiovascular mortality at low cholesterol concentrations was observed. All-cause mortality was significantly higher in the highest compared with the lowest fifth of the cholesterol distribution. Thus, total serum cholesterol concentration is a strong predictor of mortality from CAD, cardiovascular disease, and all causes in women as well as in men. Low cholesterol concentrations were not associated with mortality from noncardiovascular conditions.

Iribarren and colleagues[9] analyzed total cholesterol change over a 6-year period from the first examination (1965 through 1968) to the third examination (1971 through 1974) in Japanese-American men. The study was based on 5941 men 45–68 years of age without a history of CAD, stroke, cancer, or gastrointestinal-liver disease at the first examination who also participated in the third examination of the Honolulu Heart Program. The association of total cholesterol change with mortality was investigated with 2 different approaches, including continuous and categorical total cholesterol change with standard survival analysis techniques. Reduction in total cholesterol was associated with a subse-

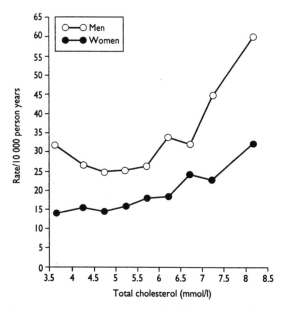

FIGURE 1-3. Mortality (per 10 000 person-years) for all-cause mortality according to category of serum total cholesterol concentration in men and women aged 30–54 years after (on average) 12 years of follow-up, adjusted for age, smoking, blood pressure, and body mass index. Reproduced with permission from Verschuren and Kromhout.[8]

quent increased risk of death caused by some cancers, including hematologic, esophageal, and prostate; noncardiovascular noncancer causes, especially liver disease; and all causes. The risk-factor–adjusted rate of all-cause mortality was 30% higher among persons with a decline from middle to low total cholesterol values than in persons remaining at a stable middle level. In contrast, there was no significant increase in all-cause mortality risk among cohort men with stable low total cholesterol levels. These results add strength to the concern about lowering total cholesterol from middle to low values and the reverse-causality proposition that in some individuals catabolic diseases cause total cholesterol to decrease.

To examine the relation of total cholesterol and HDL cholesterol to CAD mortality and the recurrence of new CAD events in persons aged 71 and older, Corti and associates[10] from Boston, Massachusetts; Iowa City, Iowa; and New Haven, Connecticut, interviewed 2527 women and 1377 men who had serum lipid determinations and survived at least 1 year. New CAD events were evaluated in persons with no CAD history of hospitalization. After adjustment for established CAD risk factors, the RR of death due to CAD for those with low HDL cholesterol (<35 mm/dL) compared with the reference group (HDL cholesterol ≥60 mm/dL) was 2.5. Elevated risk was present in subgroups aged 71–80 years (RR, 4.1) and over 80 years (RR, 1.8) and in men and women. Low HDL cholesterol predicted an increased risk of occurrence of new CAD events (RR, 1.4) with similar but nonsignificant results in subgroups of men and women. Total cholesterol was less consistently associated with CAD mortality than HDL cholesterol. When the authors compared individuals with total cholesterol of 1.61–1.99 mm/dL, a significant risk of CAD mortality was seen for women (RR, 1.8) but not for men (RR, 1.0). In the total population, for each 1 unit increase in the total cholesterol/HDL cholesterol ratio there was a 17% increase in the risk of CAD death that was statistically significant (Figure 1-4). Low HDL predicts CAD mortality and occurrence of new CAD events in persons older than 70 years. Elevated total cholesterol was not found to be associated with CAD mortality in older men but may be a risk factor of CAD in older women.

Low Values

To examine the relation between low serum total cholesterol concentrations and causes of mortality, Wannamethee and associates[11] from London, UK, studied 7735 men aged 40–59 years and selected at random from 24 general practices. During the mean follow-up period of nearly 15 years, there were 1257 deaths from all causes, 640 cardiovascular deaths, 433 cancer deaths, and 184 deaths from other causes (Figure 1-5). Low serum cholesterol concentration (<4.8 mmol/L), present in 5% (n = 410) of the men, was associated with the highest mortality from all causes, largely due to a significant increase in cancer deaths (age-adjusted RR, 1.6; <4.8 vs. 4.8–5.9 mmol/L) and in other noncardiovascular deaths (age-adjusted RR, 1.9 [1.1–3.1]). Low serum cholesterol concentration was associated with an increased prevalence of several disease and indicators of ill health and with lifestyle characteristics such as smoking and heavy drinking. After adjustment for these factors in the multivariate analysis the increased risk for cancer was attenuated (RR, 1.4 [0.9–2.0]) and the inverse association with other noncardiovascular, noncancer causes was no longer significant (RR,

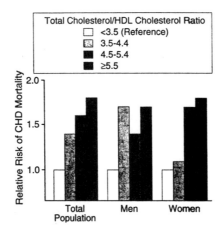

FIGURE 1-4. Relative risk of coronary heart disease (CHD) mortality according to ratio of total to high-density lipoprotein (HDL) cholesterol in total population and by sex. Estimates were calculated from proportional hazard models, adjusting for age, level of blood pressure, history of high blood pressure, diabetes, heart attack, stroke, ethanol consumption, smoking, and body mass index. The total population analysis was also adjusted for sex. Those dying during the first year of follow-up were excluded from the analysis. In tests for trend, P <0.001 for total population and women, P = 0.11 for men. Reproduced with permission from Corti et al.[10]

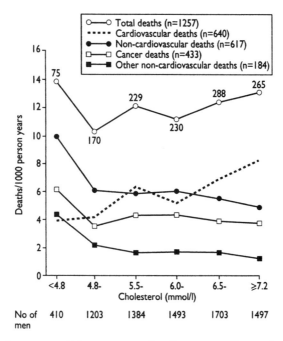

FIGURE 1-5. Death rates per 1000 person-years for all causes, cardiovascular causes, all noncardiovascular causes, and cancer and other noncardiovascular causes by 6 serum cholesterol concentration groups. Reproduced with permission from Wannamethee et al.[11]

1.5 [0.9–2.6]; <4.8 vs. 4.8–5.9 mmol/L). The excess risks of cancer and of other noncardiovascular deaths were most pronounced in the first 5 years and became attenuated and nonsignificant with longer follow-up. By contrast, the positive association between serum total cholesterol concentration and cardiovascular mortality was seen even after more than 10 years of follow-up. The association between comparatively low serum total cholesterol concentrations and excess mortality seemed to be due to preclinical cancer and other noncardiovascular diseases. This suggests that public health programs encouraging lower average concentrations of serum total cholesterol are unlikely to be associated with increased cancer or other noncardiovascular mortality.

Lipoprotein(a)

Cantin and colleagues[12] in Montreal, Canada, undertook a study to evaluate the distribution and the relation of lipoprotein(a) concentration with intermittent claudication in a cohort of men aged 35–64 years, randomly selected in 1974 and followed until 1990. In 1985, blood samples for a complete fasting lipid profile and lipoprotein(a) were obtained in 2424 men representing 62% of the living cohort. The diagnosis of intermittent claudication was made by trained nurses using a standardized questionnaire and confirmed by a cardiologist. Lipoprotein(a) distribution did not change with age and was similar to that of other Caucasian populations. Because lipoprotein(a) concentration did not vary with age, its relation to the incidence of intermittent claudication was assessed from 1974 through 1990. The incidence of intermittent claudication was 42 of 10 000 person-years. The 113 men with intermittent claudication, in contrast to men without this symptomatology, were older at entry (49 vs. 45 years) and had higher systolic pressure (144 vs. 136 mm Hg) and lipoprotein(a) levels (46 vs. 33 mg/dL). There was also a significantly greater prevalence of smoking and diabetes among men with intermittent claudication. The risk of intermittent claudication was doubled in men in the second and third tertiles of lipoprotein(a) concentration. Thus, high lipoprotein(a) levels constitute a significant risk for intermittent claudication in this population.

Apolipoprotein E

Stengård and colleagues[13] in Helsinki, Finland; Ann Arbor, Michigan; and Kuopio, Finland, evaluated the usefulness of allelic variation of the apolipoprotein E gene for predicting CAD. There is already substantial evidence from cross-sectional studies of an association between allelic variation of the gene coding for apolipoprotein E and interindividual variation in plasma lipids and the presence of CAD. In this study, 2 samples of elderly Finnish men were followed for 5 years, 1 in the east (n = 297) and the other in the southwest of Finland (n = 369). At baseline, when the apolipoprotein E genotypes were assessed, the men were 65 to 84 years old. At the end of the follow-up, the vital status of each man was determined and the cause of death was coded. Relative frequencies of the three alleles—$\epsilon 2$, $\epsilon 3$, and $\epsilon 4$—were significantly different: 0.037, 0.827, and 0.136 in the eastern and 0.062, 0.763, and 0.175 in the southwestern samples, respectively. During the 5-year follow-up, a total of 28 deaths from CAD were recorded in the eastern and 42 in the southwestern samples. Among those who died from CAD, there was a doubling of the relative $\epsilon 4$ allele frequency in both samples. Thus, allelic variation in the apolipoprotein E gene is a statistically significant predictor of CAD death in elderly Finnish men.

Ribera and associates[14] from Barcelona, Spain, examined 115 patients with xanthelasma and 105 age-matched control subjects without xanthelasma in a cross-sectional study to determine the prevalence and types of dyslipidemia associated with xanthelasma. Univariate and multivariate comparisons of lipid variables (including total cholesterol; triglycerides; VLDL, LDL, and HDL cholesterol; cholesterol of HDL subfractions 2 and 3 [HDL$_2$ cholesterol and HDL$_3$ cholesterol]; apolipoprotein A-1 and B; and apolipoprotein E phenotypes) and nonlipid coronary risk factors were made between patients with and without xanthelasma. Patients with xanthelasma had higher levels of cholesterol, LDL cholesterol, and apolipoprotein B, and lower levels of HDL$_2$ cholesterol than control subjects. The prevalence of the apolipoprotein E4/E3 phenotype was higher in cases than in controls. Patients with xanthelasma had a higher prevalence of personal and familial history of cardiovascular disease and were more overweight than control subjects. A stepwise discriminant of xanthelasma with lower HDL cholesterol, HDL$_2$ cholesterol, and HDL$_3$ cholesterol levels in men, and with higher total cholesterol and lower HDL$_2$ cholesterol levels in women. Xanthelasma appears to be associated with qualitative and quantitative abnormalities of lipid metabolism that may favor lipid deposition in the skin and arterial wall. The findings support the notion that xanthelasma is a marker of dyslipidemia and underline the need to determine a full lipid profile in these patients to detect those potentially at increased risk of cardiovascular disease.

High-Density Lipoprotein Subfractions

Although the inverse relation between HDL cholesterol concentration and the risk of CAD is well established, little is known about the relation of HDL subfractions HDL$_2$ and HDL$_3$ or lipoprotein A-1 and A-1-A-11 to extracoronary disease, particularly at its silent phase before the appearance of clinical lesions. Atger and colleagues[15] in Paris, France, investigated the potential influence of HDL subfractions as risk markers, among the other main lipid and nonlipid risk factors, by assessing early atherosclerotic plaques detected by three ultrasound imaging sites in 181 hypercholesterolemic symptom-free men. No plaques were found in 36% of the patients, but plaques were found at carotid, aortic, and femoral sites in 24%, 40%, and 46% of subjects, respectively. Data were analyzed using univariate comparisons and multiple logistic regression. According to the logistic analysis, plaques were associated (1) with BP and LDL cholesterol in the carotid arteries; (2) with age, triglycerides, and cigarette smoking at the aortic site; and (3) inversely with HDL$_3$ cholesterol and positively with cigarette smoking, and age in the femoral site. The number of arterial sites affected (0, 1, 2, and 3) by plaques was inversely associated with HDL$_3$ cholesterol and positively associated with smoking, BP, LDL cholesterol, and age. Using models of multivariate analysis, the investigators showed that HDL$_2$ and HDL$_3$ subfractions were better predictors of plaque at the femoral site and of the number of affected segments than total HDL cholesterol. Thus, in hypercholesterolemic asymptomatic middle-aged men, LDL cholesterol and HDL$_3$ cholesterol concentrations are two specific lipid parameters that strongly influence the development of arterial plaque. A significant increase in the LDL:HDL$_3$ ratio was associated with the presence of plaque at each site and also with the number of diseased sites. The investigators' data support the hypothesis of a specific protective effect of HDL_3 subfraction at the early stage of atherosclerosis, and they propose the $LDL:HDL_3$ ratio as a potential marker of the presence and extent of extracoronary plaques.

Effects of Fasting

To determine the effect of a self-selected meal on concentrations of LDL cholesterol and HDL cholesterol in a screening setting and to determine the effect of using nonfasting values to classify individuals according to National Cholesterol Education Program guidelines, Wilder and associates[16] from Baltimore, Maryland, studied 115 employees who had previously participated in a worksite total cholesterol screening. Total cholesterol, triglycerides, HDL cholesterol, and estimated LDL cholesterol were determined before subjects ate a self-selected breakfast and 3 and 5 hours after it was eaten. LDL cholesterol values determined 3 and 5 hours after breakfast were approximately 7% and 2.5% lower, respectively, than fasting values. Use of the 3-hour and 5-hour LDL cholesterol determinations to classify individuals with elevated levels resulted in false-negative rates of 20% and 14%, respectively. Three- and 5-hour HDL cholesterol values were approximately 4% and 1.5% lower, respectively, than fasting levels. Use of 3-hour HDL cholesterol values to classify individuals with low fasting levels resulted in no false negatives, whereas one in seven individuals with low fasting HDL cholesterol were misclassified when 5-hour values were used. These results support the 1993 National Cholesterol Education Program guidelines that LDL cholesterol levels should be determined only in fasting persons and that nonfasting HDL cholesterol values may be acceptable for screening purposes.

Effects of Insulin Levels

To assess whether circulating insulin is a major contributor to adverse lipid profiles during the transition from adolescence to young adulthood, Jiang and associates[17] examined in a cross-sectional survey 4136 individuals aged 5–30 years from a biracial community. Fasting insulin levels were strongly and positively correlated with serum triglyceride and VLDL cholesterol levels and negatively correlated with HDL cholesterol levels in all age groups. An increasing impact of insulin on LDL cholesterol levels was observed in adults aged 25–30 years. In multivariant analysis, fasting insulin level was associated with a VLDL cholesterol level for most of the age groups in both races independently of age, sex, glucose levels, obesity, cigarette smoking, and alcohol intake. The independent relation to LDL cholesterol level persisted in young adults aged 25–30 years. The independent and negative association with HDL cholesterol level remained in white subjects aged 5–24 years and black subjects aged 19–24 years. When individuals were divided into tertiles according to insulin concentration and subscapular skinfold thickness, the independent effect of insulin level and obesity on lipoprotein fractions was also noted. Furthermore, a stronger association of insulin level with lipoprotein fraction was observed in obese than in lean white males. These data indicate that an increasing association of insulin levels with adverse lipoprotein levels in young adults, especially obese individuals, may have adverse consequence for adult cardiovascular diseases.

In Coronary Artery Disease

Fujiwara and colleagues[18] in Fukui, Japan, investigated the association between hyperinsulinemia and changes in lipid, lipoprotein, and apolipoprotein that would increase the risk of CAD independent of glucose tolerance. A coronary angiogram was recorded in 127 male subjects, including 41 with normal glucose tolerance, 41 with impaired glucose tolerance, and 45 with non–insulin-dependent diabetes mellitus. Subjects were divided into two groups according to results: those with CAD (n = 94) and those with normal coronary arteries (n = 33). All subjects had normal lipid levels (total cholesterol, <230 mg/dL; triglycerides, <150 mg/dL). The CAD group had a significantly lower plasma level of HDL cholesterol and apolipoprotein A-1 and a higher level of apolipoprotein B than the normal group with normal glucose tolerance. In considering subjects with impaired glucose tolerance or non–insulin-dependent diabetes, the CAD group had a significantly lower plasma level of HDL cholesterol and apolipoprotein A-1 and a significantly higher plasma level of total cholesterol, triglycerides, and apolipoprotein B than the normal group. In each of the subjects with normal and impaired glucose tolerance, and non–insulin-dependent diabetes, the elevation of plasma insulin concentration during both the complete test period and the early phase of an oral glucose challenge was significantly higher in the CAD than in the normal group. In all subjects, graded reductions in HDL cholesterol and apolipoprotein A-1 and graded increases in plasma total cholesterol, triglycerides, and apolipoprotein B were observed with increasing tertiles of the postglucose challenge measurements of insulinemia. Multivariate analysis of the data confirmed the independent effect of plasma levels of apolipoprotein A-1 and apolipoprotein B on the severity of CAD. Thus, hyperinsulinemia appeared to be associated with changes in lipid and apolipoprotein that predisposed toward coronary atherosclerosis not only in nondiabetic subjects, but also in those with impaired glucose tolerance and non–insulin-dependent diabetes mellitus. The plasma levels of both apolipoprotein A-1 and apolipoprotein B, both nontraditional risk factors, were better predictors of CAD than were plasma levels of lipids in normolipidemic men.

Rubins and coinvestigators[19] in Minneapolis, Minnesota, measured fasting lipid profiles in more than 8500 community-living men with CAD to determine the distribution of lipid abnormalities in this population: 81% were white and 16% black; mean age, 63 years; mean total cholesterol, 214 mg/dL; LDL, 140 mg/dL; HDL cholesterol, 39 mg/dL; and triglycerides, 190 mg/dL. After adjusting for age, the only significant difference between blacks and whites was a higher HDL cholesterol in blacks (45 vs. 38 mg/dL). With use of cut points established by the National Cholesterol Education Program, 87% of subjects had high LDL cholesterol, 38% had low HDL cholesterol, and 33% had high triglycerides. The investigators estimated that 42% of men with CAD would be definite candidates for cholesterol-lowering medication according to the National Cholesterol Education Program guidelines and that 41% of those in whom cholesterol-lowering medication would not be definitely indicated had low levels of HDL cholesterol. The investigators concluded that (1) black men with CAD have substantially higher HDL cholesterol than white men, (2) almost 90% of male patients with CAD are candidates for dietary intervention and >40% may need medications to lower LDL cholesterol, and (3) 40% of patients without a definite indication for cholesterol-lowering medications have low levels of HDL cholesterol.

In Stroke

While serum cholesterol levels predict CAD, whether there is any association with stroke is unclear. To investigate whether lipid-lowering reduces the risk of stroke, Hebert and associates[20] from Boston and West Roxbury, Massachusetts, performed an overview of randomized trials that included more than 36 000 individuals. The mean reduction in total cholesterol levels in the treated compared with the control subjects ranged from 6% to 23%. Those assigned to treatment experienced no significant reduction in all (fatal + nonfatal) stroke or fatal stroke.

In Suicide, Parasuicide, and Trauma

Recent results from some cholesterol level-lowering trials have supported a link between low or lower serum cholesterol levels and violent death. Iribarren and associates[21] from Alhambra and Novato, California; Honolulu, Hawaii; and Bethesda, Maryland, further investigated this issue by assessing the relation of baseline serum total cholesterol levels with long-term risk of mortality due to trauma and suicide in 7309 middle-aged Japanese-American men. After 23 years of follow-up, a total of 75 traumatic fatalities and 24 deaths by suicide were documented. Rather than an inverse relation, a positive association between serum cholesterol level and risk of suicide death was observed. After controlling for potential confounders, the relative risk of suicide associated with an increment of 0.98 mmol/L (38 mg/dL) in serum cholesterol level (1 SD) was 1.46. Multivariate analysis of traumatic mortality failed to detect a relation with serum cholesterol level (RR, 0.89). Heavy alcohol consumption (>1200 mL of alcohol per month, top quintile) was an independent risk factor for trauma death relative to abstinence (RR, 1.86). These findings contradict the hypothesis of an inverse relation between serum cholesterol level and suicide, but they support the hypothesis that heavy alcohol consumption is a risk factor for traumatic fatal events.

Galerani and associates[22] from Ferrara, Italy, evaluated whether people who have committed parasuicide have a low serum cholesterol concentration. The authors did blood tests in 331 patients aged 44 ± 21 years admitted to hospitals for parasuicide compared with those of a control group of 331 nonsuicidal subjects. Serum cholesterol concentrations and possible association with parasuicide, considering sex, violence of method of parasuicide, and underlying psychiatric disorder, were measured. Lower serum cholesterol concentrations (4.96 [SD 1.16] mmol/L) were found in parasuicide subjects than in the control group (5.43 [1.30]), regardless of sex and degree of violence of parasuicide method. Both men and women with 2 sets of blood test results had lower cholesterol concentrations after parasuicide. Linear regression analysis showed that the difference in cholesterol concentrations was significantly related to the length of time between the taking of the 2 sets of blood samples. The study showed low cholesterol concentrations after parasuicide.

In Hairy-Cell Leukemia

Hypocholesterolemia is a common finding in various malignant disorders, including acute myeloid leukemia, chronic myeloproliferative disorders, and carcinoma of the colon. It is unclear whether it is a risk factor for development of malignancy or secondary to the cancer. In cases of acute myeloid leukemia, hypocholesterolemia is the result of an increased uptake of cholesterol by leukemic cells as indicated by an inverse correlation between cholesterol concentration and the activity of LDL lipoprotein receptors in leukemic cells. Hypocholesterolemia is uncommon in lymphoid tumors such as lymphoma and chronic lymphocytic leukemia, but it has been observed in patients with hairy-cell leukemia, a rare disease affecting middle-aged men and characterized by cytopenia, splenomegaly, and impaired immunity; it may be fatal after an infection. To evaluate mechanisms behind the development of hypocholesterolemia in patients with hairy-cell leukemia, Juliusson and associates[23] from Huddinge, Sweden, analyzed serial serum lipid concentrations after treatment with 2-chlorodeoxyadenosine in 24 patients with active disease. Total cholesterol, LDL cholesterol, HDL cholesterol, and triglyceride concentrations all rose significantly after treatment. The mean difference in LDL concentration from baseline values was 0.90 mmol/L in 24 patients at 3 months and 0.98 mmol/L in 18 patients at 6 months. Thus, hypolipidemia, mainly caused by low concentration of LDL cholesterol, is a frequent finding in advanced hairy-cell leukemia, but values revert to normal after successful treatment. Thus, it is a disease-related phenomenon and not a predisposing factor for tumor development. Hypocholesterolemia in patients with active disease was not caused by LDL receptors being more active in hairy cells than in normal blood lymphocytes; this indicates that the disease's mechanism is different in hairy-cell leukemia and acute myeloid leukemia, in which leukemic cells show increased uptake of cholesterol. The lipid concentrations were related to the size of the spleen, and hypocholesterolemia is more common in patients with splenomegaly than in those with normal sized spleen or in those who have had a splenectomy.

Frequency of Hypothyroidism

Treatment of hypercholesterolemia can reduce the risk of developing premature atherosclerosis. The hypercholesterolemia caused by hypothyroidism is potentially reversible by thyroid hormone therapy. Diekman and associates[24] from Amsterdam, the Netherlands, determined the prevalence of hypothyroidism in patients referred to a university lipid research clinic and studied the changes in lipid and lipoprotein levels on restoration of the euthyroid state. A retrospective follow-up study was performed. In all 1509 consecutive referrals for severe dyslipidemia, thyrotropin levels were measured. Patients with hypothyroidism were identified by means of a computed database, from January 1, 1989, to July 1, 1993, first by levothyroxine sodium medication and second by serum thyrotropin values greater than 5 mU/L. Twenty-one patients were available to evaluate the effect of restoration of the euthyroid state on plasma lipid and lipoprotein levels. The observed prevalence of hypothyroidism proved to be 4.2% (64 of 1509). The disorder was previously known in 25 patients and newly diagnosed in 39 patients (11 with overt hypothyroidism and 28 with subclinical hypothyroidism). Significant reductions in total cholesterol and

LDL cholesterol levels occurred only in patients with pretreatment thyrotropin values of 10 mU/L or more. The prevalence of newly diagnosed cases of overt hypothyroidism in patients referred to a lipid clinic is approximately two times that in the general population. The absence of significant reductions in total cholesterol and LDL cholesterol levels on levothyroxine treatment in patients with minor subclinical hypothyroidism (thyrotropin level, <10 mU/L) does not support the view that this condition is a risk factor for atherosclerosis mediated by an elevated LDL cholesterol level. All patients referred for diagnosis and treatment of dyslipidemia should be screened for hypothyroidism by measurement of thyrotropin values.

Effect of Running

To examine the association between miles run per week and HDL cholesterol levels in healthy middle-aged men, Kokkinos and associates[25] from Washington, DC, and College Park, Maryland, studied healthy, nonsmoking men (n = 2906; age, 43 ± 4 years) who completed a questionnaire on health habits and physical activities and a symptom-limited exercise test. They were then stratified on the basis of the number of miles they ran each week. Six groups, with mileages of 0, 45, 9, 12, 17, and 31 per week, were established. A gradual increase in HDL cholesterol level was observed with increased miles (0.008 mol/L [0.308 mg/dL] increase in HDL cholesterol level/mile) (Figure 1-6). Most of the changes were associated with distances of 7–14 miles per week. Levels of LDL cholesterol, triglycerides, and the ratio of total cholesterol to HDL cholesterol also improved with weekly mileage (Figure 1-7). The HDL cholesterol level correlated significantly with all exercise components, anthropometric measures, and alcohol consumption. Group comparisons disclosed significant differences in exercise time to exhaustion, miles run each week, body fat, body weight, and BMI. Age and alcohol consumption were similar across groups. These results indicate a dose-response relation between miles run each week, HDL cholesterol level, and other LDL cholesterol levels. Most changes were noted in those who ran 7–14 miles per week at mild to moderate intensities. A mileage threshold for changes in HDL cholesterol level was not observed.

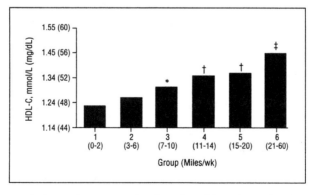

FIGURE 1-6. HDL cholesterol (HDL-C) levels and weekly mileage for all groups (n = 2906). Asterisk indicates P <0.001, group 3 vs. group 1; dagger, P <0.001, groups 3 and 4 vs. groups 1 and 2; and double dagger, P <0.01, group 6 vs. groups 1 through 5. Reproduced with permission from Kokkinos et al.[25]

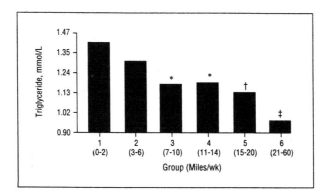

FIGURE 1-7. Triglyceride levels and weekly mileage for all groups (n = 2900). Asterisk indicates P <0.001, groups 3 and 4 vs. group 1; dagger, P <0.001, group 5 vs. groups 1 and 2; and double dagger, P <0.01, group 6 vs. groups 1 through 5. Reproduced by permission of Kokkinos et al.[25]

However, when compared with those of the nonexercising group, HDL cholesterol levels attained statistical significance at 7 or more miles per week.

Effect of Soy Protein Intake

In laboratory animals, the consumption of soy protein, rather than animal protein, decreases serum cholesterol concentrations, but studies in humans have been inconclusive. Anderson and associates[26] from Lexington, Kentucky, examined the relation between soy protein consumption and serum lipid concentrations by using a meta-analysis of 38 controlled clinical trials. In most of the studies, the intake of energy, fat, saturated fat, and cholesterol was similar when the subjects ingested control and soy-containing diets; soy protein intake averaged 47 g/d. Ingestion of soy protein was associated with the following net changes in serum lipid concentrations from the concentrations reached with the control diet: total cholesterol, a decrease of 23.2 mg/dL (0.60 mmol/L), or 9.3%; LDL cholesterol, a decrease of 21.7 mg/dL (0.56 mmol/L), or 12.9%; and triglycerides, a decrease of 13.3 mg/dL (0.15 mmol/L), or 10.5%. The changes in serum cholesterol and LDL cholesterol concentrations were directly related to the initial serum cholesterol concentration. The ingestion of soy protein was associated with a nonsignificant 2.4% increase in serum concentrations of HDL cholesterol. The authors found that the consumption of soy protein rather than animal protein significantly decreased serum concentrations of total cholesterol, LDL cholesterol, and triglycerides.

Effects of Naproxen and Nabumetone

In a 12-week controlled clinical study on the effects of two nonsteroidal anti-inflammatory drug regimens on serum lipoproteins in patents with osteoarthritis, Young and associates[27] from Palo Alto, California, treated 54 patients with naproxen (500 mg twice daily) and 45 patients with nabumetone (1000 mg once daily). In patients receiving naproxen, the mean levels of total serum cholesterol decreased by 18.3 mg/dL (7.0%) from baseline to 12 weeks, HDL cholesterol remained unchanged, and LDL cholesterol decreased by 15.4 mg/dL (8.7%). In patients who received nabumetone, mean levels of total serum cholesterol increased 10.4 mg/dL (4.0%), HDL cholesterol remained unchanged, and LDL cholesterol increased 7.2 mg/dL (4.1%). Furthermore, serum triglyceride levels tended to increase in nabumetone-treated patients and decrease in naproxen-treated patients, with a statistically significant difference between treatments. The decreases in total cholesterol and LDL cholesterol levels in patients receiving naproxen were statistically significant. These results confirm previous findings on naproxen's cholesterol-lowering effect.

Low-Fat and/or Low-Cholesterol Diet

Interventions to avoid atherosclerosis might be more successful if launched early in life when lifestyle patterns are formed, but dietary interventions have been limited by fears of diet-induced growth failure. Lapinleimu and associates[28] from Turku, Finland, investigated the effects of a diet low in saturated fat and cholesterol on serum lipid concentrations and growth in 1062 healthy 7-month-old infants in a randomized study. Every 1–3 months, families in the intervention group received dietary advice aimed at adequate energy supply, with low fat intake (30–35% energy, polyunsaturated/monounsaturated/saturated fatty acid ratio 1:1:1, and cholesterol intake <200 mg/d). Infants in control families consumed an unrestricted diet. Three-day food records were collected at ages 8–13 months. Growth was carefully monitored. Between 7 and 13 months serum cholesterol and non-HDL cholesterol concentrations did not change significantly in the intervention group (mean change, –0.03 [SD 0.72] mmol/L and 0.01 [0.67] mmol/L) but increased substantially in the control group (0.24 [0.64] mmol/L and 0.23 [0.60] mmol/L). Daily intakes of energy and saturated fat were lower in the intervention than in the control group at 13 months (4065 [796] vs. 4370 [748] kJ, and 9.3 [3.5] vs. 14.5 [4.8] g), and intake of polyunsaturated fat was higher (5.8 [2.2] vs. 4.4 [1.4] g). Growth did not differ between the groups and was as expected for children at this age. Serum cholesterol concentrations fell significantly in parents of intervention-group infants. The increases in serum cholesterol and non-HDL cholesterol concentration that occur in infants between the ages of 7 and 13 months can be avoided by individualized diets, with no effect on the children's growth.

To assess the efficacy and safety of lowering dietary intake of total fat, saturated fat, and cholesterol to decrease LDL cholesterol in children, a randomized controlled clinical trial involving six centers and 362 prepubertal boys and 301 prepubertal girls aged 8–10 years with LDL cholesterol levels ≥80th and <98th percentiles for age and sex were randomly assigned to an intervention group (n = 334) and a usual care group (n = 329).[29] Behavioral intervention to promote adherence to a diet providing 28% of energy from total fat, less than 8% from saturated fat, up to 9% polyunsaturated fat, and less than 75 mg/4200 kJ (1000 kcal) per day of cholesterol (not to exceed 150 mg/d). The primary efficacy measure was the mean LDL cholesterol level after 3 years. Primary safety measures were mean height and serum ferritin levels at 3 years. Secondary efficacy outcomes were mean LDL cholesterol levels at 1 year and mean total cholesterol levels at 1 and 3 years. Secondary safety outcomes included red blood cell folate values; serum zinc, retinol, and albumin levels; serum HDL cholesterol values, LDL cholesterol:HDL cholesterol ratio, and total triglyceride levels; sexual maturation; and psychosocial health. At 3 years, dietary total fat, saturated fat, and cholesterol levels decreased significantly in the intervention group compared with the usual care group. Levels of LDL cholesterol decreased in the intervention and usual care groups by 0.40 mmol/L (15.4 mg/dL) and 0.31 mmol/L (11.9 mg/dL), respectively. Adjusting for baseline level and sex and imputing values for missing data, the mean difference between the groups was −0.08 mmol/L (−3.23 mg/dL), −0.15 to −0.01 mmol/L (−5.6 to −0.5 mg/dL), which was significant. There were no significant differences between the groups in adjusted mean height or serum ferritin levels of other safety outcomes. The dietary intervention achieved modest lowering of LDL cholesterol levels over 3 years while maintaining adequate growth, iron stores, nutritional adequacy, and psychological well-being during the critical growth period of adolescence.

To quantify changes in size and severity of myocardial perfusion abnormalities by positron emission tomography (PET) in patients with CAD after 5 years of risk factor modification, Gould and associates[30] from Houston, Texas, and Sausalito and San Francisco, California, randomly assigned 20 patients to risk factor modification consisting of a very-low-fat vegetarian diet, mild-to-moderate exercise, stress management, and group support, and in 15 control subjects to usual care by their own physicians, consisting principally of any anginal therapy. Quantitative coronary arteriography and PET at baseline and 5 years after randomization were performed. The size and severity of perfusion abnormalities on dipyridamole PET images decreased (improved) after risk factor modification in the experimental group compared with an increase (worsening) of size and severity in controls. The percentage of LV perfusion abnormalities outside 2.5 SDs of those of normal persons (based on 20 disease-free individuals) on the dipyridamole PET image of normalized counts worsened in controls (mean ± SEM, +10.3 ± 5.6%) and improved in the experimental group (mean ± SEM, −5.1 ± 4.8%); the percentage of the left ventricle with activity <60% of the maximum activity on the dipyridamole PET image of normalized counts worsened in controls (+14 ± 3.8%) and improved in the experimental group (−4.2 ± 3.8%); and the myocardial quadrant on the PET image with the lowest average activity expressed as a percentage of maximum activity worsened in controls (−8.8 ± 2.3%) and improved in the experimental group (+4.9 ± 3.3%). The size and severity of perfusion abnormalities on resting PET images were also significantly improved in the experimental group compared with controls. The relative magnitude of changes in size and severity of PET perfusion abnormalities was comparable with or greater than the magnitude of changes in percent diameter stenosis, absolute stenosis lumen area, or stenosis flow reserve documented by quantitative coronary arteriography. Modest regression of coronary artery stenoses after risk factor modification is associated with decreased size and severity of perfusion abnormalities on rest-dipyridamole PET images. Progression or regression of CAD can be followed noninvasively by dipyridamole PET reflecting the integrated flow capacity of the entire coronary arterial circulation.

To assess the effects of a diet restricted in fat, saturated fat, and cholesterol under weight-maintenance and ad libitum conditions on body weight and plasma lipid levels in hypercholesterolemic patients, Schaefer and associates[31] from Boston, Massachusetts, studied 27 free-living, healthy middle-aged and elderly men and women with LDL cholesterol levels ≥130 mg/dL. The subjects underwent three dietary phases. Consumption of the low-fat diet under weight maintenance conditions had significant lowering effects on plasma total cholesterol, LDL cholesterol, and HDL cholesterol levels (mean change, −13%, −17%, and −23%, respectively). This diet significantly increased plasma triglyceride (+47%) and the total cholesterol/HDL cholesterol ratio (+15%). In contrast, consumption of the low-fat ad libitum diet was accompanied by a significant weight loss (−4 kg), by a mean decrease in LDL cholesterol (−24%), and by mean triglyceride levels and total cholesterol/HDL cholesterol ratio that were not significantly different from values obtained at baseline. These results indicated that a low-fat ad libitum diet promotes weight loss and LDL cholesterol lowering without adverse effects on triglycerides or the total cholesterol/HDL cholesterol ratio.

To determine the extent to which plasma lipid concentrations of individuals are consistently sensitive to changes in saturated fats; to examine whether groups that consistently have large or small responses can be defined; and to identify factors that predict response of lipids to dietary change, Cox and associates[32] from Dunedin, New Zealand, studied 67 free-living subjects with total cholesterols ranging from 5.5 to 7.9 mmol/L using a double crossover design in which 2 diets (S, providing 21% energy from saturated fat, and P, providing 10%) were followed for periods of 6 weeks in the sequences of SP or PSPS. Similar average changes in cholesterol mask a wide range of individual responses. Response was not related to compliance. In all participants the change in cholesterol observed when the nature of dietary fat was changed on the two crossovers was correlated; the degree of correlation between the two sets of responses was greater in the 46 consistent responders than in the 21 variable responders. Mean differences in cholesterol between diet S and diet P during the 2 crossovers were 1.16 mmol/L and 0.95 mmol/L for consistent hyperresponders and 0.18 mmol/L and 0.18 mmol/L for consistent minimal responders. In consistent responders, changes in total cholesterol in response to increasing saturated fats correlated with baseline levels of cholesteryl ester transfer activity, total cholesterol, triglycerides, and apolipoprotein B. There is a degree of consistency in cholesterol response to instructions to change dietary fat that is not explained by dietary compliance, and there are groups of consistent hyperresponders and minimal responders within a population of hypercholesterolemic individuals.

To determine the relative efficacy in general practice of dietary advice given by dietitian, a practice nurse, or a diet leaflet alone in reducing total and LDL cholesterol concentration, Neil and associates[33] from Oxford and South Hampton, UK, performed a randomized 6-month parallel involving 2004 subjects aged 35–64 years, including 163 men and 146 women with a repeat total cholesterol concentration of 6.0–8.5 mmol/L. At the end of the trial no significant differences were found in mean concentrations of lipid, lipoproteins, and antioxidants or body mass index between groups. After data were pooled from the three groups, the mean total cholesterol concentration fell by 2%, and LDL cholesterol also fell. The authors concluded that dietary advice was equally effective when given by a dietitian, a practice nurse, or a diet leaflet alone, but the results from this advice showed only a small reduction in levels of total and LDL cholesterol.

Denke[34] from Dallas, Texas, reviewed cholesterol-lowering large trials of dietary intervention and smaller trials of angiographic assessment of the impact of diet on CAD. Two trials of dietary therapy as intensive individualized counseling in the individuals at usual risk for CAD achieved 75% to 80% of the cholesterol lowering as predicted by the metabolic ward studies and produced a 5–14% reduction in total cholesterol levels. Four studies in high-risk individuals exceeded predictions and achieved a 4–17% reduction in total cholesterol levels. Similar efficacy was observed in 6 of the 7 trials for diet for secondary prevention. Four trials using the population approach achieved small but often significant reductions in total cholesterol levels of 1–11%. The effectiveness of diet was enhanced when individualized counseling was used, follow-up was maintained, and weight reduction is achieved.

Drug Therapy of Hyperlipidemia

Lovastatin—Cost-Effectiveness

To evaluate the lifetime cost-effectiveness of 3-hydroxy-3-methylglutaryl coenzyme A (HMG-CoA) reductase for treatment of high blood cholesterol levels, Hamilton and associates[35] from Montreal, Canada, added cost data to a validated CAD prevention computer model that estimates the benefits of lifelong risk factor modification. The updated model takes into account the cost of cholesterol reduction, the savings in CAD health care costs attributable to intervention, the additional non-CAD costs resulting from patients living longer, and the beneficial effects of reducing CAD risks by reducing total cholesterol and increasing HDL cholesterol. The authors studied men and women aged 30–70 years who were free of CAD, had total cholesterol equal to the 90th percentile of the US distribution in their age and sex group, had HDL cholesterol levels equal to the mean of the US distribution in their age and sex group, and were either with or without additional CAD risk factors. Lovastatin (20 mg/d) was given to each patient. The increase in HDL cholesterol associated with lovastatin lowered cost-effectiveness ratios by approximately 40% such that the treatment of hypercholesterolemia was relatively cost-effective for men (as low as $21 000 per year of lives saved at age 50 years) and women ($37 000 per year of lives saved at age 50 years) with additional risk factors (Table 1-4). Non-CAD costs resulting from longer life expectancy after intervention added

Table 1-4. Lifetime Cost of Lovastatin Therapy at 20 mg/d* (Undiscounted Canadian Dollars)

	Age, y				
	30	**40**	**50**	**60**	**70**
Low-Risk†					
Men	40 967	32 917	25 170	18 228	12 009
Women	46 102	37 975	30 059	22 393	15 242
High-Risk‡					
Men	34 399	26 428	19 123	13 058	8 033
Women	40 201	32 187	24 571	17 462	11 167

*Lifetime costs are based on Canadian data sources.

†Nonsmokers with diastolic blood pressure of 80 mm Hg.

‡Smokers with diastolic blood pressure of 100 mm Hg.

Reproduced with permission from Hamilton et al.[35]

at most 23% to the cost-effectiveness ratios for patients who began treatment at age 70 years and as little as 3% for patients at age 30 years. The authors concluded that the cost-effectiveness of lovastatin varied widely by age and sex and was sensitive to the presence of nonlipid CAD risk factors. The additional non-CAD costs due to increased life expectancy may be significant for the elderly.

Pravastatin

Straznicky and coworkers[36] in Heidelberg, Australia, conducted a study to examine the effects of short-term cholesterol reduction on cardiovascular reactivity in mildly hypertensive patients. Seven men and 7 women aged 34 to 68 years received pravastatin (40 mg/d) or matched placebo for 3 weeks in a randomized, double-blind, or crossover study. Cardiovascular reactivity was assessed by measurement of BP responses to incremental infusions of angiotensin II and norepinephrine, by cold pressor testing, and by isometric exercise. Compared with placebo, pravastatin caused significant reductions in plasma total cholesterol and LDL cholesterol levels, which averaged 20% and 31%, respectively, and in diastolic BP responses (expressed as the infusion rate required to raise BP by 20 mm Hg) to both angiotensin II and norepinephrine. Systolic BP responses were similar with both treatments. Body weight, resting BP, and maximal BP responses to physical stressors were similar with each treatment.

Jacobson and associates[37] from several medical centers in the USA studied the lipid-lowering efficacy and safety of pravastatin in 245 African-American patients with primary hypercholesterolemia. After 4 weeks on an American Heart Association Step-1 low-fat diet, patients were randomly assigned in a double-blind manner to either pravastatin or placebo in a 3:1 ratio. After 12 weeks of pravastatin treatment LDL cholesterol levels declined 26%, total cholesterol levels 20%, and triglyceride levels 6%, whereas HDL cholesterol levels remained essentially unchanged. Overall, 72% of pravastatin-treated patients received reductions in LDL cholesterol levels in excess of 20% and 44% attained declines in excess of 30%.

Shepherd and associates[38] for the West of Scotland Coronary Prevention Study Group randomly assigned 6596 men aged 45–64 years with a mean plasma total cholesterol level of 272 ± 23 mg/dL to receive pravastatin (40 mg each evening) or placebo. The average follow-up period was 4.9 years. None of the men had a history of AMI at any time. Pravastatin lowered plasma total cholesterol levels by 20% and LDL cholesterol levels by 26%, whereas there was no change with placebo (Figure 1-8). There were 248 definite coronary events, i.e., nonfatal AMI or death from CAD, in the placebo and 174 in the pravastatin group (relative reduction in risk with pravastatin, 31%) (Table 1-5) (Figure 1-9). There were similar reductions in the risks of definite nonfatal AMI (31% reduction), death from CAD (28% reduction), and death from all cardiovascular causes (32% reduction). There was no excess of deaths from noncardiovascular causes in the pravastatin group. The authors also observed a 22% reduction in the risks of death from any cause in the pravastatin group. Thus, treatment with pravastatin significantly reduced the instance of AMI and death from cardiovascular causes

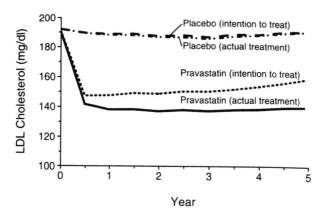

FIGURE 1-8. Effects of pravastatin therapy on plasma LDL cholesterol levels. To convert values for cholesterol to millimoles per liter, multiply by 0.026. Reproduced with permission from Shepherd et al.[38]

without adversely affecting the risk of death from noncardiovascular causes with considerable hypercholesterolemia and no history of AMI.

Fluvastatin

To determine the effects of fluvastatin combined with moderate alcohol consumption on lipid profiles and hepatic function in patients with primary hypercholesterolemia, Smit and associates[39] from Utrecht, the Netherlands, studied 31 patients with LDL cholesterol levels ≥4.2 mmol/L who had previously received a lipid-lowering diet. After a dietary baseline, 26 patients were randomly assigned to receive 6 weeks of treatment with either (1) fluvastatin, 40 mg/d, added to 20 g ethanol and diluted to 20% with orange juice or (2) fluvastatin added to orange juice alone. After a 6-week washout period, the two groups crossed over. Plasma fluvastatin levels, lipid levels, and clinical variables were determined at the end of each treatment period. Six patients left the study prematurely. The remaining patients (15 men, 5 women; mean age ± SD, 49 ± 14.5 years; mean BMI ± SD, 24.5 ± 2.2 kg/m^2) completed the study. Fluvastatin, alone and combined with alcohol, resulted in similar decreases in level of total cholesterol (22% and 23%, respectively), LDL cholesterol (28% and 29%, respectively) and apolipoprotein B (17% and 20%, respectively). HDL cholesterol and triglyceride levels were not changed. Fluvastatin with alcohol resulted in a significantly greater area under the plasma concentration curve (23.4 ± 4.7 compared with 18.2 ± 3.2 × 10^3 ng min/mL) and in a greater time to maximum concentration (187.5 ± 16.6 minutes compared with 130.9 ± 7.0 minutes) than fluvastatin alone. Terminal half-life tended to increase. No important adverse clinical effects were observed. Six weeks of daily, moderate alcohol consumption influenced the metabolism of fluvastatin but did not interfere with its lipid-lowering efficacy and had no adverse effects.

Simvastatin vs. Gemfibrozil

Bredie and coworkers[40] in Nijmegen, the Netherlands, evaluated in a double-blind, placebo-controlled, randomized trial of 45 well-defined patients with

TABLE 1-5. End Points of the Study*

Variable	Placebo (N = 3293)	Pravastatin (N = 3302)	P Value	Risk Reduction with Pravastatin (95% CI)
	no. of events (absolute % risk at 5 yr)			
Definite Coronary Events				
Nonfatal MI or death from CHD	248 (7.9)	174 (5.5)	<0.001	31 (17 to 43)
Nonfatal MI (silent MIs omitted) or death from CHD	218 (7.0)	150 (4.7)	<0.001	33 (17 to 45)
Nonfatal MI	204 (6.5)	143 (4.6)	<0.001	31 (15 to 45)
Death from CHD	52 (1.7)	38 (1.2)	0.13	28 (−10 to 52)
Definite + Suspected Coronary Events				
Nonfatal MI or death from CHD	295 (9.3)	215 (6.8)	<0.001	29 (15 to 40)
Nonfatal MI (silent MIs omitted) or death from CHD	240 (7.6)	166 (5.3)	<0.001	32 (17 to 44)
Nonfatal MI	246 (7.8)	182 (5.8)	0.001	27 (12 to 40)
Death from CHD	61 (1.9)	41 (1.3)	0.042	33 (1 to 55)
Other Events				
Coronary angiography	128 (4.2)	90 (2.8)	0.007	31 (10 to 47)
PTCA or CABG	80 (2.5)	51 (1.7)	0.009	37 (11 to 56)
Fatal or nonfatal stroke	51 (1.6)	46 (1.6)	0.57	11 (−33 to 40)
Incident cancer	106 (3.3)	116 (3.7)	0.55	−8 (−41 to 17)
Death from Other Causes				
Other cardiovascular causes (including stroke)	12	9	—	—
Suicide	1	2	—	—
Trauma	5	3	—	—
Cancer	49 (1.5)	44 (1.3)	0.56	11 (−33 to 41)
All other causes	7	7	—	—
Death from All Cardiovascular Causes	73 (2.3)	50 (1.6)	0.033	32 (3 to 53)
Death from Noncardiovascular Causes	62 (1.9)	56 (1.7)	0.54	11 (−28 to 38)
Death from Any Cause	135 (4.1)	106 (3.2)	0.051	22 (0 to 40)

*The P values are based on the log-rank test. No formal analysis was carried out for events with a low incidence. CI denotes confidence interval; CHD, coronary heart disease, MI myocardial infarction; PTCA, percutaneous transluminal coronary angioplasty; CABG, coronary artery bypass graft. Reproduced with permission from Shepherd et al.[38]

familial combined hyperlipidemia, the effect of gemfibrozil (1200 mg/d) or simvastatin (20 mg/d) on apolipoprotein B–containing lipoproteins, LDL subfraction profile, and LDL oxidizability. Although both drugs reduced plasma cholesterol and triglyceride concentrations, gemfibrozil reduced plasma triglycerides more effectively and simvastatin reduced plasma cholesterol more effectively. LDL cholesterol was reduced with simvastatin. With both drugs, total serum apolipoprotein B concentration decreased. With gemfibrozil, this was due to an exclusive reduction of very low/intermediate-density lipoprotein apolipoprotein B, whereas simvastatin decreased apolipoprotein B in both very low/intermediate-density and LDL cholesterol. Initially, a dense LDL subfraction profile was present in all patients. The decrease in LDL cholesterol with

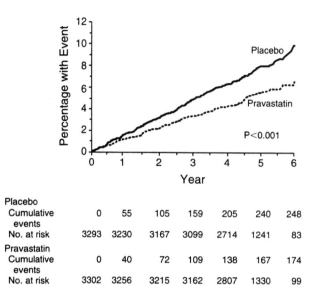

Placebo

Cumulative events	0	55	105	159	205	240	248
No. at risk	3293	3230	3167	3099	2714	1241	83

Pravastatin

Cumulative events	0	40	72	109	138	167	174
No. at risk	3302	3256	3215	3162	2807	1330	99

FIGURE 1-9. Kaplan-Meier analysis of the time to a definite nonfatal myocardial infarction or death from coronary heart disease, according to treatment group. Reproduced with permission from Shepherd et al.[38]

simvastatin was caused by a decrease in all isolated LDL subfractions except LDL$_2$; gemfibrozil increased LDL$_1$ and LDL$_2$ cholesterol and reduced LDL$_4$ cholesterol, resulting in a more buoyant LDL subfraction profile compared with simvastatin. In both groups, a predominance of small, dense LDL remained despite therapy. LDL fatty acid composition showed a shift from oleic acid to linoleic acid after gemfibrozil; arachidonic acid increased after simvastatin. Vitamin E was lower after gemfibrozil. In the measurements of LDL oxidation, only the oxidation rate was significantly reduced with simvastatin. Thus, quantitative and qualitative changes of LDL cholesterol had only a small effect on total in vitro LDL oxidizability in this population with familial combined hyperlipidemia.

Sweany associates[41] from Rahway, New Jersey; Miami, Florida; and Cincinnati, Ohio, compared the lipid-altering efficacy and safety of simvastatin with that of gemfibrozil in hypercholesterolemic patients with non–insulin-dependent diabetes mellitus. The study was a 24-week, double-blind, randomized, multicenter trial conducted at clinics and hospitals in the USA, Austria, Germany, Brazil, and New Zealand. The study population included 168 men and women aged 34–78 years with non–insulin-dependent diabetes mellitus and primary hypercholesterolemia (LDL cholesterol level at screening was ≥4.9 mmol/L with one or more other risk factors). All patients had been under moderate-to-good diabetic control (hemoglobin A$_{1c}$ [HbA$_{1c}$] ≤ 10.0%) for at least 6 months with diet alone, oral hypoglycemic agents, or insulin therapy. Patients meeting eligibility criteria were randomized to receive either simvastatin 10 mg (titrated up to 40 mg to achieve an LDL cholesterol level <3.4 mmol/L) once in the evening or gemfibrozil 600 mg twice daily. There were 81 patients in the simvastatin group and 87 patients in the gemfibrozil group. After 17 weeks of treatment, simvastatin significantly reduced levels of total cholesterol, LDL cholesterol, and VLDL cholesterol by approximately 25%, 33%, and 20%, respectively, and triglycerides by about 9%. The drug increased HDL cholesterol levels by about 6%. Gemfibrozil significantly reduced total cholesterol, VLDL cholesterol and triglyceride levels by approximately 8%, 38%, and 27%, respectively; it significantly increased HDL cholesterol values by about 12%. Gemfibrozil lowered LDL cholesterol levels by 4% but not significantly. The decreases in total cholesterol and LDL cholesterol were significantly greater in the simvastatin group, and decreases in VLDL cholesterol and triglycerides were significantly greater in the gemfibrozil group. The changes in HDL cholesterol were not significantly different between groups. LDL cholesterol values of <3.4 mmol/L were achieved in 60% of the simvastatin patients and 14% of the gemfibrozil patients. There were no significant between-group differences in fasting serum glucose or HbA$_{1c}$ at any time point. Glycemic profiles (performed at baseline and after 17 weeks of treatment) were not significantly different between treatment groups. Both drugs were generally well tolerated. In conclusion, simvastatin was more effective in reducing total cholesterol and LDL cholesterol levels, whereas gemfibrozil was more effective in reducing VLDL cholesterol and triglyceride levels. There was no deterioration of glycemic control in patients treated with simvastatin.

Colestipol

Hunninghake and associates[42] from multiple medical centers in the USA conducted a randomized, double-blind, placebo-controlled, multicenter, dose-ranging study to evaluate the efficacy and safety of a new formulation of colestipol provided in tablet form. A total of 196 patients with primary hypercholesterolemia who were following a low-fat, low-cholesterol diet (NCEP Step-1 diet), and having mean LDL cholesterol levels ≥4.14 mmol/L^{-1} and ≤6.46 mmol/L^{-1} (250 mg dL^{-1}) were studied. Study medication was taken twice daily, with breakfast and supper for 8 weeks. The 5 parallel treatment groups consisted of colestipol tablets 1, 2, 4, and 8 g twice daily, and matching placebo tablets twice daily. The main outcome measures were absolute change and percent change from baseline in selected lipid, lipoprotein, and apolipoprotein measurements; LDL cholesterol was considered primary. Statistically significant dose-dependent reductions in LDL cholesterol from 5.2% to 25.8% and in total cholesterol from 2.8% to 16.8% were observed. Colestipol tablet treatment also resulted in statistically significant dose-dependent increases in lipoprotein AI levels reaching 25.8% at 16 g day^{-1}. The treatment was well tolerated, and no serious adverse events were reported. Colestipol administered in tablet form was efficacious in lowering LDL cholesterol and total cholesterol and was well tolerated in patients with primary hypercholesterolemia.

Cholestipol + Lovastatin

Schrott and colleagues[43] in Kalamazoo Michigan, randomly assigned 96 patients with moderate elevations of LDL cholesterol to 4 different double-blind treatment regimens once a day: placebo; colestipol, 5 g, and lovastatin, 20 mg; colestipol, 10 g, plus lovastatin, 20 mg; and lovastatin, 40 mg/d. During 12 weeks of therapy, colestipol, 10 g, plus lovastatin, 20 mg, achieved the greatest reduction in total cholesterol (−32%) and LDL cholesterol (−48%) levels from baseline. This combination also exhibited significantly greater reductions in LDL cholesterol levels than the colestipol, 5 g, plus lovastatin, 20 mg, and the lovastatin, 40 mg, groups. The differences in total and LDL cholesterol reduction between the colestipol, 5 g, plus lovastatin, 20 mg, and lovastatin, 40 mg, groups were not significant. Similar changes and differences between treatments were seen in apolipoprotein B levels. Whereas mean total apolipoprotein A-1 levels increased with all treatments, lipoprotein particles A-1 were significantly increased in the colestipol, 10 g, plus lovastatin, 20 mg, group only. Results demonstrate that the combination of low-dose lovastatin (20 mg/d) with low-dose colestipol (5 or 10 g/d) produces LDL cholesterol reductions equal or greater than higher doses of lovastatin (40 mg/d). In addition, low-dose combinations are >25% more cost-effective than high-dose monotherapy.

Colestipol + Lovastatin vs. Colestipol + Niacin

To determine if lowering elevated LDL-cholesterol levels offsets the adverse effects of raised lipoprotein(a) levels on CAD levels in men, Maher and associates[44] from Seattle, Washington, studied in a randomized, double-blind, placebo-controlled trial a total of 146 men aged 62 years or younger with CAD and apolipoprotein B levels of at least 125 mg/dL. Patients received a Step-2 diet and lovastatin (40 mg/d) plus colestipol (30 g/d), niacin (4 g/d) plus colestipol, or placebo (plus colestipol if LDL cholesterol was >90th percentile) for 2.5 years. In multivariate analyses, the best correlate of baseline CAD severity was lipoprotein(a). For 36 patients with minimal LDL cholesterol reduction, CAD progression correlated only with in-treatment lipoprotein(a) levels, but for 84 patients with substantial LDL cholesterol reduction, disease regressed and its change correlated with in-treatment LDL cholesterol but not with lipoprotein(a). Lipoprotein(a) levels were not significantly altered in either group. For 40 patients with lipoprotein(a) at the 90th percentile or higher, events were frequent (39%) if reduction of LDL was minimal, but were few (9%) if reduction was substantial (RR, 0.23). In men with CAD and elevated LDL cholesterol lipoprotein(a) levels were dominant correlates of baseline disease severity, its progression, and event rate over 2.5 years. However, with substantial LDL cholesterol reductions, persistent elevations of lipoprotein(a) were no longer atherogenic or clinically threatening. This provides a possible direction for treatment in such patients with elevated lipoprotein(a) and LDL cholesterol.

Colestipol + Psyllium Mucilloid

To test whether combining psyllium mucilloid with half the usual dose of colestipol reduces the adverse effects associated with colestipol and maintains or increases its efficacy in the treatment of hyperlipidemia, Spence and associates[45] from London, Canada, in a randomized, parallel group, double-blind, controlled trial studied 120 patients with total cholesterol levels >6 mmol/L and <8 mmol/L and triglyceride levels <3 mmol/L after following a low-fat diet for 1 year. A combination of 2.5 g psyllium and 2.5 g colestipol was better tolerated and as effective as either 5 g colestipol alone or 5 g psyllium alone. The combination therapy and colestipol alone did not differ significantly with respect to changes in individual lipid values. The ratio of total cholesterol to HDL cholesterol was reduced by 18% with the combination therapy; by 11% with colestipol alone, by 6% with psyllium alone, and by 0.1% with placebo.

Combination therapy reduced the ratio of total cholesterol to HDL significantly more than colestipol alone or psyllium alone. These findings suggest that adding psyllium to half the usual dose of colestipol maintains the efficacy and improves the tolerability of these resins.

Cholestyramine vs. Cholestyramine + Lovastatin vs. Lovastatin

To test the potency of low-dose cholesterol-lowering drug therapy in patients with moderate hypercholesterolemia (LDL cholesterol levels 160–220 mg/dL and a serum triglyceride level of >200 mg/dL) and to evaluate the effectiveness of cholesterol-lowering of a safe regimen to be used in primary prevention of CAD, Denke and Grundy[46] from Dallas, Texas, tested the efficacy of 3 drug regimens (cholestyramine resin, 8 g/d; cholestyramine resin, 8 g/d, plus lovastatin, 5 mg/d; and lovastatin, 20 mg/d) in 26 men aged 31–70 years with moderate hypercholesterolemia after a Step-1 cholesterol-lowering diet. Each drug period was 3 months in duration interspersed with a 1-month period of the Step-1 diet only. Blood for lipid and lipoprotein measurement was obtained on 5 different days during the last 2 weeks of each drug and diet only. Cholestyramine resin therapy at 8 g/d achieved a significant reduction in LDL cholesterol levels from 4.47 mmol/L (173 mg/dL) to 3.90 mmol/L (151 mg/dL). The addition of 5 mg lovastatin to cholestyramine therapy achieved even lower levels, averaging 3.39 mmol/L (131 mg/dL). Lovastatin therapy at 20 mg/d produced lowering of LDL cholesterol levels similar to that of the low-dose combination. Low-dose combination drug therapy for the management of hypercholesterolemia appears to be an effective means of lowering cholesterol levels that remain persistently elevated after dietary therapy; at the same time, it should carry a low risk of toxic effects.

Niacin

To document the prevalence and nature of the side effects that occur with the use of regular and sustained-release nicotinic acid in everyday clinical practice, Gibbons and associates[47] from Dallas, Texas, studied 110 patients in a private medical clinic setting who were getting 133 separate trials of nicotinic acid during a 5-year period. Forty-three percent of individuals given regular nicotinic acid and 42% of those given sustained-release nicotinic acid were forced to discontinue the medication because of side effects. Some of the side effects necessitating discontinuing nicotinic acid did not occur until the patient had been taking the drug for 1–2 years. Thus, nicotinic acid in both regular and sustained-release forms is a powerful drug when used in doses needed to treat lipid disorders and causes disturbing side effects a very high percentage of the time. In the study by Gibbons and colleagues, nicotinic acid was not given to any patient with hepatic dysfunction, history of peptic ulcer disease, diabetes mellitus, or those with a fasting blood glucose >120 mg/dL. Liver function tests were monitored in the patients every 3–4 months, as were blood glucose and uric acid levels.

Antioxidant Vitamins

To review prospective epidemiological studies and randomized trials regarding the role of antioxidant vitamins (vitamins E and C and β-carotene) in the prevention of cardiovascular disease, with emphasis on differences in results obtained by these 2 types of studies, Jha and associates[48] from Ontario, Canada, studied epidemiological studies and randomized trials that included 100 or more participants and provided quantified estimates of antioxidant vitamin intake. All 3 large epidemiological cohort studies of vitamin E noted that high-level vitamin E intake or supplementation was associated with a significant reduction in cardiovascular disease (relative RR [RRR] range, 31–65%), as measured by various fatal and nonfatal cardiovascular end points. To obtain these reductions, vitamin E supplementation must last at least 2 years. Less consistent reductions were seen in studies of β-carotene (RRR range, −2% to 46%), and vitamin C (RRR range, −25% to 51%). Considerable biases in observational studies, such as different health behaviors of persons using antioxidants, may account for the observed benefit. By contrast, none of the completed randomized trials showed any clear reduction in cardiovascular disease with vitamin E, vitamin C, or β-carotene supplementation. The trials were not specifically designed to assess cardiovascular disease, did not provide data on nonfatal cardiovascular end points, may have had insufficient treatment durations, and used suboptimal vitamin E doses. The completed trials were of adequate size to indicate that the true therapeutic benefit of vitamin E and other antioxidants in reducing fatal cardiovascular disease (a survival benefit as long as 5 years) is probably more modest than the epidemiological data suggest. The epidemiological data suggest that antioxidant vitamins reduce cardiovascular disease, with the clearest effect for vitamin E; however, completed randomized trials do not support this finding.

Low-Density Lipoprotein Apheresis

LDL apheresis has the theoretical advantage over anion-exchange resins and hydroxymethylglutaryl coenzyme A inhibitors of decreasing lipoprotein(a) as well as LDL. To confirm this advantage, patients with heterozygous familial hypercholesterolemia and CAD were randomly assigned by Thompson and associates[49] from 4 non-US medical centers to receive LDL apheresis fortnightly (with disposable dextran sulphate/cellulose columns) plus simvastatin, 40 mg/d, or colestipol, 20 g, plus simvastatin, 40 mg/d. Quantitative coronary angiography was repeated after a mean of 2.1 years in 20 patients undergoing apheresis and in 19 on combination drug therapy. Changes in serum lipoproteins were similar in both groups apart from greater lowering by apheresis of LDL cholesterol (3.2 vs. 3.4 mmol/L in drug group) and lipoprotein(a) (geometric means, 14 vs. 21 mg/dL). There were no significant differences in primary angiographic end points per patient but lesion-based and segment-based secondary end points were biased in favor of the drug group (change in minimum lumen diameter of lesions, 0.07 vs. −0.004 mm; change in mean lumen diameter of segments, 0.02 vs. −0.06 mm). None of the angiographic changes correlated with lipoprotein(a) concentrations. Per patient changes in percent diameter stenosis and minimum lumen diameter in the 2 groups were as or more favorable than those observed in 5 published trials that assessed lipid-lowering drug therapy by quantitative coronary angiography. Although LDL apheresis with simvastatin was more effective than colestipol plus simvastatin in reducing LDL cholesterol and lipoprotein(a), it was less beneficial in influencing coronary atherosclerosis and should be reserved for patients unresponsive to drugs. Decreasing lipoprotein(a) seems to be unnecessary if LDL is reduced to 3.4 mmol/L or less.

Heparin-induced extracorporeal LDL precipitation treatments selectively remove LDL with minimal effects on HDL but limited data are available on effects between treatments. The levels of factors associated with increased CAD risk among treatments may have therapeutic significance, especially for combined heparin-induced precipitation and lipid-lowering drug therapy. Lane and colleagues[50] in Oklahoma City, Oklahoma, treated hypercholesterolemic and combined hyperlipidemic patients resistant to diet/drug therapy with biweekly heparin-induced extracorporeal LDL precipitation therapy. Hypercholesterolemic patients received either lovastatin or no drug, whereas combined hyperlipidemic patients received gemfibrozil. Plasma lipid (total cholesterol, triglycerides, LDL cholesterol, and HDL cholesterol) and apolipoprotein A-I, A-II, B, C-III, and E levels were measured before treatment, then immediately and 2, 4, 7, and 14 days after treatments. Atherogenic factor (LDL cholesterol, total cholesterol, and apolipoprotein B) levels decreased >50% with treatment, gradually increasing over 14 days to pretreatment levels. Factors associated with reduced CAD risk (HDL and apolipoproteins A-I and A-II) decreased 8% to 16% but recovered by 2 days. Components of triglyceride-rich lipoproteins (triglycerides and apolipoproteins C-III and E) decreased 38% to 55% with variable post-treatment recoveries. Lovastatin reduced pretreatment levels of atherogenic and triglyceride-rich lipoprotein components and slowed post-treatment increases compared with no drug therapy. Gemfibrozil produced changes similar to lovastatin. Drug therapy had little effect on factors associated with reduced CAD risk. Heparin-induced extracorporeal LDL precipitation apheresis produced large reductions in plasma atherogenic factor levels with gradual return to pretreatment levels over 14 days, whereas antiatherogenic factors were minimally reduced and recovered rapidly. Lipid-lowering drug therapy reduced pretreatment levels and delayed post-treatment increases of both cholesterol- and triglyceride-rich lipoproteins.

Obesity, Body Fat, Body Weight, and Weight Change

The 1990 US weight guidelines for women support a substantial gain in weight at approximately 35 years of age and recommend a range of BMI (defined as weight in kilograms divided by the square of height in meters) from 21 to 27 kg/m². To test its validity in terms of CAD risk in women, during a 14-year follow-up period, Willett and associates[51] from Boston, Massachusetts, studied 1292 women with clinical evidence of CAD. All women were 30–55 years old in 1976 and were registered nurses in the United States. After controlling for age, smoking, menopausal status, postmenopausal hormone use, and parental history of CAD and using as a reference women with a BMI of <21 kg/m², RR and 95% confidence intervals (CIs) for CAD were 1.19 for a BMI of 21–22.9 kg/m², 1.46 for a BMI of 23–24.9 kg/m², 2.06 for a BMI of 25 to 28.9 kg/m², and 3.56 for a BMI of 29 kg/m² or more. Women who gained weight from 18 years of age were compared with those with stable weight (±5 kg) in analyses that controlled for the same variables as well as BMI at 18 years of age. The RRs and CIs were 1.25 for a 5- to 7.9-kg gain, 1.64 for an 8- to 10.9-kg gain, 1.92 for an 11- to 19-kg gain, and 2.65 for a gain of 20 kg or more. Among women within the BMI range of 18 to 25 kg/m^2, weight gain after 18 years of age remained a strong predictor of CAD risk. Higher levels of body weight within the "normal" range, as well as modest weight gains after 18 years of age, appear to increase risks of CAD in middle-aged women. These data provide evidence that current US weight guidelines may be falsely reassuring to the large proportion of women older than 35 years who are within the current guidelines but have potentially avoidable risks of CAD.

To test the hypothesis that a single measurement—waist circumference—might be used to identify people at health risk both from being overweight and from having a central fat distribution, Lean and associates[52] from Glasgow, UK, studied 904 men and 1014 women as a first sample and then 86 men and 202 women as a validation sample. Waist circumference ≥94 cm for men and ≥80 cm for women identified subjects with high BMI (≥25 kg/m^2) and those with lower BMI but high waist-to-hip ratio (≥0.95 for men, ≥.80 for women) with a sensitivity of >96% and specificity >97.5%. Waist circumference ≥102 cm for men or ≥88 cm for women identified subjects with BMIs ≥30 and those with a lower BMI but high waist-to-hip ratio with a sensitivity of >96% and specificity >98%, with only about 2% of the sample being misclassified. Waist circumference could be used in health promotion programs to identify individuals who should seek and be offered weight management. Men with waist circumference ≥94 cm and women with waist circumference ≥80 cm should gain no further weight; men with waist circumference ≥102 and women with waist circumference ≥88 should reduce their weight.

To determine the frequency of cardiovascular risk factors in people categorized by previously defined "action levels" of waist circumference, Han and associates[53] from Glasgow, UK, studied 2183 men and 2698 women aged 20–59 years selected randomly from the civil registry of Amsterdam and Maastricht, the Netherlands. A waist circumference exceeding 94 cm in men and 80 cm in women correctly identified subjects with a BMI of ≥25 and waist-to-hip ratios ≥.95 in men and ≥.80 in women with a sensitivity and specificity of ≥96%. Men and women with at least one cardiovascular risk factor (total cholesterol, ≥6.5 mmol/L; HDL-C, ≤0.9 mmol/L; systolic BP, ≥160 mm Hg, diastolic BP, ≥95 mm Hg) were identified with sensitivities of 57% and 67% and specificities of 72% and 62%, respectively. Compared with those with waist measurements below action levels, age- and lifestyle-adjusted odds ratios for having at least one risk factor were 2.2 in men with a waist measurement of 94–102 cm and 1.6 in women with a waist measurement of 80–88 cm. Larger waist circumference identifies people at increased cardiovascular risk.

Manson and associates[54] from Boston, Massachusetts, examined the association between BMI (defined as the weight in kilograms divided by the square of the height in meters) and both overall mortality and mortality from specific causes in a cohort of 115 195 US women enrolled in the prospective Nurses' Health Study. These women were 30–55 years of age and free of known cardiovascular disease and cancer in 1976. During 16 years of follow-up, we documented 4726 deaths, of which 881 were from cardiovascular disease, 2586 from cancer, and 1259 from other causes. In analyses adjusted only for age, we observed a J-shaped relation between BMI and overall mortality. When women who had never smoked were examined separately, no increase in risk was observed among the leaner women, and a more direct relation between weight and mortality emerged. In multivariate analyses of women who had never smoked and had recently had stable weight, in which the first 4 years of follow-up were excluded, the relative risks of death from all causes for increasing categories of BMI were as follows: for BMI, <19.0 (the reference category), RR was 1.0; BMI, 19.0–21.9, RR, 1.2; BMI, 22.0–24.9, RR, 1.2; BMI, 25.0–26.9, RR, 1.3; BMI, 27.0–28.9, RR, 1.6; BMI, 29.0–31.9, RR, 2.1; and BMI, ≥32.0, RR, 2.2. Among women with BMIs of 32.0 or higher who had never smoked, the RR value of death from cardiovascular disease was 4.1, and that of death from cancer was 2.1, as compared with the risk among women with BMIs below 19.0. A weight gain of 10 kg (22 lb) or more since the age of 18 was associated with increased mortality in middle adulthood. Body weight and mortality from all causes were directly related among these middle-aged women. Lean women did not have excess mortality. The lowest mortality rate was observed among women who weighed at least 15% less than the US average for women of similar age and among those whose weight had been stable since early adulthood.

Iribarren and associates[55] from Minneapolis, Minnesota; Bethesda, Maryland; and Manoa, Hawaii, examined the long-term relation of weight change and fluctuation in weight with mortality over a 6-year period in 6537 middle-aged Japanese-American men enrolled in the Honolulu Heart Program, a prospective study with a mean follow-up of 14.5 years. Men who had a weight loss of 4.5 kg or more or who had large fluctuations in weight 9 or (both) over a 6-year period were, on average, in poorer health than their peers whose weight was more stable. After the exclusion of subjects who died during the first 5 years of follow-up and after adjustment for confounding factors, a weight loss of more than 4.5 kg was associated with the risk of death from all causes, with the exception of death from cancer. The subjects whose weight fluctuated the most had a significantly higher risk of death from cardiovascular causes (RR, 1.41), death from noncardiovascular and noncancerous causes (RR, 1.53), and death from all causes (RR, 1.25). However, the associations of weight loss and variation in weight with death from noncancerous causes were not found among healthy men who had never smoked. The associations between weight loss or fluctuation and mortality were partially explained by confounding factors and the presence of preexisting disease. However, weight loss and weight fluctuation were unrelated to death among healthy men who had never smoked. Thus, concern about the health hazards of weight loss and variation may not be applicable to otherwise healthy people.

Walton and associates[56] from London, UK, investigated the relation between the amount and distribution of body fat and fasting serum lipids and lipoproteins to explore whether CAD risk may be mediated through effects on the serum lipid profile. The authors determined serum total cholesterol and triglyceride, LDL cholesterol, HDL cholesterol and HDL subfractions 2 and 3 in 103 healthy men, aged 21–77 years (mean, 48.7). The amount and distribution of fat were determined directly by dual energy X-ray absorptiometry. Adiposity was determined as the ratio between total body fat tissue and total body lean tissue, whereas fat distribution was taken as the ratio between the mass of fat tissue in the android (central) and gynoid (hip and thigh) regions. Univariate analysis showed both adiposity and fat distribution to be correlated with total serum cholesterol and triglyceride concentrations (adiposity $r = 0.20, 0.21$; fat distribution, $r = 0.25, 0.38$, respectively). Fat distribution was also negatively correlated with HDL_2 cholesterol ($r = -0.20$). In multiple linear regression analysis, neither age nor adiposity was significantly correlated with any serum lipid or lipoprotein concentration, whereas increasing the android-to-gynoid ratio was independently associated with elevated total serum triglyceride ($r = 0.40$) and decreased HDL_2 ($r = -0.25$) concentrations. The associations of both age and overall adiposity with the fasting serum lipid profile are mediated via their correlations with body fat distribution. In men, the distribution, rather than the amount, of body fat is related to adverse changes in serum lipids and lipoproteins, and hence potentially to increased CAD risk.

To compare the effects of weight loss vs. aerobic exercise training on CAD risk factors in healthy sedentary, obese, middle-aged and older men, Katzel and associates[57] from Baltimore, Maryland, studied 170 obese men (BMI, 30 ± 1 kg/m²) (average age, 61 ± 1 years) on a 9-month diet-induced weight loss intervention, a 9-month aerobic exercise training program, and a weight maintenance control group. Forty-four of the 73 men randomly assigned to weight loss completed the intervention and had a 10% weight reduction, with no change in oxygen consumption. Forty-nine of 71 men randomly assigned to aerobic exercise completed the intervention, increased their oxygen consumption by a mean of 17%, and did not change their weight, whereas the 18 men in the control group had no significant changes in body composition or oxygen consumption. Weight loss decreased fasting glucose concentrations by 2%, insulin by 18%, and glucose and insulin areas during the oral glucose tolerance test by 8% and 26%, respectively. By contrast, aerobic exercise did not improve fasting glucose or insulin concentrations or glucose responses during the oral glucose tolerance test but decreased insulin areas by 17%. In analysis of variance, the decrement in fasting glucose and insulin levels and glucose areas with intervention differed between weight loss and aerobic exercise when compared with the control group. Similarly, weight loss but not aerobic exercise increased HDL cholesterol levels (+13%) and decreased BP compared with the control group. In multiple regression analyses, the improvement in lipoproteins and glucose metabolism was related primarily to the reduction in obesity. These results suggest that weight loss is the preferred treatment to improve CAD risk factors in overweight, middle-aged, and older men.

To determine if individuals who are overall obese but have a low waist-to-hip ratio have unfavorable lipid profiles, BP, and glucose statuses, Young and Gelskey[58] interviewed 2792 adults aged 18–74 years; 2339 of them underwent clinical examination. Their population with noncentral obesity tended to occupy positions between those of the nonobese and the centrally obese in terms of the effect on BP, plasma lipids, and glucose. Both BMI and waist-to-hip ratio proved to be significant predictors of most metabolic variables. The recognition of the epidemiological significance of waist-to-hip ratio as a centrality measure of obesity should not divert attention from the metabolic risk status of noncentrally obese individuals who require continued health education to reduce weight.

Physical Activity and Fitness

To evaluate the relation between changes in physical fitness and risk of mortality in men, Blair and associates[59] from Dallas, Texas; Stanford, California; and Columbia, South Carolina, assessed change or lack of change in physical fitness as associated with risk of mortality during follow-up after the subsequent examination (mean follow-up from subsequent examination, 5.1 years). The participants were 9777 men given 2 preventive medical examinations (mean interval between examinations, 4.9 years), each of which included assessment of physical fitness by maximal exercise tests and evaluation of health status. The highest age adjusted all-cause death rate was observed in men who were unfit at both examinations (122/10 000 man-years); the lowest death rate was in men who were physically fit at both examinations (39.6/10 000 man-years). Men who improved from unfit to fit between the first and subsequent examinations had an age-adjusted death rate of 67.7/10 000 man-years. This is a reduction in mortality risk of 44% relative to men who remained unfit at both examinations. Improvement in fitness was associated with lower death rates after adjusting for age, health status, and other risk factors of premature mortality. For each minute increase in maximal treadmill time between examinations, there was a corresponding 7.9% decrease in risk of mortality. Similar results were seen when the group was stratified by health status, and for cardiovascular disease mortality. Men who maintained or improved adequate physical fitness were less likely to die from all causes and from cardiovascular disease during follow-up than persistently unfit men.

To examine the independent associations of vigorous (≥ 6 resting metabolic rate [MET] score) and nonvigorous (<6 MET score) physical activity with longevity, Lee and associates[60] from Boston, Massachusetts, and Stanford, California, studied 17 321 Harvard University alumni without self-reported physician-diagnosed cardiovascular disease, cancer, or chronic obstructive pulmonary disease. Men with a mean age of 46 years reported their physical activities on questionnaires at baseline. Total energy expended and energy expenditure from vigorous activities, but not energy expenditure from nonvigorous activities, related inversely to mortality. After adjustment for potential confounders, the relative risks of dying associated with increasing quintiles of total energy expenditure were 1.00 (referent), 0.94, 0.95, 0.91, and 0.91, respectively. The RR values of dying associated with <630, 630 to <1 680, 1 680 to <3 150, 3 150 to <6 300, and 6 300 or more kJ/week expended on vigorous activities were 1.00 (referent), 0.88, 0.92, 0.87, and 0.87, respectively. Analyses of vigorous and nonvigorous activities were mutually adjusted. Among men who reported only vigorous activities (259 deaths), we observed decreasing age-standardized mortality rates with increasing activity; among men who reported only nonvigorous activities (380 deaths), no trend was apparent. These data demonstrate a graded inverse relation between total physical activity and mortality. Furthermore, vigorous activities but not nonvigorous activities were associated with longevity. These findings pertain only to all-cause mortality; nonvigorous exercise has been shown to benefit other aspects of health.

To determine whether participation in physical activity during leisure time decreases the risk of AMI in postmenopausal women, Lemaitre and associates[61] from Seattle, Washington, analyzed 268 postmenopausal women with nonfatal AMI during the period 1986–1991 and also 925 controls. Participation in physical activity during leisure time in each group was assessed from a telephone interview. After adjustment for potential confounding factors, the odds ratio for nonfatal AMI for women in the second, third, and fourth quartile of total energy expenditure, relative to women in the first quartile, were 0.52, 0.40,

0.26, and 0.40, respectively. Similar odds ratios were associated with the energy expended in nonstrenuous leisure-time physical activity, and with walking for exercise. This case-control study suggests that the risk of AMI among postmenopausal women is decreased by 50% with modest leisure-time energy expenditures, equivalent to 30–45 minutes of walking for exercise 3 times a week.

Cigarette Smoking

Prevalence in the United States

The annual prevalence of cigarette smoking among adults in the United States declined 40% from 1965 to 1990 (from 42.4% to 25.5%) but was virtually unchanged 1990–1992. A survey (1993 National Health Interview Survey) collected self-reported information of cigarette smoking from a random sample of civilian, noninstitutionalized adults aged ≥18 years.[62] The response rate for the survey was 81%. For 1993, current smoking status was determined through two questions: (1) Have you smoked at least 100 cigarettes in your entire life? and (2) Do you now smoke cigarettes every day, some days, or not at all? "Ever smokers" were persons who reported having smoked at least 100 cigarettes during their entire lives. Current smokers were defined as those who had smoked 100 cigarettes and now smoked either every day (daily smokers) or some days (some day smokers). Former smokers had smoked at least 100 cigarettes in their lives but did not currently smoke. The prevalence of cessation was the percent of former smokers among ever smokers. In 1993, an estimated 46 million (25%) adults in the USA were current smokers: 24.4% were daily smokers, and 4.6% were occasional smokers. Smoking prevalence was higher among men (28%) than women (22%). Twenty-four million men smoked and 22 million women smoked. The ratio/ethnic group–specific prevalence was highest among American Indians/Alaskan Natives (39%) and lowest among Asians/Pacific Islanders (18%). The prevalence among persons with ≤8 years of education was significantly higher than among persons with 9–15 years of education; among persons with ≥9 years of education, prevalence is varied in virtually with education level. For all groups, the prevalence of smoking was highest among males who had dropped out of high school (42%). Smoking prevalence was higher among persons living below the poverty level (32%) than among those living at or above the poverty level (24%). The prevalence of current smokers in 1993 was unchanged statistically from 1992. The prevalence of daily smoking in 1993 (20.4%) was significantly lower than in 1992 (22.3%). In addition, prevalence estimates for current smokers during 1993 were lower overall for women, persons with a college education or higher, total persons living at or above the poverty level, and women living at or above the poverty level. Of current smokers, an estimated 32 million persons (70%) reported that they wanted to quit smoking completely. In 1993, an estimated 46 million adults were former smokers (50% of ever smokers). The prevalence of cessation was higher among men (52%), whites (52%), and persons living at or above the poverty level (52%), and increased directly with age.

Nicotine Therapy

To determine the effectiveness of the 4-mg and 2-mg dosages of nicotine polacrilex vs. placebo through the first 6 weeks of treatment in assisting high-dependent smokers to stop smoking when instructed to use a fixed amount (12 pieces) of medication daily, Sachs[63] from Stanford, California, studied 90 high-dependent healthy male and female smokers, highly motivated to quit smoking, and enrolled them in a 6-week randomized, double-blind, placebo-controlled trial in which they were instructed to use 12 pieces per day of their assigned dosage formulation: 4 mg, 2 mg, or 0.5 mg (placebo) of nicotine polacrilex. For 55 of the 90 smokers who met the originally planned definition of high dependence, results were 63% in the 4-mg group, 25% in the 2-mg group, and 25% in the placebo group. In addition, the 4-mg dose produced a statistically significantly higher abstinence rate in compliant subjects. Thus, it appears that the 4-mg dose of nicotine polacrilex is the drug and dose of choice for the initial phase of tobacco-dependent treatment in high-dependent smokers. The 2-mg dose was no better than placebo.

To compare the efficacy and safety of 22-mg and 44-mg doses of transdermal nicotine therapy paired with minimal, individual, or group counseling to improve smoking cessation rates, Jorenby and associates[64] from Madison, Wisconsin, and Rochester, Minnesota, conducted an 8-week clinical trial (*r* weeks double-blind followed by 4 weeks open label) using random assignment of participants to both dose (22 or 44 mg) and counseling (minimal, individual, or group) conditions. Treatment included 4 weeks of 22- or 44-mg transdermal nicotine therapy followed by 4 weeks of dosage reduction (2 weeks of 22 mg followed by 2 weeks of 11 mg). Counseling consisted of a self-help pamphlet (minimal); a self-help pamphlet, a brief physician motivational message, and three brief (<15 minutes) follow-up visits with a nurse (individual); or the pamphlet, the motivational message, and 8 weekly 1-hour group smoking cessation counseling visits (group). All participants returned weekly to turn in questionnaires and for assessment of their smoking status. A total of 504 daily cigarette smokers (≥15 cigarettes a day for at least 1 year) were enrolled at two sites. Abstinence from smoking was based on self-report, confirmed by an expired carbon monoxide concentration lower than 10 ppm. Withdrawal severity was assessed by means of an eight-item self-report questionnaire completed daily. Smoking cessation rates for the two nicotine patch doses and three levels of counseling did not differ significantly at either 8 weeks or 26 weeks following the quit date. Among those receiving minimal contact, the 44-mg dose produced greater abstinence at 4 weeks than did the 22-mg dose (68% vs. 45%). Participants receiving minimal-contact adjuvant treatment were less likely to be abstinent at the end of 4 weeks than those receiving individual or group counseling (56% vs. 67%). The 44-mg dose decreased the desire to smoke more than did the 22-mg dose, but this effect was not related to success in quitting smoking. Transdermal nicotine therapy at doses of 44 mg produced a significantly greater frequency of nausea (28%), vomiting (10%), and erythema with edema at the patch site (30%) than did a 22-mg dose (10%, 2%, and 13%, respectively). Three serious adverse events occurred during use of the 44-mg patch dose. There does not appear to be any general, sustained benefit of initiating transdermal nicotine therapy with a 44-mg dose or of providing intense adjuvant smoking cessation treatment. The 2 doses and all adjuvant treatments produced equivalent effects at the 26-week follow-up, and the higher treatments produced more adverse effects. Higher-dose (44-mg) nicotine replacement does not appear to be indicated for general clinical populations, although it may provide short-term benefit to some smokers attempting to quit with minimal adjuvant treatment.

Cessation and Weight Gain

The proportion of US adults 35–74 years of age who are overweight increased 9.6% for men and 8.0% for women between 1978 and 1990. Since the prevalence of smoking declined over the same period, smoking cessation has been suggested as a factor contributing to the increasing prevalence of overweight. To estimate the influence of smoking cessation on the increase in the prevalence of overweight, Flegal and associates[65] from Hyattsville, Maryland, analyzed data on current and past weight and smoking status for a national sample of 5247 adults 35 years of age or older who participated in the third National Health and Nutrition Examination Survey, conducted from 1988–1991. The results were adjusted for age, sociodemographic characteristics, level of physical activity, alcohol consumption, and (for women) parity. The weight gain over a 10-year period that was associated with the cessation of smoking (i.e., the gain among smokers who quit that was in excess of the gain among continuing smokers) was 4.4 kg for men and 5.0 kg for women. Smokers who had quit within the past 10 years were significantly more likely than respondents who had never smoked to become overweight (odds ratios, 2.4 for men and 2.0 for women). For men, about a quarter (2.3 of 9.6% points) and for women, about a sixth (1.3 of 8.0% points) of the increase in the prevalence of overweight could be attributed to smoking cessation within the past 10 years. Although its health benefits are undeniable, smoking cessation may nevertheless be associated with a small increase in the prevalence of overweight.

Effects on Endothelial Function

Zeiher and colleagues[66] in Frankfurt, Germany, investigated whether long-term is smoking associated with impaired endothelial vasodilator function of epicardial conductance vessels irrespective of the presence or absence of atherosclerotic lesions. Using quantitative coronary angiography, they measured epicardial artery diameter at baseline, after maximal increases in coronary blood flow that caused flow-mediated dilation, and after intracoronary injection of nitroglycerin in 96 patients. Endothelium-dependent, flow-mediated dilation was significantly blunted in smokers compared with nonsmokers. The ratio of flow-dependent dilation to nitroglycerin-induced dilation was significantly lower in smokers compared with nonsmokers, indicating that the blunted dilator response to increased blood flow was out of proportion to the mildly impaired dilator response to nitroglycerin in smokers. In the presence of angiographically visible atherosclerosis, flow-dependent dilation was essentially absent in smokers (Figure 1-10). Multivariate analysis revealed that luminal irregularities by angiography and smoking were the only variables to be independently associated with a reduced flow-dependent dilator response of epicardial arteries. Intracoronary ultrasound showed that flow-dependent dilation progressively decreased with increasing atherosclerotic plaque load. Segments from smokers exhibited a significantly impaired flow-dependent dilator response compared with those of nonsmokers. Thus, long-term cigarette smoking

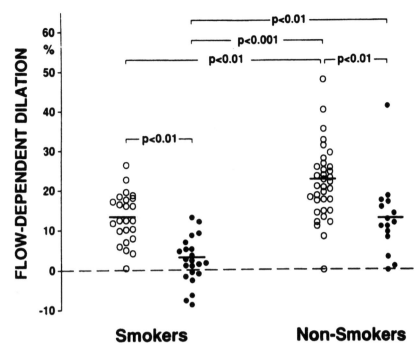

FIGURE 1-10. Plot showing flow-dependent dilation of angiographically normal (○) and angiographically irregular segments (●) in smokers and nonsmokers. Reproduced with permission from Zeiher et al.[66]

is associated with impaired endothelium-dependent coronary vasodilation irrespective of the presence or absence of coronary atherosclerosis.

Effect on Myocardial Blood Flow

Czernin and colleagues[67] in Los Angeles, California, examined the effect of short-term and long-term smoking on coronary vasodilator capacity and myocardial flow reserve in 12 smokers and 12 sex- and age-matched nonsmokers serving as controls. Myocardial blood flow was quantified at rest and during dipyridamole-induced hyperemia under baseline conditions and during short-term cigarette smoking with ^{13}N-ammonia and positron emission tomography. Smoking significantly increased the rate-pressure product at rest, which was paralleled by a proportional increase in myocardial blood flow at rest. However, hyperemic blood flow declined from baseline during smoking (Figure 1-11). The myocardial flow reserve also declined in smokers from baseline during smoking. Myocardial blood flow and flow reserve were similar in young, long-term smokers and young, healthy nonsmokers. However, short-term smoking increased coronary vasomotor tone during dipyridamole-induced hyperemia and markedly reduced myocardial flow reserve. Long-term smoking did not attenuate the coronary vasodilator capacity in young individuals with a relatively short smoking history. Short-term reduction in the coronary vasodilator capacity during smoking may lower the ischemic threshold in smokers with coronary disease and contribute to the risk of coronary heart disease.

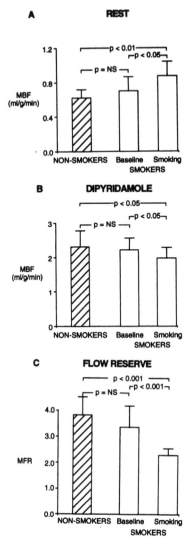

Figure 1-11. Bar graphs show rest and hyperemic blood flows in the study and control groups. A, Myocardial blood flow (MBF) at rest did not differ between smokers and nonsmokers under baseline conditions. Short-term smoking induced a significant increase in myocardial blood flow in proportion to the increase in rate-pressure product. B, MBF during intravenous dipyridamole did not differ between smokers and nonsmokers under baseline conditions. Short-term smoking induced a significant decrease in hyperemic MBF (P <0.05 vs. baseline and control). C, The increase in resting blood flow together with the decline in hyperemic blood flow resulted in a marked reduction in the myocardial flow reserve (MFR) during short-term smoking (P <0.0001 vs. nonsmokers; P <0.001 vs. baseline). Reproduced with permission from Czernin et al.[67]

Passive Smoking

Recent clinical, laboratory, and epidemiological evidence that passive smoking causes atherosclerotic heart disease was reviewed, with particular emphasis on understanding the underlying physiological and biochemical mechanisms. Glantz and Parmley[68] from San Francisco, California, reviewed publications in peer-reviewed journals on passive smoking. They concluded that passive smoking reduces the blood's ability to deliver oxygen to the heart and compromises the myocardium's ability to use oxygen to create adenosine triphosphate. These effects are manifested as reduced exercise capability in people breathing secondhand smoke. Secondhand smoke increases platelet activity, accelerates atherosclerotic lesions, and increases tissue damage following ischemia or AMI. The effects of secondhand tobacco smoke on the cardiovascular system are not caused by a single component of the smoke but by the effects of many elements, including carbon monoxide, nicotine, polycyclic aromatic hydrocarbons, and other, not fully specified, elements in the smoke. Nonsmokers exposed to secondhand smoke in everyday life exhibit an increased risk of both fatal and nonfatal cardiac events.

Diabetes Mellitus

Nahser and colleagues[69] in Iowa City, Iowa, studied 24 diabetic and 31 nondiabetic patients during cardiac catheterization to evaluate coronary microvascular function in patients with diabetes mellitus. A Doppler catheter or guidewire was used to measure changes in coronary blood flow velocity in a nonstenotic artery. Maximal coronary blood flow reserve was determined through the use of intracoronary adenosine or papaverine. Coronary dilation in response to an increase in myocardial metabolic demand was assessed through the use of rapid atrial pacing. Maximal vasodilator responses to papaverine and adenosine were compared in 12 diabetic patients. Maximal pharmacological coronary flow reserve was depressed in diabetic patients compared with nondiabetic patients. During atrial pacing, the decrease in coronary vascular resistance was lessened in the diabetic compared with nondiabetic patients. Differences in coronary microvascular function between diabetic and nondiabetic patients were not attributable to differences in drug therapy, resting hemodynamics, or the presence or absence of hypertension. In 12 diabetic patients, the maximal coronary vasodilator responses to papaverine and adenosine were similar. Thus, these data indicate that both reduced maximal coronary vasodilation and impairment in the regulation of coronary flow in response to submaximal increases in myocardial oxygen demand are present in patients with diabetes mellitus.

The Diabetes Control and Complications Trial, a multicenter, randomized, controlled clinical trial, demonstrated that intensive diabetes therapy delays the onset and slows the progression of retinopathy, nephropathy, and neuropathy in patients with insulin-dependent diabetes mellitus. A study by the group in Bethesda, Maryland, presented the effect of intensive therapy on atherosclerosis-related events and associated risk factors.[70] Patients (n = 1441) between the ages of 13 and 39 years with insulin-dependent diabetes mellitus were randomly assigned to conventional or intensive diabetes treatment. The patients were free of cardiovascular disease at baseline. Patients with hypertension, hypercholesterolemia, or obesity were excluded. Average length of follow-up was 6.5 years. The study used standardized definitions of macrovascular events, verification of such events, and central laboratories for determination of lipids and the grading of electrocardiograms. The number of combined major macrovascular events was almost twice as high in the conventionally treated group (40 events) as in the intensive-treatment group (23 events), although the differences were not statistically significant. There were no differences in the cumulative incidence of hypertension. Mean total serum cholesterol, calculated LDL cholesterol, and triglycerides were significantly reduced in the intensive-treatment group, as was the development of LDL cholesterol levels >160 mg/dL. Weight gain was significantly increased in the intensive-treatment group. There were no differences in cigarette smoking habits, consumption of alcohol, or aspirin use between treatment groups. The reduction in some, but not all, cardiovascular risk factors suggests a potential beneficial effect of intensive therapy on macrovascular disease in insulin-dependent diabetes mellitus.

Endothelial-Cell Dysfunction

Patients with hypercholesterolemia have impaired endothelium-dependent vasodilation. However, previous human studies have invariably used muscarinic agents to assess endothelial function. Casino and coworkers[71] in Bethesda, Maryland, designed a study to determine whether impaired endothelium-dependent vasodilation of hypercholesterolemic patients is related to a specific and isolated defect of the muscarinic receptor, or to a broader abnormality of the endothelial cells. The forearm vascular responses to the endothelium-dependent agents acetylcholine and substance P, and to the direct smooth muscle dilator sodium nitroprusside were studied in 16 hypercholesterolemic patients (eight men and eight women; mean age, 50 years; serum cholesterol >250 mg/dL) and 16 normal volunteers (eight men and eight women; mean age, 47 years; serum cholesterol <200 mg/dL). Drugs were infused into the brachial artery and the response of the forearm vasculature was measured by strain-gauge plethysmography. The vasodilator response to acetylcholine was reduced in hypercholesterolemic patients compared with normal controls; at the highest dose the increase in forearm blood flow was 14 mL/min per 100 mL in the control group and 8 in patients. The response to substance P was also blunted in hypercholesterolemic patients; at the highest dose the increase in forearm blood flow was 12 mL/min per 100 mL in the control group and 8 in patients. A significant correlation was found between the highest blood flow responses with acetylcholine and with substance P. No difference was found between the two groups in their response to sodium nitroprusside. These findings indicate that impaired endothelium-dependent vasodilation in hypercholesterolemia is not due to an isolated defect of the muscarinic receptor, and suggest either a more generalized endothelial abnormality or a defect in the final common pathway that regulates the endothelial modulation of vascular tone.

Goode and colleagues[72] in Manchester, UK, conducted a study to investigate the effects of cholesterol reduction on the in vitro function of human peripheral small arteries in middle-aged patients with hypercholesterolemia. Subcutaneous gluteal fat biopsies were taken from 18 hypercholesterolemic patients with a total serum cholesterol of 9.7 mmol/L and 16 age- and sex-matched control subjects with a mean serum cholesterol of 4.69 mm/L. Subcutaneous small arteries with an internal diameter of <330 μm were dissected and mounted on a wire myograph for isometric tension measurements. The hypercholesterolemic patients showed impaired relaxation to acetylcholine after preconstriction with a thromboxane A_2 analogue compared with the control subjects. Incubation with the nitric oxide substrate, L-arginine, improved the endothelium-dependent vasorelaxation responses to acetylcholine in patients, but not in control subjects. There was a small but significant difference in responses to the endothelium-independent vasodilator, sodium nitroprusside, between the hypercholesterolemic group and normal individuals. In 10 patients with a second gluteal skin biopsy and repeat functional studies after successful cholesterol-lowering therapy at a mean of 10 months later, there was a significant improvement in vasorelaxation in response to acetylcholine and sodium nitroprusside. Although both groups were normotensive, there were higher blood pressures in the patients with hypercholesterolemia than in the control group. Blood pressure fell to control values after serum cholesterol reduction. These results indicate that abnormalities of both endothelium-dependent and independent relaxation occur in peripheral small arteries in patients with hypercholesterolemia.

DuBois-Randé and coworkers[73] in Creteil, France, designed the study to assess the vasomotor response of coronary arteries to exercise in the cold pressure test, and its relation with endothelium-mediated dependent mechanism. Twenty-two patients were entered in the study. Group 1 was composed of 12 patients with a total cholesterol level less than 200 mg/dL associated with angiographically smooth, normal coronary arteries. Group 2 consisted of 10 patients with both a cholesterol level greater than 200 mg/dL and angiographic luminal irregularities of the left anterior descending coronary artery. Coronary blood flow was assessed by a 0.018-inch–tip guidewire Doppler ultrasonography; an analysis of the coronary arterial dimension of the mid portion of the left anterior descending coronary artery was performed by quantitative coronary angiography. Catecholamine concentrations were assessed at different stages of the protocol. Rate pressure product increased during both the cold pressure test and exercise. Coronary blood flow velocity increased in the cold pressure and exercise test by 25% to 72%, respectively, and by 127% after administration of papaverine. In group 1 the cold pressure test had a more pronounced vasodilating effect on epicardial coronary arteries compared with group 2. Similarly, exercise had a vasodilating action in group 1 compared with group 2. Both responses were highly correlated. The papaverine administration had a vasodilating action in patients from group 1 (12%) compared with group 2 (–1%). Both the vasomotor responses to the cold pressure test and exercise were correlated to the response to papaverine administration. Noradrenaline concentration increased both during the cold pressure test and exercise, but not after papaverine administration. These results show that the endothelium modulates response of epicardial coronary arteries and sympathetic stimulation mainly by a flow-mediated mechanism.

Estrogen and Estrogen-Replacement Therapy

To assess pairwise differences between placebo, unopposed estrogen, and each of 3 estrogen/progestin regimens on selected heart disease risk factors in healthy postmenopausal women, the Writing Group for the Postmenopausal Estrogen/Progestin Interventions (PEPI) Trial performed a 3-year, multicenter, randomized, double-blind placebo control study involving 875 healthy, postmenopausal women ages 45–64 years who had no known contraindication to hormone therapy.[74] Participants were randomly assigned in equal numbers to the following groups: (1) placebo; (2) conjugated equine estrogen (CEE), 0.625 mg/d; (3) CEE, 0.625 mg/d, plus cyclic medroxyprogesterone acetate (MPA), 10 mg/d, for 12 d/mo; (4) CEE, 0.625 mg/d, plus consecutive MPA, 2.5 mg/d; or (5) CEE, 0.625 mg/d, plus cyclic micronized progesterone (MP), 200 mg/d, for 12 d/mo. Four end points were chosen to represent four biological systems related to the risk of cardiovascular disease: (1) LDL cholesterol (HDL cholesterol), (2) systolic BP, (3) serum insulin, and (4) fibrinogen. Mean changes in HDL cholesterol segregated treatment regimens into three statistically distinct groups: (1) placebo (decrease of 0.03 mmol/L [1.2 mg/dL]); (2) MPA regimens (increases of 0.03 to 0.04 mmol/L [1.2 to 1.6 mg/dL]); and (3) CEE with cyclic MP (increase of 0.11 mmol/L [4.1 mg/dL]) and CEE alone (increase of 0.14 mmol/L [5.6 mg/dL]). Active treatments decreased mean LDL cholesterol (0.37 to 0.46 mmol/L [14.5 to 17.7 mg/dL]) and increased mean triglyceride (0.13 to 0.15 mmol/L [11.4 to 13.76 mg/dL]) compared with placebo. Placebo was associated with a significantly greater increase in mean fibrinogen than any active treatment (0.10 g/L compared with −0.02 to 0.06 g/L); differences among active treatments were not significant. Systolic BP increased and postchallenge insulin levels decreased during the trial, but neither varied significantly by treatment assignment. Compared with other active treatments, unopposed estrogen was associated with a significantly increased risk of adenomatous or atypical hyperplasia (34% vs. 1%) and of hysterectomy (6% vs. 1%). No other adverse effect differed by treatment assignment or hysterectomy status. Estrogen alone or in combination with a progestin improves lipoproteins and lowers fibrinogen levels without detectable effects on postchallenge insulin or BP. Unopposed estrogen is the optimal regimen for elevation of HDL cholesterol, but the high rate of endometrial hyperplasia restricts use to women without a uterus. In women with a uterus, CEE with cyclic MP has the most favorable effect on HDL cholesterol and no excess risk of endometrial hyperplasia.

Hormone-replacement therapy is associated with a reduction in cardiovascular events in postmenopausal women. Gilligan and coworkers[75] in Bethesda, Maryland, recently found that acute 17β-estradiol administration improves endothelium-dependent vasodilation in both the peripheral and coronary circulations of postmenopausal women. A study was undertaken in 33 estrogen-deficient postmenopausal women (mean age, 59 years) to determine if short-term estrogen-replacement therapy also improves endothelium-dependent vasodilation in peripheral circulation. Acute intra-arterial infusion of estradiol, which increased forearm venous estradiol levels from 16 to 345 pg/mL, potentiated forearm vasodilation induced by the endothelium-dependent vasodilator acetylcholine by 49%. Acute estradiol also potentiated vasodilation induced by the endothelium-independent vasodilator nitroprusside by 5%. However, after 3 weeks of transdermal estradiol administration (0.1 mg/d), which achieved an estradiol level of 120 pg/mL, the vasodilator responses to acetylcholine and to sodium nitroprusside were unchanged from initial measurements obtained before acute administration of estradiol. Repeat intra-arterial infusion of estradiol in eight women, while receiving transdermal estradiol, increased forearm venous estradiol levels to 268 pg/mL and again potentiated the vasodilator response to acetylcholine to a similar degree as that observed in the initial study after acute administration of estradiol. Thus, although acute intra-arterial infusion of 17β-estradiol potentiates endothelium-dependent vasodilation in the forearms of postmenopausal women, this effect was not maintained with a 3-week cycle of systemic estradiol administration. The different effects of acute and chronic estradiol may be due to the lower plasma levels achieved with chronic estrogen administration.

Gebara and colleagues[76] in Boston, Massachusetts, determined the relation between estrogen status and fibrinolytic potential in postmenopausal women. The investigators determined levels of plasminogen activator inhibitor (PAI-1) antigen and tissue plasminogen activator (TPA) antigen in 1431 subjects from the Framingham Offspring Study. Fibrinolytic potential was compared between subjects with high estrogen status (premenopausal women and postmenopausal women receiving hormone-replacement therapy) and low estrogen status (men and postmenopausal women not receiving hormone-replacement therapy). Subjects with high estrogen status had greater fibrinolytic potential, including lower PAI-1 levels than subjects with low estrogen status. Postmenopausal women receiving estrogen-replacement therapy had lower levels of PAI-1 than those not receiving therapy. Premenopausal women had lower levels of PAI-1 than men of a similar age, but this sex difference diminished when postmenopausal women not receiving hormone-replacement therapy were compared with men of a similar age. Premenopausal women had markedly lower levels of PAI-1 antigen than postmenopausal women not receiving estrogen therapy. Thus, in each of these comparisons, there is evidence that the cardioprotective effects of estrogen may be mediated, at least in part, by an increase in fibrinolytic potential.

To test the lipid-lowering effects of continuous combined hormone-replacement therapy in hypercholesterolemic postmenopausal women, Denke[77] from Dallas, Texas, identified 32 postmenopausal women through health fair and cholesterol screening records whose ad libitum LDL cholesterol level (mean of two measurements) was >130 mg/dL and whose fasting triglycerides were <250 mg/dL. Women with a history of uterine fibroids, thrombophlebitis, family or personal history of breast cancer, or recent hormone use were excluded. After a 1-month period to standardize baseline dietary intake (Hi-Sat), patients were taught a cholesterol-lowering, Step-1 diet, which they followed for the remainder of the study. After 3 months, patients supplemented the Step-1 diet with daily placebo tablets for 3 months, followed by supplementation with conjugated estrogens (0.625 mg/d) plus medroxyprogesterone (2.5 mg/d) for 3 months. The means of 5 fasting lipid and lipoprotein values at the end of each 3-month supplementation period were compared. Total cholesterol fell from 261 mg/dL to 250 mg/dL to 233 mg/dL, with LDL reduction from 181 mg/dL to 173 mg/dL to 150 mg/dL, on diet and diet plus continuous combined hormone-replacement therapy, respectively. Although 26 of the 32 women had LDL values above 160 mg/dL during the Hi-Sat diet, only 10 of the 32 women remained with LDL values in this range during Step-1 diet plus hormone therapy. Besides improving LDL cholesterol levels, continuous combined hormone-replacement therapy was associated with an increase in HDL cholesterol levels from 51 to 54 mg/dL. The 2 women whose HDL cholesterol levels were <35 mg/dL during the Step-1 diet plus placebo achieved HDL cholesterol levels >35 mg/dL during hormone therapy. Nevertheless, continuous combined hormone-replacement therapy was associated with a high frequency of side effects, including breast tenderness and uterine bleeding. Most bothersome side effects dissipated after an initial adjustment period. Continuous combined hormone-replacement therapy can produce significant and therapeutic reductions in LDL cholesterol levels in hypercholesterolemic postmenopausal women. After internists become familiar with the expected side effects and their time course, this regimen may provide an effective approach in the management of hypercholesterolemia in postmenopausal women who have not undergone a hysterectomy.

To study whether vascular dysfunction in hypercholesterolemia is reversible, Stroes and associates[78] from Utrecht, the Netherlands, investigated patients without overt arterial disease who were taking maintenance treatment for hypercholesterolemia. Medication was stopped for 2 weeks, reinstituted for 12 weeks, and again stopped for 6 weeks. During both maintenance treatment and the 12 weeks of step-up medication the lipid profile was improved but did not return to normal. Dose-response curves for serotonin-induced vasodilatation, an index of nitric oxide–dependent vasodilatation, showed a comparable and significant rightward shift after a medication-free period of 2 and 6 weeks compared with control subjects, indicating endothelial dysfunction, which was already maximum after 2 weeks. After 12 weeks of lipid-lowering medication, the difference in endothelial function between the control group and patients had disappeared. Coinfusion of L-arginine, the substrate for nitric oxide synthase, returned the impaired serotonin response during hypercholesterolemia to normal but had no effect on this response in controls or in patients while on lipid-lowering medication. Neither endothelium-independent vasorelaxation, assessed by sodium nitroprusside infusion, nor vasoconstriction induced by the nitric oxide blocker L-NMMMA, were different between the control group and the patients, whether the latter were on or off lipid-lowering medication. The authors' results show an L-arginine–sensitive, impaired nitric-oxide-mediated vascular relaxation of forearm resistance vessels in hypercholesterolemia that is reproducible and reversible after short-term lipid-lowering therapy.

To ascertain the prevalence and duration of use of hormone-replacement therapy by menopausal women doctors in the UK, Isaacs and associates[79] from London, UK, studied a sample of women doctors in the UK who obtained full registration between 1952 and 1976. Overall, 46% (436 out of 954) of women physicians aged 45–65 years had ever used hormone-replacement therapy. When the results from women still menstruating regularly were excluded, 55% (428) were former users and 41% (319) current users. The cumulative probability of remaining on hormone-replacement therapy was 0.707 at 5 years and 0.576 at 10 years. Women doctors have a higher prevalence of use of hormone-replacement therapy than has been reported for other women in the UK, and most users seem to be taking hormone-replacement therapy for more than 5 years. The results may become useful for a wider population as information on the potential benefits of hormone-replacement therapy is disseminated.

Homocysteine

In 482 patients sequentially referred for diagnosis and therapy of hyperlipidemia, Glueck and associates[80] in Cincinnati, Ohio, determined the prevalence of homocysteinemia to assess whether it was independently associated with atherosclerotic vascular disease and to determine how effectively high homocysteine could be treated with folic acid and pyridoxine. Of the 482 patients,

18 had high homocysteine (≥16 μmol/L), 31 had high cystathionine (≥342 nmol/L) with normal homocysteine, and 433 had normal cystathionine and homocysteine. Of the 18 patients with high homocysteine, 13 had atherosclerotic vascular disease, much higher than the 44% with normal homocysteine. In the 18 kindreds with homocysteinemic proband, 14 had one or more first-degree relatives with atherosclerotic vascular disease before age 65 compared with 50% of the families where the proband had normal homocysteine. In the 482 patients already at high risk for atherosclerotic vascular disease by virtue of hyperlipidemia, when assessed by logistic regression, homocysteine was an independent positive predictor of atherosclerotic vascular disease; RR values for atherosclerotic events was three times higher in patients with top than with bottom quintile homocysteine. After 15 weeks of folic acid (5 mg/d) and pyridoxine (100 mg/d) therapy in 10 patients with high homocysteine, median homocysteine normalized, decreasing from 18 to 11 μmol/L. To best quantitate and ameliorate risk for atherosclerotic vascular disease, homocysteine should routinely be measured at least once in hyperlipidemic patients at high risk for atherosclerosis and, if high, should be treated.

Several studies have shown a relation between hyperhomocysteinemia and arterial vascular disease. Den Heijer and associates[81] from the Hague and Leiden, the Netherlands, looked at the association between hyperhomocysteinemia and venous thrombosis, which could be clinically important because hyperhomocysteinemia is easily corrected by vitamin supplementation. The authors studied 185 patients with a history of recurrent venous thrombosis and 220 control subjects from the general population. Homocysteine concentrations were measured before and 6 hours after oral methionine loading. The authors defined hyperhomocysteinemia as the homocystein concentration above the fasting or the postmethionine value found for the 90th percentile of the control subjects. Of the 185 patients with recurrent thrombosis, 46 (25%) had fasting homocysteine concentrations above the 90th percentile or the control level (odds ratio, 3.1). After adjusting for age, sex, and menopausal status the odds ratio was 2.0 (1.5–2.7). Similar results were found for the postmethionine value (unadjusted odds ratio, 3.1; adjusted 2.6). Hyperhomocysteinemia is a common risk factor for recurrent venous thrombosis and can lead to a 2-fold or 3-fold increase in risk.

Dalery and coworkers[82] in Montreal, Canada, determined plasma levels of homocysteine in 584 healthy subjects (380 men and 204 women) from a major utility company in the province of Québec, Canada, and in 150 subjects (123 men and 27 women) with angiographically documented CAD (age <60 years). Plasma levels of vitamins B_{12}, B_6, pyridoxal phosphate (a vitmain B_6 derivative), and folate were also determined. Mean homocysteine levels were higher in the bottom quartiles for folate, vitamin B_{12}, and pyridoxal phosphate. A significant correlation was noted between homocysteine levels and folate and vitamin B_{12} levels. No significant correlation was found between plasma homocysteine levels and age, lipids and lipoprotein cholesterol, glucose, and the presence of hypertension or cigarette smoking in healthy subjects or in patients with CAD. Control men had higher homocysteine levels than control women. Men and women with CAD had higher levels of homocysteine than controls (12 vs. 10 nmol/mL and 12 vs. 8 nmol/mL, respectively). Women and men with CAD had similar homocysteine levels. The proportion of patients with CAD having homocysteine levels >90th percentile of controls was 18% for men and 44%

for women. Significantly lower pyridoxal phosphate levels were seen in subjects with CAD, men and women combined. No significant differences were observed for B_{12}, folate, or total B_6. Multivariate analysis revealed that an elevated homocysteine level is a risk factor for CAD in French Canadian men and women and that reduced levels of pyridoxal phosphate, folate, and vitamin B_{12} may contribute to elevated plasma homocysteine levels. The investigators concluded that in their subjects of French Canadian descent, plasma levels of homocysteine are influenced by levels of folate, vitamin B_{12}, and pyridoxal phosphate. In healthy men, mean homocysteine levels are higher than in healthy women. Men and women with CAD had significantly higher homocysteine levels than controls and this elevation is independent of traditional risk factors.

To determine the risk of elevated total homocysteine levels for atherosclerosis, estimate the reduction of total homocysteine by folic acid, and calculate the potential reduction of CAD mortality by increasing folic acid intake, Boushey and associates[83] from Seattle, Washington, did a MEDLINE search for meta-analysis of 27 studies relating homocysteine to atherosclerosis and 11 studies of folic acid effects on total homocysteine levels. Three prospective and 6 population-based case control studies were considered of high quality. Five cross-sectional and 13 other case control studies were also included. Elevation of total homocysteine was considered an independent graded risk factor for atherosclerosis. The odds ratio for CAD of a 5-μmol/L total homocysteine increment is 1.6 for men and 1.8 for women. A total of 10% of the population's CAD risk appears attributable to total homocysteine. The odds ratio for cerebrovascular disease (5-μmol/L total homocysteine increment) is 1.5. Peripheral arterial disease also showed a strong association. Increased folic acid intake (approximately 200 μg/d) reduces total homocysteine levels by approximately 4 μmol/L. Assuming that lower total homocysteine levels decrease CAD mortality, the authors calculated the effect of (1) increased dietary folate, (2) supplementation by tablets, and (3) grain fortification. Under different assumptions, 13 500 to 50 000 CAD deaths annually could be avoided; fortification of food had the largest impact. A 5-μmol/L total homocysteine increment elevates CAD risk by as much as cholesterol increases of 0.5 mmol/L (20 mg/dL). Higher folic acid intake by reducing total homocysteine levels promises to prevent arteriosclerotic vascular disease. Clinical trials are urgently needed. Concerns about masking cobalamin deficiency by folic acid could be lessened by adding 1 mg cobalamin to folic acid supplements.

To estimate the relation between established cardiovascular risk factors and total homocysteine in plasma, Nygard and associates[84] from Bergen, Norway, examined 7591 men and 8585 women aged 40–67 years of age with no history of hypertension, diabetes, CAD, or cerebrovascular disease. The level of plasma homocysteine was higher in men than in women and increased with age. In subjects 40–42 years old, geometric means were 10.8 μmol/L for 5918 men and 9.1 μmol/L for 6348 women. At age 65–67 years, the corresponding homocysteine level increased markedly with the daily number of cigarettes smoked in all age groups. Its relation to smoking was particularly strong in women. The combined effect of age, sex, and smoking was striking. Heavy-smoking men aged 65–67 years had a mean homocysteine level 4.8 μmol/L higher than never-smoking women aged 40–42 years. Plasma homocysteine level also was positively related to total cholesterol level, BP, and heart rate and inversely related to physical activity. The relations were not substantially changed by multivariate adjustment, including intake of vitamin supplements, fruits, and vegetables. Elevated plasma homocysteine level was associated with major components of the cardiovascular risk profile, i.e., male sex, old age, smoking, high BP, elevated cholesterol level, and a lack of exercise.

Left Ventricular Hypertrophy

To evaluate the effect of echocardiographically determined LV hypertrophy on survival in comparison with number of narrowed coronary arteries and LV systolic dysfunction, Liao and associates[85] from Maywood and Chicago, Illinois, and Nashville, Tennessee, studied 1089 consecutive black patients in a single intercity hospital who underwent both coronary angiography and M-mode cardiography as a part of a diagnostic evaluation. Nonstenosed coronary arteries, single-vessel disease, and multivessel disease were found in 48%, 16%, and 36% of patients, respectively; LV hypertrophy (LV mass index >131 g/m^2 in men and >100 g/m^2 in women) was detected in 50% of patients. Hypertrophy without coexistent obstructive coronary disease was associated with a lower survival rate than that observed for single-vessel CAD and was similar to multivessel CAD. When LV hypertrophy, number of diseased vessels, and LV dysfunction were subjected to multivariate analysis, hypertrophy conferred an RR of 2.4. By comparison, the presence of a single stenosed vessel did not increase the risk of death. Multivessel disease and ejection fraction less than 45% were associated with an RR of 1.6 and 2.0, respectively. Calculation of the attributable risk fraction demonstrated that for every 100 deaths in this cohort, LV hypertrophy independently accounted for 37. The corresponding attributable risk fractions were 1%, 22%, and 9% for single-vessel disease, multivessel disease, and ventricular dysfunction, respectively. LV hypertrophy was associated with a greater RR and attributable risk than the traditional measures of coronary disease severity. The high prevalence and powerful risk of LV hypertrophy make an important contribution to the adverse survival rates among black patients with heart disease and may account for much of the black-white differential.

Liao and colleagues[86] in Nashville, Tennessee, determined whether there is a sex differential in the impact of LV hypertrophy on mortality in women versus men. This study enrolled 436 consecutive patients: 163 men and 273 women free of angiographic evidence of CAD from a hospital registry. LV mass/body surface area ≥117 g/m^2 in men and ≥104 g/m^2 in women was found in 84 men and 119 women. During a mean of 5 years' follow-up, 49 patients died, including 26 men and 23 women. The mortality rate was 5.4 per 100 patient-years in men with LV hypertrophy and 2.58 in men without LV hypertrophy, and 3.21 and 0.66, respectively, in women. Using Cox regression analysis, adjusting for age, hypertension, and LV ejection fraction, the RR for LV hypertrophy was 2.0 in men and 4.3 in women. For cardiac death, the RR was 1.3 and 7.5 in men and women, respectively. Analyses using LV mass indexed by height or height using different LV hypertrophy cut points, comparing patients in the highest and lower 2 tertiles and the use of LV mass indexes as continuous variables, still demonstrate a greater increase in risk of either fatal end point among women than men. Thus, these findings indicate a sex difference in the contribution of LV mass risk in women.

Miscellaneous Topics

Fetal and Infant Growth

To examine whether cardiovascular risk factors in women are related to fetal and infant growth, Fall and associates[87] from South Hampton, Cambridge, and London, UK, performed a follow-up study of women born from 1923–1930 whose birth weights and heights at 1 year had been recorded. The subjects included 297 women born and living in East Herfordshire. Fasting plasma concentrations of glucose, insulin, and 32–33 split proinsulin fell with increasing birth weight when current body mass index was allowed for. Glucose and insulin concentrations 120 minutes after an oral glucose load showed similar trends. Systolic BP, waist-to-hip ratio, and serum triglyceride concentrations also fell with increasing birth weight while serum HDL cholesterol concentration rose. At each birth weight, women who currently had a higher body mass index had higher levels of risk factors. The authors concluded that in women, as in men, reduced fetal growth leads to insulin resistance and the associated disorders: raised BP and high serum triglycerides and low serum HDL cholesterol concentrations. The highest values of these coronary risk factors occurred in people who were small at birth and had become obese. In contrast to men, low rate of infant growth did not predict levels of risk factors in women.

Risk Factors in Black and White Men

Epidemiological studies begun in the southeastern USA in the 1960s indicated that the prevalence of CAD was 2 to 3 times greater among white men than black men and also showed an excess incidence of CAD among white men, although systemic hypertension was twice as prevalent among blacks. Keil and associates[88] from Charleston, South Carolina; Claxton, Georgia; and Chapel Hill, North Carolina, conducted a study to see if racial differences exist in CAD mortality and coronary risk factors. Data from the 2 population-based cohorts of the Charleston, South Carolina, and Evans County, Georgia, heart studies were pooled to make comparisons of CAD mortality and its risk factors. A total of 726 black men and 1346 white men aged 35 years or older in 1960 in the combined cohort were followed up for 30 years. There were 125 deaths among the black men and 323 deaths among the white men attributable to coronary disease; the age-adjusted rates were 5.0/1000 person-years in the black men and 6.5/1000 person-years in the white men. Black-white coronary mortality risk ratios were 0.8 when age-adjusted and 0.7 when also adjusted for other cardiovascular risk factors. Elevated systolic BP and cigarette smoking were significant predictors of coronary mortality in black and white men. Serum total cholesterol level was a statistically significant risk factor only in white men. Higher education level was significantly protective in black and white men. Black men experienced significantly less coronary disease mortality than white men. Except for cholesterol level, the risk factors for coronary mortality in black and white men were similar.

French Paradox

The low rate of CAD in France compared with other developed countries with comparable dietary intake has been called the French paradox. Criquui and Ringel[89] from La Jolla, California, explored this paradox by looking at alcohol, diet and mortality data from 21 developed, relatively affluent countries in the years 1965, 1970, 1980, and 1988. The authors assessed wine, beer, and spirits intake separately. France had the highest wine intake and the highest total alcohol intake and the second lowest CAD mortality rate. In univariate analyses, ethanol in wine was slightly more inversely correlated with CAD than total wine volume. In multivariate analyses, animal fat tended to be positively correlated and fruit consumption inversely correlated with CAD. Beer and spirits were only weakly inversely correlated with CAD. The strongest and most consistent correlation was the inverse association with wine ethanol with CAD. However, wine ethanol was unrelated to total mortality. The authors conclude that ethanol, particularly wine ethanol, is inversely related to CAD but not to longevity in populations. Although light to moderate alcohol consumption may improve longevity, alcohol abuse, which sharply reduces longevity, is correlated with average alcohol consumption in populations. Thus, while the risk-to-benefit ratio varies for individuals, the use of alcohol for cardioprotective purpose should not be encouraged as a public health measure.

Fibrinolytic Parameters

Salomaa and the ARIC Investigators[90] studied the association of PAI-1 antigen, TPA antigen, and D-dimer with early atherosclerosis in a cross-sectional, case-control study involving 457 pairs chosen from the biracial cohort of the Atherosclerosis Risk in Communities Study (ARIC). As examined by B-mode ultrasound, patients had intima-media thickness of carotid arteries above the 90th percentile and control subjects had thickness below the 75th percentile of the ARIC cohort. Patients with a history of heart disease, stroke, or claudication were excluded from the case-control selection. In this study, PAI-1, TPA, and D-dimer were higher in patients than in control subjects. In conditional logistic regression analysis, the odds ratio of carotid atherosclerosis were for PAI-1, 1.22, 1.54, and 1.60 in the second, third, and fourth quartiles compared with the first quartile test of linear-trend, adjusted for age, systolic BP, total cholesterol, aspirin use, and method of obtaining the blood sample. Corresponding tests for D-dimer and TPA also showed an increase in trend. Thus, these findings support the hypothesis that thrombosis and fibrinolysis play a role in the early stage of the atherosclerotic process.

Dietary Fish and Mercury

Salonen and colleagues[91] in Kuopio, Finland, studied the relation of the dietary intake of fish and mercury, as well as hair content and urinary excretion of mercury to the risk of AMI and death from CAD, cardiovascular disease, and any cause in 1833 men 42 to 60 years of age who had no clinical evidence of CAD, stroke, claudication, or cancer. Among these individuals, 73 had an AMI in the next 2 to 7 years. Of the 78 deceased men, 18 died of CAD and 24 died of cardiovascular disease. Men who had consumed local nonfatty fish species had elevated hair mercury contents. In Cox models with the major cardiovascular risk factors as covariates, dietary intakes of fish and mercury were associated with significantly increased risks of AMI and death from CAD, cardiovascular disease, and any death. Men in the highest tertile of hair mercury content had a 2-fold age and CAD-adjusted risk of AMI and a 3-fold adjusted risk of cardiovascular death compared with those with a lower hair mercury content. In nested case-control subsamples, the 24-hour urinary mercury excretion had a significant independent association with the risk of AMI. Both the hair and urinary mercury associated significantly with titers of immune complexes containing oxidized LDL. These data suggest that a high intake of mercury from nonfatty fresh water fish and the consequent accumulation of mercury in the body are associated with excess risk of AMI as well as death from CAD, cardiovascular disease, and any cause in Eastern Finnish men, and this increased risk may be due to the promotion of lipid peroxidation by mercury.

It has been hypothesized that a diet containing n-3 fatty acids from fish reduces the risk of CAD, but few large epidemiological studies have examined this question. Ascherio and associates[92] from Boston, Massachusetts, did a 6-year follow-up of 44 895 male health professionals, 40–75 years of age when examined in 1986 who were at that time free of known cardiovascular disease and who completed detailed and validated dietary questionnaires as part of the Health Professionals Follow-up Study. The authors documented 1543 coronary events in the group: 264 deaths from CAD, 547 nonfatal AMI, and 732 having CABG or PTCA. After controlling for age and several coronary risk factors, the authors observed no significant association between dietary intake of n-3 fatty acids or fish intake in the risk of CAD. For men in the top fifth of the group in terms of intake of n-3 fatty acids (median, 0.58 g/d), the multivariate relative risk of CAD was 1.12 compared with the men in the bottom fifth (median, 0.07 g/d). For men who consumed 6 or more servings of fish per week compared with those who consumed 1 serving per month or less, the multivariate RR of CAD was 1.14. The risk of death due to CAD among men who ate any amount of fish compared with those who ate no fish was 0.74, but the risk did not decrease as fish consumption increased. Although the possibility of residual confounding by unmeasured factors cannot be entirely excluded, these data suggest that increasing fish intake from 1 to 2 servings per week to 5 to 6 servings per week does not substantially reduce the risk of CAD among men who are initially free of cardiovascular disease.

Shift Work

Kawachi and colleagues[93] in Boston, Massachusetts, examined prospectively the relation of shift work to risk of CAD in a cohort of women. An ongoing prospective cohort of US female nurses initially evaluated in 1988 for the total number of years during which they were rotating night shifts included 79 109 women, 42–67 years of age in 1988 who were without recognized CAD and stroke. Incident CAD was defined as nonfatal AMI and fatal CAD. From 1988 to 1992, 292 cases of incident CAD, including 248 nonfatal AMIs and 44 CAD-related deaths occurred. The age-adjusted relative risk of CAD was 1.38 in women who reported ever doing shift work compared with those who had never done so. The excess risk persisted after adjustment for cigarette smoking and a variety of other cardiovascular risk factors. Compared with women who had never done shift work, the multivariate adjusted RR of CAD was 1.2 among women reporting less than 6 years and 1.5 among those reporting 6 or more years of rotating night shifts. These data are compatible with the possibility that 6 or more years of shift work may increase the risk of CAD in women.

Anti-Cardiolipid Antibodies

Vaarala and colleagues[94] in Helsinki, Finland, determined whether the presence of antiphospholipid antibodies, in particular, anti-cardiolipin antibodies carries a risk for AMI in a nested case-control design with 133 patients and 133 control subjects matched for treatment and geographical area. The sera to be studied were taken from middle-aged dyslipidemic men participating in the Helsinki Heart Study, a 5-year coronary primary prevention trial with gemfibrozil. Individuals studied had a non-HDL cholesterol ≥5.2 mmol/L. The study population was selected by screening from a cohort of 19 000 male employees in private and government-owned industries. A total of 140 of 4081 subjects in the Helsinki Heart Study population had a cardiac end point, either cardiac death or nonfatal AMI during the double-blind study period. Sera drawn at baseline in 1981 through 1982 and preserved at −20°C was available in 133 patients with cardiac end points. A control subject without an end point was selected for each patient using drug treatment and the clinic in the study organization as matching variables. Samples were tested for IgG-class antibodies to cardiolipin. Anti-cardiolipin antibody level, as expressed in optimal density units, was significantly higher in patients than in control subjects (0.417 compared with 0.361). Subjects with the antibody level in the highest quartile of distribution had a relative risk for AMI of 2.0 compared with the remainder of the population. This risk was independent of other factors, including age, smoking, systolic BP, LDL, and HDL. There was a correlation between the levels of anti-cardiolipin antibodies and antibodies to oxidized LDL and their combined effect was additive for the risk of AMI. Thus, these data obtained from healthy middle-aged men with elevated serum cholesterols indicate that a high anti-cardiolipin antibody level is an independent risk factor for AMI or cardiac death.

Mutation in Gene Coding or Coagulation Factor V

A specific point mutation in the gene coding for coagulation factor V is associated with resistance to degradation by activated protein C, a recently described abnormality of coagulation that may be associated with an increased risk of venous thrombosis. Whether this mutation also predisposes patients to arterial thrombosis is unknown, as is the value of screening for the mutation to define the risk of venous thrombosis among unselected healthy patients. Among 14 916 apparently health men in the Physicians' Health study who provided baseline blood samples, 374 had AMI, 209 had strokes, and 121 had deep venous thrombosis, pulmonary embolism, or both, during a mean follow-up of 8.6 years. Ridker and associates[95] from Boston, Massachusetts, and St. Louis, Missouri, determined whether a mutation at nucleotide position 1691 of the factor V gene was present or absent in these 704 men and in an equal number of matched participants who remained free of vascular disease. The

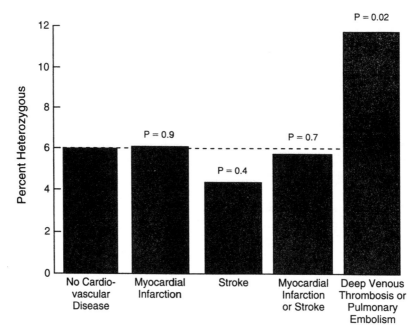

FIGURE 1-12. Prevalence of heterozygosity for the factor V mutation among 1408 apparently healthy men in the physicians' Health Study. Data shown are for cardiovascular disease occurring during follow-up. No subject was homozygous for the mutated *1691A* allele. *P* values shown are for the comparison with the reference value (dashed line). Reproduced with permission from Ridker et al.[95]

prevalence of heterozygosity for the mutation among men who had AMI (6.1%) or strokes (4.3%) was similar to that among men who remained free of vascular disease (6.0%) (Figure 1-12). However, the prevalence of the mutation was significantly higher among men who had venous thrombosis, pulmonary embolism, or both (11.6%). In adjusted analyses, the relative risk of venous thrombosis among men with the mutation was 2.7. This increased risk was seen with primary venous thrombosis (RR, 3.5) but not with secondary venous thrombosis (RR, 1.7). Specifically, the prevalence of the mutation among men over the age of 60 in whom primary venous thrombosis developed was 25.8% (RR, 7.0). In a large cohort of apparently healthy men, the presence of a specific point mutation in the factor V gene was associated with an increased risk of venous thrombosis, particularly primary venous thrombosis. The presence of the mutation was not associated with an increased risk of myocardial infarction or stroke. This mutation appears to be the most common inherited factor thus far recognized that predisposes patients to venous thrombosis.

Angiotensin-Converting Enzyme Gene Polymorphism

In a previous study, men with a history of AMI were found to have an increased prevalence of homozygosity for the deletional allele (D) of the angiotensin-converting enzyme (ACE) gene. The D allele is associated with higher levels of ACE, which may predispose a person to CAD. Lindpaintner and associates[96] from Boston, Massachusetts, investigated the association between the ACE genotype and the incidence of AMI and other manifestations of CAD in a large prospective cohort of US male physicians. In the Physicians' Health Study, CAD as defined by angina, coronary revascularization by 1992. They were matched with 2340 controls according to age and smoking history. Zygosity for the deletion-insertion (D-I) polymorphism of the ACE gene was determined by an assay based on the polymerase chain reaction. Data were analyzed for both matched pairs and unmatched samples, with adjustment for the effects of known or suspected risk factors by conditional and nonconditional logistic regression, respectively. The ACE genotype was not associated with the occurrence of either CAD or AMI. The adjusted RR associated with the D allele was 1.07 for CAD and 1.05 for AMI, if an additive mode of inheritance is assumed. Additional analyses assuming dominant and recessive effects of the D allele also failed to show any association, as did the examination of low-risk subgroups. In a large, prospectively followed population of US male physicians, the presence of the D allele of the ACE gene conferred no appreciable increase in the risk of CAD or AMI.

Green Tea

To investigate the association between consumption of green tea and various serum markers in a Japanese population, with special reference to preventive effects of green tea against cardiovascular disease and disorders of the liver, Imai and Nakachi[97] from Komuro, Japan, studied 1371 men over 40 years of age who were residents in Yoshimi and surveyed their living habits including daily consumption of green tea. Increased consumption of green tea was associated with significantly decreased serum concentrations of total cholesterol and triglyceride and an increased proportion of HDL cholesterol together with a decreased proportion of LDL and VLDL cholesterol, which resulted in a decreased atherogenic index. Moreover, increased consumption of green tea, especially more than 10 cups a day, was related to decreased concentrations of hepatological markers in serum, aspartate aminotransferase, alanine transferase, and ferritin. The inverse association between consumption of green tea and various serum markers shows that green tea may act protectively against cardiovascular disease and disorders of the liver.

1. Nieto FJ, Alonso J, Chambless LE, Zhong M, Ceraso M, Romm FJ, Cooper L, Folsom AR, Szklo M: Population awareness and control of hypertension and hypercholesterolemia. Arch Intern Med 1995 (April 10);155:677–684.
2. Goldberg RJ, Burchfiel CM, Benfante R, Chiu D, Reed DM, Yano K: Lifestyle and biologic factors associated with atherosclerotic disease in middle-aged men. Arch Intern Med 1995 (April 10);155:686–694.
3. Prospective Studies Collaboration: Cholesterol, diastolic blood pressure, and stroke: 13,000 strokes in 450,000 people in 45 prospective cohorts. Lancet 1995 (December 23/30);346:1647–1653.
4. Bhatnagar D, Anand IS, Durrington PN, Patel DJ, Wander GS, Mackness MI, Creed F, Tomenson B, Chandrashekhar Y, Winterbotham M, Britt RP, Keil JE, Sutton GC: Coronary risk factors in people from the Indian subcontinent living in West London and their siblings in India. Lancet 1995 (February 18);345:405–409.
5. Iribarren C, Reed DM, Burchfiel CM, Dwyer JH: Serum total cholesterol and mortality: Confounding factors and risk modification in Japanese-American men. JAMA 1995 (June 28);273:24:1926–1932.
6. Verschuren WMM, Jacobs DR, Bloemberg BPM, Kromhout D, Menotti A, Aravanis C, Blackburn H, Buzina R, Dontas AS, Fidanza F, Karvonen MJ, Nedeljkovic S,

Nissinen A, Toshima H: Serum total cholesterol and long-term coronary heart disease mortality in different cultures. JAMA 1995 (July 12);274:131–136.

7. Burchfiel CM, Laws A, Benfante R, Goldberg RJ, Hwang L-J, Chiu D, Rodriguez BL, Curb JD, Sharp DS: Combined effects of HDL cholesterol, triglyceride, and total cholesterol concentrations on 18-year risk of atherosclerotic disease. Circulation 1995 (September);92:1430–1436.

8. Verschuren WMM, Kromhout D: Total cholesterol concentration and mortality at a relatively young age: Do men and women differ? Br Med J (September 23);311:779–783.

9. Iribarren C, Reed DM, Chen R, Yano K, Dwyer JH: Low serum cholesterol and mortality: Which is the cause and which is the effect? Circulation 1995 (November);92:2396–2403.

10. Corti MC, Guralnik JM, Salive ME, Harris T, Field TS, Wallace RB, Berkman LF, Seeman TE, Glynn RJ, Hennekens CH, Havlik RJ: HDL cholesterol predicts coronary heart disease mortality in older persons. JAMA 1995 (August 16);274:539–544.

11. Wannamethee G, Shaper AG, Whincup PH, Walker M: Low serum total cholesterol concentrations and mortality in middle aged British men. Br Med J 1995 (August 12);311:409–413.

12. Cantin B, Moorjani S, Dagenais GR, Lupien PJ: Lipoprotein(a) distribution in a French Canadian population and its relation to intermittent claudication (the Quebec Cardiovascular Study). Am J Cardiol (June 15);75:1224–1228.

13. Stengård JH, Zerba KE, Pekkanen J, Ehnholm C, Nissinen A, Sing CF: Apolipoprotein E polymorphism predicts death from coronary heart disease in a longitudinal study of elderly Finnish men. Circulation 1995 (January);91:265–269.

14. Ribera M, Pintó X, Argimon JM, Fiol, C, Pujol R, Ferrándiz C: Lipid metabolism and apolipoprotein E phenotypes in patients with xanthelasma. Am J Med 1995 (November);99:485–490.

15. Atger V, Giral P, Simon A, Cambillau M, Levenson J, Gariepy J, Megnien JL, Moatti N, and the PCVMETRA Group: High-density lipoprotein subfractions as markers of early atherosclerosis. Am J Cardiol 1995 (January 15);75:127–131.

16. Wilder LB, Bachorik PS, Finney CA, Moy TF, Becker DM: The effect of fasting status on the determination of low-density and high-density lipoprotein cholesterol. Am J Med 1995 (October);99:374–377.

17. Jiang X, Srinivasan SR, Webber LS, Wattigney WA, Berenson GS: Association of fasting insulin level with serum lipid and lipoprotein levels in children, adolescents, and young adults: The Bogalusa Heart Study. Arch Intern Med 1995 (January 23);155:190–196.

18. Fujiwara R, Kutsumi Y, Hayashi T, Nishio H, Kashino Y, Shimada Y, Nakai T, Miyabo S: Relation of angiographically defined coronary artery disease and plasma concentrations of insulin, lipid, and apolipoprotein in normolipidemic subjects with varying degrees of glucose tolerance. Am J Cardiol 1995 (January 15);75:122–126.

19. Rubins HB, Robins SJ, Collins D, Iranmanesh A, Wilt TJ, Mann D, Mayo-Smith M, Faas FH, Elam MB, Rutan GH, Anderson JW, Kashyap MD, Schectman G, for the Department of Veterans Affairs HDL Intervention Trial Study Group: Distribution of lipids in 8,500 men with coronary artery disease. Am J Cardiol (June 15);75:1196–1201.

20. Hebert PR, Gaziano JM, Hennekens CH: An overview of trials of cholesterol lowering and risk of stroke. Arch Intern Med 1995 (January 9);155:50–55.

21. Iribarren C, Reed DM, Wergowske G, Burchfiel CM, Dwyer JH: Serum cholesterol level and mortality due to suicide and trauma in the Honolulu heart program. Arch Intern Med 1995 (April 10);155:695–700.

22. Galerani M, Manfredini R, Caracciolo S, Scapoli C, Molinari S, Fersini C: Serum cholesterol concentrations in parasuicide. Br Med J 1995 (June 24);310:1632–1636.

23. Juliusson G, Vitols S, Liliemark J: Mechanisms behind hypocholesterolaemia in hairy cell leukaemia. Br Med J 1995 (July 1);311:27.

24. Diekman T, Lansberg PJ, Kastelein JJP, Wiersinga WM: Prevalence and correcting of hypothyroidism in a large cohort of patients referred for dyslipidemia. Arch Intern Med 1995 (July 24);155:1490–1495.

25. Kokkinos PF, Holland JC, Narayan P, Colleran JA, Dotson CO, Papademetriou V: Miles run per week and high-density lipoprotein cholesterol levels in healthy, middle-aged men. Arch Intern Med 1995 (February 27);155:415–420.

26. Anderson JW, Johnstone BM, Cook-Newell ME: Meta-analysis of the effects of soy protein intake on serum lipids. N Engl J Med 1995 (August 3);333(5):276–282.

27. Young D, Peterson C, Basch C, Halladay SC: Effects of naproxen and nabumetone on serum cholesterol levels in patients with osteoarthritis. Clin Ther 1995;17:2:231–240.

28. Lapinleimu H, Viikari J, Jokinen E, Salo P, Routi T, Leino A, Ronnemaa T, Seppanen R, Valimaki J, Simell O: Prospective randomised trial in 1062 infants of diet low in saturated fat and cholesterol. Lancet 1995 (February 25);345:471–476.

29. The Writing Group for the DISC Collaborative Research Group: Efficacy and safety of lowering dietary intake of fat and cholesterol in children with elevated low-density lipoprotein cholesterol: The intervention study in children (DISC). JAMA 1995 (May 10);273:18:1429–1438.

30. Gould KL, Ornish D, Scherwitz L, Brown S, Edens P, Hess MJ, Mullani N, Bolomey L, Dobbs F, Armstrong WT, Merritt T, Ports T, Sparler S, Billings J: Changes in myocardial perfusion abnormalities by positron emission tomography after long-term, intense risk factor modification. JAMA 1995 (September 20);274:894–901.

31. Schaefer EJ, Lichtenstein AH, Lamon-Fava S, McNamara JR, Schaefer MM, Rasmussen H, Ordovas JM: Body weight and low-density lipoprotein cholesterol changes after consumption of a low-fat ad libitum diet. JAMA 1995 (November 8);274:1450–1455.

32. Cox C, Mann J, Sutherland W, Ball M: Individual variation in plasma cholesterol response to dietary saturated fat. Br Med J 1995 (November 11);311:1260–1264.

33. Neil HAW, Roe L, Godlee RJP, Moore JW, Clark GMG, Brown J, Thorogood M, Stratton IM, Lancaster T, Mant D, Fowler GH: Randomised trial of lipid lowering dietary advice in general practice: The effects on serum lipids, lipoproteins, and antioxidants. Br Med J 1995 (March 4);310:569–574.

34. Denke MA: Cholesterol-lowering diets: A review of the evidence. Arch Intern Med 1995 (January 9);155:17–26.

35. Hamilton VH, Racicot FE, Zowall H, Coupall L, Grover SA: The cost-effectiveness of HMG-CoA reductase inhibitors to prevent coronary heart disease. JAMA 1995 (April 5);273:13:1032–1038.

36. Straznicky NE, Howes LG, Lam W, Louis WJ: Effects of pravastatin on cardiovascular reactivity to norepinephrine and angiotensin II in patients with hypercholesterolemia and systemic hypertension. Am J Cardiol 1995 (March 15);75:582–586.

37. Jacobson TA, Chin MM, Curry CL, Miller V, Papademetriou V, Schlant RC, LaRosa JC: Efficacy and safety of pravastatin in African Americans with primary hypercholesterolemia. Arch Intern Med 1995 (September 25);155:1900–1906.

38. Shepherd J, Cobbe SM, Ford I, Isles CG, Lorimer AR, Macfarlane PW, McKillop JH, Packard CJ, for the West of Scotland Coronary Prevention Study Group: Prevention of coronary heart disease with pravastatin in men with hypercholesterolemia. N Engl J Med 1995 (November 16);333:1301–1307.

39. Smit JW, Wijnne HJ, Schobben F, Sitsen A, DeBruin TW, Erkelens DW: Effects of alcohol and fluvastatin on lipid metabolism and hepatic function. Ann Intern Med 1995 (May 1);122:9:678–680.

40. Bredie SJH, de Bruin TWA, Demacker PNM, Kastelein JJP, Stalenhoef AFH: Comparison of gemfibrozil versus simvastatin in familial combined hyperlipidemia and effects on apolipoprotein-B-containing lipoproteins, low-density lipoprotein subfraction profile, and low-density lipoprotein oxidizability. Am J Cardiol 1995 (February 15);75:348–353.

41. Sweany AE, Shapiro DR, Tate AC, Goldberg RB, Stein EA, the NIDDM Study Group: Effects of simvastatin versus gemfibrozil on lipids and glucose control in patients with non–insulin-dependent diabetes mellitus. Clin Ther 1995;17:2:186–203.

42. Hunninghake DB, Stein EA, Bremner WF, Greenland P, Demke DM, Oliphant TH: Dose-response study of colestipol tablets in patients with moderate hypercholesterolemia. Am J Ther 1995 (May);2:180–189.

43. Schrott HG, Stein EA, Dujovne CA, Davidson MH, Goris GB, Oliphant TH, Phillips JC, Shawaryn GG: Enhanced low density lipoprotein cholesterol reduction and cost-effectiveness by low-dose colestipol plus lovastatin combination therapy. Am J Cardiol 1995 (January 1);75:34–39.
44. Maher VMG, Brown BG, Marcovina SM, Hillger LA, Zhao XQ, Albers JJ: Effects of lowering elevated LDL cholesterol on the cardiovascular risk of lipoprotein(a). JAMA 1995 (December 13);274:1771–1774.
45. Spence JD, Huff MW, Heidenheim P, Viswanatha A, Munoz C, Lindsay R, Wolfe B, Mills D: Combination therapy with colestipol and psyllium mucilloid in patients with hyperlipidemia. Ann Intern Med 1995 (October 1);123:493–499.
46. Denke MA, Grundy SM: Efficacy of low-dose cholesterol-lowering drug therapy in men with moderate hypercholesterolemia. Arch Intern Med 1995 (February 27);155:393–399.
47. Gibbons LW, Gonzalez V, Gordon N, Grundy S: The prevalence of side effects with regular and sustained-release nicotine acid. Am J Med 1995 (October);99:378–385.
48. Jha P, Flather M, Lonn E, Farkouh M, Yusuf S: The antioxidant vitamins and cardiovascular disease. Ann Intern Med 1995 (December 1);123:860–872.
49. Thompson GR, Maher VMG, Matthews S, Kitano Y, Neuwirth C, Shortt MB, Davies G, Rees A, Mir A, Prescott RJ, DeFeyter P, Henderson A: Familial hypercholesterolaemia regression study: A randomised trial of low-density-lipoprotein apheresis. Lancet 1995 (April 1);345:811–816.
50. Lane DM, Alaupovic P, Knight-Gibson C, Dudley VS, Laughlin LO: Changes in plasma lipid and apolipoprotein levels between heparin-induced extracorporeal low-density lipoprotein precipitation (HELP) treatments. Am J Cardiol (June 1);75:1124–1129.
51. Willett WC, Manson JE, Stampfer MJ, Colditz GA, Rosner B, Speizer FE, Hennekens CH: Weight, weight change, and coronary heart disease in women. JAMA 1995 (February 8);273:6:461–465.
52. Lean MEJ, Han TS, Morrison CE: Waist circumference as a measure for indicating need for weight management. Br Med J 1995 (July 15);311:158–161.
53. Han TS, van Leer EM, Lean MEJ: Waist circumference action levels in the identification of cardiovascular risk factors: Prevalence study in a random sample. Br Med J 1995 (November 25);311:1401–1404.
54. Manson JE, Willett WC, Stampfer MJ, Coldtiz GA, Hunter DJ, Hankinson SE, Hennekens CH, Speizer FE: Body weight and mortality among women. N Engl J Med 1995 (September 14);333:677–685.
55. Iribarren C, Sharp DS, Burchfiel CM, Petrovitch H: Association of weight loss and weight fluctuation with mortality among Japanese American men. N Engl J Med 1995 (September 14);333:686–692.
56. Walton C, Lees B, Crook D, Worthington M, Godsland IF, Stevenson JC: Body fat distribution, rather than overall adiposity, influences serum lipids and lipoproteins in healthy men independently of age. Am J Med 1995 (November);99:459–464.
57. Katzel LI, Bleecker ER, Colman EG, Rogus EM, Sorkin JD, Goldberg AP: Effects of weight loss vs aerobic exercise training on risk factors for coronary disease in healthy, obese, middle-aged and older men. JAMA 1995 (December 27);274:1915–1921.
58. Young TK, Gelskey DE: Is noncentral obesity metabolically benign? JAMA 1995 (December 27);274:1939–1941.
59. Blair SN, Kohl HW III, Barlow CE, Paffenbarger RS Jr, Gibbons LW, Macera CA: Changes in physical fitness and all-cause mortality. JAMA 1995 (April 12);273:14:1093–1098.
60. Lee IM, Hsieh CC, Paffenbarger RS Jr: Exercise intensity and longevity in men. JAMA 1995 (April 19);273:15:1179–1184.
61. Lemaitre RN, Heckbert SR, Psaty BM, Siscovick DS: Leisure-time physical activity and the risk of nonfatal myocardial infarction in postmenopausal women. Arch Intern Med 1995 (November 27);155:2302–2308.
62. Morbidity and Mortality Weekly Report 1994;43:925–930: Cigarette smoking among adults—United States, 1993. JAMA 1995 (February 1);273:5:369–372.

63. Sachs DPL: Effectiveness of the 4-mg dose of nicotine polacrilex for the initial treatment of high-dependent smokers. Arch Intern Med 1995 (October 9);155:1973–1980.

64. Jorenby DE, Smith SS, Fiore MC, Hurt RD, Offord KP, Croghan IT, Hays JT, Lewis SF, Baker TB: Varying nicotine patch dose and type of smoking cessation counseling. JAMA 1995 (November 1);274:1347–1352.

65. Flegal KM, Troiano RP, Pamuk ER, Kuczmarski RJ, Campbell SM: The influence of smoking cessation on the prevalence of overweight in the United States. N Engl Med 1995 (November 2);333:1167–1170.

66. Zeiher AM, Schächinger V, Minners J: Long-term cigarette smoking impairs endothelium-dependent coronary arterial vasodilator function. Circulation 1995 (September);92:1094–1100.

67. Czernin J, Sun K, Brunken R, Böttcher M, Phelps M, Schelbert H: Effect of acute and long-term smoking on myocardial blood flow and flow reserve. Circulation 1995 (June);91:2891–2897.

68. Glantz SA, Parmley WW: Passive smoking and heart disease. JAMA 1995 (April 5);273:1047–1053.

69. Nahser PJ, Brown RE, Oskarsson H, Winniford MD, Rossen JD: Maximal coronary flow reserve and metabolic coronary vasodilation in patients with diabetes mellitus. Circulation 1995 (February);91:635–640.

70. The Diabetes Control and Complications Trial (DCCT) Research Group: Effect of intensive diabetes management on macrovascular events and risk factors in the Diabetes Control and Complications Trial. Am J Cardiol (May 1);75:894–903.

71. Casino PR, Kilcoyne CM, Cannon RO III, Quyyumi AA, Panza JA: Impaired endothelium-dependent vascular relaxation in patients with hypercholesterolemia extends beyond the muscarinic receptor. Am J Cardiol 1995 (January 1);75:40–44.

72. Goode GK, Heagerty AM: In vitro responses of human peripheral small arteries in hypercholesterolemia and effects of therapy. Circulation 1995 (June);91:2898–2903.

73. Dubois-Randé JL, Dupouy P, Aptecar E, Bhatia A, Teiger E, Hittinger L, Berdeaus A, Castaigne A, Geschwind H: Comparison of the effects of exercise in cold pressor test on the vasomotor response of normal and atherosclerotic coronary arteries and their relation to the flow-mediated mechanism. Am J Cardiol 1995 (September 1);76:467–473.

74. The Postmenopausal Estrogen/Progestin Interventions (PEPI) Group: Effects of estrogen or estrogen/progestin regimens on heart disease risk factors in postmenopausal women. JAMA 1995 (January 18);273(3):199–208; 240–241.

75. Gilligan DM, Badar DM, Panza JA, Quyyumi AA, Cannon RO III: Effects of estrogen replacement therapy on peripheral vasomotor function in postmenopausal women. Am J Cardiol 1995 (February 1);75:264–268.

76. Gebara OCE, Mittleman MA, Sutherland P, Lipinska I, Matheney T, Xu P, Welty FK, Wilson PWF, Levy D, Muller JE, Tofler GH: Association between increased estrogen status and increased fibrinolytic potential in the Framingham offspring study. Circulation 1995 (April);91:1952–1958.

77. Denke MA: Effects of continuous combined hormone-replacement therapy on lipid levels in hypercholesterolemic postmenopausal women. Am J Med 1995 (July);99:29–35.

78. Stroes ESG, Koomans HA, deBruin TWA, Rabelink TJ: Vascular function in the forearm of hypercholesterolaemic patients off and on lipid-lowering medication. Lancet 1995 (August 19);36:467–471.

79. Isaacs AJ, Britton AR, McPherson K: Utilisation of hormone replacement therapy by women doctors. Br Med J 1995 (November 25);311:1399–1401.

80. Glueck CJ, Shaw P, Lang JE, Tracy T, Sieve-Smith L, Wang Y: Evidence that homocysteine is an independent risk factor for atherosclerosis in hyperlipidemic patients. Am J Cardiol 1995 (January 15);75:132–136.

81. Den Heijer M, Blom HJ, Gerrits WBJ, Rosendaal FR, Haak HL, Wijermans PW, Bos GMJ: Is hyperhomocysteinaemia a risk factor for recurrent venous thrombosis? Lancet 1995 (April 8);345:882–885.

82. Dalery K, Lussier-Cacan S, Selhub J, Davignon J, Latour Y, Genest J Jr: Homocysteine and coronary artery disease in French Canadian subjects: Relation with vitamins B_{12}, B_6, pyridoxal phosphate, and folate. Am J Cardiol (June 1);75:1107–1111.

83. Boushey CJ, Beresford SAA, Omenn GS, Motulsky AG: A quantitative assessment of plasma homocysteine as a risk factor for vascular disease. JAMA 1995 (October 4);274:1049–1057.

84. Nygard O, Vollset SE, Refsum H, Stensvold I, Tverdal A, Nordrehaug JE, Ueland PM, Kvale G: Total plasma homocysteine and cardiovascular risk profile. JAMA 1995 (November 15);274:1526–1533.

85. Liao Y, Cooper RS, McGee DL, Mensah GA, Gahli JK: The relative effects of left ventricular hypertrophy, coronary artery disease, and ventricular dysfunction on survival among black adults. JAMA 1995 (May 24/31);273:20:1592–1597.

86. Liao Y, Cooper RS, Mensah GA, McGee DL: Left ventricular hypertrophy has a greater impact on survival in women than in men. Circulation 1995 (August);92:805–810.

87. Fall CHD, Osmond C, Barker DJP, Clark PMS, Hales CN, Stirling Y, Meade TW: Fetal and infant growth and cardiovascular risk factors in women. Br Med J 1995 (February 18);310:428–432.

88. Keil JE, Sutherland SE, Hames CG, Lackland DT, Gazes PC, Knapp RG, Tyroler HA: Coronary disease mortality and risk factors in black and white men. Arch Intern Med 1995 (July 24);155:1521–1527.

89. Cruqui MH, Ringel BL: Does diet or alcohol explain the French paradox? Lancet 1994 (December 24/31);344:1719–1723.

90. Salomaa V, Stinson V, Kark JD, Folsom AR, Davis CE, Wu KK: Association of fibrinolytic parameters with early atherosclerosis. The ARIC study. Circulation 1995 (January);91:284–290.

91. Salonen JT, Seppänen K, Nyyssönen K, Korpela H, Kauhanen J, Kantola M, Tuomi-lehto J, Esterbauer H, Tatzber F, Salonen R: Intake of mercury from fish, lipid peroxidation, and the risk of myocardial infarction and coronary, cardiovascular, and any death in Eastern Finnish men. Circulation 1995 (February);91:645–655.

92. Ascherio A, Rimm EB, Stampfer MJ, Giovannucci EL, Willett WC: Dietary intake of marine n-3 fatty acids, fish intake, and the risk of coronary disease among men. N Engl J Med 1995 (April 13);332:15:977–982.

93. Kawachi I, Colditz GA, Stampfer MJ, Willett WC, Manson JE, Speizer FE, Hennekens CH: Prospective study of shift work and risk of coronary heart disease in women. Circulation 1995 (December);92:3178–3182.

94. Vaarala O, Mänttäri M, Manninen V, Tenkanen L, Puurunen M, Aho K, Palosuo T: Anti-cardiolipin antibodies and risk of myocardial infarction in a prospective cohort of middle-aged men. Circulation 1995 (January);91:23–27.

95. Ridker PM, Hennekens CH, Lindpaintner K, Stampfer MJ, Eisenberg PR, Miletich JP: Mutation in the gene coding or coagulation factor V and the risk of myocardial infarction, stroke, and venous thrombosis in apparently healthy men. N Engl J Med 1995 (April 6);332:912–917.

96. Lindpaintner K, Pfeffer MA, Kreutz R, Stampfer MJ, Grodstein F, LaMotte F, Buring J, Hennekens CH: A prospective evaluation of an angiotensin-converting-enzyme gene polymorphism and the risk of ischemic heart disease. N Engl J Med 1995 (March 16);332:11:706–711.

97. Imai K, Nakachi K: Cross-sectional study of effects of drinking green tea in cardiovascular and liver diseases. Br Med J 1995 (March 18);310:693–700.

2

Coronary Artery Disease

Miscellaneous Topics

Modifying Risk Factors After Events

This study by the Clinical Quality Improvement Network Investigators[1] in Edmonton, Canada, defined the patterns of investigation and treatment of serum lipids and other modifiable risk factors for atherosclerosis among 3304 hospitalized patients at high risk for future cardiovascular events. There were 2161 men and 1143 women; 1955 were younger than 70 years and 1349 were older than 70 years. Acute (61%) and chronic (65%) cardiac ischemia was the most prevalent reason for high-risk status, followed by cardiac revascularization and diabetes. Only 28% of patients had lipid measurements recorded during their hospital stay or recorded at any time between 1988 and 1993. A lipid-lowering diet or drugs were prescribed for 22% and 8% of all patients, respectively, and an adjustment in lifestyle in only 5% of all patients. Moreover, measurement and therapy of lipid risk were recorded less frequently in older patients and less often in women. Logistic regression analysis revealed admission for revascularization, preadmission lipid-lowering or lifestyle therapy, and a history of hyperlipidemia or diabetes to be associated with increased likelihood of in-hospital measurements; age greater than 70 years was associated with reduced likelihood of lipid determination. The overall investigation in therapy of serum lipids and other risk factors in acute care patients at high risk for cardiovascular events appear less than optimal. Moreover, there are significantly fewer measurements and less treatment of risk factors in women and older patients.

Preoperative Assessment

Dennis T. Mangano and Lee Goldman[2] provided a superb review of current concepts regarding preoperative assessment of patients with known or suspected coronary artery disease in the December 28, 1995, issue of *The New England Journal of Medicine*.

To determine whether preoperative angiography and revascularization improves short-term outcomes in patients undergoing noncardiac vascular surgery, Mason and associates[3] from Palo Alto, California, utilized a decision analysis for patients undergoing elective vascular surgery who either had no or mild angina and a positive dipyridamole-thalium scan result. Three strategies were compared. The first strategy was to proceed directly with vascular surgery. The second was to perform coronary angiography, followed by selective coronary revascularization, before proceeding to vascular surgery and to cancel vascular surgery in patients with severe, inoperable CAD. The third was to perform coronary angiography followed by selective coronary revascularization, before proceeding to vascular surgery and to perform vascular surgery in pa-

61

tients with inoperable CAD. Mortality, nonfatal AMI, stroke, uncorrected valvular disease, and cost were assessed within 3 months. Proceeding directly to vascular surgery led to lower morbidity and cost in the base case analysis. The coronary angiography strategy led to higher mortality if vascular surgery would proceed in patients with inoperable CAD, but led to slightly lower morality if vascular surgery were canceled in patients with inoperable CAD. The coronary angiography strategy also led to lower mortality when vascular surgery was particularly risky. Decision analysis indicates vascular surgery without preoperative coronary angiography generally leads to better outcomes. Preoperative coronary angiography should be reserved for patients whose estimated mortality from vascular surgery is substantially higher than average.

Lee and associates[4] from Durham, North Carolina, performed continuous 12-lead digital electrocardiographic monitoring before, during, and after gastroendoscopy and found that myocardial ischemia occurred during the periprocedural period in 16% of hospitalized patients with severe CAD. Women experienced more periprocedural myocardial ischemia than did men (31% vs. 11%).

American vs. Canadian Functional Status

Coronary angiography and revascularization are used more often in the United States than Canada although the rates of mortality and myocardial infarction are similar. To further evaluate this issue, quality of life was measured in patients enrolled in 7 American and 1 Canadian site in the bypass angioplasty revascularization investigation.[5] Quality of life was generally better in the 934 Americans compared with the 278 Canadians, with overall health rated as excellent or very good in 30% of the Americans vs. 20% of the Canadians. Results were essentially unchanged after statistical adjustment for potential confounding factors. These authors concluded that although the functional status of patients without prior symptoms of heart disease is similar in Americans and Canadians, among patients with previous symptomatic heart disease, functional status is higher in Americans than in Canadians. They postulate that this difference may be due to different patterns of medical management of heart disease in the 2 countries.

Survival in Various Time Periods

Ramanathan and associates[6] from Memphis, Tennessee, retrospectively reviewed long-term survival in patients with documented CAD who had cardiac catheterization at their hospital from 1972 to 1982. Risk factors and survival of patients who underwent cardiac catheterization from 1972 through 1982 were followed up for at least 5 years. Cohort A included 1821 patients studied from 1972 through 1977; cohort B included 5369 patients studied between 1977 and the end of 1982. Each cohort was subdivided based on type of therapy (medical or surgical) that the patients received. The 30-day (short-term) and 5-year (long-term) survival rates were compared by life-table methods. Short-term survival improved significantly in both medical (from 94.9% to 97.5%) and surgical (from 95.5% to 97.5%) groups from cohort A to cohort B. Long-term survival, however, did not differ significantly between the 2 cohorts. In the medical group, 5-year survival in cohort A was 86.3% and 86.9% in cohort B.

In the surgical group, the 5-year survival in cohort A was 89.1% and 89.4% in cohort B. Prevalence of both cigarette smoking and hypercholesterolemia declined significantly from cohort A to cohort B in both surgical and medical groups. However, advanced age, female gender, and previous myocardial infarction were significantly more common in cohort B than in cohort A for both treatment groups. These results indicate that during the study period, a significant decline in short-term mortality occurred for patients with angiographically documented coronary artery disease. Long-term survival did not, however, improve, possibly due to a complex interplay between factors that promote CAD, e.g., cigarette abuse and hypercholesterolemia, and factors that determine survival, such as increases in age and history of prior infarction and advances in medical and surgical therapy.

Heart Rate Variability and Depression

Decreased heart rate variability is an independent risk factor for mortality in the cardiac populations. Clinical depression has also been associated with adverse outcome in patients with CAD. A study by Carney and coinvestigators[7] in St. Louis, Missouri, tested the hypothesis that depressed patients with CAD have decreased heart rate variability compared with nondepressed CAD patients. Nineteen patients with angiographically documented CAD and either major or minor depression were compared with a sample of nondepressed CAD patients according to age, sex, and smoking status. All patients underwent 24-hour Holter monitoring, and the standard deviation of all normal-to-normal intervals was used as the primary index of heart rate variability. Heart rate variability was significantly lower in depressed than nondepressed patients (90 vs. 117 msec) even after adjusting for relevant covariants. Thus, decreased heart rate variability may help explain the increased risk of cardiac mortality and morbidity in depressed CAD patients.

Costs of Psychological Distress

To determine the effect of psychological distress, measured with a commonly used screening questionnaire, on 6-month morbidity and rehospitalization costs in CAD patients, Allison and associates[8] from Rochester, Minnesota, studied 381 patients (311 men and 70 women) referred for cardiac rehabilitation after an index hospitalization for unstable angina, AMI, PTCA, or CABG. Patients with a symptom checklist-90-Revised score above the 90th percentile for outpatient adults were considered distressed (n = 41); patients with scores below this level were considered nondistressed (n = 340). The 6-month follow-up was complete in all but one of the 381 patients. Distressed patients had significantly higher rates of cardiovascular rehospitalization, any recurrent events, and recurrent "hard events" (cardiac death, AMI, or cardiac arrest and resuscitation) within 6 months after dismissal from their index hospitalization in comparison with nondistressed patients. Adjustment for other factors associated with a risk of early rehospitalization and recurrent events did not reduce the strength or significance of the association between psychological distress and early cardiovascular rehospitalization or recurrent events. The mean rehospitalization costs were significantly higher in the distressed than in the nondistressed patients ($9504 vs.

$2146). These data add support to the hypothesis that psychological distress adversely affects the prognosis in CAD patients, confirm the added morbidity and rehospitalization costs attributable to psychological distress, and suggest the potential for improving the prognosis in selected CAD patients by identification and appropriate treatment of psychological distress.

Dilatation of Atherosclerotic Arteries

McPherson and coinvestigators[9] in Iowa City, Iowa, evaluated the vasodilating responses of atherosclerotic coronary arteries through the use of intraoperative high-frequency (12 MHz) epicardial echocardiography. The investigators obtained continuous high-frequency epicardial echocardiographic recordings during surgery, and determined cross-sectional lumen area from 17 coronary artery segments in 12 patients. Nitroglycerin was administered intravenously to reduce mean arterial pressure an average of 14 mm Hg. The cross-sectional arterial images were classified using 3 different parameters: arterial lumen area, percentage of the arterial wall circumference that was atherosclerotic, and presence of an eccentrically shaped arterial lumen. Nine arterial segments had small (<5.0 mm^2) lumens. With nitroglycerin, the luminal area increased 0.8 mm^2 (39%). The remaining 8 segments had larger (≥5.0 mm^2) lumens. With nitroglycerin, the luminal area increased 4.3 mm^2 (51%). Seven arterial segments had eccentric lumens; mean maximal-to-minimal ratio was 1.8. The area increased 39% with nitroglycerin. In the 10 concentrically shaped lumens, nitroglycerin increased luminal area by 48%. With regard to the percent arterial wall circumference that was atherosclerotic, 11 segments had 75% to 100% involvement of the arterial circumference. Nitroglycerin increased luminal area by 48%. Similar variability was seen in segments having primarily normal wall thickness, where luminal area increased 38%. Thus, severely atherosclerotic coronary arteries retained vasodilating ability. However, the absolute and/or percent increase in luminal areas was often small, especially in the most severely diseased arteries.

Myocardial Bridges

In this investigation by Juillière and associates[10] from Vandoeuvre-les-Nancy, France, among 7467 consecutive coronary angiograms performed during an 8-year period, 61 patients had a myocardial bridge of the LAD coronary artery. The overall prevalence of myocardial bridges was 0.82% (from 0.41% to 1.16% per year). Among these patients, 26 had CAD, four had valvular heart disease, and three had cardiomyopathy. The investigators studied the long-term outcome (11 ± 3 years) of the other 28 patients with isolated milking at baseline. Two groups were constituted according to the percentage of systolic reduction of the LAD coronary artery lumen: group A, <50% (15 patients), and group B, ≥50% (13 patients). During follow-up, 1 group A patient (cancer) and 2 group B patients (1 cancer and 1 suicide) died. None of the patients sustained a myocardial infarction during follow-up. In group A patients, 71% felt very well or well and 50% had clinical symptoms; 64% took antianginal medications. In group B patients, 50% felt well and 70% had clinical symptoms; 50% took antianginal drugs. The long-term prognosis of isolated myocardial bridges of the LAD coronary artery is good and is independent of the severity of systolic narrowing of internal lumen diameter.

In Heterozygous Familial Hypercholesterolemia

Ferrières and colleagues[11] in Montreal, Canada, studied the association between CAD and common risk factors in 263 French Canadian familial hyper-cholesterolemia patients, including 147 women and 116 men carrying the same >10-kb deletion of the LDL receptor gene. Thirty-five women and 54 men had CAD. The mean age of onset of CAD was 45 years in women and 39 years in men. Multiple logistic regression analyses were performed to test the association between CAD and age, tendonxanthomas, cigarette smoking, hyper-tension, diabetes mellitus, apolipoprotein E polymorphism, total plasma choles-terol, triglycerides, VLDL cholesterol, LDL cholesterol, HDL cholesterol, and lipoprotein(a). In women with familial hypercholesterolemia, significant multi-variate predictors were age, VLDL cholesterol, and LDL cholesterol. In men with familial hypercholesterolemia, age, and HDL cholesterol were significant predictors of disease. The lipoprotein(a) was not a significant predictor in univariate or multivariate analyses. This study suggests that increased risk of CAD in familial hypercholesterolemia is not related solely to elevated choles-terol levels and demonstrates a sex-specific lipoprotein influence on CAD in the patients with familial hypercholesterolemia carrying the same LDL receptor gene defect.

Cocaine-Associated Myocardial Ischemia—Review

A superb review of management of cocaine-associated myocardial ischemia was provided in the November 9, 1995, issue of *The New England Journal of Medicine* by Dr. Judd E. Hollander.[12]

Waiting Times for Cardiovascular Procedures

A recurrent criticism of national health care systems is long waiting times for high-technology procedures. Carroll and associates[13] from Maywood, Illinois; Salt Lake City, Utah; and Orebro, Sweden, mailed a questionnaire to directors of cardiac catheterization laboratories in the United States, the Veterans' Administration (VA) system, Canada, the UK, and cardiology clinics in Sweden (Figure 2-1). Significant differences in waiting times were found among the systems for 4 scenarios (elective and urgent angiography and elective and urgent bypass surgery). For example, for elective coronary angiography, the median time was 24–72 hours in the United States, 72 hours to 2 weeks in the VA system, 2–6 weeks in Canada and 6 weeks to 3 months in both Sweden and the UK. For urgent coronary angiography, in the US non-VA and VA systems all patients would obtain angiography within 2 weeks. Many responders indi-cated waiting times >2 weeks (Canada, 16%; Sweden, 46%; and the UK, 36%). Overall, the longest waiting times for all 4 procedures were reported in the UK, Sweden, and Canada with some waiting times for elective procedures > 9 months. These authors concluded that differences in health care systems can result in significantly longer waits for cardiac catheterization and CABG.

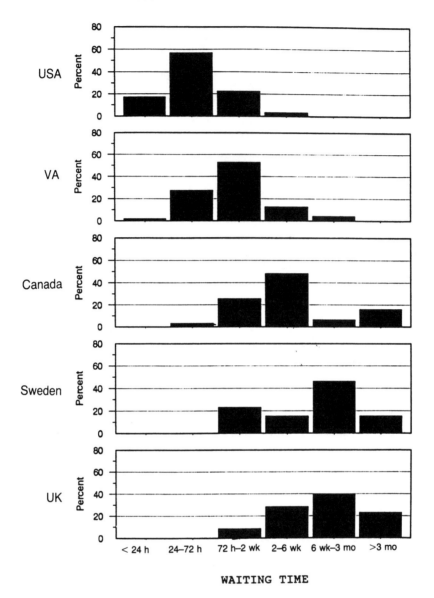

FIGURE 2-1. Frequency distribution of waiting times by country for elective coronary angiography. Reproduced with permission of Carroll et al.[13]

Intravascular Ultrasound in Coronary Aneurysms

Coronary artery aneurysms are usually diagnosed by contrast coronary angiography, which portrays the silhouette of the lumen but cannot distinguish true and false aneurysms. To differentiate true and false aneurysms and to study the morphologic changes of the vessel wall, intravascular ultrasound was performed by Ge[14] and associates from Essen, Germany, and Edinburgh, Scotland, in patients with angiographic signs of coronary artery aneurysms. These investigators used a 4.8F or 3.5F, 20-MHz intravascular ultrasound catheter for ultrasound examination. Fourteen patients (12 men and 2 women ranging in age from 43 to 73 years) with angiographic signs of coronary aneurysms were enrolled. Intravascular ultrasound imaging was optimally obtained in all patients. The vessel area, lumen area, and plaque area of the aneurysm segment and of the proximal and distal segments were determined. Intravascular ultrasound showed that both the proximal and distal reference segments were severely affected by atherosclerotic lesions in all the patients and by calcium deposits in 6 patients. The percent stenoses were 63 ± 14% and 61 ± 18% in the proximal and distal reference segments, respectively. In nine patients the walls of the aneurysms showed signs of atherosclerosis. Three angiographically indicated aneurysms were found to be plaque ruptures. Although the lumen and the vessel areas of the aneurysm segments were larger than those of the proximal and distal segments, no significant differences in plaque area and plaque composition were found between the aneurysm segment and adjacent vessel segments. In conclusion, intravascular ultrasound allows detailed characterization of coronary aneurysms. Atherosclerosis seems to play an important role in the formation of acquired coronary aneurysms.

Energy Expenditure From Household Tasks

Wilke and coworkers[15] in Milwaukee, Wisconsin, determined the energy expenditure for and heart rate responses to common household tasks in 26 older (mean age, 62 years) women with CAD. Each activity was performed at a self-determined pace for 6 or 8 minutes. The average oxygen uptake (mL/kg per minute) for each task evaluated was 6.5 for washing dishes, 6.8 for ironing, 7.2 for scrubbing pans, 8.6 for unpacking groceries, 9.5 for vacuuming, 9.8 for sweeping, 10.1 for mopping, 12.0 for changing bed linens, and 12.4 for washing the floor (hands and knees) (Figure 2-2). None of the subjects reported angina. Mean relative oxygen uptake (i.e., percentage of peak response with treadmill testing) ranged from 31% for washing dishes to 62% for changing the bed linens and washing the floor. Percentage of peak treadmill heart rate ranged from 62% for washing dishes to 73% for washing the floor. In four of the more physically demanding household activities (vacuuming, mopping, washing the floor, and changing bed linens), the responses of 10 age-matched normal women were evaluated. The absolute and relative demands of the tasks were similar between the CAD and normal groups. These results indicate that the mean energy expenditure rate of common household tasks evaluated in this study range from 2 to 4 METs, suggesting that most women with CAD who are able to achieve ≥5 METs during a treadmill exercise test without adverse signs or symptoms should be able to resume these activities.

Detection

Costs of Diagnostic Tests

Patterson and colleagues[16] in Atlanta, Georgia, compared exercise ECG, stress single-photon emission computed tomography (SPECT), positron emission tomography (PET), and coronary angiography to determine the cost-effectiveness and utility of these 4 methods used to diagnose CAD. The effectiveness of each technique was defined as the number of patients with diagnosed CAD,

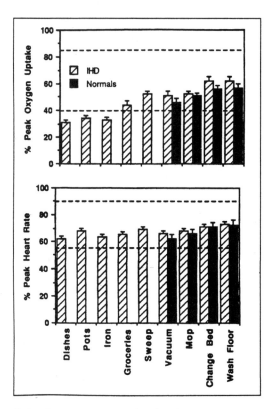

FIGURE 2-2. Mean relative (i.e., percentage of each subject's peak treadmill response) oxygen uptake and heart rate reponses for each household task. The areas between the *broken lines* represent work intensities recommended for aerobic exercise training by the American College of Sports Medicine. Reproduced with permission of Wilke et al.[15]

and utility was defined as the clinical outcome, i.e., the number of quality-adjusted life-years extended by therapy after the diagnosis of CAD. The model used published values for cost, accuracy, and complication rates of tests. Analysis of the model used indicates the following results: (1) The direct cost or fee for each test differs considerably from total cost per quality-adjusted life-years. (2) As pretest likelihood of CAD increased, there was a linear increase in cost per patient tested, but a hyperbolic decrease in cost per effect and cost per utility unit. (3) At lower pretest likelihood of CAD, stress PET was the most cost-effective test with the lowest cost per utility followed by SPECT, exercise ECG, and angiography, in that order. (4) With a higher pretest likelihood of CAD, proceeding directly to angiography as the first test had the lowest cost. Thus, these data indicate that the estimation of total cost for diagnostic tests for CAD requires consideration of the direct costs of the test and also the indirect and induced costs of management algorithms based on the test. It is important to consider the clinical history of CAD when selecting the clinical algorithm to make a diagnosis with the lowest cost. Stress PET has the lowest cost in patients with a pretest CAD likelihood <70%. Angiography has the lowest cost in patients with pretest CAD likelihood >70%.

Coronary Calcium by Ultrafast Computed Tomography

Ultrafast computed tomography has been shown to be a sensitive method for detection of coronary calcium. Devries and associates[17] from Chicago, Illinois, evaluated the influence of age and gender on the presence of coronary calcium. Seventy men and 70 women were studied with ultrafast computed tomography for analysis of coronary calcium and also underwent coronary angiography. Significant obstructive CAD was defined as a lumen diameter narrowing >70%. Coronary calcium had a sensitivity of 80% for identification of patients with atherosclerotic disease and 97% for those with obstructive disease. The sensitivity of coronary calcium for detection of atherosclerotic disease in women <60 years old was 50% compared with 97% sensitivity in women older than 60 years, and 87% sensitivity in men <60 years. Logistic regression revealed a 1.81-fold increase in the likelihood of detecting coronary calcium in the atherosclerotic lesions of men compared with those in women. These authors concluded that atherosclerotic lesions in women are less likely to have coronary calcium than men in lesions with a similar degree of lumen narrowing.

Rumberger and colleagues[18] in Rochester, Minnesota, studied 50 women and 89 men with electron-beam computed tomography an average of 1 day after coronary arteriography to determine the effect of a patient's sex on the diagnostic ability of the computed tomography to detect coronary atherosclerosis. Maximum arteriographic percent luminal diameter stenosis of any artery was paired with the total electron-beam computed tomography coronary calcium score for each subject. The women were older than the men (mean, 56 vs. 47 years), but the subjects were matched for indications for arteriography and extent of disease as assessed by arteriography. Sensitivity, specificity, and positive and negative predictive values for coronary calcium were nearly identical for men and women, regardless of the degree of arteriographic disease. Electron-beam computed tomography was highly sensitive to the presence of arteriographic disease (range, 94–100%), but had only moderate specificity (57–66%) for significant disease defined as ≥50% stenosis and low specificity (35–38%) for any arteriographic disease (>0% stenosis) (Figure 2-3 and Table 2-1). Negative predictive values in men and women ranged

Table 2-1. Sensitivity, Specificity, and Predictive Values for EBCT Detection of Coronary Calcium and Arteriographic Disease Severity

EBCT and coronary calcium	Any arteriographic disease		Significant arteriographic disease	
	Women	Men	Women	Men
Sensitivity	97 ± 3%	94 ± 3%	100 ± 0%	98 ± 2%
Specificity	38 ± 12%	35 ± 10%	66 ± 8%	57 ± 8%
Positive predictive value	85 ± 6%	89 ± 4%	46 ± 8%	66 ± 6%
Negative predictive value	91 ± 9%	79 ± 9%	100 ± 0%	95 ± 5%

EBCT, electron-beam computed tomography.

Data are presented as mean±SEM.

Reproduced with permission of Rumberger et al.[18]

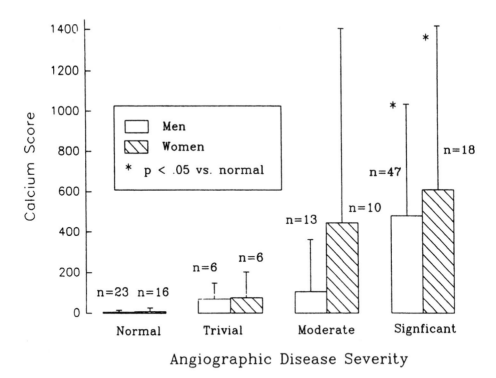

FIGURE 2-3. Mean calcium scores for men and women in each of the 4 categories of arteriographic disease severity (normal [normal coronary arteriogram, 0% stenosis], trivial [>0% but ≤20% stenosis], moderate [>20% but <50% stenosis], and significant [≥50% stenosis]). Reproduced with permission of Rumberger et al.[18]

from 79–91% for any arteriographic disease and from 95–100% for significant disease, respectively. Numerical calcium scores were significantly different between those with normal arteriograms and those with significant disease, but calcium score had limited ability to separate trivial, moderate, and significant disease. Thus, in middle-aged populations, noninvasive definition of coronary calcium by electron-beam computed tomography has similar predictive value for arteriographic CAD in men and women.

To determine the prevalence and quantity of coronary artery calcium in asymptomatic subjects from the general population, to identify asymptomatic subjects without risk factors for CAD with coronary artery calcium scores in the top quartile of the distribution, and to compare coronary artery calcium scores in patients who underwent angiography with percentiles in asymptomatic subjects of the same age and sex, Kaufmann and associates[19] from Rochester, Minnesota, and Ann Arbor, Michigan, studied 2 samples from Rochester consisting of 772 asymptomatic subjects from the general population and 145 patients who underwent angiography, all of whom were 20–59 years of age. Asymptomatic subjects were classified on the basis of their CAD risk profile. All subjects in both study samples underwent electron-beam computed tomography. Age- and sex-specific calcium score percentiles were calculated in the asymptomatic sample. Coronary artery calcium prevalence in the asymptomatic subjects was lower in female than in male subjects and increased with advancing age. Of the asymptomatic sample, 8% had a low-risk profile with calcium scores in the top quartile of the distribution. More patients than expected in the angiography sample had calcium scores above the 50th through 95th score percentiles. The quantity of coronary artery calcium was substantially increased in patients who underwent angiography. Subjects with large amounts of coronary artery calcium but without known CAD risk factors may be a valuable subset of the population to investigate for previously unidentified CAD risk factors.

Pharmacological Stress Testing

To compare the hemodynamic responses and adverse effects associated with two coronary vasodilators used for pharmacological stress testing, Johnston and associates[20] from Rochester, Minnesota, retrospectively studied the results of adenosine- and dipyridamole-perfusion imaging in 2000 patients who underwent pharmacological stress radionuclide-perfusion imaging. One thousand patients given dipyridamole between April 1989 and April 1991 (before adenosine became available) were compared with 1000 patients given adenosine between April 1991 and October 1992. A standard protocol was used to infuse the drugs before myocardial perfusion imaging with thallium-201 or technitium-99m sestamibi. Peak heart rate was higher (85 vs. 83 beats/min) and systolic BP was lower (129 vs. 133 mm Hg) with adenosine than with dipyridamole. More patients had a decrease in systolic BP of 30 mm Hg or more with adenosine than with dipyridamole. Horizontal or downsloping ST-segment depression of 1 mm or more occurred in 9% of patients who received adenosine and in 8% of those who received dipyridamole. Adverse effects occurred in 78% of the adenosine study group and in 50% of the dipyridamole group. Chest pain was the most common symptom with both drugs. AV block occurred in 76 patients who received adenosine but in none who received dipyridamole. Because of adverse effects, 28% of patients who received dipyridamole required extra monitoring time (mean, 6 ± 5 minutes beyond the standard protocol). Aminophylline was administered to 163 and 6 patients, respectively, in the dipyridamole and adenosine study groups. Adenosine causes slightly greater systemic vasodilation than does dipyridamole. Adverse effects occur less often with dipyridamole but, in comparison with adenosine, are more difficult to manage and necessitate more monitoring time as well as fairly frequent intravenous use of aminophylline for reversal.

Arbutamine is an agent designed to simulate exercise and has been used with a closed-loop delivery system that modulates the rate of administration on the basis of physiological feedback. Two hundred ten patients with symptoms and angiographic evidence of coronary artery disease were studied.[21] In the 210 patients the mean increase in heart rate and blood pressure evoked by arbutamine and exercise was similar. Arbutamine detected ischemia more often than exercise with each of 3 ischemic end points (angina, and/or the presence of ST depression). For angina alone, sensitivity was 73% for arbutamine and 64% for exercise. For ST segment alone, sensitivity was 47% for arbutamine and 44% for exercise. These authors concluded that in patients with documented coronary artery disease, the sensitivity of arbutamine testing was equal to that of exercise for the end point of ST change alone and was superior to exercise testing for either ST change or angina or for angina alone.

Stress thallium using a closed-loop arbutamine system was evaluated in 184 patients of whom 122 had angiographically defined CAD.[22] The sensitivity for detecting CAD using arbutamine was 87%. In patients completing both arbutamine and exercise stress testing, thallium sensitivity for detecting CAD was 94% and 97%. These authors concluded that arbutamine administered by closed-loop feedback system was a safe and effective pharmacological stress agent. Arbutamine stress ^{201}Tl SPECT appeared to be accurate for the diagnosis of CAD with a diagnostic efficacy similar to that of treadmill exercise thallium-201 studies.

Stress Echocardiography

To describe the techniques and applications of exercise echocardiography, Roger and associates[23] from Rochester, Minnesota, reviewed pertinent and experimental clinical studies previously published and their own experiences with the first 2000 patients having exercise echocardiography in their laboratory. Exercise echocardiography proved to have considerable accuracy in the diagnosis of CAD (mean sensitivity, 84%; mean specificity, 87%). In high-volume laboratories, feasibility studies have shown success rates between 90% and 99%; thus far, reproducibility has been satisfactory.

To describe the rationale, methods, and clinical applications for dobutamine stress echocardiography, Pellikka and associates[24] from Rochester, Minnesota, reviewed their experiences with the first 1000 Mayo clinic patients who underwent this procedure. They found the test to be valuable in the noninvasive diagnosis of CAD and to have an accuracy comparable to that of tomographic perfusion imaging. Other indications for dobutamine stress echocardiography in their view included risk stratification to report nonsurgical procedures, risk stratification after AMI, and identification of viable myocardia in patients with LV dysfunction. The authors found dobutamine stress echocardiography to be accurate, safe, cost-effective, and a portable procedure for the noninvasive diagnosis of CAD and for the preoperative assessment of patients with CAD, especially those who are unable to perform adequate exercise tests.

Transesophageal Echocardiography

Dobutamine stress testing in combination with standard two-dimensional echocardiography has been widely used as a diagnostic test in patients at risk for CAD. Frohwein and colleagues[25] from Atlanta, Georgia, evaluated the feasibility, safety, sensitivity, and specificity of transesophageal dobutamine stress echocardiography for the detection of CAD. Fifty-one male patients were enrolled in the study. Of 27 patients with significant CAD, 22 had positive study results (sensitivity, 82%). Of 13 patients without significant obstructive CAD, one had a false-positive study result (specificity, 93%). There were no adverse outcomes or complications. These authors concluded that transesophageal dobutamine stress echocardiography is a feasible, safe, and accurate technique for the detection of myocardial ischemia. There is an inherent limitation, however, since not all individuals can have successful placement of the transesophageal probe.

To evaluate the clinical impact of transesophageal echocardiography on subsequent management outcome in hemodynamically unstable patients with suspected cardiovascular conditions, Sohn and associates[26] from Rochester,

Minnesota, reviewed data on patients with hemodynamic instability (hypotension, shock, or pulmonary edema) who underwent transesophageal echocardiography between December 1987 and May 1994 at the Mayo Clinic. A total of 127 patients, (70 male and 57 female patients with a mean age of 68 years) underwent transesophageal echocardiography at our institution as part of the diagnostic procedures used to evaluate unstable hemodynamics. No clinically significant complication was encountered during the procedure; transesophageal echocardiographic imaging was inadequate in three patients (2%). Of the 124 patients with adequate images, transesophageal echocardiography disclosed a severe cardiovascular abnormality responsible for the unstable hemodynamics in 65 patients (52%), and 26 patients (21%) underwent urgent pericardiocentesis or a cardiac surgical procedure, primarily based on transesophageal echocardiograhic findings. Transesophageal echocardiography can be safely performed in hemodynamically unstable patients, produces a high diagnostic yield, and provides important information for prompt therapeutic decision making. Therefore, the authors recommend transesophageal echocardiography as one of the initial diagnostic procedures in critically ill patients suspected of having an underlying cardiovascular disorder.

Intravascular Ultrasonography

Mintz and colleagues[27] in Washington, DC, evaluated 1155 native-vessel target lesions in 1117 patients using intravascular ultrasound and coronary angiography to determine presence and distribution of target lesion calcium. The presence, magnitude, location, and distribution of intravascular ultrasound calcium were analyzed and compared with the detection and classification by angiography. Angiography detected calcium in 440 of 1155 lesions in which 306 had moderate calcium and 134 severe. Intravascular ultrasound detected lesion calcium in 841 of 1155. Target lesion calcium was only superficial in 48%, only deep in 28%, and both superficial and deep in 24%. Three hundred seventy-five of 1155 reference segments contained calcium. Angiographic detection and classification of calcium depended on arcs, lengths, location, and distribution of lesion and reference segment calcium. By discriminant analysis, the classification function for predicting angiographic calcium included the arc of target lesion calcium, the arc of superficial calcium, the length of reference segment calcium, and the location of calcium within the lesion. This model correctly predicted the angiographic detection of calcification in 74% of lesions and the angiographic classification of calcium in 63% of lesions. Thus, intravascular ultrasound detected calcium in >70% of lesions and more often than standard angiography.

Pathological studies indicate that the extent of coronary atherosclerosis is underestimated by visual analysis of angiographically normal coronary artery segments. Intravascular ultrasound was used to study angiographically normal coronary artery reference segments in 884 patients evaluated for transcatheter therapy for symptomatic CAD.[28] Only 7% of 884 angiographically normal reference segments were normal by intravascular ultrasound. Reference segment percent cross-sectional narrowing measured 51% and correlated poorly with target lesion percent cross-sectional narrowing, which was 1 cm away. Reference segment disease was not an independent predictor of subsequent angiographic restenosis or clinical events within 12 months of follow-up. These authors concluded that atherosclerosis is ubiquitous in angiographically normal coronary artery reference segments. Reference segment disease parallels the severity of target lesion disease. Because of insensitivity in detecting atherosclerosis in angiographically normal reference segments, intravascular ultrasound should enhance the study of risk factors for atherosclerosis and the results of therapies to control disease progression.

Lee and associates[29] from Los Angeles, California, determined the effect of intravascular ultrasound imaging on decision making in the performance of coronary interventions. One hundred lesions were assessed in 87 patients undergoing balloon or laser angioplasty, atherectomy, stent placement, and additional diagnostic examination. Angiographically acceptable results were deemed inadequate by intravascular ultrasound in 29% of angioplasties and 30% of stent deployments, and planned procedures subsequently were altered. Abnormalities commonly identified by intravascular ultrasound and not by angiography were 13 coronary dissections after the procedure and 14 significant stenoses in apparently normal angiograms. Significant stenoses were excluded in 7 patients with ambiguous angiograms. The apparent contribution of coronary intravascular ultrasound imaging led to its significantly increased use over a 1-year period: coronary interventional decisions on the basis of intravascular ultrasound findings increased from 4 (17%) of 19 to 60 (74%) of 81. These data suggest that intravascular ultrasound is a useful adjunct to angiography in selected patients for (1) identification or exclusion of dissection, (2) assessment of the adequacy of balloon angioplasty, (3) identification or exclusion of thrombus, (4) measurement of the depth of tissue removal, (5) determination of stent size and the result of stent deployment, and (6) assessment of the severity of stenoses, especially at ostial sites.

Coronary vasospasm is manifested by either focal or diffuse pattern in clinical settings. To examine the differences in vessel wall morphologic appearance between the sites of focal and diffuse vasospasm, Koyama and associates[30] from Osaka, Japan, studied 29 patients with chest pain at rest, during exertion, or both by intravascular ultrasound. By angiography, focal vasospasm with diameter reduction of 90% ± 3% was provoked by intracoronary ergonovine (0.01 to 0.04 mg) in 15 patients. Diffuse vasospasm with diameter reduction of 79% ± 5% was provoked in 7 patients, and the remaining 7 patients served as the control group. By ultrasonography, a significantly thickened intimal leading edge with sonolucent zone was observed in 55 sites from 22 coronary arteries with either focal or diffuse vasospasm (0.61 ± 0.32 mm), although these sites were normal or minimally narrowed by angiography. Seven segments from the control group exhibited a thin intimal leading edge with sonolucent zone (0.23 ± 0.08 mm). When the thickness of the intimal leading edge with sonolucent zone was compared between the abnormal sites with focal and diffuse vasospasm, this was significantly greater at focal spasm, 1.01 ± 35 mm (n = 40). At the sites with diffuse spasm, some of the lesions lay scattered along the coronary vessels, although the lesions were localized at the sites of focal vasospasm. These results indicate that atherosclerosis is present at sites with both focal and diffuse vasospasm even in the absence of angiographically significant coronary artery disease. Thus, the differences in severity of underlying atherosclerosis, disease distribution, or both can be related to the pattern of vasospasm in clinical settings.

Maheswaran and colleagues[31] from Irvine, California, performed intravascular ultrasound imaging in vitro on 6 histologically normal and 104 minimally diseased arteries in patients aged 13 to 83 years. This study tested the hypothesis that normal coronary arteries produce a 3-layer image that corresponds to the histological layers of intima, media, and adventitia. The results showed a very good correlation between area of the echolucent ultrasound layer with the media and the inner echogenic layer with intimal area. In addition, a 3-layer appearance was consistently seen when the internal elastic membrane was present with or without intimal hyperplasia. If the internal elastic membrane was absent, a 3-layer appearance was still seen if the collagen content of the media was low. However, a 2-layer appearance was observed when there was absence of the internal elastic membrane as well as a high collagen content of the media.

Angiographic Predictors of New Narrowings

To determine whether coronary angiography is predictive of the future site of coronary occlusion, Pétursson and associates[32] from Reykjavík, Iceland, analyzed the coronary angiograms of 246 consecutive patients having 2 or more angiograms without therapeutic invasive intervention in the interval between angiograms. The average interval between studies was 46 months. Of 2183 normal segments at the first angiogram, 51 (2.3%) were occluded at the second angiogram, whereas in segments with minimal disease (1% to 25% diameter stenosis) 33 (8%) of 411 were occluded. There was a further stepwise increase in the occlusion ratio, with increasing stenosis reaching a 31% occlusion ratio in lesions with critical (91% to 99%) stenosis at the first angiogram. For any given degree of stenosis, the occlusion ratio of long lesions (5 to 20 mm) was on the average more than twice that of short lesions (<5 mm), except in lesions with critical stenosis (91% to 99%), where length was no longer important. Occlusion of segments judged free of disease on the first angiogram was 4.7% in the right coronary artery vs. 2.7% in the LAD and 0.6% in the left circumflex (LC). History of recent myocardial infarction was a good clinical predictor of occlusion and deterioration of ventricular function.

Angioscopy in "Normal" Coronary Arteries

Compared with pathological studies, coronary angiography is a relatively insensitive technique to detect early atherosclerosis. Coronary angioscopy is a new technique providing direct information on luminal vessel surface. To determine whether coronary angioscopy may detect the presence of atherosclerotic disease on angiographically normal coronary segments, 52 patients underwent coronary angioscopy before coronary angioplasty in this study by Alfonso and associates[33] from Madrid, Spain. The mean age was 59 ± 10 years; 46 patients were men and 6 were women. The cause of coronary angioplasty was unstable angina in 36 patients, stable angina in 8 patients, and silent ischemia in 8 patients. In 7 patients angiography revealed luminal irregularities on the coronary segment proximal to the culprit lesion, and all these patients also had proximal disease as demonstrated by coronary angioscopy. In the remaining

45 (87%) patients angiography revealed a smooth-vessel contour proximal to the target lesion. On quantitative angiography these "normal" coronary segments measured 2.8 ± 0.4 mm in luminal diameter. In 30 (67%) of these patients angioscopy revealed proximal disease on the vessel wall, but in 15 (33%) patients the luminal surface of these segments also appeared normal on angioscopy. Disease as detected by angioscopy in angiographically normal segments included yellow plaques in 19 patients, mural thrombus in 5, mixed plaques in 4, and small flaps in 2 patients. In 8 patients coronary angioscopy detected that atherosclerotic disease extended proximally from the target lesion, but in the remaining 22 patients the angioscopic findings appeared to be discrete and well separated from the angiographic lesion. All these plaques were relatively small and did not protrude into the coronary lumen. Thus, in patients with CAD (1) coronary angioscopy is sensitive enough to visualize atherosclerotic disease at sites angiographically normal; (2) these parietal plaques are heterogeneous, small, and do not disrupt luminal contour; and (3) coronary angioscopy confirms that atherosclerotic involvement of the arterial wall extends beyond the angiographic lesion site.

Left Main "Equivalent" Disease

Caracciolo and colleagues[34] in the Coronary Artery Surgery Study (CASS) evaluated 912 patients with left main equivalent disease, defined as combined stenoses of ≥70% in the proximal LAD before the first septal perforator and proximal LC coronary artery before the first obtuse marginal branch, initially treated with either surgical or nonsurgical therapy. The 15-year cumulative survival estimates were 44% for the 630 patients in the surgical group and 31% for the 283 patients in the medical group (Figure 2-4). Median survival in the surgical

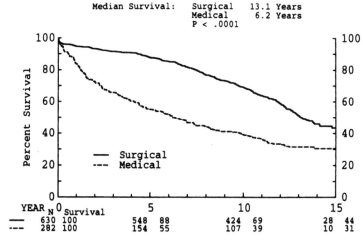

FIGURE 2-4. Graph showing 15-year cumulative survival estimates in 912 Coronary Artery Surgery Study Registry patients with left main equivalent disease, defined as combined stenoses of ≥70% in the proximal left anterior descending coronary artery before the first septal perforator and proximal circumflex coronary artery before the first obtuse marginal branch, who were initially treated with coronary artery bypass graft surgery (630 patients) and nonsurgical therapy (282 patients). The number of patients at risk for each follow-up interval is depicted next to the cumulative survival. Reproduced with permission of Caracciolo et al.[34]

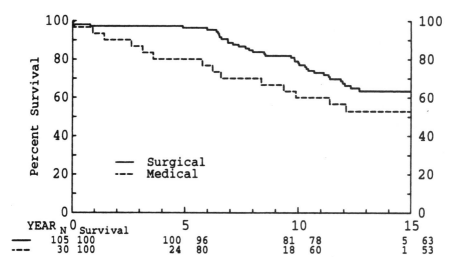

FIGURE 2-5. Graph showing 15-year cumulative survival estimates in patients with right coronary artery (RCA) stenosis ≥70% with normal left ventricular (LV) systolic function (LV score, 5). Cumulative survival was similar in the two treatment groups and better than the 41% and 28% survival rates for the surgical and medical groups, respectively, in the overall group with an RCA stenosis ≥70%. Reproduced with permission of Caracciolo.[34]

group was 13 years compared with only 6 years in the medical group. Median survival was also significantly longer in the surgical group stratified by age, sex, anginal class, LV function, and coronary anatomy. However, CABG did not prolong median survival in patient subgroups with (1) normal LV systolic function, even if a right coronary artery stenosis was present, and (2) mildly abnormal LV systolic function. The 15-year cumulative survival in patients with normal LV systolic function in the surgical and medical groups was 63% and 54%, respectively (Figure 2-5). Median survival was >15 years in both the surgical and medical groups. In patients with normal LV systolic function and right coronary stenosis, the 15-year cumulative survival was also similar in the surgical and medical groups. Median survival was >15 years in both the surgical and medical groups. The 15-year cumulative survival in all subgroups were affected by convergence of the surgical and medical groups survival. Twenty-six percent of patients in the medical group ultimately had CABG. If all medical group patients had survived long enough, approximately 65% would be estimated to have had CABG by 15 years. Thus, these data demonstrate CABG prolongs life in most clinical angiographic subgroups of patients with left main equivalent coronary lesions. However, median survival is not prolonged by CABG in patients with normal LV systolic function even if a significant right coronary artery stenosis was present or in patients with an LV ejection fraction ≥50%.

Prognosis

Exercise Testing

Many prior studies involving a predominantly male population have demonstrated the importance of exercise test results in determining the outcome of patients with CAD. The prognostic significance of exercise testing in women is unknown. In the Coronary Artery Surgery Study Registry, Weiner and colleagues[35] in Boston, Massachusetts, examined a total of 3086 men and 747 women who underwent maximal treadmill exercise testing, coronary angiography, and were prospectively followed for up to 16 years. The patients were divided into 3 groups (high, intermediate, and low risk) on the basis of exercise testing. Sixteen-year survival based on exercise test groups ranged from 38% to 61% in men and from 44% to 79% in women. Among men, 12-year survival was enhanced by CABG vs. medical therapy in the high-risk subgroup (69% vs. 55%, respectively), but the 2 therapies were similar in the intermediate- and low-risk subgroups. Among women, neither medical nor surgical therapy resulted in improved 12-year survival rates in any of the 3 subgroups. These results suggest that exercise testing is helpful in assessing long-term survival in men and women. However, only exercise testing in men could identify a high-risk subset whose survival was enhanced by CABG.

Heart Rate Response to Mental Stress

Krittayaphong and associates[36] in Chapel Hill, North Carolina, assessed the relation between hemodynamic data during a standardized mental stressor and ambulatory ischemia to determine if laboratory-induced responses could predict the magnitude of daily-life ischemia. Forty-two men and 11 women, aged 46 to 79 years, with CAD- and exercise-induced ischemia were studied. All patients underwent 24–48-hour ambulatory electrocardiographic monitoring and laboratory-induced mental stress using a public speaking task. Hemodynamic data were obtained at rest and every minute during mental stress. Thirty-three of 53 patients (62%) had at least 1 ischemic episode during electrocardiographic monitoring. In patients who had ambulatory ischemia, there was a mean number of 8 episodes. Significant positive correlations were found for peak heart rate and changes in heart rate during mental stress and ambulatory ischemia in patients who had ambulatory ischemia. There was no correlation between systolic BP during mental stress and ambulatory ischemia. Results of this study demonstrated that heart rate response during laboratory-induced mental stress correlates with magnitude of ischemia on ambulatory electrocardiographic monitoring in patients with CAD.

Coronary Patency

McCully and coworkers[37] in Memphis, Tennessee, examined the relative importance of patency of the LAD coronary artery on long-term survival when the LAD is the only significantly narrowed coronary artery. From a cardiac disease registry of 21 786 patients, 826 medically treated patients with isolated LAD disease were identified. These patients were followed for >5 years. Patients were divided into those with open vs. those with closed arteries. With the use of univariate and multivariate analysis, the relative importance of the patency of the LAD was determined. All patients with previous anterior wall AMI were analyzed as a separate group, and those with and without a patent LAD were compared. Overall, survival was significantly better in patients with an open LAD. However, multivariate analysis of either the entire study group or the group with AMI showed that coronary artery patency was not an independent predictor of long-term survival. Analysis of patients with prior anterior AMI showed significantly improved 5-year survival in younger patients (<70 years) who had an open (but stenosed) vs. a closed LAD without angiographic collateral formation. Furthermore, this survival difference was most striking in patients with LV dysfunction. Survival in younger patients with an open LAD was similar to that of patients with a closed LAD with collateral formation. No differences in survival were observed in the groups without infarction. This study implies that an open LAD improves long-term survival for younger patients with a previous anterior wall AMI and no collateral support to the ischemic or infarcted myocardium.

Unstable Angina Pectoris

Cardiologist vs. Internist Management

In the changing health care environment, there are sparse data on a comparison of the care of patients by generalists and specialists. Schreiber and colleagues[38] from Royal Oak, Michigan, reviewed a prospectively collected cohort of patients discharged with the diagnosis of unstable angina. Of 890 consecutive patients, 225 were treated by internists and 665 by cardiologists. They compared these 2 groups with respect to patterns of use of established pharmacotherapies for unstable angina, diagnostic testing, and clinical outcome. Internists were less likely to use aspirin (68% vs. 78%), heparin (67% vs. 84%), or β-adrenergic blocking agents (18% vs. 30%) in their initial management. Exercise tests were performed more frequently by internist-treated patients (37% vs. 22%), but catheterization (27% vs. 61%) and angioplasty (7% vs. 40%) were utilized less frequently. The incidence of AMI was similar (11% vs. 9%) in the two groups but the mortality rate tended to be higher (4% vs. 1.8%, $P = 0.06$) in the internists group. These authors concluded that patients with unstable angina treated by internists were less likely to receive effective medical therapy or revascularization procedures and experienced a trend to poorer outcome. This provocative study does not support a positive gatekeeper role for generalists in the treatment of unstable angina.

Risk Stratification

To validate the Braunwald classification of unstable angina pectoris as a predictor of in-hospital cardiac complications, to determine which factors of the Braunwald classification contributed significantly to this prediction, and to devise a method for combining these predictive factors into an overall odds ratio for complications, Calvin and associates[39] from Chicago, Illinois, studied 393 patients admitted consecutively to the coronary care and intermediate care units of their hospital with unstable angina. Multiple logistic regression analysis identified four clinical factors used in the Braunwald classification that predicted the in-hospital occurrence of major cardiac complications: (1) AMI within >14 days (OR, 5.72); (2) need for intravenous nitroglycerin (OR, 2.33); (3) lack of β-blocker or calcium antagonist therapy before admission (OR, 3.83); and (4) baseline ST depression (OR, 2.81). Two other clinical factors, diabetes mellitus and age, also were significant predictors. Thus, the classification of unstable angina proposed by Braunwald includes four factors that predict risk of major in-hospital cardiac complications. Specific factors used in the classification can be combined with diabetes and age to better stratify risk of major cardiac complications in this disorder using a simpler model.

Stratmann and coinvestigators[40] in St. Louis, Missouri, assessed the prognostic value of predischarge maximal exercise stress testing with technetium-99m sestamibi myocardial tomography in 126 consecutive men hospitalized with a diagnosis of unstable angina pectoris who were medically stabilized. None had coronary revascularization for ≤6 months after testing. Over a mean follow-up of 12 months, 35 patients (28%) had a cardiac event: nonfatal AMI (n = 6), cardiac death (n = 5), or rehospitalization for unstable angina (n = 24). Any type of cardiac event occurred in 12% of patients with normal sestamibi scans compared with 39% of those with an abnormal sestamibi scan and 60% of those with a reversible perfusion defect. Only 2% of patients with normal scans had either a nonfatal AMI or cardiac death compared with 14% of those with abnormal sestamibi scans and 25% with a reversible defect. A fixed perfusion defect was not associated with increased cardiac risk. With use of multivariate Cox proportional-hazards modeling, the only scintigraphic variable with independent predictive value was the presence of a reversible sestamibi defect, with an RR of 3.8 for any cardiac event and 19.2 for a nonfatal AMI or cardiac death. Cardiac event-free survival was also significantly decreased in patients with a reversible perfusion defect. Thus, exercise-stress sestamibi tomography provides long-term prognostic information in patients with unstable angina who can be medically stabilized before hospital discharge. A normal sestamibi scan is associated with a low risk of subsequent cardiac events, whereas a reversible perfusion defect is an independent predictor of increased cardiac risk despite continued medical therapy.

Angiographic Narrowing Compared with Other Coronary Subsets

Cianflone and coworkers[41] in Rome, Italy, compared coronary angiographic findings in patients who presented with AMI (n = 75), unstable angina pectoris (n = 36), or stable angina pectoris (n = 36) for ≥2 years without evidence of any previous acute event and with an angiogram within 2 years of the initial symptoms. Angiograms were evaluated blindly for severity, extent (depending on the percentage of each coronary segment showing atherosclerosis), and pattern (discrete: three or fewer loci of narrowings involving <50% of any segment; diffuse: anything exceeding this). Patients in the stable angina pectoris group had more narrowed arteries (2.4 vs. 1.3 and 1.4), more stenoses (6.0 vs. 2.1 and 2.6) and occlusions (1.3 vs. 0.7 and 0.3), and a greater extent index (0.9 vs. 0.5 and 0.5) than those in the AMI and unstable angina pectoris groups. Furthermore, a discrete pattern was less prevalent in patients with unstable angina than in those with stable angina or AMI. In conclusion, patients who present with acute coronary syndromes have less extensive atherosclerosis than those who present with chronic stable angina. Therefore, in the former group, coronary atherosclerosis appears to be more susceptible to ischemic stimuli responsible for acute coronary syndromes. Conversely, whether acute ischemic stimuli result in AMI or unstable angina does not appear to depend on the severity of coronary atherosclerosis.

TABLE 2-2. Clinical Features in 28 Patients Who Showed Disease Progression and 56 Patients Who Did Not Show Disease Progression

	All Patients (n = 85)*	Nonprogressors (n = 56)	Progressors (n = 26)	P
Age, y	56±10	57±10	55±10	NS
Sex				
Male	68 (80%)	44 (79%)	23 (82%)	NS
Risk factors				
Hypertension	22 (26%)	15 (27%)	7 (25%)	NS
Smoking	45 (53%)	29 (52%)	16 (57%)	NS
Diabetes	9 (11%)	5 (9%)	3 (11%)	NS
Family history	26 (31%)	15 (27%)	11 (39%)	NS
Cholesterol, mmol/L	6.3±1.4	6.2±1.3	6.5±1.4	NS
History of myocardial infarction	27 (32%)	17 (30%)	10 (36%)	NS
Coronary artery disease				
Single-vessel	52 (61%)	35 (63%)	17 (61%)	
Multivessel	33 (39%)	21 (37%)	11 (39%)	NS
Antianginal medication				
β-Blockers	64 (75%)	41 (73%)	22 (79%)	NS
Calcium antagonists	60 (71%)	39 (70%)	21 (75%)	NS
Long-acting nitrates	56 (66%)	37 (66%)	18 (64%)	NS
Aspirin	77 (92%)	51 (91%)	25 (89%)	NS

*Including 1 patient who died of acute myocardial infarction before repeat angiography.

Reproduced with permission of Chen et al.[42]

Angiographic Progression

Chen and colleagues[42] in London, UK studied 85 consecutive patients with unstable angina who stabilized on medical therapy but were found to require PTCA for treatment of CAD. Angiography was performed at admission and patients were reevaluated 8 months after the first angiogram. Ischemia-related stenoses were identified and classified as "complex," including having irregular borders and overhanging edges, or thrombus or "smooth" when there was an absence of the complex features. Stenosis progression ≥20% diameter reduction or new total occlusion was assessed. At initial angiography, there were 198 stenoses of which 85 were ischemia-related (54 complex and 31 smooth). At reevaluation, 21 ischemia-related stenoses and eight non–ischemia-related stenoses progressed (Table 2-2). Seventeen of the 21 ischemia-related stenoses that progressed developed into total occlusions compared with three of the eight non–ischemia-related stenoses. Changes in average stenosis severity and in absolute stenosis diameter were larger in ischemia-related stenoses than in non–ischemia-related stenoses. Eighteen complex stenoses progressed compared with three smooth lesions. During follow-up, 1 patient died and 25 patients had nonfatal coronary events associated with progression of ischemia-related stenoses in 14. Thus, in patients with unstable angina who stabilize medically, short-term stenosis progression and coronary events are common. The complex coronary stenoses in patients with unstable CAD are often not stabilized and continue to progress over the subsequent months.

Kaski and colleagues[43] in London, UK, studied the role of complex stenosis morphology and rapid disease progression in 94 consecutive patients awaiting

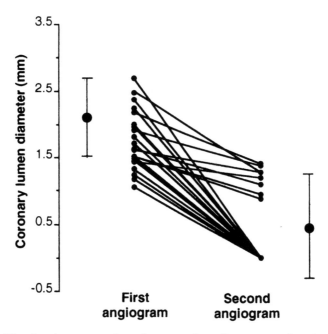

FIGURE 2-6. Plot showing progression of stenoses from first to second angiogram. Twenty-three coronary artery stenoses had progressed on restudy. Of these, 15 (65%) progressed to total occlusion. Reproduced with permission of Kaski et al.[43]

routine PTCA. Coronary arteriography was repeated at 8 months' follow-up, immediately preceding PTCA (68 patients), or after an acute coronary event (26%). Disease progression of 217 stenoses of which 79 (36%) were "complex" and 138 (64%) were "smooth" was assessed by computerized angiography. At presentation, 63 patients had stable angina and 31 had unstable angina that resolved with medical therapy. At follow-up, 23 patients (24%) had progression of preexisting stenoses and 71 (76%) had no progression (Figure 2-6). Patients with progression were younger (55 years) than those without (58 years), but they did not differ with regard to risk factors, previous AMI, or severity and extent of CAD. Twenty-three lesions (11%) progressed, 15 to total occlusion, including 11 complex and 4 smooth. Progression occurred in 17 of the 79 complex stenoses (22%) and in 6 of the 138 smooth lesions (4%). Mean stenosis diameter reduction was also significantly greater in complex than in smooth lesions. Acute coronary events occurred in 57% of patients with progression compared with 18% of those without progression and were more frequent in patients who presented with unstable angina. These data indicate that rapid stenosis progression is not uncommon among patients with unstable angina and complex stenoses are more at risk for rapid progression than smooth lesions.

Angiography in Octogenarians

To determine the risks and consequences of coronary angiography on octogenarians with symptomatic CAD, Ricou and associates[44] from Geneva, Switzerland, retrospectively evaluated 115 consecutive patients with angina pectoris aged 80 or above who underwent coronary angiography at their hospital from 1988–1992. In all, 115 patients (68 men) aged 82 ± 2 years, 70% with unstable angina, underwent coronary angiography, accounting for 1.4% of all the coronary angiography procedures performed during the 4-year period. Three-vessel or left main CAD, or both, was found in 42% of the patients, but this proportion decreased over the years. Revascularization by means of PTCA or CABG followed angiography in 54% of cases. Use of revascularization has markedly increased, from 33% in 1988 to 64% in 1992, and now tends to be performed more often by PTCA. Eight patients (7%) suffered minor periprocedural complications and eight (7%) died in the hospital, but none of the deaths was directly related to the diagnostic procedure itself. At follow-up (28±16 months), 68% and 44% of the survivors were free of angina after revascularization and medical treatment, respectively, and there was a nonsignificant trend for better survival after revascularization. Of the survivors, 80% were able to pursue an independent life. Coronary angiography may be done in symptomatic octogenarians with an acceptably low complication rate. After diagnostic evaluation, revascularization procedures are performed in an increasing proportion of patients, and despite a relatively high procedural complication rate, they result in definite symptomatic improvement.

Intracoronary Angioscopy and/or Ultrasonography

de Feyter and colleagues[45] in Rotterdam, the Netherlands, assessed the characteristics of the ischemia-related lesions with coronary angiography and intracoronary angioscopy and determined their compositions with intracoronary ultrasound in 44 patients with unstable and 23 patients with stable angina. The angiographic images were classified as noncomplex (smooth borders) or complex (regular borders, multiple lesions, or thrombus). Angioscopic images were classified as either stable (smooth surface) or thrombotic (red thrombus). Ultrasound characteristics of the lesion were classified as poorly echoreflective, highly echoreflective with shadowing, or highly echoreflective without shadowing. There was a poor correlation between clinical status and angiographic findings. The angiographic complex lesion (n = 33) was found in 55% of patients with unstable angina and a noncomplex lesion (n = 34) was found in 61% of patients with stable angina. There was a good correlation between clinical status and angioscopic findings. An angioscopic thrombotic lesion (n = 34) correlated with unstable angina in 68% of patients and a stable lesion was found in 83% of patients with stable angina (Table 2-3). The ultrasound-obtained information was similar in patients with stable and unstable angina. Thus, in this study, angioscopy demonstrated that plaque rupture and thrombosis were present in 17% of patients with stable angina and 68% of unstable angina patients. Currently available ultrasound technology does not discriminate stable from unstable plaques.

Silva and colleagues[46] in New Orleans, Louisiana, performed coronary angioscopy in 55 consecutive patients with unstable angina. They observed plaque color, texture, and the incidence of intracoronary thrombus associated with the culprit lesions in these patients. The population consisted of 17 diabetic and 38 nondiabetic patients. The presence of coronary risk factors was not significantly different between the 2 populations. Ulcerated plaque was found in 16 of 17 diabetic patients vs. 23 of 38 nondiabetic patients. Intracoronary thrombi were seen in 16 of 17 diabetic patients vs. 21 of 38 nondiabetic patients. Thus, the

TABLE 2-3. Angioscopic Characteristics of Ischemia-Related Lesions

	Unstable Angina (n = 44)	Stable Angina (n = 23)	P
Thrombus, n (%)	30 (68)	4 (17)	<0.001
Occlusive	2	0	
Protruding	8	1	
Mural	20	3	
Surface lesion, n			
Ulcerated	20	3	<0.05
Rough	11	6	
Smooth	13	14	
Yellow plaque, n (%)	29 (66)	16 (69)	

Reproduced with permission of de Feyter et al.[45]

results of the angioscopic examination demonstrate that diabetic patients with unstable angina have a higher incidence of plaque ulceration and intracoronary thrombosis than nondiabetic patients. The increased frequency of complex lesion morphology is consistent with a higher risk for development of coronary syndromes in these patients.

Acute Thrombotic Reactant Markers

Gurfinkel and colleagues[47] in Buenos Aires, Argentina, recorded ischemic electrocardiographic changes within 2 hours of admission using a 12-lead electrocardiographic continuous monitor with a 20-second scanning interval and an alarm mode for asymptomatic events. Blood samples were obtained at admission and at the moment of asymptomatic events (group A). In the other patients who did not develop ischemia, a second blood sample was taken 12 hours later (group B). The investigators determined prothrombin time, activated partial thromboplastin time, clotting factor VIII activity, t-PA activity, t-PA inhibitor-1, cross-linked fibrin degradation product, and thrombin-antithrombin III complexes. There was a statistically significant difference between group A and B patients when the basal samples were analyzed for thrombin-antithrombin III and D-dimer. Prothrombin fragment 1+2 were significantly reduced, and D-dimer was elevated when basal blood samples were compared with the second sample in patients who developed silent events. A plasma concentration of thrombin-antithrombin III complex was also significantly decreased when sample 2 was compared with the basal blood sample. In group A, 5 recurrent episodes of angina and 2 nonfatal infarctions occurred, and 4 urgent revascularization procedures were performed. In group B, there was only 1 nonfatal infarction. The results of this study suggest that a time-dependent thrombotic process is detectable in the blood stream as a cyclic movement. Further studies are needed to determine if some other factors, such as intensive shear stress in the vessel wall, may activate plaque instability during asymptomatic episodes.

Early Morning Ischemic Threshold

Ischemic threshold was assessed in patients with unstable angina by atrial pacing from 7:00 to 8:00 AM and 12:00 to 1:00 PM in 46 individuals.[48] In the 34 with a positive pacing response, including ST-segment shift >1.0 mm, the

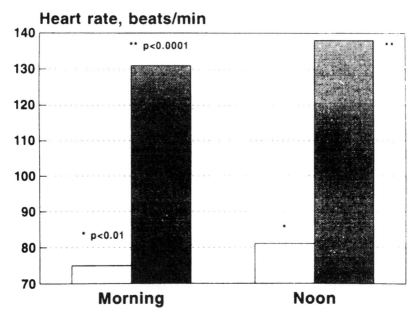

FIGURE 2-7. Bar graph shows heart rate at control prepacing and at ischemic threshold in the morning and at noon in patients with positive pacing. Both control (*$P < 0.01$) and ischemic threshold (**$P < 0.0001$) values were significantly lower in the morning than at noon. Reproduced with permission of Figueras and Lidón.[48]

ischemic threshold was lower from 7:00 to 8:00 AM than at 12:00 to 1:00 PM; in the remaining 12 patients, pacing response was negative (Figure 2-7). Four patients presented ST-segment elevation during pacing in the morning, but only one at noon and at a higher threshold. Baseline heart rate and diastolic BP were higher at noon than in the morning. The morning lowering of ischemic threshold in the absence of increases in baseline BP or heart rate suggest that a reduced coronary vasodilator capacity or an increased coronary tone may favor the increased incidence of ischemic events during this interval.

P-Selectin

Ikeda and colleagues[49] in Kurume, Japan, measured plasma P-selectin levels by a monoclonal antibody-based enzyme immunoassay on plasma samples taken from 12 patients with unstable angina, 11 patients with stable angina, and 15 healthy volunteers. Patients with unstable angina had angina at rest with electrocardiographic changes. In patients with unstable angina, plasma P-selectin levels within 1 hour and at 3 hours after angina were significantly higher than those in volunteers. Plasma P-selectin levels did not differ from those in volunteers. In patients with stable angina, the plasma P-selectin did not change before and 1 hour after exercise. These data suggest that plasma P-selectin levels after angina increase significantly in patients with unstable angina but do not change in patients with stable effort angina. These findings may contribute to better understanding of the pathophysiology of the acute coronary syndrome and suggest new therapeutic alternatives.

Diltiazem vs. Glyceryl Trinitrate

The effect of dihydropyridines in patients with unstable angina is discouraging. To discern the effect of the nondihydropyridine-like calcium antagonist diltiazem, Göbel and associates[50] from Groningen, the Netherlands, conducted a double-blind trial of diltiazem with glyceryl trinitrate both given intravenously in 129 patients with unstable angina pectoris. Refractory angina alone or together with AMI was significantly less frequent in the diltiazem group. While taking the trial drugs the number of patients with refractory angina were 6 (10%) in the diltiazem group vs. 17 (28%) in the glyceryl trinitrate group, and the numbers with refractory angina and AMI were 9 (15%) vs. 23 (38%). Over 48 hours 8 (13%) patients in the diltiazem group had refractory angina vs. 18 (30%) in the glyceryl trinitrate group and 12 (20%) in the diltiazem group had refractory angina and AMI vs. 25 (41%) in the glyceryl trinitrate group. Patients in the diltiazem group had better event-free survival while taking the drugs. Heart-rate pressure product was reduced significantly only by diltiazem (Figure 2-8). The incidence of bradyarrhythmias did not differ significantly. AV conduction disturbances occurred in 5 (8%) patients in the diltiazem group but were not seen in the glyceryl trinitrate group. These disturbances could be reversed by decreasing the dose of the drug or withdrawing it. No temporary pacemakers were required. Headache requiring an analgesic or dose adjustment occurred significantly less in the diltiazem group: 3 (5%) vs. 15 (25%). These results indicate that intravenous diltiazem, compared with intravenous glyceryl trinitrate, significantly reduces ischemic events and can be used safely in patients with unstable angina.

Subcutaneous Heparin vs. Intravenous Heparin vs. Aspirin

Intravenous heparin has been used in the control of myocardial ischemia in patients with unstable angina pectoris. Serneri and associates[51] of the SESAIR group assessed the efficacy of subcutaneous heparin in reducing myocardial ischemia in patients with unstable angina: 343 of 399 patients with unstable angina were monitored for 24 hours and 108 were refractory to conventional antianginal treatment and were entered into a randomized multicenter trial. Thirty-seven patients were assigned to heparin infusion (partial thromboplastin time 1.5–2 times baseline), 35 to subcutaneous heparin (adjusted dose with partial thromboplastin time 1.5–2 times baseline), and 36 to aspirin (325 mg/ d). All had additional conventional antianginal therapy. After the run-in patients were monitored for 3 days. The primary end point was reduced myocardial ischemia assessed by the number of anginal attacks, silent ischemic episodes, and duration of ischemia per day. At 1 week and 1 month we accounted for anginal attacks and other clinical events (myocardial infarction, revascularization procedures, and death). Aspirin did not significantly affect the incidence of myocardial ischemia. On the first 3 days, infused and subcutaneous heparin significantly decreased the frequency of angina (on average by 91% and 86%, respectively), episodes of silent ischemia (by 56% and 46%), and the overall duration of ischemia (66% and 61%) vs. run-in day and aspirin. The favorable effects of heparin therapy remained evident during follow-up. Only minor bleeding complications occurred. Subcutaneous heparin is effective in the control of myocardial ischemia in patients with unstable angina.

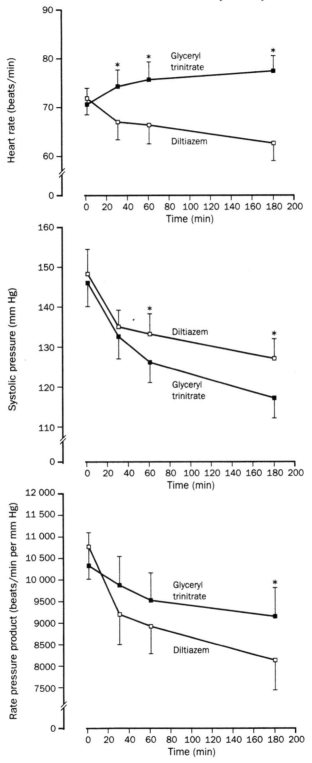

FIGURE 2-8. Changes in heart rate, systolic blood pressure, and rate-pressure product during first 180 min on study drug. Asterisks denote significant ($P < 0.05$) differences between diltiazem and glyceryl trinitrate groups. Values are means with bars indicating the standard deviation. HR indicates heart rate. Reproduced by permission of Göbel et al.[50]

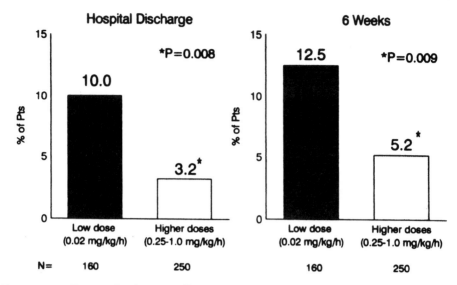

FIGURE 2-9. Bar graphs showing effect on mortality and nonfatal myocardial infarction at hospital discharge and 6 weeks. N indicates number of patients (Pts). Reproduced by permission of Fuchs et al.[52]

Hirulog Treatment

Fuchs and colleagues[52] in Boston, Massachusetts, and the TIMI Investigators evaluated the protective effects of direct thrombin inhibitors utilizing hirulog, a synthetic peptide based on the leech-derived compound, hirudin, which is a highly specific, direct inhibitor of free and clot-bound thrombin. These studies were done in the TIMI 7 trial, a randomized, double-blind study of hirulog given with 325 mg/d of aspirin to 410 patients with unstable angina. Patients received a constant infusion of hirulog for 72 hours at 1 of 4 doses: 0.02 (n = 160), 0.25 (n = 81), 0.5 (n = 88), and 1.0 (n = 81) mg/kg^{-1} per hour. The primary efficacy end point was "unsatisfactory outcome," defined as death, nonfatal AMI, rapid clinical deterioration, or recurrent ischemic pain at rest with electro-cardiographic changes by 72 hours. Unsatisfactory outcome was not different among the 4 dose groups. However, the secondary end points of death or nonfatal AMI through hospital discharge occurred in 10% of patients treated with 0.02 mg/kg^{-1} per hour compared with 3% of patients treated with the three higher doses of hirulog (Figure 2-9). Major hemorrhage attributable to hirulog occurred in only two of 410 patients (0.5%). Thus, the direct thrombin inhibitor hirulog appears to be a promising new antithrombotic agent that deserves further evaluation and the results of the TIMI 7 trial provide support for the use of a direct antithrombin with aspirin in the treatment of patients with unstable angina.

Stable Angina Pectoris

Patient Preferences in Treatment

Although practice guidelines sometimes make recommendations based on symptom severity, they rarely account for how patients feel about their symptoms. To investigate the possible importance of patient preferences in treatment of CAD, Nease and associates[53] for the Ischemic Heart Disease Patient Outcomes Research Team assessed attitudes toward symptoms in patients with angina pectoris. They studied a total of 220 subjects selected from 589 patients with chronic stable angina referred from cardiologists to achieve patient samples balanced for sex, race, and angina severity. Although the mean responses followed the expected patterns (those with more severe Canadian Cardiovascular Society scores chose lower utilities), attitudes toward symptoms varied substantially among patients with similarly severe angina. For example, there was a 33% chance that a patient with class II angina had a time trade-off utility that was lower (i.e., more bothered by symptoms) than a patient with more severe angina (class III/IV). This variation in utilities was not due to random error in the assessments. Angina patients with similar functional imitation vary considerably in their tolerance for their symptoms, as measured by utilities. These findings suggest that guidelines for the management of CAD should be based on the preferences of the individual patient rather than on symptom severity alone.

Risk of Infarction or Sudden Death

Increased levels of certain hemostatic factors may play a part in the development of acute coronary syndromes and may be associated with an increased risk of coronary events in patients with angina pectoris. Thompson and associates[54] for the European Concerted Action on Thrombosis and Disabilities Angina Pectoris Study Group conducted a prospective multicenter study of 3043 patients with angina pectoris who underwent angiography and were followed for 2 years. Baseline measurements included the concentrations of selected hemostatic factors indicative of a thrombophilic state or endothelial injury. The results were analyzed in relation to the subsequent incidence of AMI or sudden coronary death. After adjustment for the extent of CAD and other risk factors, an increased incidence of AMI or sudden death was associated with higher baseline concentrations of fibrinogen (mean ± SD, 3.28 ± 0.74 g/L in patients who subsequently had coronary events, as compared with 3.00 ± 0.71 g/L in those who did not), von Willebrand factor antigen (138 ± 49% vs. 125 ± 49%), and t-PA antigen (11.9 ± 4.7 ng/mL vs. 10.0 ± 4.2 ng/mL). The concentration of C-reactive protein was also directly correlated with the incidence of coronary events, except when the authors adjusted for the fibrinogen concentration (Figure 2-10). In patients with high serum cholesterol levels, the risk of coronary events rose with increasing levels of fibrinogen and C-reactive protein, but the risk remained low even given high serum cholesterol levels in the presence of low fibrinogen concentrations. In patients with angina pectoris, the levels of fibrinogen, von Willebrand factor antigen, and t-PA antigen are independent predictors of subsequent acute coronary syndromes. In addition, low fibrinogen concentrations characterize patients at low risk for coronary events despite increased serum cholesterol levels. The authors' data are consistent with a pathogenetic role of impaired fibrinolysis, endothelia-cell injury, and inflammatory activity in the progression of CAD.

Narrowing Progression

Progression of coronary stenosis has prognostic significance and may be influenced by stenosis morphology. Chester and associates[55] from London, UK,

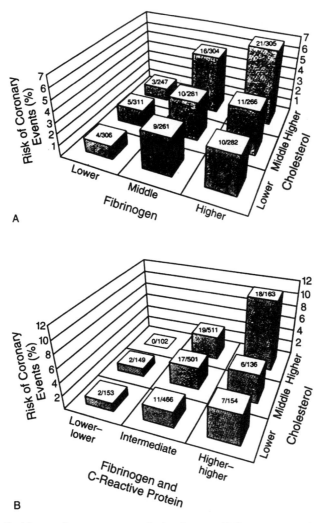

FIGURE 2-10. Incidence of coronary events during 2 years of follow-up, according to concentrations of fibrinogen, C-reactive protein, and total cholesterol. Panel A: the risk of coronary events according to fibrinogen and total cholesterol concentrations. Panel B: the risk according to fibrinogen and C-reactive protein concentrations combined, as compared with total cholesterol concentrations. The concentrations of these variables are divided into 3 categories (lower, middle, and higher), each containing a third of the sample, according to their respective distributions. Panel B: "intermediate" refers to all combinations of fibrinogen and C-reactive protein concentrations other than lower-lower or higher-higher. The values used to divide the sample into thirds were 2.71 and 3.31 g/L for fibrinogen, 5.79 and 6.80 mmol per liter (224 and 263 mg per deciliter) for cholesterol, and 0.88 and 2.17 mg/L for C-reactive protein. The number of coronary events and the number of patients at risk are shown for each group. Only patients for whom data on both fibrinogen and total cholesterol concentrations were available are included in the analysis. Reproduced by permission of Thompson et al.[54]

studied 50 men with stable angina who (1) had 1 complex coronary stenosis and 1 smooth stenosis in different noninfarct-related coronary vessels at initial coronary angiography, and (2) had a second angiogram after a median interval of 9 months. All patients remained in stable condition during follow-up. Progression, defined as an increase in diameter stenosis by >15%, was seen in only 8 complex stenoses (16%) but in no smooth lesions. On average, the annual rate of growth was 11% and 1.5% for complex and smooth lesions, respectively. These authors concluded that few coronary stenoses progressed rapidly in stable angina. Complex stenosis morphology, however, is an important determinant of more rapid progression of stenosis in patients with apparently clinically stable CAD.

Percutaneous Coronary Angioscopy

To pinpoint the link between plaque characteristics and acute coronary syndromes, Uchida and associates[56] from Tokyo and Funsbashi, Japan, performed a 12-month prospective follow-up study in 157 patients with stable angina pectoris in whom coronary plaques were observed by percutaneous coronary angioscopy. Acute coronary syndromes (unstable angina or AMI) occurred more frequently in patients with yellow plaques than in those with white plaques (11 of 39 vs. 4 of 118). Moreover, the syndromes occurred more frequently in patients with glistening yellow plaques than in those with nonglistening yellow plaques (9 of 13 vs. 2 of 26). Thrombus arising from ruptured plaques was confirmed by angioscopy as the culprit lesion of the syndromes. The results indicate that acute coronary syndromes occur frequently and in a short time in patients with glistening yellow plaques and that angioscopy but not angiography is feasible for prediction of the syndromes.

Circadian Variation in Coronary Tone

El-Tamimi and colleagues[57] in Gainesville, Florida, evaluated the role of the coronary endothelium in modulating the effects of circadian variations in coronary tone in 72 nonstenotic coronary segments in 12 patients with chronic stable angina. Responses of these nonstenotic coronary segments to acetylcholine and nitroglycerin were evaluated at 6:00 AM and 1:00 PM. Following baseline angiography, 3 infusions of acetylcholine (10^{-6}, 10^{-5}, and 10^{-4}mol/L) were administered selectively into the left coronary artery followed by nitroglycerin. Diameters in millimeters of proximal, middle, and distal segments were measured by quantitative techniques. Forty-seven segments showed a constrictor response to acetylcholine (group 1, dysfunctional endothelium) and 25 other segments showed a dilator response (group 2, normally functioning endothelium). In group 1, the constrictor response to acetylcholine was greater in the morning than in the afternoon and the dilator response to nitroglycerin was also significantly greater in the morning than in the afternoon (Figure 2-11). In group 2 patients, the dilator response to acetylcholine did not differ significantly between the morning and afternoon and the dilator response to nitroglycerin was also similar at both times of the day. These data indicate that coronary segments with dysfunctional endothelium exhibit an early morning exaggeration in vasomotor activity, whereas segments with normally functioning endothelium do not show circadian variations. These observations suggest a potential protective role for the endothelium in modulating variations in coronary tone that may contribute to the increased incidence of cardiovascular events in the early morning hours.

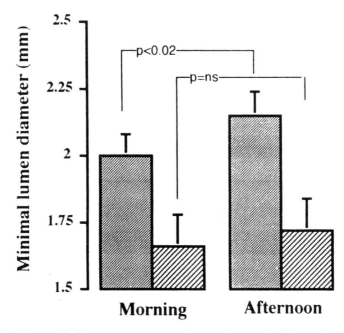

FIGURE 2-11. Bar graph shows mean coronary lumen diameter (millimeters) at two times of day in groups 1 and 2 segments. There is a significant increase in segment diameter in group 1 (shaded boxes) in the afternoon compared with the morning that is not seen in group 2 segments (striped boxes). Reproduced by permission of El-Tamimi et al.[57]

Intensive Exercise and Low-Fat Diet

Niebauer and associates[58] in Heidelberg, Germany, performed a randomized study to assess the effects of more than 3 hours of physical exercise per week and a low-fat diet on collateral formation in nonselected patients with CAD. Results were compared with those of patients in a control group (n = 57) who received usual care by their private physicians. Coronary lesions were assessed by quantitative coronary angiography at the beginning and 1 year of study (n = 92). As previously reported after 1 year, there was a significant retardation of progression of CAD in the intervention group compared with the control group. In this study, evaluation of collateral formation revealed no significant difference between both groups and changes in hemodynamic and metabolic variables or leisure time physical activity were not related to changes in collateral formation. Although progression of the disease was significantly related to an increase in collateral formation, regression was significantly related to a decrease in collateral formation. Because patients in the intervention group exercised more than 3 hours per week, and patients with regression of CAD even dedicated 5 to 6 hours to leisure time physical activity per week, these findings question whether an exercise program within the safety tolerance of patients will be able to induce coronary collateralization.

Silent Myocardial Ischemia

With Mental Stress

To evaluate the relation of mental stress-induced ischemia to silent ischemia on ambulatory monitoring, 46 patients with stable CAD underwent standardized laboratory mental stress and exercise treadmill testing by Legault and colleagues[59] in Toronto, Canada, according to National Institutes of Health protocol during which LVEF was determined using the nuclear VEST. Life stress, type A behavior, and hostility were determined using standard interviews. Subsequently, 48-hour ambulatory electrocardiographic monitoring was performed. Twenty-three patients (50%) had an ischemic response (LVEF decrease ≥5%) to mental stress, which was associated with ambulatory ischemia (13 of 19 with ambulatory ischemia had mental stress-induced ischemia vs. 10 of 27 without ambulatory ischemia). LVEF response to mental stress was a significant predictor of ambulatory ischemia independent of EF response to exercise. Patients with mental stress-induced ischemia had longer total duration (31 vs. 8 minutes) and more frequent episodes of ambulatory ischemia (3 vs. 1 episodes). Life stress, type A behavior, and hostility were not associated with prevalence or severity of ambulatory ischemia. In conclusion, an ischemic response to mental stress is significantly associated with higher prevalence, longer duration, and more frequent episodes of ambulatory ischemia.

Thirty patients with stable angina pectoris and ischemia on stress perfusion imaging underwent continuous ambulatory LV function monitoring by Jain and colleagues[60] in New Haven, Connecticut. Mental stress was induced by mental arithmetic. Fifteen patients developed transient LV dysfunction during mental arithmetic. Patients were followed for 2 years for adverse cardiac events. Twelve patients had cardiac events over 1 year (AMI in 4, and unstable angina in 8). Nine of 15 patients with and only 3 of 15 without mental stress-induced LV dysfunction developed cardiac events. A higher proportion of patients with cardiac events were taking β-blockers and had lower resting heart rates than those without cardiac events. There was no difference in the baseline characteristics between the groups with and without cardiac events. At 2-year follow-up, 10 of 15 patients with mental stress-induced LV dysfunction had adverse events compared with only 4 of 15 with no mental stress-induced LV dysfunction. Thus, in this cohort of patients with stable angina pectoris, mental stress-induced LV dysfunction was associated with higher cardiac events on follow-up. The exact mechanism of this association is not clear. Mental stress may be a trigger for adverse cardiac events in these patients. Transient LV dysfunction in response to mental stress may be a marker of abnormal cardiovascular reactivity to emotional and psychological stimuli in patients with CAD and may be useful for risk stratification.

With Exercise Testing

Matsubara and associates[61] from Nagoya and Obu, Japan, compared cardiohemodynamic response to dynamic exercise in 32 patients with exercise-induced silent or symptomatic myocardial ischemia. All patients had CAD without prior myocardial infarction and LV hypertrophy. Patients underwent supine leg-exercise testing and received right-heart catheterization. All patients exhibited ischemic ST-segment depression on electrocardiogram during exercise testing. They were classified retrospectively into two groups according to the absence (n = 10, group 1) or presence (n = 22, group 2) of chest pain induced by exercise. There was no significant difference between groups in the magnitude of peak ST-segment depression. PA wedge pressure at peak exercise was significantly lower and the cardiac index was significantly higher in group 1 vs. group 2. These results indicate that the exercise-induced LV dysfunction is less severe in patients with silent myocardial ischemia than in those with symptomatic ischemia.

To evaluate the significance of silent myocardial ischemia during exercise testing in women compared with men, Weiner and associates[62] from Boston, Massachusetts; Seattle, Washington, St. Louis, Missouri: Birmingham, Alabama; and Milwaukee, Wisconsin, analyzed the data on 1087 women and 3834 men who underwent exercise testing and coronary angiography from the CASS registry. The patients were divided into 3 groups on the basis of the results of exercise testing: group 1, silent ischemia (253 women and 853 men); group 2, symptomatic ischemia (156 women and 1250 men); and group 3, no ischemia (678 women and 1731 men). The survival rate at 12 years for women was 80% for group 1, 75% for group 2, and 86% for group 3; the survival rate for men was 69% for group 1, 69% for group 2, and 76% for group 3. In both men and women with silent ischemia, the 12-year survival rate was related to the severity of CAD and ranged from 79% for women with 1-vessel CAD to 46% for men with 3-vessel CAD. Survival at 12 years was enhanced by CABG compared with medical treatment in patients with silent ischemia and 3-vessel CAD for men but not for women. These data suggest that silent ischemia in women and men adversely affects survival rate and that men may gain more benefit from CABG than women when 3-vessel CAD is present.

Magnitude of Myocardial Dysfunction

The functional significance of painless vs. painful demand-driven ischemia remains controversial. Nihoyannopoulos and colleagues[63] from London, UK, evaluated the presence and extent of inducible myocardial dysfunction during painful and painless ischemia in a homogeneous patient cohort with CAD and no previous AMI. Exercise echocardiography was performed in 89 patients with significant CAD and positive stress test results. Fifty-eight patients had painful and 31 painless myocardial ischemia. Patients with painless ischemia achieved better exercise performance with greater exercise duration, and higher maximal rate pressure product, than those with painful ischemia. New wall motion abnormalities were seen 93% with painful vs. 55% with painless ischemia. These authors concluded that patients with painless ischemia frequently have regional myocardial dysfunction on exertion detected by echocardiography, but painful episodes are accompanied by a greater magnitude of myocardial dysfunction.

Outcome

The ACIP study assessed the ability of 3 treatment strategies to suppress ambulatory electrocardiographic ischemia to determine whether a large-scale trial studying the impact of these strategies on clinical outcomes was feasible.[64] This report discusses the outcome at 1 year of patients in the ACIP trial: 558 patients with coronary anatomy amenable to revascularization, at least one episode of asymptomatic ischemia on the 48-hour ambulatory electrocardiograph, and ischemia on treadmill exercise testing were randomly assigned to 1 of 3 treatment strategies: (1) medication to suppress angina (n = 183); (2) medication to suppress both angina and ambulatory ischemia (n = 183); or

% with Death, MI, Non-protocol PTCA/CABG or Hospitalization

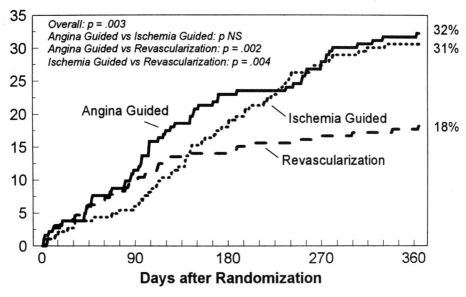

Days after Randomization

FIGURE 2-12. Reproduced by permission of Rogers et al.[64]

(3) revascularization strategy with angioplasty or bypass surgery (n = 192). Medication was titrated atenolol-nifedipine or diltiazem-isosorbide dinitrate. Frequency of AMI, unstable angina, stroke, and CHF was not significantly different among the 3 strategies. The revascularization group had significantly fewer hospital admissions and nonprotocol revascularization at 1 year (Figure 2-12). At 1 year, the mortality rate was 4.4% in the angina-guided group, 1.6% in the ischemia-guided group, and 0% in the revascularization group. These authors concluded that after 1 year, revascularization was superior to both angina-guided and ischemia-guided medical strategies in suppressing symptomatic ischemia and was associated with better outcome. These findings require confirmation by a larger trial.

Variant, Spastic, or Microvascular Angina

Kaski and associates[65] from London, UK evaluated the course of 99 patients with syndrome X over an average period of 7 years. The syndrome was more common in women (78 women and 21 men) and 62% of the women were postmenopausal before the onset of chest pain. The average duration of episodes of chest pain was >10 min in 53% of patients. Sublingual nitrate was effective for relief of pain in 42% of patients. During follow-up, no deaths or myocardial infarctions occurred and LV function was unchanged. Heart failure developed in one patient; systemic hypertension occurred in 8 patients, and conduction disturbances in 4. Symptoms lessened in 11 patients, were variable or unchanged in 64, and worsened in 24. These authors concluded that syndrome X occurs predominantly in postmenopausal women. Conventional and antianginal treatment was often not successful. Myocardial perfusion abnormalities occurred in only a small proportion of patients. Long-term survival was not adversely affected and deterioration of cardiac function rarely occurred.

Patients with typical angina pectoris but normal coronary angiographic findings are not uncommon. The long-term prognosis of such patients, however, has been uncertain. Lichtlen and colleagues[66] from Hannover, Germany, followed 176 patients (mean age, 48.3 years) who had angina-like chest pain but normal coronary angiography and LV angiograms for an average of 9.3 years. Exercise tests were positive in 31. Eight percent (14 patients) had a coronary event (0.65%/yr). Two of the 14 died of a coronary event (0.09%/yr). Four patients had a nonfatal myocardial infarction at an average of 8.1 years and 8 had severe angina pectoris after an average of 10.3 years, confirmed by a second angiogram with positive findings. Chest pain persisted in 81% of the survivors and disappeared in 19%. These authors concluded that patients with typical angina or angina-like chest pain and normal coronary angiograms have a good long-term prognosis despite persistence of pain for many years. Coronary morbidity and mortality are similar to those of the overall population and seem to be due to the development of coronary artery disease, mainly in patients with elevated risk factors.

Kaikita and colleagues[67] in Kumamoto City, Japan, examined plasma soluble P-selectin levels in the coronary sinus and aortic root simultaneously in 16 patients with coronary spasm before and after left coronary artery spasm was induced by intracoronary injection of acetylcholine and in 15 patients with stable exertional angina before and after AMI induced by rapid atrial pacing. Ten control patients with chest pain but normal coronary arteries and no coronary spasm received intracoronary acetylcholine. Plasma soluble P-selectin levels were increased significantly in the coronary sinus and in the aortic root after the attacks in the coronary spasm group, but remained unchanged in the stable exertional anginal group after the attack and in the control group after the administration of acetylcholine. Furthermore, the coronary sinus-arterial difference of soluble P-selectin increased significantly after the attacks of coronary artery spasm. These data indicate that soluble P-selectin is released into the coronary circulation after coronary artery spasm. The authors conclude that coronary artery spasm may induce leukocyte adhesion in the coronary circulation and lead to myocardial damage.

Shinozaki and colleagues[68] investigated the association of hyperinsulinemia and insulin resistance with vasospastic angina. The study population consisted of 60 patients with vasospastic angina and 42 control subjects, including 62 with normal glucose tolerance and 40 with impaired glucose tolerance. Insulin sensitivity was determined by the steady-state plasma glucose method for nondiabetic, normotensive, nonobese subjects. Compared with the control groups, the 2-hour insulin area under the plasma insulin concentration-time curve during a 75-g oral glucose tolerance test was significantly higher in both vasospastic angina groups with normal and impaired glucose tolerance. Vasospastic angina was found in subjects with clustered risk factors for insulin resistance, suggesting a close association of vasospastic angina with this syndrome. In stepwise discriminant analysis, the 2-hour insulin area was significantly associated with vasospastic angina independent of other risk factors. Steady-state plasma glucose levels were significantly elevated in patients with vasospastic angina and obstructive CAD compared with normal individuals. These data indicate that hyperinsulinemia is associated with insulin resistance and both may play a role as risk factors for vasospastic angina in the early atheromatous lesion.

Ozaki and colleagues[69] in Rotterdam, the Netherlands, measured changes in coronary luminal diameter in 30 patients with vasospastic angina at intervals 45 months apart. Quantitative coronary arteriography was used in conjunction with ergonovine provocation. All patients had vasospastic anginal symptoms and coronary spasm on the initial provocative test. Among 30 patients, 16 had persistent symptoms of angina and showed coronary spasm at the same site on the follow-up angiogram (group 1), whereas the remaining 14 patients whose vasospastic anginal symptoms disappeared at follow-up demonstrated a negative response to ergonovine on the follow-up tests (group 2). There were no significant differences in patients' baseline characteristics between the 2 groups. Long-term changes in minimal luminal diameter and mean luminal diameter were measured in millimeters after administration of isosorbide dinitrate in 19 vasospasm and 93 nonvasospasm segments in group 1 and in 17 segments with previous vasospasm and 81 segments without vasospasm in group 2. Both minimal luminal diameter and mean luminal diameter were measured in 210 coronary segments of the 30 patients at baseline and after administration of ergonovine and isosorbide dinitrate using a computer-based quantitative coronary arteriographic system. Stenosis progression and regression of individual lesions were defined as a change in minimal luminal diameter of ≥0.4 mm. In group 1, both the minimal luminal diameter and mean luminal diameter of 19 vasospastic segments were smaller at follow-up compared with the initial angiogram, whereas the mean luminal diameters of 93 segments without vasospasm in group 1 were not significantly different between the initial and follow-up angiograms. In group 2, the minimal luminal diameter of the 17 previously vasospastic segments improved at follow-up, and the mean and minimal luminal diameters of the 81 segments without vasospasm were not significantly different between the two studies. In group 1, significant stenosis progression of individual lesions was observed more frequently at sites of vasospasm than at those without, whereas stenosis regression was observed in no segments with vasospasm and in only three segments without vasospasm. In group 2, stenosis progression was observed at one segment with previous vasospasm and four segments without previous vasospasm. Thus, these results demonstrate an association between persistent segmental vasospasm and progression of atherosclerosis and an association between cessation of vasospastic activity and regression of atherosclerosis.

In patients with variant angina, changing electrocardiographic locations have suggested that the location of vasospastic activity may change over time. Ozaki and colleagues[70] from Rotterdam, the Netherlands, evaluated this question in 29 patients with vasospastic angina by doing coronary angiography and ergonovine provocation tests at an interval of 43 months apart. In 13 patients coronary spasm was observed in the same 16 coronary segments at both the initial and follow-up tests. In 16 patients angiographic changes occurred between the initial and follow-up tests in 48 major vessels. Some segments that developed spasm initially did not have spasm at follow-up, whereas others that did not demonstrate spasm initially did demonstrate follow-up spasm. Thus, in 46% of 48 vessels fluctuation of spastic location was observed at the follow-up. These authors concluded that quantitative coronary angiography

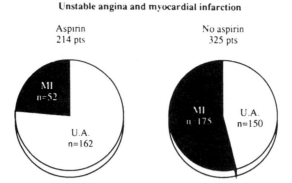

FIGURE 2-13. Diagrams showing (top) proportions of patients with a diagnosis of unstable angina vs. myocardial infarction by the previous use or nonuse of aspirin. The odds ratio for developing myocardial infarction was reduced by 72% (95% Cl, 59% to 90%) with aspirin. Bottom, proportions of patients with a diagnosis of non–Q-wave vs. Q-wave myocardial infarction by the previous use or nonuse of aspirin. The odds ratio for developing Q-wave infarction with aspirin was reduced by 49% (95% Cl, 25% to 103%). Reproduced by permission of Garcia Dorado.[71]

and repeat ergonovine tests reveal that some patients with persistent vasospastic angina demonstrate fluctuation of vasospastic location whereas others exhibit a fixed location of vasospasm.

Diet and Drugs for Myocardial Ischemia

Aspirin

Garcia-Dorado and colleagues[71] investigated whether the prior use of aspirin could influence the severity of the manifestation of acute CAD syndromes, given the well-documented observation that aspirin may prevent AMI, stroke, and death. A series of 539 consecutive patients admitted to the coronary care unit of the General Hospital was carefully characterized in a study with an ambidirectional design with regard to previous medical history, aspirin use, and subsequent hospital diagnosis. Among 214 patients previously taking aspirin, the hospital diagnosis was AMI in 24% and unstable angina in 76% compared with 54% and 46%, respectively, among the 325 not taking aspirin, for a reduction of 72% in the OR of AMI with aspirin. (Figure 2-13). The decrease

TABLE 2-4. Pharmacokinetics and Recommended Doses of Available Nitrates*

Nitrate	Usual Dose, mg	Onset of Action, min	Effective Duration of Action
Sublingual			
NTG	0.3–0.8	2–5	20–30 min
ISDN	2.5–10.0	5–20	45–120 min
Buccal NTG	1–3 prn or TID	2–5	30–300 min†
Oral			
ISDN	10–60 BID or TID	15–45	2–6 h
ISDN-SR	80–120 QD	60–90	10–14 h
ISMN	20 BID‡	30–60	3–6 h
ISMN-SR	60–120 QD	60–90	10–14 h
NTG-SR	6.5–19.5	20–45	2–6 h
NTG			
Ointment (2%)	0.5–2.0 inches TID	15–60	3–8 h
Patch	0.4–0.8 mg/h§	30–60	8–12 h

*ISDN indicates isosorbide dinitrate; ISMN, isosorbide mononitrate; NTG, nitroglycerin; SR, sustained release; prn, as needed; TID, three times daily; BID, twice daily; and QD, daily.

†Effect persists only when tablet is intact.

‡Two daily doses 7 hours apart, e.g., 8:00 AM and 2:00PM.

§Patch should be removed daily for 10 to 12 hours.

Reproduced by permission of Abrams.[72]

in odds was homogeneous in all subsets studied and independent of age, sex, previous angina, or previous AMI. The AMIs were of a Q-wave type in 62% of aspirin users compared with 76% of nonusers. By multivariate analysis, previous aspirin use was a strong predictor of unstable angina versus AMI and the only independent predictor of non–Q-wave vs. Q-wave AMI. This study suggests a shift to less severe manifestations of acute coronary syndromes with aspirin use, implying that the failure of the drug in many patients with an acute coronary syndrome is only partial and that aspirin has the potential of attenuating the severity of acute thrombotic disease processes.

Nitrates

Abrams[72] from Albuquerque, New Mexico, provided a fine review on the role of nitrates in patients with symptomatic myocardial ischemia. Pharmacokinetics and recommended doses of the available nitrates are shown in Table 2-4.

Parker and colleagues[73] in Kingston, Canada, examined the effect of nitroglycerin patch removal on anginal threshold in 12 patients with stable angina enrolled in a randomized, double-blind, placebo-controlled crossover study. These patients had reproducible treadmill walking times and were taking no other long-acting antianginal medications. They received 0.8 mg/hr transdermal nitroglycerin or wore a matching placebo patch for 5 to 7 days and then crossed over to the other treatment arm of the study. Transdermal nitroglycerin was applied at 8:00 PM and removed at 8:00 AM each day. On the last day of each treatment period, patients underwent treadmill exercise testing at 8:00 AM before patch removal and at 2, 4, and 6 hours after patch removal. The primary end point was the treadmill walking time until moderate angina. Other end points included the treadmill walking time until onset of angina, the amount of ST segment depression, and treadmill walking time until the development of 1-mm ST-depression. Heart rate, systolic BP, and the rate-pressure product were determined at rest before exercise and with the development of angina. Removal of the active transdermal nitroglycerin patch was associated with significant decrease in the time to onset of angina at 2, 4, and 6 hours after patch removal compared with placebo. There was also a decrease in the time to development of moderate angina after active patch removal that was significant when compared with placebo at 2 and 4. There were no differences in heart rate, BP, or amount of ST depression after active compared with placebo patch removal. Therefore, in patients with stable angina, intermittent transdermal nitroglycerin therapy is associated with a decrease in angina threshold for 4 to 6 hours after patch removal.

Nitroglycerin patches require a nitrate-free interval in order to minimize the tolerance or attenuation of the therapeutic effect. Freedman and associates[74] from Sydney, Australia, evaluated whether rebound ischemia occurred during nitrate-free periods in patients with angina who were receiving background antianginal therapy. Fifty-two patients with stable effort angina taking either a β-adrenergic blocking agent (n = 25) or diltiazem (n = 22) or their combination (n = 5) completed a randomized, double-blind, placebo-controlled crossover study of cutaneous nitroglycerin patches (50 mg). Active or placebo patches were worn for 1 week, applied at 8:00 AM and removed at 10:00 PM, to provide a 10-hour daily nitrate-free (or placebo-free) period. During the last 48 hours of each study phase, a Holter monitor was used to detect ischemia. Only 31 patients experienced ischemia during either phase of the study. A total of 463 ischemic episodes were recorded; 246 during placebo and 217 during nitroglycerin. The majority (88%) of ischemic episodes were silent. There was an increase in duration of ischemia with active therapy during the patch-off period (47 min vs. 22.5 min for placebo). There was also a decrease in the patch-on period (27.5 min for active therapy vs. 34.5 min/24 hours for placebo). There was also a change in the pattern of diurnal distribution of ischemic episodes. During placebo there was a nadir in the incidence of ischemia in the overnight patch-off period between midnight and 6:00 AM. During the nitroglycerin patch-off period there was a loss of this overnight nadir with the same incidence of ischemia between midnight and 6:00 AM as the other 6-hour periods. These authors concluded that the majority of patients taking background antianginal therapy experienced no ischemia during the nitroglycerin patch-off period. In the 44% of patients with ischemia during the patch-off period there was an increase in the duration of ischemia with active therapy and a change in the distribution of diurnal ischemia. This provides suggestive evidence that rebound ischemia may be a problem with regard to intermittent cutaneous nitroglycerin.

Parker and colleagues[75] in Kingston, Canada, assessed the antianginal and anti-ischemic effects of 3 dose levels of transdermal nitroglycerin patches applied for 12 hours daily for 30 days. The study also assessed the development of tolerance and rebound. Intermittent transdermal nitroglycerin therapy with a patch-free period of 10 to 12 hours each day has documented clinical benefits during the period of patch application, but studies have failed to document clearly prolonged exercise duration for the entire period of patch application. In this study, a multicenter, randomized, double-blind, placebo-controlled parallel design with treadmill exercise tests at days 0, 1, 7, 15, and 30 days were carried out up to 12 hours after patch application. There was a significant treatment effect with increases in treadmill walking time to moderate angina in each nitroglycerin patch group compared with placebo at various time points up to 12 hours throughout the 30-day study period. There was an increased treatment effect as evidenced by increases in treadmill walking time to moderate angina in each nitroglycerin patch group throughout the 30-day study period. There were also consistent increases in times to 1-mm ST-segment depression. There was no evidence of tolerance or rebound. Thus, intermittent transdermal nitroglycerin therapy increases exercise duration and maintains anti-ischemic effects for 12 hours after patch application throughout 30 days of therapy without evidence of tolerance or rebound.

Fallen and colleagues[76] in Hamilton, Canada, used positron-emission tomography to examine the effect of transdermal nitroglycerin on global and regional myocardial perfusion in patients with angiographically proven CAD. Myocardial perfusion with [13N]ammonia was estimated from dynamic time-activity curves at baseline and 3 hours after application of either a 0.4 mg/hr nitroglycerin skin patch (n = 10) or a placebo patch (n = 10) in a double-blind parallel design. From resliced cross-sectional images, regional flow, expressed as [13N]ammonia retention was estimated from 216 myocardial sectors. Ischemia was defined as a significant reduction >2 standard deviations in [13N]ammonia retention within 10 contiguous myocardial sectors coupled with an increase or no change in counts derived from [18F]fluorodeoxyglucose. There was no change in global myocardial blood flow as expressed by [13N]ammonia retention following either placebo or nitroglycerin. However, there was a significant increase in the proportion of blood flow to the ischemic zones with nitroglycerin. No change in the distribution of blood flow to either ischemic or nonischemic zones was observed with placebo. Thus, these data suggest that under resting conditions, topical nitroglycerin decreases myocardial perfusion by preferentially increasing flow to areas of reduced perfusion with little or no change in global myocardial perfusion.

The relief of anginal pain with nitroglycerin may not correspond to the disappearance of ischemia. To evaluate the possible lack of the elimination of ischemia with sublingual nitroglycerin, Khosla and colleagues[77] in North Chicago, Illinois, studied 25 male patients with stable angina pectoris who underwent exercise stress testing with recording of BP, pulse, and ST-segment displacement. The stress test was repeated 30 minutes after administration of 0.4 mg of sublingual nitroglycerin. All 25 patients had angina and ischemic ST-segment changes in the first stress test. On repeat stress testing, 15 patients had angina and ST-segment changes, two patients had angina but no ST-segment changes, and four patients had no ST-segment changes and no angina. Four patients, however, had no angina but persistent ischemic ST-segment changes suggesting that angina was converted into silent ischemia. The mean exercise duration was 311 seconds before and 421 seconds after the nitroglycerin test. Peak heart rate and systolic BP before the nitroglycerin stress test were 109 and 155 mm Hg; in the repeat stress test, they increased to 123 and 162 mm Hg, respectively.

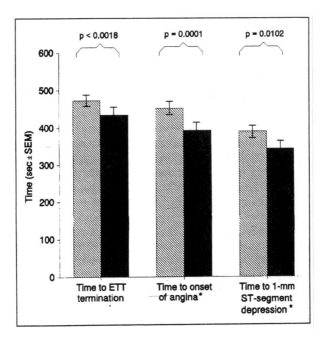

Figure 2-14. Comparison of end of 3-month open-label treatment *(slashed bars)* to end of the 1-week, randomized placebo phase *(shaded bars)* for exercise tolerance test (ETT) efficacy variables (n = 47). *If angina or 1-mm ST-segment depression did not occur, the time to termination was used. Reproduced with permission from Nadeau et al.[78]

Diltiazem

The 3-month efficacy and safety of a once-daily controlled formulation of diltiazem (180 to 360 mg/d) were assessed by Nadeau and colleagues[78] in Montreal, Canada, in a study of 54 patients with angina pectoris. This multicenter study was a nonrandomized, placebo run-in, open-label, 3-month trial followed by a 1-week, double-blind, randomized period during which most patients (89%) received placebo. There were only minimal changes in the time to termination, time to onset of angina, and the time to 1-mm ST-segment depression from the end of the titration phase to the end of the open-label study. There were, however, statistically significant differences between the end of the 3-month treatment phase and the end of the 1-week randomized placebo phase for those three efficacy parameters (Figure 2-14). Diltiazem significantly decreased the frequency of anginal attacks and nitroglycerin use at the end of the 3-month treatment phase compared with results at the end of the randomized double-blind placebo phase. No new or unusual adverse events were reported during treatment. The present results suggest that there is no loss of efficacy of once-a-day diltiazem when administered for a long period to patients with chronic unstable angina pectoris.

Metoprolol vs. Diltiazem

Brouwer and colleagues[79] in Groningen, the Netherlands, investigated whether analysis of heart rate variability may be used to predict the efficacy of drug treatment of myocardial ischemia. In a double-blind crossover study, 28 patients with stable angina pectoris, proven CAD, and myocardial ischemia during Holter monitoring received control-release metoprolol, 200 mg once daily, and diltiazem, 60 mg 4 times daily. After a placebo run-in phase and after each treatment, 72-hour Holter recordings were obtained for heart rate variability and ST-segment analyses. At baseline, the total duration of myocardial ischemia was 11.4 minutes, and the total number of episodes was 2.2. Metoprolol significantly reduced the total duration of ischemia by minus 8.7 minutes and the total number of episodes by −1.9 in patients with a low standard deviation of normal-to-normal intervals at baseline, using the median value of 50 msec as a cut-off value. In contrast, significant treatment effects were not observed in patients with a higher standard deviation of normal-to-normal intervals at baseline. Similar results were obtained using baseline total power of low-frequency power or low-frequency power but not when using baseline heart rate. Diltiazem reduced the total duration of ischemia by minus 4.9 minutes but not the number of episodes. Moreover, in contrast to metoprolol, efficacy of diltiazem was not related to baseline of heart rate variability. In conclusion, patients with reduced heart rate variability at baseline responded to treatment with metoprolol. This differential pattern was not observed with diltiazem. These results therefore suggest that analysis of heart rate variability may be useful in selecting patients who will benefit from treatment with β-blockers.

Metoprolol vs. Nifedipine

Little information is available on how the characteristics of anginal symptoms and the results of exercise testing can be used in selecting medical treatment in patients with chronic stable angina pectoris. Ardissino and colleagues[80] from Pavia, Italy, evaluated these characteristics relative to the favorable anti-ischemic effect of the β-adrenergic blocking agent metoprolol and the calcium antagonist nifedipine in patients with stable angina pectoris. Two hundred eighty patients with stable angina were enrolled in 25 European centers. The patients were randomly allocated to double-blind treatment for 6 weeks with either metoprolol (controlled-release, 200 mg once daily) or nifedipine (retard, 20 mg twice daily). At the end of this period exercise tests were repeated 1 to 4 hours after drug intake. Both metoprolol and nifedipine prolonged exercise tolerance over baseline levels with the improvement being greater in the patients receiving metoprolol. Multivariate analysis revealed that low exercise tolerance was the only variable associated with a more favorable effect within each treatment group. These authors concluded that the results of a baseline exercise test, but not the characteristics of anginal symptoms, may offer useful information for selecting medical treatment in patients with stable angina pectoris.

Metoprolol vs. Verapamil (on Platelet Aggregability)

Wallen and coinvestigators[81] in Stockholm, Sweden, studied the effects of 1 month of treatment with either verapamil or metoprolol on several aspects of platelet function at rest and during physical exercise or mental stress in patients with stable angina pectoris participating in the Angina Prognosis Study in Stockholm. Platelet aggregability was measured by filtragometry ex vivo, which reflects platelet aggregability in vivo and by Born aggregometry in vitro. Platelet secretion in vivo was assessed by measurements of β-thromboglobulin in plasma. Verapamil reduced plasma norepinephrine levels and attenuated platelet aggregability at rest. Aggregability in platelet-rich plasma was not influenced. Metoprolol did not significantly affect filtragometry readings or aggregability in vitro. However, there was a tendency toward enhanced adenosine diphosphate sensitivity. β-Thromboglobulin levels were low and not influenced by either treatment. Physical exercise (bicycle ergometry) increased platelet aggregability in vivo both before and after drug treatment. Verapamil also attenuated platelet aggregability after exercise, whereas metoprolol had no such effect. Platelet function was not seriously altered by mental stress despite significant effects on hemodynamics and plasma catecholamines either before or after treatment with either drug. Thus, verapamil attenuates platelet aggregability in patients with stable angina pectoris, whereas metoprolol has no such effect.

Nitroglycerin vs. Nitroprusside (on Platelet Aggregability)

Diodati and coworkers[82] Bethesda, Maryland, assessed the inhibitory effect of nitroglycerin and sodium nitroprusside on platelet aggregation in a model of platelet activation across coronary circulation. Platelet aggregation is believed to contribute to the precipitation of acute ischemic syndromes. The investigators had previously shown that rapid atrial pacing in patients with stable CAD causes platelet hyperaggregability during blood passage in coronary circulation. Because nitroglycerin and sodium nitroprusside have been shown to inhibit platelet aggregation, the investigators examined the effect of these drugs on this model of platelet activation. During catheterization of 19 patients with CAD (>50% diameter narrowing of epicardial coronary arteries), the investigators measured platelet aggregation (using whole blood platelet aggregometry) on blood samples obtained simultaneously from the coronary sinus and aorta at rest and 2 minutes after onset of rapid atrial pacing. This procedure was repeated during an intravenous infusion of either nitroglycerin or sodium nitroprusside. There was no arteriovenous difference in platelet aggregation under resting conditions. Atrial pacing caused an increase in platelet aggregation in coronary sinus blood but not in arterial blood. This increase was transient and returned toward baseline 10 minutes after termination of pacing. Although resting platelet aggregation was not affected by nitroglycerin or sodium nitroprusside, activation of platelets with atrial pacing across the coronary bed was stopped by pretreatment with therapeutic doses of nitroglycerin or sodium nitroprusside. When coronary blood flow increases in patients with CAD, platelets are activated and aggregate more easily. This activation can be blunted by pretreatment with nitroglycerin or sodium nitroprusside. This mechanism may in part explain the beneficial effect of nitrovasodilators in acute ischemic syndromes, and may contribute to the therapeutic value of these agents in stable CAD.

Amlodipine vs. Atenolol vs. Amlodipine + Atenolol

There may be different pathophysiological differences between ischemia which occurs during ambulatory monitoring that observed during exercise treadmill testing. Davies and colleagues[83] from Ottawa, Canada, evaluated the effects of amlodipine, atenolol, and their combination on myocardial ischemia during treadmill exercise and ambulatory monitoring in the CASIS trial. One hundred patients with stable CAD and ischemia during both treadmill testing and ambulatory monitoring underwent a counterbalanced, crossover evaluation of single drug and placebo, followed by evaluation of the combination. Ischemia during treadmill testing was more effectively suppressed by amlodipine, whereas ischemia during ambulatory monitoring was more effectively suppressed by atenolol. The combination was more effective than either single drug in both settings. These authors concluded that there may be important differences in the pathophysiology of ischemia in these 2 settings.

Low–Molecular Weight Heparin vs. Regular Heparin or Aspirin

Unstable angina is associated with plaque disruption and thrombosis. Gurfinkel and colleagues[84] from Buenos Aires, Argentina, evaluated the effects of a low–molecular weight heparin as a therapeutic agent. It has the potential advantage of not requiring laboratory monitoring. A total of 219 patients with unstable angina were randomly assigned to receive aspirin (200 mg/d), aspirin plus regular heparin (400 IU/kg body wt per day intravenously and titrated by activated partial thromboplastin time), or aspirin plus low–molecular weight heparin (214 UIC/kg twice daily subcutaneously). Recurrent angina in these 3 groups occurred respectively in 37%, 44%, and 21% of patients. Nonfatal AMI was respectively present in 7 patients, 4 patients, and none. Urgent revascularization was performed in 9 patients, 7 patients, and 1 patient, respectively. Two major episodes of bleeding occurred in the group receiving aspirin plus heparin. Silent myocardial ischemia was present respectively in 38%, 41%, and 25% of the patient groups. These authors concluded that treatment with aspirin plus a high dose of low–molecular weight heparin during the acute phase of unstable angina was significantly better than treatment with aspirin alone or aspirin plus regular heparin.

Lovastatin

Impaired endothelium-mediated relaxation contributes to vasospasm and myocardial ischemia in patients with CAD. Treasure and associates[85] from Atlanta, Georgia; Louisville, Kentucky, Rahway, New Jersey; and Charlotte, North Carolina, hypothesized that cholesterol-lowering therapy with lovastatin could improve endothelium-mediated responses in patients with coronary atherosclerosis. In a randomized, double-blind, placebo-controlled trial, we studied coronary endothelial responses in 23 patients randomly assigned to either lovastatin (40 mg twice daily; 11 patients) or placebo (12 patients) plus a lipid-lowering diet (American Heart Association Step-1 diet). Patients were studied 12 days after randomization and again at 5.5 months. These patients had total cholesterol levels ranging from 160–300 mg/dL (4.1–7.8 mmol/L) and were undergoing coronary angioplasty. At the initial and follow-up studies, patients received serial intracoronary infusions (in a coronary artery not undergoing angioplasty) of acetylcholine to assess endothelium-mediated vasodilatation. The responses of the coronary vessels were analyzed with quantitative angiography. The patients in the placebo and lovastatin groups had similar responses to acetylcholine at a mean of 12 days of therapy (expressed as the percentage of change in diameter in response to acetylcholine doses of 10^{-9}, 10^{-8}, 10^{-7}, and 10^{-6} M. In the placebo group, the respective mean (±SE) changes were 1 ± 2%, 0 ± 2%, −2 ± 4%, and −19 ± 4%; in the lovastatin group, they were −2 ± 2%,

$-4 \pm 4\%$, $-12 \pm 5\%$, and $-16 \pm 7\%$. (Coronary artery constriction is reflected by negative numbers.) The responses to acetylcholine in the placebo group after a mean of 5.5 months of therapy were $-3 \pm 3\%$, $-1 \pm 2\%$, $-8 \pm 4\%$, and $-18 \pm 5\%$, respectively; there was significant improvement in the lovastatin group, which had responses of $3 \pm 3\%$, $3 \pm 3\%$, $0 \pm 2\%$, and $0 \pm 3\%$. Cholesterol lowering with lovastatin significantly improved endothelium-mediated responses in the coronary arteries of patients with atherosclerosis. Such improvement in the local regulation of coronary arterial tone could potentially relieve ischemic symptoms and signal the stabilization of the atherosclerotic plaque.

In a double-blind, placebo-controlled trial, Waters and colleagues[86] in Hartford, Connecticut, studied 62 women with diffuse but not necessarily severe CAD documented on a coronary angiogram and with fasting serum cholesterol values between 220 and 300 mg/dL. More than one half had a history of increased BP, approximately 25% were diabetics, and one third were current smokers. All women received dietary counseling. Lovastatin or placebo was begun at 20 mg/d and was titrated, if necessary, to 40 mg/d and then 80 mg/d during the first 16 weeks to attain a fasting LDL cholesterol ≤130 mg/dL. The mean lovastatin dose was 34 mg/d. Total and LDL cholesterol decreased by 24% and 32%, respectively, in lovastatin-treated women but by <3% in women receiving placebo. Coronary arteriography repeated after 2 years in 54 women (87%) evaluated their 394 lesions "blindly" on pairs of films with an automated computerized quantitative system. Progression, defined as worsening in minimum diameter of one or more stenoses by ≥0.4 mm was found in seven of 25 lovastatin-treated women and 17 of 29 placebo-treated women (28% vs. 59%). New coronary lesions developed in 1 lovastatin-treated woman and 13 placebo-treated women (4% vs. 45%). The outcome for each of the angiographic end points was not significantly different between the women and the 245 men who completed the trial. Thus, these data indicate that lovastatin slows the progression of coronary atherosclerosis and reduces the frequency of development of new lesions in women.

Lovastatin + Cholestyramine vs. Lovastatin + Probucol

Patients with CAD and abnormalities at the serum lipid levels often have endothelial vasodilated dysfunction, which may contribute to ischemic cardiac events. Whether cholesterol-lowering or antioxidant therapy can restore endothelium-dependent coronary vasodilation is unknown. Anderson and associates[87] from Boston, Massachusetts, randomly assigned 49 patients (mean serum cholesterol, 209 ± 33 mg/dL) to receive one of 3 treatments: an American Heart Association Step-1 diet (the diet group, 11 patients), lovastatin and cholestyramine (the LDL cholesterol-lowering group, 21 patients), or lovastatin and probucol (the LDL cholesterol-lowering-antioxidant group, 17 patients). Endothelium-dependent coronary-artery vasomotion in response to an intracoronary infusion of acetylcholine (10^{-8}–10^{-6}M) was assessed at baseline and after 1 year of therapy. Vasoconstrictor responses to these doses of acetylcholine are considered to be abnormal. Treatment resulted in significant reductions in LDL cholesterol levels of $41 \pm 22\%$ in the LDL cholesterol-lowering group. The maximal changes in coronary-artery diameter with acetylcholine at baseline and at follow-up were -19% and -2% in the diet group. (The negative numbers indicate vasoconstriction.) Thus, the greatest improvement in the vasoconstrictor response was seen in the LDL cholesterol-lowering antioxidant group. The improvement in endothelium-dependent vasomotion with cholesterol-lowering and antioxidant therapy may have important implications for the activity of myocardial ischemia and may explain in part the reduced incidence of adverse coronary events that is known to result from cholesterol-lowering therapy.

Pravastatin

Jukema and colleagues[88] in Leiden, the Netherlands, evaluated the effects of cholesterol lowering on progression and regression of coronary atherosclerosis in 885 patients with a serum cholesterol between 155 and 310 mg/dL by quantitative coronary angiography. In the Regression Growth Evaluation Statin Study (REGRESS), a double-blind, placebo-controlled multicenter approach was used to evaluate the effects of 2 years of treatment with pravastatin, a 3-hydroxy-3-methylgultaryl coenzyme A (HMG CoA) reductase inhibitor, on progression and regression of coronary heart disease. Primary end points were 1) changes in average mean segment diameter per patient and 2) changes in average minimum obstruction diameter per patient. Clinical events were also analyzed. Among 885 patients, 778 (88%) had an evaluable final angiogram. Mean segment diameter decreased 0.10 mm in the placebo group vs. 0.06 mm in the pravastatin group. The mean difference between treatment groups was 0.04 mm. The median minimum obstruction diameter decreased 0.09 mm in the placebo group compared with 0.03 mm in the pravastatin group. At the end of the follow-up period, 89% of the pravastatin patients and 81% of the placebo patients were without new cardiovascular events (Figure 2-15). Thus, these data indicate that in symptomatic men with significant CAD and normal to moderately elevated serum cholesterol, pravastatin may lead to less progression of coronary atherosclerosis and fewer new cardiovascular events.

Byington and colleagues[89] pooled clinical data from four atherosclerosis regression trials that evaluated pravastatin for a predetermined analysis of the effect of that agent on the risk of coronary events. All trials were double-masked, placebo-controlled designs that used pravastatin as monotherapy for 2 to 3 years. The 1891 participants in the trials had evidence of atherosclerosis and mildly to moderately elevated serum lipid values. For fatal or nonfatal AMI, there was a 62% reduction in events attributable to pravastatin. This effect was evident in younger and older patients, men and women, and patients with and without histories of hypertension and prior AMI. There was a 46% reduction in all-cause mortality and a 62% reduction in the risk of fatal or nonfatal stroke (Figures 2-16, 2-17, and 2-18). These pooled data provide additional strong support to indicate that pravastatin (and probably other HMG CoA reductase inhibitors) reduce the risk of cardiovascular events in patients with atherosclerotic disease and mildly to moderately elevated serum lipid values. The benefit for reducing the risk of AMI is evident in older and younger patients, men and women, and patients with and without histories of increased BP and prior AMI.

Four hundred eighty-eight patients with coronary artery disease and an LDL cholesterol level >130 were randomly assigned in a 3-year study to receive pravastatin or placebo.[90] Atherosclerosis progression was evaluated by quantitative coronary arteriography. Pravastatin decreased total and LDL cholesterol

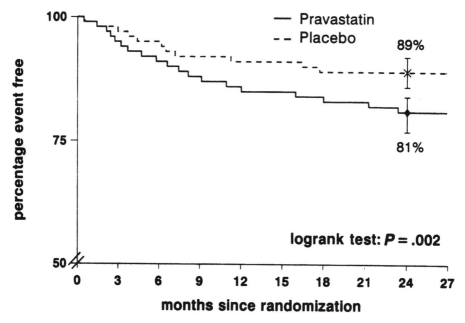

FIGURE 2-15. Kaplan-Meier curves for time to first clinical event for the 2 treatment groups. All events: myocardial infarction, death, coronary artery bypass graft surgery/percutaneous transluminal coronary angioplasty, cerebral vascular accident. Reproduced with permission from Jukema et al.[88]

by 19% and 28%. HDL cholesterol was increased by 7%. Progression of atherosclerosis was reduced by 40% for minimum vessel diameter compared with placebo. There were also fewer lesions in those assigned pravastatin. AMI was reduced during the active treatment (eight in the pravastatin group and 17 in the placebo group), with the benefit emerging after 1 year. These authors concluded that in patients with CAD and mild to moderate cholesterol elevations, pravastatin reduced the progression of CAD and myocardial infarction. This is consistent with other data that indicate that lipid-lowering therapy is very effective in reducing clinical events in patients with known CAD.

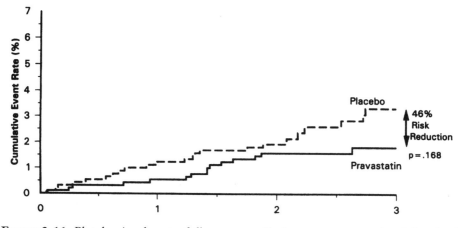

FIGURE 2-16. Plot showing the rate of all-cause mortality by treatment group (pooled analysis). Reproduced with permission from Byington et al.[89]

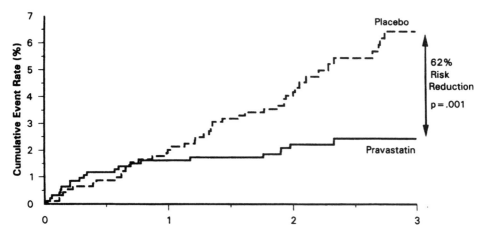

FIGURE 2-17. Plot showing the rate of nonfatal or fatal MI by treatment group (pooled analysis). Reproduced by permission of Byington et al.[89]

Lacoste and colleagues[91] in Perth, Australia, and Montreal, Canada, measured mural platelet thrombus formation on an injured arterial wall in a model simulating vessel stenosis and plaque rupture in hypercholesterolemic CAD patients before and after cholesterol reduction. Thirty-two patients with stable CAD were evaluated. Platelet thrombus formation and serum lipids were measured in 16 hypercholesterolemic patients with a serum cholesterol >5.2 mmol/L before and after a mean of 2.5 months of pravastatin therapy (40 mg/d) and in 16 normocholesterolemic control patients. Thrombus formation was assessed by exposing porcine aortic media to the patient's flowing venous blood for 3 minutes at a shear rate of 754 or 2546/sec at 37°C in an ex vivo superfusion chamber. Quantitative morphometric platelet thrombus formation at baseline was higher in the hypercholesterolemic patients at both the high and low shear rates (Figure 2-19). Pravastatin decreased total serum cholesterol from 6.5 to 4.5 mmol/L and LDL cholesterol from 4.5 to 2.8 mmol/L. Platelet thrombus formation at high and low shear rates decreased to 2 and 1.3 μm^2/mm, respec-

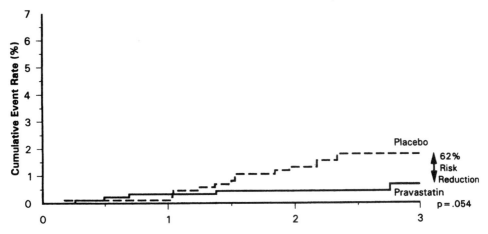

FIGURE 2-18. Plot showing rate of stroke by treatment group (pooled analysis). Reproduced by permission of Byington et al.[89]

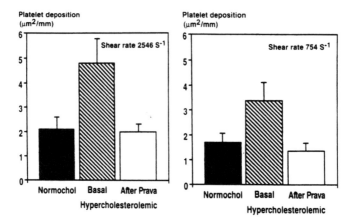

FIGURE 2-19. Bar graphs showing platelet deposition at the high shear rate of 2546/sec (left) and at the low shear rate of 754/sec (right) in normocholesterolemic (Normochol) and hypercholesterolemic patients at baseline (Basal) and after treatment with pravastatin (After Prava). Reproduced by permission of Lacoste et al.[91]

tively. These data suggest that hypercholesterolemia is associated with increased platelet thrombus formation on an injured artery, increasing the possibility of acute thrombosis. Reductions in serum cholesterol appear to reduce platelet thrombus formation at both high and low shear rates.

Simvastatin

Pedersen and associates[92] of the Scandinavian Simvastatin Survival Study Group examined the relation between the risk of major coronary events (coronary death and non-AMI) and baseline cholesterol levels in patients with CAD randomly assigned to placebo or simvastatin therapy. The RR reduction in the simvastatin group was 35% in the lowest quartile of baseline LDL cholesterol and 36% in the highest (Table 2-5). Simvastatin significantly reduced the risk of major coronary events in all quartiles of all baseline total, HDL cholesterol, LDL cholesterol, by a similar amount in each quartile.

n-3 vs. n-6 Fatty Acids

Epidemiological studies of populations whose intake of oily fish is high have suggested that fish oil is antiatherogenic. Sacks and colleagues[93] from Boston, Massachusetts, conducted a randomized clinical trial to test whether fish oil supplements can improve human coronary atherosclerosis. Patients with angiographically documented CAD and normal plasma lipid levels were randomly assigned to receive either fish oil capsules (n = 31) or olive oil capsules (n = 28) for 28 months. Coronary atherosclerosis was quantified by computer-assisted image analysis. Mean minimal diameter of atherosclerotic coronary arteries decreased by 0.104 and 0.138 mm in the fish oil and control groups, respectively. These authors concluded that fish oil treatment for 2 years does not promote major favorable changes in the diameter of atherosclerotic coronary arteries.

The influence of dietary supplementation with n-3 vs. n-6 fatty acid on plasma lipoprotein(a) levels was studied by Herrmann and associates[94] in Re-

TABLE 2-5. Quartile Limits of Baseline Lipids and Frequency of Major Coronary Events

	Quartile			
	1	2	3	4
Total cholesterol (mmol/L)	≤6–24	6.25–6.74	6.75–7.24	≥7.25
Placebo, n(%)	134(25.7)	162(27.9)	156(27.9)	171(30.4)
Simvastatin, n(%)	107(19.9)	106(18.3)	104(18.9)	114(20.6)
Relative risk (95% CI)	0.76(0.59–0.97)	0.62(0.49–0.80)	0.64(0.50–0.82)	0.65 (0.51–0.82)
LDL-cholesterol (mmol/L)	≤4.39	4.40–4.84	4.85–5.34	≥5.35
Placebo, n(%)	135(25.4)	158(29.6)	153(25.9)	175(31.1)
Simvastatin, n(%)	89(17.2)	122(20.7)	108(18.4)	118(20.9)
Relative risk (95% CI)	0.65(0.50–0.85)	0.67(0.52–0.85)	0.68(0.53–0.87)	0.64(0.51–0.81)
HDL-cholesterol (mmol/L)	≤0.99	1.00–1.14	1.15–1.34	≥1.35
Placebo, n(%)	177(32.1)	143(28.0)	154(27.4)	144(24.4)
Simvastatin, n(%)	121(22.5)	110(20.4)	97(16.6)	96(17.7)
Relative risk (95% CI)	0.67(0.53–0.84)	0.71 (0.55–0.91)	0.57 (0.44–0.74)	0.70 (0.54–0.90)
LDL-cholesterol/HDL-cholesterol	≤3.51	3.52–4.26	4.27–5.14	≥5.15
Placebo, n(%)	125 (22.2)	156(28.3)	164(30.3)	173(30.9)
Simvastatin, n(%)	87(16.2)	102(18.7)	115(20.2)	120(21.7)
Relative risk (95% CI)	0.71(0.54–0.93)	0.62(0.49–0.80)	0.64(0.50–0.81)	0.67(0.53–0.84)

Reproduced with permission of Scandinavian Simvastatin Survival Study Group.[92]

gensburg, Germany. Thirty-five male hospitalized patients with CAD were treated for 4 weeks with 12 g/d of fish oil (8.5 g of n-3 fatty acids) in combination with a 5000-kJ, 30%-fat diet and moderate exercise. Eighteen control patients given the same dietary and training program were treated with 12 g/d of rapeseed oil. Plasma lipoprotein(a), in addition to several lipids and lipoproteins, blood clotting factors, and platelet activity, were measured before and at the end of therapy. Total cholesterol, LDL cholesterol, and apolipoprotein B levels decreased significantly in both rapeseed oil and fish oil groups. Triglycerides decreased 20%, and HDL cholesterol increased 8%, significant only in patients treated with fish oil. Plasma lipoprotein(a) levels were reduced by 14% in the fish oil group but were unaffected in the rapeseed oil group. The patients treated with fish oil could be categorized in 2 subgroups: "responders," with a reduction in lipoprotein(a) by 24% and "nonresponders," with a small nonsignificant increase in serum lipoprotein(a). Responders and nonresponders exhibited a marked reduction in cholesterol, LDL cholesterol, apolipoprotein B, and triglycerides and an increase in HDL_3 cholesterol. There was a large reduction in t-PA in the fish oil group, which correlated significantly with a reduction in lipoprotein(a). Platelet number and aggregation behavior would not significantly change in either group. No physiological differences were seen between responders and nonresponders.

Estrogen

Collins and colleagues[95] in London UK; New Haven, Connecticut; and Novo Nordisk, Bagsvaerd, Denmark, studied 9 postmenopausal women (mean age, 59 years) and 7 men (mean age, 52 years) with proven CAD. The patients had measurements of coronary artery diameter and coronary blood flow before and after the intracoronary administration of acetylcholine 1.6 and 16 µg/min before and 20 minutes after the intracoronary administration of 2.5 µg of 17β-estradiol into atherosclerotic, nonstenotic coronary arteries. Changes in coronary artery diameter were measured by quantitative coronary arteriography and changes in coronary blood flow were measured with an intracoronary Doppler catheter. In female patients, acetylcholine 1.6 and 16 µg/min caused vasoconstriction before the administration of 17β-estradiol (Figure 2-20). Administration of 17β-estradiol converted the constriction to dilatation. However, in males, the administration of the estrogen did not change the vasoconstriction associated with acetylcholine infusion. 17β-Estradiol alone had no significant effect on coronary diameter or coronary blood flow. Isosorbide dinitrate caused dilatation of the coronary arteries. The data demonstrate that 17β-estradiol modulates acetylcholine-induced coronary artery responses in postmenopausal females with CAD but not in males with similar atherosclerosis. These human data confirm reports from studies in cynomolgus monkeys that estrogen modulates the responses of atherosclerotic coronary arteries in postmenopausal females.

Zatebradine

Heart rate reduction is considered to be the primary mechanism whereby many drugs reduce angina in patients with CAD. It is difficult, however, to distinguish between the heart rate–lowering effect and other effects of various antianginal agents. Frishman and colleagues[96] examined the effect of zatebrad-

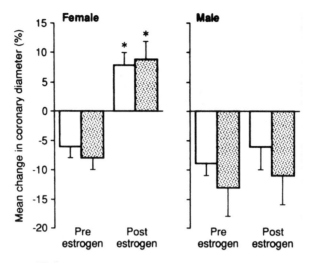

Figure 2-20. Bar graphs showing change in the diameter of female coronary arteries (left) produced by an intracoronary infusion of acetylcholine (1.6 μmol/min, open bars; 16 μmol/min, stippled bars) before and after 2.5 μmol of intracoronary 17β-estradiol. Net constriction before estrogen was converted to dilatation after estrogen (*$P < 0.01$ before vs. after estrogen). Change in the diameter of male coronary arteries (right) produced by an intracoronary infusion of acetylcholine (1.6 μmol/min, open bars; 16 μmol/min, stippled bars) before and after 2.5 μmol of intracoronary 17β-estradiol (P = NS before vs. after estrogen). Reproduced with permission of Collins et al.[95]

ine, a direct sinus node inhibitor, in patients with angina who were taking extended-release nifedipine. In this single-blind, placebo run-in, randomized double-blind, placebo-controlled, multicenter study, patients were randomized to receive zatebradine (5 mg twice a day, n = 64), or placebo (n = 60). Zatebradine reduced heart rate both at rest and at the end of exercise (13 and 17 beats per minute). However, there were no additional benefits of zatebradine in measurements of total exercise duration, time to 1-mm ST-segment depression, or time to onset of angina. These authors concluded that zatebradine seems to provide no additional antianginal benefit to patients already receiving nifedipine. The data raise questions regarding the benefit of heart rate reduction alone as an antianginal approach to patients with chronic stable angina.

Coronary Angioplasty vs. Bypass

The Coronary Angioplasty vs. Bypass Revascularisation Investigation (CABRI) is a multinational, multicenter, randomized trial comparing the strategies of revascularization by CABG and PTCA in patients with symptomatic multivessel CAD; 1054 patients (220 men and 234 women) were recruited from 26 European cardiac centers.[97] The average age was 60 years, and 62% presented with angina of class 3 or greater. Five hundred thirteen patients were randomly assigned to CABG and 541 to PTCA, and 93% and 96%, respectively, of those randomized underwent the allocated procedure. This first report presents data analyzed by intention to treat and documents all deaths, major cardiac events, and the symptom status of the patients 1 year after randomization (Figure 2-21, Table 2-6). After 1 year of follow-up, 14 (2.7%) of those assigned to CABG and 21 (3.9%) of those assigned to PTCA had died. The PTCA group's RR of

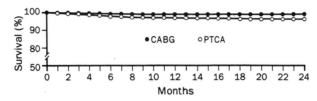

FIGURE 2-21. Cumulative survival after randomization. Reproduced with permission of CABRI Trial Participants.[97]

death was 1.42. Patients randomly assigned to CABG (RR, 5.23 [3.90–7.03]). The patients in the PTCA group took significantly more medication at 1 year (RR, 1.30 [1.18–1.43]). They were also more likely to have clinically significant angina (RR, 1.54 [1.09–2.16]); this association was present in both sexes but was significant only in females. CABRI is the largest trial of CABG vs. PTCA to be reported so far. Its findings are consistent with previous studies and add to the weight of information that clinicians need to discuss with patients when options for the management of severe angina are under consideration.

A patient with severe angina will often be eligible for either PTCA or CABG. Results from eight published randomized trials were combined by Pocock and associates[98] from several international medical centers in a collaborative meta-analysis of 3371 patients (1661 CABG and 1710 PTCA) with a mean follow-up of 2.7 years (Figure 2-22, Table 2-7). The total deaths in the CABG and PTCA groups were 73 and 79, respectively, with an RR value of 1.08 (95%). The combined end point of cardiac death and nonfatal AMI occurred in 169 PTCA patients and 154 CABG patients (RR, 1.10) (Table 2-8). Among patients randomly assigned to PTCA, 17.8% required additional CABG within 1 year, whereas in subsequent years the need for additional CABG was around 2% per annum. The rate of additional nonrandomized interventions (PTCA and/or CABG) in the first year of follow-up was 33.7% and 3.3% in patients randomly assigned to PTCA and CABG, respectively. The prevalence of angina after 1 year was considerably higher in the PTCA group (RR, 1.56), but at 3 years this difference had attenuated (RR, 1.22). Overall, there was substantial similarity in outcome across the trials. Separate analyses were performed for the 732 cases of single-vessel disease. The combined evidence comparing PTCA with CABG shows no difference in prognosis between these 2 initial revascularization strategies. However, the treatments differ markedly in the subsequent requirement for additional revascularization procedures and in the relief of angina.

Table 2-6. Initial and Subsequent Revascularization

	CABG (n = 513)	PTCA (n = 541)
Initial intervention CABG	478 (93.2%)	15 (2.8%)
Subsequent PTCA	11 (2.1%)	4 (0.7%)
Subsequent CABG	0 (0.0%)	1 (0.2%)
Initial procedure only	467 (91.0%)	11 (2.0%)
Initial intervention PTCA	20 (3.9%)	522 (96.3%)
Subsequent PTCA	3 (0.6%)	109 (20.1%)
Subsequent CABG	4 (0.8%)	84 (15.5%)
Initial procedure only	13 (2.5%)	348 (64.3%)

Reproduced with permission of CABRI Trial participants.[97]

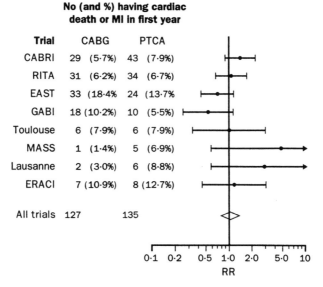

No (and %) having cardiac death or MI in first year

Trial	CABG	PTCA
CABRI	29 (5·7%)	43 (7·9%)
RITA	31 (6·2%)	34 (6·7%)
EAST	33 (18·4%	24 (13·7%
GABI	18 (10·2%)	10 (5·5%)
Toulouse	6 (7·9%)	6 (7·9%)
MASS	1 (1·4%)	5 (6·9%)
Lausanne	2 (3·0%)	6 (8·8%)
ERACI	7 (10·9%)	8 (12·7%)
All trials	127	135

FIGURE 2-22. Cardiac death and myocardial infarction for PTCA group compared with CABG group in first year since randomization. Shown as RR (PTCA:CABG) with 95% CI. Reproduced with permission of Pocock et al.[98]

These results will influence the choice of revascularization procedure in future patients with angina.

Sim and coworkers[99] in Stanford, California, performed a meta-analysis of randomized trials that compared PTCA with CABG in patients with multivessel CAD. The outcomes of death, combined death, nonfatal AMI, repeat revascularization, and freedom from angina were analyzed. The overall risk of death in nonfatal AMI was not different over a follow-up of 1–3 years. (CABG:PTCA OR, 1.03; 95% CI, 0.81 to 1.32). Patients randomly assigned to CABG tended to have a high risk of death or AMI in the early periprocedural period, but a lower risk in subsequent follow-up. CABG patients were much less likely to undergo another revascularization procedure and were more likely to be angina free. Thus, CABG and PTCA patients have similar overall risk of death and nonfatal AMI at 1–3 years of follow-up, but RR differences and mortality of up to 25% cannot be excluded. CABG patients have significantly less angina and fewer repeat revascularizations than PTCA patients.

Weintraub and colleagues[100] and the EAST Investigators engaged in a randomized trial that compared, by intention to treat, the clinical outcomes and costs of PTCA and CABG for multivessel CAD. The primary end point was a composite of death, Q-wave AMI, and a large reversible thallium defect at 3 years. Hospital charges were reduced to cost through step-down accounting methods. All costs and charges were deflated to 1987 dollars. Costs were assessed for the initial hospitalization and the cumulative costs of the initial hospitalization and additional revascularization procedures for up to 3 years. Patients were randomized from 1987 through 1990. There were 198 patients in the PTCA group and 194 in the surgery group. The clinical characteristics of these patients were similar (Table 2-9). In this study, there was no difference in mortality or the primary end points between the 2 modalities of treatment.

Table 2-7. Characteristics of Eight Randomised Trials Comparing PTCA and CABG

Trial	Country	Principal investigator	Single or multi vessel	Number of patients		Follow-up
				CABG	PTCA	
Coronary Angioplasty versus Bypass Revascularisation Investigation[1] (CABRI)	Europe	A F Rickards	Multi	513	541	1 yr
Randomised Intervention Treatment of Angina trial[2] (RITA)	UK	J R Hampton	Single (n = 456) and multi (n = 555)	501	510	4.7 yr
Emory Angioplasty versus Surgery Trial[3] (EAST)	USA	S B King	Multi	194	198	3 yr
German Angioplasty Bypass Surgery Investigation[4] (GABI)	Germany	C W Hamm	Multi	177	182	1 yr+
The Toulouse trial[5] (Toulouse)	France	J Puel	Multi	76	76	2.8 yr
Medicine Angioplasty or Surgery study[6] (MASS)	Brazil	W Hueb	Single	70	72	3.2 yr
The Lausanne trial[7] (Lausanne)	Switzerland	J-J Goy	Single	66	68	3.2 yr
Argentine Trial of PTCA versus CABG[8] (ERACI)	Argentina	A Rodriquez	Multi	64	63	3.8 yr

Reproduced with permission of Poock et al.[98]

Table 2-8. Mortality Results by Study, by Cause of Death, and by Time Since Randomisation

Study	No of deaths		No (and %) dying in first year	
	CABG	PTCA	CABG	PTCA
CABRI	14	21	14 (2.7%)	21 (3.9%)
RITA	26	24	6 (1.2%)	9 (1.8%)
EAST	12	14	4 (2.1%)	7 (3.5%)
GABI	9	4	9 (5.1%)	4 (2.2%)
Toulouse	7	5	2 (2.6%)	3 (3.9%)
MASS	1	1	0	1 (1.4%)
Lausanne	1	4	0	1 (1.5%)
ERACI	3	6	3 (4.7%)	3 (4.8%)
Cause of death			**RR(95% Cl)**	
All causes	73	79	1.08 (0.79, 1.50)	
Cardiac	46	46	1.00 (0.65, 1.54)	
Other cardiovascular	4	10	2.50 (0.72, 10.90)	
Noncardiovascular	23	23	1.00 (0.54, 1.86)	
Time since randomization				
During initial hospital period	21	17	0.81 (0.40, 1.61)	
First year*	38	49	1.29 (0.83, 2.02)	
Subsequent follow-up	35	30	0.86 (0.51, 1.44)	

*Including initial hospital period and before randomised procedure could be done.

Reproduced with permission of Pocock et al.[98]

TABLE 2-9. Clinical Characteristics

	PTCA Group, %	CABG Group, %	P
Patients, n	198	194	
Age, y	62 ± 10	61 ± 10	NS
Male, n (%)	148 (75)	141 (73)	NS
Diabetes, n (%)	49 (25)	41 (21)	NS
Systemic arterial hypertension, n (%)	106 (54)	100 (52)	NS
Prior MI, n (%)	81 (41)	79 (41)	NS
Class III–IV angina, n (%)	147 (77)	155 (72)	NS
	(n = 189)	(n = 190)	
Congestive heart failure, n (%)	5 (2.5)	8 (4.1)	NS
Two-vessel disease, n (%)	119 (60)	117 (60)	NS
Three-vessel disease, n (%)	79 (40)	77 (40)	NS
Ejection fraction	61 ± 12	62 ± 12	NS
Initial treatment received as randomized, n (%)	196 (99)	193 (99)	NS
In-hospital deaths, n (%)	2 (1.0)	2 (1.0)	NS
In-hospital Q-wave MI, n (%)	6 (3.0)	20 (10.3)	.005
3-Year mortality, n (%)	14 (7.1)	12 (6.2)	NS
3-Year Q-wave MI, n (%)	29/173 (14.6)	38/172 (19.6)	NS
Primary end point, n/total (%)	58/177 (28.8)	53/171 (27.3)	NS

PTCA indicates percutaneous transluminal coronary angiography; CABG, coronary artery bypass graft surgery; and MI, myocardial infarction.

Reproduced with permission of Weintraub et al.[100]

Mean initial hospital charges were $12 654 for the PTCA patients and $20 214 for the patients treated by CABG (Figure 2-23). Professional charges were $4538 for PTCA and $9426 for CABG. Three-year hospital charges were $19 047 for

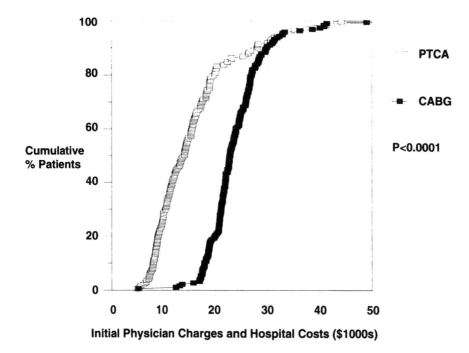

Figure 2-23. Plot showing initial hospitalization costs and professional charges by assigned treatment group. The data are presented as cumulative number of patients scaled to 100%. PTCA indicates percutaneous transluminal coronary angioplasty; CABG, coronary artery bypass graft surgery. Reproduced with permission of Weinstraub et al.[100]

PTCA and $21 174 for patients undergoing CABG. Three-year professional charges were $6412 for PTCA and $9861 for CABG. Three-year total charges were $25,458 for PTCA and $31,033 for CABG. Total 3-year costs were $23 734 for PTCA and $25 310 for CABG. There were more hospitalizations for angina and more antianginal medications used in the PTCA group, further narrowing the differences in cost. There were no differences in the primary end points or their components at 3 years. Thus, the primary procedural cost of CABG is higher than for PTCA, but this cost advantage for PTCA is largely lost by 3 years because of the more frequent additional procedures and other resource consumption after PTCA.

PTCA and bypass surgery are often performed in patients with a single proximal stenosis of the LAD coronary artery. However, it is unclear whether revascularization offers greater clinical benefit than medical therapy alone. Hueb and colleagues[101] from Sao Paulo, Brazil, randomly assigned 214 patients with stable angina, normal ventricular function, and a proximal stenosis of the LAD coronary artery to mammary CABG alone, PTCA, or medical therapy. At an average follow-up period of 3 years, a primary end point (cardiac death, AMI, or refractory angina requiring revascularization) had occurred in 3% assigned to CABG compared with 24% assigned to PTCA and 17% assigned to medical therapy. No patient assigned to CABG needed additional revascularization compared with eight assigned to PTCA and seven assigned to medical treatment. Both revascularization techniques resulted in greater symptomatic relief and a lower incidence of ischemia on the treadmill, although all 3 strategies eventually resulted in the abolition of limiting angina. These authors concluded that the more aggressive therapeutic approach with initial CABG for patients with single, severe proximal stenosis of the LAD coronary artery is associated with a lower incidence of medium-term adverse events than PTCA or medical treatment. All 3 strategies resulted in a similar incidence of death and infarction during an average follow-up period of 3 years.

Percutaneous Transluminal Coronary Angioplasty

Transradial Approach

Kiemeneij and associates[102] from Amsterdam, the Netherlands, explored the feasibility and safety of PTCA with miniaturized PTCA equipment via the radial artery. PTCA via the femoral or brachial arteries may be associated with vascular complications such as bleeding and damage to the artery and adjacent structures. It was postulated that PTCA via the radial artery with miniaturized angioplasty equipment is feasible and that no major puncture site–related complications occur because hemostasis is obtained easily and no major structures are near the radial artery. With double blood supply to the hand, radial artery occlusion is well tolerated. In 100 patients with collateral blood supply to the right hand, PTCA was attempted with 6F guiding catheters and rapid-exchange balloon catheters for exertional angina (87 patients) or nonexertional angina (13 patients). Angioplasty was attempted in 122 lesions (type A, n = 67 [55%]; type B, n = 37 [30%], and type C, n = 18 [15%]). Pre- and post-PTCA computerized quantitative coronary analysis was performed. Radial artery function and structure were assessed clinically and with Doppler and two-dimensional ultrasound on the day of discharge. Coronary catheterization via the radial artery was successful in 94 patients (94%). The 6 remaining patients had successful PTCA via the femoral artery (n = 5) or the brachial artery (n = 1). Procedural success (120 of 122 lesions) was achieved in 92 patients (98%) via the radial artery and in 98 patients of the total study population. Minimal luminal diameter increased from 0.9 ± 0.3 to 2.0 ± 0.5 mm, and diameter stenosis was reduced from 74 ± 11% to 24 ± 11%. In 3 patients a coronary stent was implanted via the radial artery because PTCA results were suboptimal. Of 98 patients with a successful PTCA, 4 (4%) had acute myocardial ischemia 1 to 24 hours after the procedure. In these patients an emergency second PTCA procedure via the femoral artery was performed successfully, but in 2 patients AMI could not be prevented. No other major cardiac complications were encountered. No major entry site–related complications were seen, and no patient required vascular surgery or blood transfusions. In 10 patients radial artery pulsations were absent at discharge, and all 10 were asymptomatic. Of these 10 patients, late recanalization was evident in 5, and in 3 patients pulsations remained absent. PTCA via the radial artery is effective and safe and minimizes major puncture site–related complications.

In Rest Angina Pectoris

In the TAUSA trial (Thrombolysis and Angioplasty in Unstable Angina) 469 patients were randomly assigned to receive either intracoronary urokinase or placebo during coronary PTCA of the culprit lesion in patients with ischemic rest angina with or without recent AMI.[103] This report analyzed the role of complex lesion morphology on the acute results of PTCA. Complex lesions were associated with a higher abrupt closure rate (10.6% vs. 3.3%) and also a higher recurrent in-hospital rate of angina and emergent CABG. Abrupt closure was particularly high in the urokinase group (15.0%) vs. the placebo group (5.9%). These authors concluded that complex lesions increased the acute complication rate after PTCA. In particular, urokinase had significant adverse effects, especially in complex lesions.

For Saphenous Venous Graft Narrowing

Holmes and colleagues[104] in Rochester, Minnesota; Cleveland, Ohio; Durham, North Carolina; Chicago, Illinois; Royal Oaks, Michigan; Louisville, Kentucky; Portland, Maine; Brooklyn, New York; Philadelphia, Pennsylvania; Toronto, Canada; and Indianapolis, Indiana, compared outcomes after directional coronary atherectomy and angioplasty and PTCA in patients with de novo bypass graft stenoses. Investigators at 54 North American and European sites randomly assigned 305 patients with de novo vein graft lesions to atherectomy (n = 149) or angioplasty (n = 156). Quantitative coronary arteriography assessed initial and 6-month results. Initial angiographic success was greater with atherectomy (89% vs. 79%) and luminal gain was also greater. Distal embolization was increased with atherectomy, and there was a trend toward a more frequent non–Q-wave AMI. Although the 6-month net minimal luminal diameter gain was 0.68 mm for atherectomy and 0.50 mm for PTCA, the restenosis rates were similar (46% for atherectomy and 51% for PTCA). At 6 months, there was a greater trend toward decreased repeated target-vessel intervention for atherectomy. Thirteen percent of patients treated with atherectomy vs. 22% of the PTCA patients required repeat percutaneous intervention of the initial target lesion. Thus, these data suggest that atherectomy of de novo vein graft lesions is associated not only with improved initial angiographic success and luminal diameter but also with increased distal embolization. There were no differences in 6-month restenosis rates, but primary atherectomy patients tended to require fewer target-vessel revascularization procedures.

In Men vs. Women

Bell and colleagues[105] from Rochester, Minnesota, performed a retrospective analysis in 3027 consecutive patients, including 824 women and 2203 men, who underwent successful PTCA and who had been followed continuously for a mean of 5.5 years. The follow-up was 100% completed. Event-free survival was assessed by the Kaplan-Meier method, and clinical end points were examined by Cox proportional-hazards models to account for important baseline differences when appropriate. There was a trend toward lower survival among women during follow-up, but it was not significant. No significant sex differences in the occurrence of Q-wave AMI were observed. Women were less likely to remain free of angina after 10 years (34% vs. 37%, respectively), but after adjustment for baseline differences, this difference was not significant. Women tended to have less CABG performed during follow-up, and adjustment for baseline differences made this finding significant. Among patients who were not treated during AMI, no sex differences in survival and freedom from AMI were noted.

These data indicate that after successful PTCA, the long-term prognosis for women is good and similar to that in men. However, although risk-adjusted survival did not differ between the sexes, there was less frequent use of subsequent CABG in women.

Sixty-Millimeter Balloon

To report preliminary clinical experience with a new 60-mm-long angioplasty balloon, Harris and Holmes[106] of Rochester, Minnesota, reviewed the results in patients who underwent this type of angioplasty between May and October 1993 at their institution. The study group consisted of 14 high-risk patients (57% with rest-related angina) and 19 treated coronary segments—52% in native coronary arteries and 48% in saphenous vein grafts (mean age, 9 years). Often, long-balloon angioplasty was used in conjunction with laser or transluminal extraction atherectomy. Angiographic success (40% or more visual reduction in diameter stenosis) was achieved in all patients. Intimal dissection occurred in 4 of the 19 treated segments (21%), but each was less than 50% obstructive. No patient required intracoronary stenting. Clinical success was achieved in 13 patients (93%). The 1 death that occurred was from vein graft distal embolization. At a mean follow-up of 9 months, 3 patients had required reinterventional procedures and 1 patient had undergone CABG. No AMI or death occurred during this period. Preliminary clinical experience with a 60-mm–long angioplasty balloon to treat complicated coronary lesions in high-risk patients suggests that when used alone or in combination with other devices, this new balloon results in high initial success and low complication rates.

Gender Bias?

It has been suggested that women with CAD are less likely to be referred for coronary angiography and CABG than men. Bell and colleagues[107] from Rochester, Minnesota, evaluated whether a referral bias exists once angiography has been performed. They retrospectively analyzed over 22 000 patients with suspected CAD who underwent angiography between 1981 and 1991 and compared the numbers of women and men who underwent either CABG or PTCA within 30 days of coronary angiography. More women tended to have PTCA but fewer had CABG than men. When the 2 revascularization strategies were considered together, however, there was no significant gender difference. These authors concluded that once diagnostic coronary angiography had been performed, no major differences in the overall utilization of revascularization procedures were noted for women compared with men.

In-Laboratory Closure

Abdelmeguid and colleagues[108] in Cleveland, Ohio, studied 4863 consecutive patients who underwent successful PCTA or directional coronary atherectomy. Eighty-eight patients who had an uncomplicated, successfully reversed transient in-laboratory vessel closure (group 2) were compared with 4775 patients who had a successful procedure not associated with transient in-laboratory closure (group 1). Clinical follow-up was available in 4839 patients (99.5%) with a mean duration of 41 months. Survival analysis demonstrated that successfully treated, uncomplicated transient vessel closure itself does not have an adverse effect on long-term prognosis, including death, AMI, or need for repeat coronary intervention. However, when the procedure, angioplasty or atherectomy, was associated with an increase in creatine kinase-MB, there was a significant adverse effect on long-term outcome. By multivariate logistic regression, an increase in postprocedure creatine kinase-MB was the most significant predictor of cardiac death and of major ischemic complication, including AMI or need for future coronary intervention on follow-up. Thus, transient, uncomplicated in-laboratory vessel closure itself does not have an adverse long-term effect unless there is an associated increase in creatine kinase-MB isoenzyme. An increase in creatine kinase-MB isoenzyme is associated with an adverse event on prognosis.

Abrupt closure with coronary angioplasty has been associated with an adverse outcome. The results from the Coronary Angioplasty Versus Excisional Atherectomy Trial (CAVEAT) I, a randomized trial of PTCA versus directional coronary atherectomy, were analyzed.[109] This multicenter trial enrolled more than 1000 patients. Abrupt closure occurred in 60 patients (5.9%) and was associated with a significantly longer hospital stay. Abrupt closure was associated with a marked increase in subsequent complications (AMI, 47% vs. 2%; emergency CABG, 38% vs. 0.3%; deaths, 33% vs. 0%) and occurred more frequently in the directional coronary atherectomy group (8% vs. 3.8%). These authors concluded that abrupt closure remains the principal determinant of adverse outcome after PTCA. Although abrupt closure is more common with directional atherectomy than angioplasty, the results are similar.

Danchin and colleagues[110] from Vandoeuvre-les-Nancy, France, compared the incidence and management of acute closure complicating PTCA in three historic populations of patients having undergone the procedure at the same center: group 1 (n = 146 of 881; early years of angioplasty, 1980 to 1986), group 2 (n = 113 of 1781; bailout stenting learning curve, 1990 to 1992), and group 3 (n = 34 of 525; 1993). The incidence of acute closure decreased from group 1 (146 [17%] of 881) to groups 2 and 3 (147 [6%] of 2306). Management of the occlusion changed over the years, with less emergency CABG (52 [36%] of 146, 15 [13%] of 113, and 3 [9%] of 34, respectively), and more repeat PTCA (70 [48%] of 146, 87 [78%] of 113, and 30 [88%] of 34, respectively). The use of prolonged inflations (>10 minutes) and stenting increased from group 2 (15 [13%] of 113 and 16 [14%] of 113, respectively) to group 3 (12 [35%] of 34, and 10 [30%] of 34, respectively). In-hospital death occurred in 18 (12%) of 146, 7 (6%) of 113, and 2 (6%) of 34 patients in the three groups. AMI decreased from 64% to 46% and 27%, respectively. Overall, the number of patients free of events at hospital discharge increased from 38 (26%) of 146 to 53 (47%) of 113 and to 23 (68%) of 34. In group 3, 80% of the patients treated with prolonged balloon inflations or stenting were free of events compared with 50% of the others. Improvement in the management of acute occlusion complicating PTCA results from increased experience in this difficult setting and also from the use of new angioplasty techniques such as bailout stenting or prolonged balloon inflations.

Platelet IIb/IIIa Inhibition Therapy

The activated clotting time has been used during PTCA to monitor the extent of thrombin inhibition and anticoagulation from heparin in an attempt to minimize untoward thrombotic events and hemorrhagic complications. With the introduction of potent platelet inhibitors, such as the chimeric monoclonal antibody c7E3, to interventional cardiology, the utility of measuring and regulating procedural activated clotting time has not been examined. To investigate the possible influence of platelet IIb/IIIa antagonism on procedural activated clotting time, Moliterno and coworkers[111] in Cleveland, Ohio, reviewed data from the Evaluation of c7E3 Fab in the Prevention of Ischemic Complications (EPIC) trial. In this trial, 2099 patients undergoing PTCA with a high risk of abrupt vessel closure were randomly assigned to receive placebo or the IIb/IIIa platelet receptor antagonist c7E3 Fab. Despite receiving less procedural heparin, and fewer patients receiving very high heparin doses (>14 000 U) than the placebo, those receiving c7E3 Fab had a higher mean (401 vs. 367 seconds) activated clotting time when corrected for body weight. The activated clotting time is increased approximately 35 seconds by the platelet IIb/IIIa receptor antagonist c7E3 Fab. This has important implications for dosing conjunctive heparin therapy and performing PTCA or directional coronary atherectomy in the setting of IIb/IIIa-directed therapy.

Tcheng and colleagues[112] determined whether Integrelin, a synthetic cyclic heptapeptide with high affinity and marked specificity for platelet integrin glycoprotein IIb/IIIa, effectively blocks ADP-induced platelet aggregation. One hundred fifty patients undergoing elective PTCA were evaluated with random assignment made to one of three treatment regimens: placebo; a 90 µg/kg bolus of Integrelin before angioplasty followed by a 1 µg/kg per minute infusion of Integrelin for 4 hours; or a 90 µg/kg bolus followed by a 1 µg/kg per minute infusion of Integrelin for 12 hours. Patients were followed to 30 days for the composite occurrence of AMI, stent placement, repeat urgent or emergent PTCA or CABG, or death. Administration of a 90 µg/kg bolus of Integrelin achieved an 86% inhibition of platelet aggregation that was maintained by a 1.0 µg/kg per minute infusion. There was a trend toward reduction in end-point events from 12% for placebo to 10% for 4-hour infusion to 4% for 12-hour infusion, although these differences were not statistically significant for the 12-hour group compared with placebo. Major bleeding occurred in 8%, 8%, and 2% of patients, whereas minor bleeding was observed in 14%, 33%, and 47% of patients, respectively. There was no difference in bleeding index among groups defined as a change in hematocrit divided by 3 plus red blood cell units transfused. Thus, these data suggest that during routine, elective, low- and high-risk coronary intervention, the Integrelin may provide some efficacy in preventing untoward clinical events.

Aguirre and colleagues[113] for the EPIC investigators reviewed the bleeding complications and described clinical and procedural variables associated with increased bleeding following the administration of a chimeric antibody to the platelet glycoprotein IIb/IIIa receptors. In this study, the periprocedural use of aspirin, heparin, and the chimeric antibody c7E3 Fab in 2099 patients reduced postprocedural ischemic complications and 6-month clinical evidence of restenosis, but was also associated with increased procedural bleeding complications. Patients with high-risk clinical or lesion morphologic characteristics were randomly to receive placebo bolus plus placebo infusion, c7E3 Fab bolus plus placebo infusion, or c7E3 Fab bolus and c7E3 Fab infusion. All patients received periprocedural aspirin and intravenous heparin continued for a minimum of 12 hours after the procedure. The need for transfusions, decreased hemoglobin, and an index including both variables were used in these evaluations. Major bleeding complications unrelated to CABG occurred in 3%, 9% and 11% and blood product transfusions were used in 8%, 14%, and 17% of patients treated with placebo, bolus 7E3 Fab, and bolus plus infusion 7E3 Fab, respectively. Most bleeding complications occurred at the femoral access site regardless of treatment. Intracranial hemorrhage (0.3%) and death (0.09%) attributable to major bleeding complications were rare. Multivariable regression analyses identified several variables as being related to major bleeding complications or greater blood loss, including greater age, female sex, lower weight, c7E3 Fab therapy, and duration and complexity of the index procedure. Major bleeding complications and blood loss in patients receiving bolus plus infusion 7E3 Fab were not significantly greater than in those receiving bolus therapy alone. Thus, bleeding complications unrelated to CABG were 2 to 3 times more frequent in patients receiving c7E3 Fab than in those receiving placebo, but most bleeding was transient and well tolerated.

Treatment with Bivalirudin (Hirulog) Afterwards

Bittl and associates[114] for the Hirulog Angioplasty Study Investigators studied whether closure of dilated coronary arteries at sites of coronary angioplasty could be prevented when the direct thrombin inhibitor bivalirudin (hirulog) was used in place of heparin. The authors performed a double-blind, randomized trial in 4098 patients undergoing coronary angioplasty for unstable or postmyocardial infarction angina. Patients were assigned to receive either heparin or bivalirudin immediately before angioplasty. The primary end point was death in the hospital, AMI, abrupt vessel closure, or rapid clinical deterioration of cardiac origin. In the total study group, bivalirudin did not significantly reduce the incidence of the primary end point (11.4% vs. 12.2% for heparin) but did result in a lower incidence of bleeding (3.8% vs. 9.8%). In the prospectively stratified subgroup of 704 patients with postinfarction angina, bivalirudin therapy resulted in a lower incidence of the primary end point (9.1% vs. 14.2%) and a lower incidence of bleeding (3.0% vs. 11.1%), but in a similar cumulative rate of death, AMI, and repeated revascularization in the 6 months after angioplasty (20.5% vs. 25.1%). Bivalirudin was at least as effective as high-dose heparin in preventing ischemic complications in patients who underwent angioplasty for unstable angina, and it carried a lower risk of bleeding. Bivalirudin, as compared with heparin, reduced the risk of immediate ischemic complications in patients with postinfarction angina, but this difference was no longer apparent after 6 months.

Novel Hemostatic Device

Cardiac catheterization procedures are associated with the risk of complications at the arterial access site. Kussmaul and colleagues[115] for a multicenter group evaluated the safety and efficacy of a novel bioabsorbable hemostatic puncture closure device deployed through an arterial sheath. In a randomized multicenter trial in 435 patients undergoing cardiac catheterization or PTCA at eight participating centers, hemostasis was achieved with the device in 218 patients; 217 patients were assigned to the manual pressure control group. Time to hemostasis was considerably shorter in the device group (2.5 vs. 15.3 min). The deployment success rate for the device was 96%, and 76% of this group experienced immediate hemostasis. Complication rates were lower in the device group for bleeding, hematoma, and occurrence of any complication. Ultrasound follow-up studies 60 days after device deployment revealed complete absorption of the device in all cases. These authors concluded that the sheath-deployed, bioabsorbable device provided a safe and effective means of obtaining rapid arterial hemostasis after cardiac catheterization procedures. It appears to be particularly useful in those patients most at risk for access site complications.

Intravascular Ultrasonic Findings Afterwards

van der Lugt and coinvestigators[116] in Rotterdam, the Netherlands, investigated whether vascular damage and quantitative changes observed with intravascular ultrasound at the most stenotic site are representative of the ultimate outcome after coronary balloon angioplasty. Atherosclerotic coronary arteries (n= 40) were studied in vitro with intravascular ultrasound. From each vascular specimen, 10 corresponding intravascular ultrasound cross-sections obtained before and after balloon angioplasty were selected for comparison with their histological counterpart. Morphologic and quantitative data obtained from all cross sections were compared with data derived from the most stenotic site. The incidence of vascular damage (dissection, plaque rupture, and media rupture) at the most stenotic site was lower than that seen for each vascular specimen. The sensitivity of intravascular ultrasound in detecting these morphologic features for each vascular specimen was higher for dissection and media rupture (79% and 76%, respectively) and low for plaque rupture (37%). After balloon angioplasty, quantitative changes seen at the most stenotic site were greater than those in all cross-sections: free lumen area +58% vs. +29%, media bound area +17% vs. +12%, and plaque area reduction −9% vs. −6%, respectively. The increase in free lumen area was caused predominantly by media bound area increase (81%) and to a less extent by plaque area decrease (19%). This study revealed that a higher incidence of vascular damage is found when the whole segment is analyzed rather than one single cross-section at the most stenotic site. Quantitative effects of coronary balloon angioplasty seen with intravascular ultrasound were greater at the most stenotic site than in all cross-sections.

In-Hospital Costs

Ellis and colleagues[117] at the Cleveland Clinic analyzed 65 clinical, angiographic, physician, and outcome variables as potential correlates of total cost, including hospital and physician costs. Information was obtained from a consecutive series of 1258 procedures with attempted percutaneous transluminal coronary revascularization. Direct and indirect costs, for both hospital and physician, were determined on the basis of resource utilization using "top-down" methodology and were available for 1237 procedures in 1086 patients. Mean patient age was 62 years, 76% were male, 3% had AMI, 71% had unstable angina, 58% had

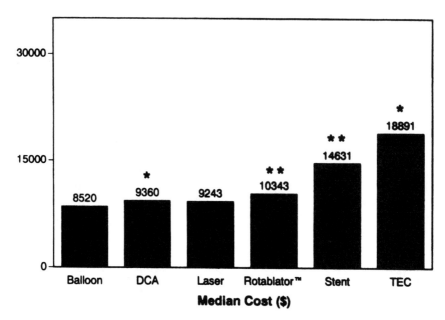

FIGURE 2-24. Bar graph showing median unadjusted in-hospital costs for patients treated with the devices noted. $*P \leq 0.05$, $**P \leq 0.01$ compared with balloon angioplasty in multivariate modeling. DCA indicates directional coronary atherectomy; TEC, transluminal extraction coronary atherectomy. Reproduced with permission of Ellis et al.[117]

multivessel CAD, and mean LVEF was 54%. Twenty-six percent of the patients had at least one nonballoon revascularization device used, and median length of hospital stay was 4 days. Procedural success was obtained in 89% of patients and major complications, including death, CABG, or Q-wave AMI, occurred in 4%. Median cost was $9176, but it was asymmetrically distributed and the inter-quartile and total ranges were wide ($7333 to $13 845 and $3422 to $193 474, respectively) (Figure 2-24). Analyses of independent correlates of cost and $\log_e$ (cost) were performed using multivariate linear regression in training and test populations. Modeling found 15 independent preprocedural correlations of $\log_e$ (cost). Preprocedural variables most predictive of $\log_e$ (cost) included presentation with AMI, decision delay, weekend delay, use of IABP, intention to start, creatinine ≥ 2 mg/dL, and lesion complexity (Table 2-10).

Relation Between Procedure Volume and Length of Hospital Stay, and Complications

Wolfe and colleagues[118] identified factors responsible for prolonged hospital stay after PTCA in 591 consecutive patients undergoing PTCA at 9 medical centers in North America. Major or minor complications occurred in 91 patients (15%) and were observed to be related to several baseline characteristics, including unstable angina, multivessel CAD, patient age, and lesion complexity. Compared with a median length of hospital stay of 2 days after PTCA for the entire cohort of patients, the length of stay was increased in patients with unstable angina, multivessel CAD, age >65 years, complex lesions, and filling defects. Length of stay was more strikingly increased in patients who had major or minor PTCA complications, including emergent CABG, Q-wave or non–Q-wave

Table 2-10. Cost Effects of Preintervention and Postintervention Risk Factors Including Delays but Not Including Total Length of Stay (n = 1214)

	Cost Effect, %	95% CI	*P*
Rise in creatinine ≥1 mg%	88	(64, 114)	<0.001
Urgent CABG	83	(59, 112)	<0.001
Blood product transfusion	64	(52, 77)	<0.001
Decision delay	61	(43, 81)	<0.001
Q-wave MI	57	(38, 77)	0.002
Weekend delay	52	(35, 70)	<0.001
Acute MI	51	(35, 68)	<0.001
IABP use	42	(19, 71)	<0.001
TEC	40	(11, 77)	0.004
Procedure failed without complications	34	(19, 51)	<0.001
Noncardiac death	32	(2, 71)	0.032
Non-Q-wave MI	29	(18, 41)	<0.001
Rotablator	25	(14, 36)	<0.001
Stent	25	(14, 37)	<0.001
Hematoma	23	(12, 35)	<0.001
Recent MI	20	(13, 27)	<0.001
Heparin use before intervention	15	(9, 21)	<0.001
Diabetes	12	(5, 19)	<0.001
Perfusion balloon	12	(−5, 33)	0.173
DCA	10	(4, 16)	0.002
Laser	7	(−6, 21)	0.338
Hospital transfer	7	(2, 13)	0.008
Per unit lesion complexity score	7	(3, 10)	<0.001
Per diseased vessel	7	(4, 9)	0.002
Hospital transfer and weekend delay	−23	(−33, −11)	<0.001

CABG indicates coronary artery bypass graft surgery; MI, myocardial infarction; IABP, intra-aortic balloon pump; TEC, transluminal extraction catheter; and DCA, directional coronary atherectomy.

End point is $\log_e$(cost). R^2 = 0.65. Postprocedural variables not independently correlated with $\log_e$ (cost): arteriovenous fistula, physician/interventionalist, pseudoaneurysm, retroperitoneal hemorrhage, stroke.

Reproduced with permission of Ellis et al.[117]

AMI, transfusion unrelated to CABG, or abrupt vessel closure. On stepwise multiple linear regression, PTCA complications appeared to be the greatest predictors of length of hospital stay. Thus, although PTCA complications were correlated with baseline variables, including unstable angina, multivessel CAD, advanced age, complex lesions, and filling defects, excess length of stay after PTCA was most strongly influenced by the development of minor and major PTCA complications. In patients with several baseline risk factors, there was a significantly prolonged hospitalization.

To assess the relation between the volume of PTCAs performed in a cardiac catheterization laboratory and major complications after adjusting for case mix, Kimmel and associates[119] from Philadelphia, Pennsylvania, analyzed 19 594 consecutive patients without an AMI undergoing a first PTCA. There was a significant decrease in the rates of in-hospital mortality, emergency CABG, and major complications (defined as 1 of these 3 complications) with increasing cardiac catheterization volume (Figure 2-25). After adjustment for case mix using multivariable analyses, these associations persisted. There was no significant difference in outcomes in laboratories performing at least 200 vs. fewer

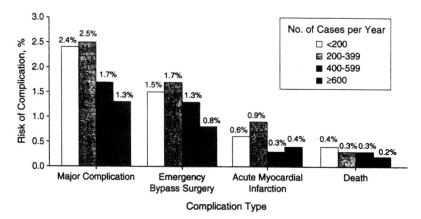

FIGURE 2-25. Rates of each complication in laboratories with different volumes of procedures. Numbers above each bar represent the rate of complications in that category of laboratory volume. P values for test for trend, $P < 0.001$ for major complications, $P < 0.001$ for emergency bypass surgery, $P = 0.001$ for acute myocardial infarction, and $P = 0.04$ for mortality. Reproduced with permission of Kimmel et al.[119]

than 200 procedures per year, the currently recommended minimal laboratory volume. A statistically significant decrease in major complications, however, was observed in laboratories performing more than 400 procedures per year vs. laboratories performing 400–599 procedures and at least 600 procedures, respectively, when compared with those laboratories performing <200 procedures per year. Thus, an inverse association between cardiac catheterization laboratory procedure volume and major complications during PTCA exists independent of differences in patients' risk profiles. These data suggest that the currently recommended minimum laboratory volume may be too low to distinguish high-risk from low-risk laboratories.

Quality of Life Afterwards

Strauss and colleagues[120] in West Roxbury, Massachusetts, reported on changes in self-assessed quality of life among patients randomly assigned to treatment by PTCA or medical therapy and related these measurements to changes in exercise performance and coronary angiograms. Patients with stable angina, a positive exercise tolerance test, and at least 70% stenosis in the proximal two thirds of one major coronary artery were randomly assigned to receive PTCA or medical therapy. Six months after randomization, each patient underwent repeat exercise testing and coronary arteriography. Before randomization and at the 6-month visit, patients completed a self-administered quality-of-life questionnaire that measured physical functioning and psychological well-being. The authors compared the changes in quality of life with changes between the baseline and 6-month exercise tests, stratified by terciles, and in patients in whom there was more or less than 2 standard deviation changes in diameter stenosis of the index lesion in the initial minus follow-up angiogram. These variables were related to changes in quality-of-life measurements. One hundred eighty-two patients with 1-vessel disease completed baseline and 6-month questionnaires. At baseline, there were no differences in any quality-of-life measurements between treatment groups. At the 6-month follow-up visit,

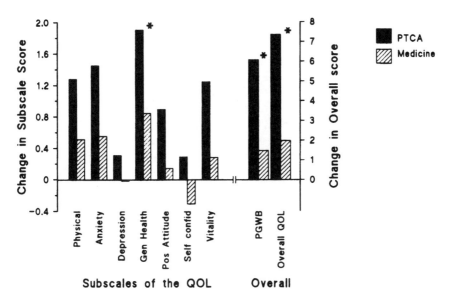

FIGURE 2-26. Bar graphs of changes in quality of life (QOL) at 6 months: individual subscales and summed mean values at 6-month follow-up minus baseline score. *P = < 0.05. PGWB indicates Psychologic General Well-Being Index; PTCA, percutaneous transluminal coronary angioplasty. Reproduced by permission of Strauss et al.[120]

there was greater improvement in both physical functioning and psychological well-being scores for patients receiving PTCA (Figure 2-26). Improvement in quality-of-life variables was noted only in patients demonstrating an increase in exercise and ability. Patients assigned to either treatment whose angiograms demonstrated >19% improvement in index lesion percent stenosis had a significant increase in the quality-of-life scores. Thus, this was the first study of the relative changes in quality-of-life measures assessed with the use of previously validated and standardized instruments in patients randomly assigned to medical therapy or treatment with PTCA. Patients assigned to receive PTCA had a significantly greater improvement in both physical and psychological measures.

Long-term Follow-up

To determine long-term angiographic prognosis after successful angioplasty (<50% residual stenosis, ≥20% reduction of stenosis, and no major complications), coronary angiography was performed by Kitazume and associates[121] from Tokyo, Japan, 2 to 4 years after angioplasty in patients who were ≤70 years old at the time of treatment and who showed patency (≤50% stenosis) 6 months after the initial procedure. Among 407 lesions that were dilated in 333 patients between 1983 and 1989, 298 (73%) lesions were reviewed by long-term angiography after 177 ± 34 weeks. At long-term follow-up, 4 (1.3%) lesions were totally occluded, 3 (1.0%) had severe stenosis (≥75% stenosis), 9 (3.0%) had mild stenosis (>50% to <75% stenosis), and 282 (95%) were patent (≤50% stenosis). The percentage of stenosis of patent lesions decreased from 24 ± 14% at 6 months to 21 ± 13% at long-term follow-up. No specific clinical or angiographic characteristics were identified in patients with severe stenosis at long-term follow-up. These findings indicate that when patency is obtained 6 months after angioplasty, a 95% long-term patency rate with regression of stenosis can be expected.

Detre and colleagues[122] for the Investigators of the National Heart, Lung, and Blood Institute's Percutaneous Transluminal Coronary Angioplasty Registry compared the effects of early and more recent management with PTCA with a 5-year follow-up of 1345 consecutive patients with their first PTCA between 1977 and 1981 (registry 1) and 2136 consecutive patients with PTCA between 1985 and 1986 (registry 2). Sixteen participating centers entered consecutive patients who had PTCA for the first time between 1977 and 1981 and between 1985 and 1986. Patients with recent AMI were excluded. Vessel disease was defined according to the CASS study. Successful dilatation required ≥20% reduction in luminal narrowing and <50% luminal diameter stenosis after intervention. Routine annual follow-up was conducted by telephone interview. Cox regression analysis to model relative risk, adjusted relative risk of events between the 2 registries, and logistic regression when the exact time of outcome was not known were used for analysis. Long-term event rates were computed by vessel disease for all patients and for the cohort of patients with initially successful PTCA. After adjustment for extent of disease, diabetes, prior CABG, hypertension, age, and sex, 5-year risk of death was similar in the 2 registry cohorts. However, the rates of AMI, CABG, and a combined outcome measure of death, AMI, and/or CABG were significantly lower in the registry 2 cohort for all patients and for patients who were initially treated successfully. Use of repeat PTCA was higher and freedom from symptoms without adverse events was better in the latter cohort. These data demonstrate that the management of the registry 2 cohort resulted in lower 5-year morbid event rates and reduced CABG operations. Mortality rates remained similar. When symptomatic status was considered in combination with events, a significantly better outcome was found overall and in the initially successful cohort. In registry 2, repeat PTCA was used with much greater frequency early after the initial procedure.

Influence of Diabetes on Outcome

Stein and colleagues[123] in Atlanta, Georgia, used data from 1133 diabetic and 9300 nondiabetic patients undergoing elective PTCA from 1980 to 1990 to evaluate outcomes in patients with diabetes mellitus. Diabetics were older and had more cardiovascular comorbidity. Insulin-requiring diabetics had diabetes for a longer duration and worse renal and ventricular function compared with non–insulin-dependent subjects. Angiographic and clinical successes after PTCA were high and similar in diabetics and nondiabetics. In-hospital major complications were infrequent with a trend toward higher death or AMI in insulin-requiring diabetics. Five-year survival and freedom from AMI were lower and CABG and additional PTCA were required more often in diabetics. In diabetics, only 36% survived free of AMI or additional revascularization compared with 53% of nondiabetics with a marked attrition in the first year after PTCA, when restenosis is most common (Figure 2-27). Using multivariate analysis, the correlates of decreased 5-year survival were patients that were older, had reduced LVEF, history of CHF, multivessel CAD, and diabetes. Insulin-receiving diabetics had a poorer long-term survival and AMI-free survival than non–insulin-receiving diabetics. PTCA in diabetics is associated with high

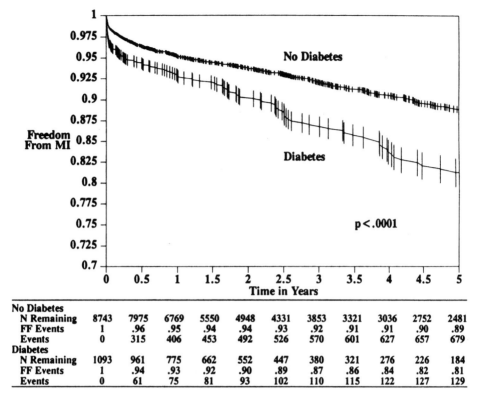

No Diabetes										
N Remaining	8743	7975	6769	5550	4948	4331	3853	3321	3036	2752	2481
FF Events	1	.96	.95	.94	.94	.93	.92	.91	.91	.90	.89
Events	0	315	406	453	492	526	570	601	627	657	679
Diabetes										
N Remaining	1093	961	775	662	552	447	380	321	276	226	184
FF Events	1	.94	.93	.92	.90	.89	.87	.86	.84	.82	.81
Events	0	61	75	81	93	102	110	115	122	127	129

FIGURE 2-27. Graph showing 5-year freedom from (FF) myocardial infarction (MI) after initial angioplasty in diabetics compared with nondiabetics. Reproduced with permission of Stein et al.[123]

success and low complication rates. Although long-term survival is acceptable, diabetics have a higher rate of future AMI and a greater need for additional revascularization procedures, probably because of early restenosis and late progression of CAD.

Restenosis

de Groote and colleagues[124] in Lille Cedex, France, identified 67 consecutive patients with unstable angina in whom 2 lesions, in different vessels, were dilated during the same procedure. They attempted to identify the relative contributions of local and systemic factors to the excess risk of restenosis by comparing changes in minimal lumen diameter and the incidence of restenosis, determined by quantitative coronary arteriography, after coronary angioplasty at culprit and nonculprit lesions dilated in the course of a single procedure in patients with unstable angina. Lesions were designated as culprit or nonculprit on the basis of the location of electrocardiographic changes during chest pain combined with assessment of the angiographic characteristics of the lesion. Using these criteria, 43 patients had identifiable culprit lesions. Stenosis severity before and immediately after PTCA and at follow-up were assessed with quantitative angiography. Angiographic follow-up was performed in 91% of these patients. Culprit lesions were more severe than nonculprit lesions. The

Table 2-11. Quantitative Angiographic Data for Study Population

	Lesion		
	Culprit	**Nonculprit**	**P**
Minimal lumen diameter, mm			
Before PTCA	0.63 ± 0.36	0.84 ± 0.35	0.02
After PTCA	1.84 ± 0.4	1.77 ± 0.45	NS
Acute gain	1.2 ± 0.5	0.9 ± 0.42	<0.01
Follow-up angiography	0.97 ± 0.64	1.42 ± 0.53	<0.01
Late loss	0.87 ± 0.75	0.33 ± 0.69	<0.01
Loss index	0.75 ± 0.6	0.37 ± 0.8	0.01
Reference diameter, mm			
Before PTCA	2.92 ± 0.73	2.75 ± 0.73	NS
After PTCA	2.92 ± 0.73	2.77 ± 0.69	NS
Follow-up angiography	2.86 ± 0.69	2.83 ± 0.68	NS
Stenosis, %			
Before PTCA	76.2 ± 13.6	69.2 ± 9.6	0.01
After PTCA	33 ± 9.96	32.1 ± 10.9	NS
Follow-up angiography	63.3 ± 23	47 ± 17.9	<0.01

PTCA indicates percutaneous transluminal coronary angioplasty.

Reproduced with permission of de Groote et al.[124]

late loss at culprit lesions was significantly greater than the equivalent value for nonculprit lesions (Table 2-11). Using a definition of >50% stenosis at follow-up to identify restenosis lesions, restenosis occurred at 67% of culprit lesions and at 32% of nonculprit lesions. The greater loss in minimal luminal diameter and the consequent higher rate of restenosis at culprit compared with nonculprit lesions suggests that local "lesion-related" factors are a more important determinant of the high rate of restenosis when PTCA is performed in patients with unstable angina.

Many interventions have been tried in an attempt to reduce restenosis after PTCA. Faxon and associates[125] evaluated the effects of the ACE-inhibitor *cilazapril* on restenosis. Patients received either 1 or 2.5 mg cilazapril after successful coronary angioplasty and 1, 5 or 10 mg twice daily for 6 months vs. matched placebo. Coronary angiograms before and after angioplasty and at 6-month follow-up were quantitatively analyzed. A total of 1436 patients with successful PTCA were recruited. Results showed no beneficial effect of cilazapril. Thus, both high and low doses of cilazapril did not prevent restenosis and did not favorably influence the overall clinical and angiographic outcome after PTCA.

Desmet and associates[126] from Leuven, Belgium, studied the diagnostic value of exercise electrocardiographic testing in 191 patients who were completely asymptomatic 6 months after a successful PTCA procedure. With >70%- and >50%-diameter stenosis at follow-up as restenosis criteria, the sensitivities of exercise electrocardiographic testing were 29% and 21%; the specificities, 89% and 91%; the positive predictive values, 20% and 52%; the negative predictive values, 93% and 70%; the accuracies, 83% and 68%; and the risk ratios, 2.8 and 1.7, for prevalence of 9% and 33%, respectively. There were no significant differences in the diagnostic value of exercise electrocardiographic testing between men and women, patients receiving or not receiving β-blocking agents, and the presence or absence of pathological Q waves. In conclusion, the diagnostic value of exercise electrocardiographic testing for silent restenosis is low, and supplementation with other techniques seems to be warranted.

Itoh and colleagues[127] in Osaka, Japan, used coronary angioscopy to determine whether the visual appearance of plaque provides new insight into the risk of restenosis after PTCA. Forty-seven patients with stable angina were studied. Angioscopy was performed before and after PTCA with a 0.68-mm angioscope and with a double-guiding catheter system. Patients who were successfully evaluated by angioscopy were divided into two groups according to the color of the lesion: group 1, mainly yellow, and group 2, white. Angiographic, angioscopic, and clinical variables in the 2 groups were compared. Detailed angioscopic findings were obtained in 36 of the 47 patients before PTCA and in 24 of the 47 patients after PTCA. Yellow plaque was found in 13 of 36 (36%). Age, sex, presence of coronary risk factors, serum cholesterol level, and duration of angina showed no correlation with plaque color. The incidence rates of dissection and thrombi after PTCA were not different. Successful dilatation was achieved in 13 of 13 patients in group 1 and in 21 of 23 patients in group 2. However, the restenosis rate of group 1 was significantly lower than in group 2 (17% vs 58%). Cox proportional hazards model revealed that plaque color was the independent variable associated with restenosis after PTCA.

Desmarais and colleagues[128] in Charlottesville, Virginia, assessed 240 consecutive patients undergoing PTCA and obtained measurements of serum lipoprotein(a), total cholesterol, triglycerides, HDL cholesterol, LDL cholesterol, apolipoprotein A-I, and apolipoprotein B-100. Patients were evaluated 4 to 6 months after PTCA for clinical recurrence by repeat angiography if angina had returned or by maximal exercise treadmill testing with thallium-201 imaging if patients remained asymptomatic. Ninety-seven patients (40%) had clinical recurrence; 143 (60%) did not. Patients with recurrence had significantly greater lipoprotein(a) concentrations compared with those without. Each patient quintile stratified by increasing lipoprotein(a) concentrations had incrementally greater recurrence rates ranging from 27% to 60%. Multivariate logistic regression analysis demonstrated that the lipoprotein(a) concentration was the only predictor of recurrence. These data suggest that an elevated lipoprotein(a) concentration is a risk factor for clinical recurrence of coronary artery narrowing after PTCA.

Violaris and colleagues[129] in Rotterdam, the Netherlands, examined long-term restenosis after successful balloon dilatation of coronary occlusions at a predetermined time interval with quantitative angiography and compared this with a control population of stenoses. The study population consisted of 2950 patients and 3583 lesions prospectively enrolled in and successfully completed four major restenosis trials. The quantitative angiographic follow-up was 86%. Cineangiographic films were processed and analyzed at a central core laboratory with the use of an automated edge detection technique. The study population compared 266 occlusions (7%) defined as total when there was absent antegrade filling beyond the lesion (109 lesions) and functional (157 lesions) when faint, late anterograde opacification of the distal segment was seen in the absence of a discernible luminal continuity. Three thousand three hundred seventeen lesions were defined as stenoses (93%). Restenosis was significantly higher after successful dilatation of occlusions than of stenoses. The restenosis rate was 45% in occlusions compared with 34% in stenoses. The absolute loss, defined as a change (in millimeters) in minimal luminal diameter between post-coronary angioplasty and follow-up was significantly greater in occlusions than in stenoses. The higher restenosis rate in the occlusion group was due predominantly to an increased number of occlusions at follow-up angiography in this group (19% vs. 5% for stenosis). Within the occlusion group, there were no significant differences in long-term outcome between total and functional occlusions. These data indicate that successfully dilated coronary occlusions, both total and functional, have a higher rate of angiographic restenosis at 6 months than stenoses. This appears to be primarily due to a higher rate of occlusion at follow-up angiography in this group of lesions.

Montalescot and colleagues[130] in Paris, France, studied 107 consecutive patients undergoing PTCA and measured plasma levels of t-PA, plasminogen activator inhibitor (PAI-1), von Willebrand factor, and fibrinogen before and immediately after PTCA and at a 6-month follow-up. Individual changes of intraluminal diameter were measured by quantitative coronary arteriography and patients were classified into four definitions of restenosis: (1) a final stenosis >50%; (2) a loss of minimal luminal diameter during the follow-up period greater than the measured variability in the laboratory (>0.52 mm); (3) a loss of at least 50% of the gain in luminal diameter achieved by PTCA; and (4) the combination of definitions 1 and 2. Angiographic follow-up was obtained in 92% of patients with a primary success of PTCA. Global restenosis rates were 38%, 43%, 48%, and 30% for definitions 1 through 4, respectively. Plasma levels of t-PA and PAI-1 were not associated with any of the four definitions of restenosis. Multivariate analysis demonstrated that von Willebrand factor measured immediately after PTCA predicted restenosis according to definitions 2 and 3. Fibrinogen measured within 6 months of follow-up was significantly increased in all restenosis groups for 4 definitions. Patients with a fibrinogen concentration >3.5 g/L at follow-up had higher restenosis rates than patients with a concentration <3.5 g/L. The measurements of fibrinogen and von Willebrand factor levels were made from platelet-poor plasma obtained after centrification of a peripheral blood sample for 20 minutes at 10°C. Fibrinogen was measured by a thrombin time method; von Willebrand factor levels were measured with a commercial kit. Loss index was lower and the net gain higher in patients with a fibrinogen level <3.5 g/L. There was a significant correlation between fibrinogen level and angiographic loss index. Multivariate analysis confirmed that the fibrinogen level predicted restenosis for all definitions. Thus, there is an independent relation between von Willebrand factor measured immediately after PTCA and restenosis. In this study, an elevated plasma fibrinogen level during follow-up was a strong biochemical predictor of restenosis after PTCA.

Angiopeptin, a somatostatin analogue, inhibits intimal hyperplasia after PTCA in several animal models. This pilot study by Eriksen and associates[131] from Aarhus, Gentofte, Copenhagen, and Odense, Denmark; Gothenburg, Sweden; Washington, D.C.; and Boston, Massachusetts, sought to determine the effect of subcutaneous infusion of angiopeptin on clinical events and restenosis in patients undergoing successful PTCA. One hundred twelve patients were randomly assigned to receive continuous subcutaneous angiopeptin (750 μg/d) or placebo infusion from the day before PTCA and for the following 4 days in a double-blind study. An additional subcutaneous injection of 375 μg angiopeptin or saline was given immediately before PTCA. Eighty patients had a successful PTCA, and 75 of these patients with 94 lesions underwent angiography 6 ± 2 months after PTCA. All 112 patients underwent a 12-month clinical follow-up examination. Age, sex, smoking, diabetes, hypertension, hyperlipidemia, and morphologic features of stenosis were similar in both groups. The hierarchical 12-month event rate (death, AMI, CABG, and repeated PTCA) was reduced from 34% to 25% by angiopeptin by intention-to-treat analysis. Restenosis (≥50% diameter stenosis) was significantly reduced in lesions treated with angiopeptin (12% vs. 40%). Late lumen loss also was significantly reduced after angiopeptin treatment (0.12 ± 0.46 vs. 0.52 ± 0.64 mm). In conclusion, continuous subcutaneous angiopeptin infusion for 5 days tended to decrease clinical events and restenosis after PTCA.

Serrruys and associates[132] for the Helvetica Investigators studied whether hirudin, a highly selective inhibitor of thrombin with irreversible effects would prevent restenosis after coronary angioplasty. The authors randomly assigned 1141 patients with unstable angina who were scheduled for coronary angioplasty to receive 1 of 3 regimens: 1) a bolus dose of 10 000 IU of heparin followed by an intravenous infusion of heparin for 24 hours and subcutaneous placebo twice daily for 3 days (382 patients), 2) a bolus dose of 40 mg hirudin followed by an intravenous infusion of hirudin for 24 hours and subcutaneous placebo twice daily for 3 days (381 patients), or 3) the same hirudin regimen except that 40 mg hirudin was given subcutaneously instead of placebo twice daily for 3 days (378 patients). The primary end point was event-free survival at 7 months. Other end points were early cardiac events (within 96 hours), bleeding and other complications of the study treatment, and angiographic measurements of coronary diameter at 6 months of follow-up. At 7 months, event-free survival was 67.3% in the group receiving heparin, 63.5% in the group receiving intravenous hirudin, and 68.0% in the group receiving both intravenous and subcutaneous hirudin. However, the administration of hirudin was associated with a significant reduction in early cardiac events, which occurred in 11.0%, 7.9%, and 5.6% of patients in the respective groups (combined relative risk with hirudin, 0.61). The mean minimal luminal diameters in the respective groups on follow-up angiography at 6 months were 1.54, 1.47, and 1.56 mm. Although significantly fewer early cardiac events occurred with hirudin than with heparin, hirudin had no apparent benefit with longer-term follow-up.

The SHARP trial was undertaken to determine whether 12 500 IU of unfractionated heparin given subcutaneously twice daily for 4 months after PTCA could influence the subsequent rate of angiographic restenosis and the incidence of clinical events.[133] Three hundred thirty-nine patients were randomly assigned to receive heparin or no heparin. Repeat catheterization was performed in 90% of randomized patients. Results showed that long-term treatment with high-dose subcutaneous heparin for 4 months did not favorably influence angiographic or clinical outcome after PTCA.

Bauters and colleagues[134] in Lille Cedex, France, studied 117 consecutive patients who underwent successful PTCA and who had coronary angioscopy before and immediately after the procedure. The angioscopic evaluation attempted to determine whether there were morphologic features that predict subsequent restenosis. Angiographic follow-up was performed in 99 (85%) of the patients. The relation between angioscopic variables at the time of PTCA and the occurrence of restenosis was assessed by quantitative coronary arteriography. Plaque shape and color had no effect on late loss and luminal diameter. However, a protruding thrombus at the PTCA site was associated with significantly greater loss in luminal diameter. Dissection assessed by angioscopy immediately after PTCA had no effect on late loss and luminal diameter. These results indicate that coronary angioscopy may be helpful in predicting the risk of restenosis after PTCA. The high rate of angiographic recurrence observed when PTCA is performed at thrombus-containing lesions supports a role for thrombus in the process of luminal renarrowing after PTCA.

To evaluate serum levels of lipoprotein(a) as a predictor of restenosis after PTCA, Yamamoto and colleagues[135] from Hiroshima, Japan, evaluated 71 patients who underwent elective single-vessel angioplasty. Patients were divided into 2 groups according to the presence (n = 24 [34%]; group R) or absence (n = 47 [66%]; group N) of restenosis. Serum insulin levels were similar before and after the glucose challenge test in both groups. The median level of serum lipoprotein(a) was 35 mg/dL in group R compared with 19 mg/dL in group N. The frequency of the apo E4 allele was 4 (17%) in group R and 4 (9%) in group N. The incidence of restenosis was significantly higher in patients with lipoprotein(a) levels ≥30 mg/dL than in those with lipoprotein(a) levels <30 mg/dL (65% vs. 26%). These results indicate that a serum lipoprotein(a) level ≥30 mg/dL is a risk factor for restenosis.

Directional Coronary Atherectomy

Coronary embolization is a complication of coronary intervention procedures. In this study by Waksmann and associates[136] from Atlanta, Georgia, the incidence, predictors, and clinical significance of coronary embolization during directional atherectomy were examined in 111 consecutive patients who underwent directional atherectomy to 120 lesions. Distal embolization occurred in 31 (28%) of the patients. It was noted mainly in the saphenous vein graft group of patients (12 [48%] of 25) vs. the native coronary group (19 [22%] of 86). Clinical predictors were age and de novo lesions. Morphologic predictors were larger artery size, larger postprocedure minimal luminal diameter, calcific lesions, and type C lesions. The only difference in clinical outcome was a longer hospitalization in the distal embolization group with 3.9 ± 3.7 days vs. the rest of the patients 2.4 ± 2.4 days. In the majority of patients there was no significant adverse clinical outcome.

Arbustini and colleagues[137] in Pavia, Italy, investigated the incidence of the histopathological lesions and of growth factor expression in a consecutive series of directional coronary atherectomy samples from 40 unstable angina pectoris patients without prior AMI and compared the findings with those obtained in directional coronary atherectomy samples from 18 patients with stable angina without previous infarction and 18 patients with restenosis. The group investigated coronary thrombosis, neointimal hyperplasia, and inflammation. For unstable angina, they correlated the angiographic Ambrose plaque subtypes with the histopathological findings. The immunophenotype of plaque cells and the growth factor expression were assessed with specific antibodies for cell characterization and for the expression of basic fibroblast and platelet-derived AA and AB growth factors and receptors. The incidence of coronary thrombosis was 35% in patients with unstable angina, 17% in those with stable angina, and 11% in patients with restenosis. Neointimal hyperplasia was found in 38% of unstable angina cases, in 17% of stable angina cases, and in 83% of restenosis cases. Inflammation without thrombus or accelerated progression occurred in 20% of unstable angina and 6% of stable angina samples. In 52% of unstable angina cases, inflammation coexisted with thrombosis and/or neointimal hyperplasia. In the unstable angina group, 71% of all plaques with thrombus had a corresponding angiographic pattern of complicated lesions. The growth factor expression, reported as percentage of cells immunostaining with different growth factor antibodies, was highest in restenosis, followed by unstable angina and stable angina lesions. The investigators concluded that inflammation, thrombosis, and neointimal hyperplasia likely constitute the pathological substrates of increasing coronary obstruction that causes unstable angina. Further studies are vital to elucidate whether accelerated progression results from organizing thrombosis, from inflammatory cell-derived growth factors, or from both and the extent to which inflammation and thrombosis exert reciprocal influences.

Elliott and colleagues[138] at the Cleveland Clinic, St. Elizabeth's Hospital in Boston, Massachusetts, Emory University School of Medicine in Atlanta, Georgia, and Duke University Medical Center in Durham, North Carolina, examined whether directional atherectomy results in a favorable long-term outlook compared with PTCA in 1012 patients enrolled in the CAVEAT I trial. The patients were followed for at least 1 year after randomization. Analyses of predetermined end points were performed, including a detailed analysis of the 14 patients who died. At 1 year, 11 patients had died in the atherectomy group compared with 3 in the PTCA group (2% vs. 0.6%) with an excess of out-of-hospital deaths (2% vs. 0.2%) and late cardiac deaths (2% vs. 0%) (Table 2-12). Univariate predictors of death included age, abrupt closure, periprocedural enzyme elevation, and peripheral vascular complications. There was no evidence that the excess of death after atherectomy was linked to perforation, ectasia, or deep resection. Cumulative rates of AMI were higher in those who had been randomly assigned to atherectomy than in those randomly assigned to PTCA (9% vs. 4%) with a trend toward excess Q wave and non–Q wave AMI. By multivariate analysis, atherectomy was the only variable predictive of the combined end point of death or AMI. No clinical or angiographic characteristics enhanced this insight. Rates of repeat percutaneous intervention at the target site were 24% after atherectomy and 26% after PTCA and for CABG 9% after atherectomy vs. 9% after PTCA, respectively. Rehospitalization and stroke were not significantly different between the two groups. Thus, in the long-term follow-up of the 1012 patients randomly assigned to atherectomy or PTCA, there was a statistically significant excess of death after directional atherectomy that was not evident at 6 months. This raises concern about atherectomy as an interventional procedure and suggests the need to improve the safety of this procedure further.

Balloon angioplasty of ostial coronary artery lesions has been associated with a lower procedural success rate and a higher rate of complications and of restenosis than angioplasty of nonostial stenoses. Directional coronary atherectomy has been proposed as an alternative therapy for ostial lesions. In the CAVEAT I trial, 1012 patients were randomly assigned to undergo either procedure.[139] 563 patients had proximal LAD lesions, of which 74 were ostial. Direc-

TABLE 2-12. One-Year Cumulative* Event Rates in CAVEAT I

	Atherectomy n (%)	Angioplasty n (%)	P
Death	11 (2.2)	3 (0.6)	0.035
MI			
Q wave	15(2.9)	6(1.2)	0.053
Non–Q wave	30 (5.9)	16(3.2)	0.041
Total	45 (8.9)	22 (4.4)	0.005
Coronary bypass surgery	47 (9.3)	45 (9.1)	0.862
Repeat target lesion percutaneous intervention	123 (24.4)	129 (25.9)	0.467
Stroke	5 (1.0)	5 (1.0)	0.978
Hospitalization	251 (50)	232 (47.1)	0.584
Composite end points			
Death or MI	53(10.4)	23 (4.6)	<0.001
Death, MI, bypass surgery, or target lesion intervention	186 (36.5)	168 (33.9)	0.324
Death, MI, bypass surgery, or percutaneous intervention	216 (42.4)	193 (38.7)	0.223

MI indicates myocardial infarction.

Values are given as numbers (percentage). Rates were calculated using Kaplan-Meier survival techniques, with P value based on log rank test.

*Each patient may have more than one different event.

Reproduced by permission of Elliott et al.[138]

tional atherectomy led to an initially higher gain in minimum lumen diameter for ostial lesions (1.13 vs. 0.56 mm) but a higher rate of non–Q wave myocardial infarction (24% vs. 13%) than balloon angioplasty. There was no improvement in restenosis rates (average 47%). In nonostial proximal LAD lesions, angiographic restenosis was reduced (51% vs. 66%), but this was also associated with a high rate of periprocedural MI (8% vs. 2%). There was no difference in the need for subsequent CABG or repeat PTCA. These authors concluded that for ostial LAD stenoses, both procedures yielded similar rates of initial success and restenosis, but atherectomy was associated with more non–Q wave AMI. The predominant angiographic benefit of atherectomy occurred in proximal nonostial lesions of the LAD coronary artery but the tradeoff was more in-hospital MIs and no decrease in clinical restenosis.

The rate of restenosis after directional coronary atherectomy is higher than expected. To elucidate why, the current study by Nakamura and associates[140] from Irvine, California, used intravascular ultrasound imaging to investigate the mechanism of directional coronary atherectomy. To determine the accuracy of the measurement of plaque removal by intravascular ultrasound, directional coronary atherectomy was performed in 8 human atherosclerotic artery segments. The volume of removed plaque was measured by water displacement and was compared with the volume calculated from intravascular ultrasound images. A clinical study of directional coronary atherectomy was performed in 32 lesions; intravascular ultrasound was performed in 28 lesions after successful directional coronary atherectomy. Measurements of lumen dimensions from digital angiograms before and after directional coronary atherectomy were compared with observations of lumen and plaque size from the cross-sectional intravascular ultrasound images. In the vessel segment study, the mean plaque volume removed by directional coronary atherectomy was 19.9 ± 8.5 μL. The calculated estimate of removed plaque volume by intravascular ultrasound was 18.6 ± 7.9 μL and correlated closely with the volume by water displacement. The calculated volume of plaque removed from histological sections was 14 ± 6.0 μL and was linearly correlated with plaque volume by water displacement. In the clinical study, the angiographic mean minimum lumen diameter increased from 1.0 ± 0.4 to 2.7 ± 0.5 mm and the percentage stenosis decreased from 70% to 19%. The intravascular ultrasound images before and after directional coronary atherectomy showed that the lumen directional coronary atherectomy improved from 2.9 ± 1.5 to 7.0 ± 1.5 mm². In addition, the vessel cross-sectional area increased from 17 ± 5.9 to 19 ± 5.5 mm². The atheroma cross-sectional area was reduced from 14 ± 5.0 to 12 ± 4.8 mm². This combined effect of reduction in atheroma cross-sectional area and stretching of the outer vessel diameter resulted in an improvement in percentage plaque area stenosis from 83 ± 7% to 61 ± 9%. It is concluded that despite a successful angiographic appearance, directional coronary atherectomy removed an average of 2.5 mm² from the atheroma, which corresponds to only 18% of the atheroma cross-sectional area. The total lumen cross-sectional area increased 4.1 mm²; 61% of the new lumen was created by cutting and removal of plaque, whereas 39% of the new lumen was made by stretching the external wall of the artery. Despite an excellent angiographic result, intravascular ultrasound imaging reveals that after directional coronary atherectomy a significant amount of residual atheroma remains. As in balloon dilatation, a stretching effect is a significant component of directional coronary atherectomy.

In this report by Farb and associates[141] from Washington, DC, the coronary arteries and myocardium from two patients who died after coronary rotational atherectomy were analyzed to gain insights into the mechanisms of lumen enlargement and to document embolization of calcified plaque. Rotational atherectomy resulted in sharp cuts in plaque, producing a relatively smooth luminal surface. When extensive nodular calcific atherosclerosis was present, the luminal surface was focally uneven with exposure of jagged calcified plaque to blood flow. Deep plaque fissures and medial dissections were also seen. These fissures may have been created by the rotoblator or by adjunctive balloon angioplasty. Multiple calcific atheroemboli were present after rotoblator use in plaques containing extensive nodular calcification; in moderately calcified plaque only one small atheroembolus was found. Thus, embolization of calcified plaque can occur after rotational atherectomy and may correlate with the severity of plaque calcification. Rotational atherectomy produces a focally smooth, sharp-edged, luminal surface, a lumen enlargement mechanism different from balloon angioplasty.

Umans and associates[142] from Rotterdam, the Netherlands, used the complementary information of angiography, intravascular ultrasound, and intracoronary angioscopy before and after directional atherectomy to characterize the postatherectomy appearance of vessel wall contours and the mechanisms of lumen enlargement. Directional coronary atherectomy aims at debulking rather than dilating a coronary artery lesion. The selective removal of the plaque may potentially minimize the vessel wall damage and lead to subsequent better late outcome. Whether plaque removal is the main mechanism of action can only be assessed indirectly by angiography and warrants further investigation with detailed analysis of luminal changes and vessel wall damage by ultrasound and direct visualization with angioscopy. Twenty-six patients were investigated by quantitative angiography, intravascular ultrasound, and intracoronary angioscopy (n = 19) before and after atherectomy. In addition, all retrieved specimens were microscopically examined. Ultrasound imaging showed an increase in lumen area from 1.95 ± 0.70 to 7.86 ± 2.16 mm^2 at atherectomy. The achieved gain mainly resulted from plaque removal because plaque plus media area decreased from 18.2 ± 4.47 to 13.1 ± 3.10 mm^2. Vessel wall stretching (change in external elastic lamina area) accounted for only 15% of lumen area gain. Luminal gain was higher in noncalcified (6.52 ± 2.2 mm^2) lesions than in lesions containing deeply located calcium (5.19 ± 0.99 mm^2) and lowest in superficially calcified lesions (5.41 ± 2.41 mm^2). Ultrasound imaging identified an atherectomy bite in 85% of the cases, whereas angioscopy revealed such a crevice in 74%. The complementary use of the 3 techniques revealed an underestimation of the presence of dissection/tear and new thrombus by angiography (10% and 4%) and ultrasound imaging (12% and 0%) compared with angioscopy (26% and 21%). The combined use of angiography, ultrasound, and angioscopy reveals that the postatherectomy luminal lining is not as regular and smooth as that seen by angiography. Luminal enlargement with atherectomy is achieved by plaque excision rather than arterial expansion.

Complex lesions on coronary arteriography are seen commonly in patients with unstable angina and have been considered to be evidence of ruptured plaque with or without thrombus. To investigate the cause of complex lesions the histological findings in atherectomy-derived specimens in 111 patients were correlated with lesion morphologic appearance on coronary arteriography in this report by Haft and associates[143] from Newark, New Jersey. Among 91 patients with complex lesions, 81% had thrombus and 57% had evidence of plaque rupture. Of 20 patients with smooth lesions, 15% had thrombus and 10% had plaque rupture on histological evaluation. On clinical correlation in 86 (83%) patients unstable angina was associated with thrombus, or plaque rupture (63%), or both on histological evaluation. Complex lesions not associated with thrombus or plaque rupture occurred mainly (83%) in patients with stable angina. These findings support the concept that complex lesions are usually due to recent thrombus, plaque rupture, or both in patients with unstable coronary syndromes but may be due to remote plaque disruption in patients with stable angina.

Marsico and associates[144] from Pavia, Italy, conducted a study to correlate the acute luminal enlargement achieved by 3 different nonsurgical revascularization procedures in 79 patients (32 treated by balloon angioplasty, 29 by directional atherectomy, and 18 by coronary stenting) with the morphologic characteristics of coronary plaques assessed by preprocedure intravascular ultrasound. The absolute luminal gain was 2.41 ± 1.54 mm^2 for balloon angioplasty, 3.17 ± 1.8 mm^2 for directional atherectomy, and 4.56 ± 1.45 mm^2 for coronary stenting. However, when luminal gain was corrected for the external vessel area (luminal gain index), such difference was no longer present (0.22 ± 0.12 for balloon angioplasty, 0.24 ± 0.15 for directional atherectomy, and 0.30 ± 0.12 for coronary stenting). Concentric plaques treated by coronary stenting had a higher luminal gain index than eccentric plaques. A comparison of the three devices showed that a similar luminal gain index was achieved in soft plaques, whereas coronary stenting was superior to directional atherectomy (0.41 ± 0.10 vs. 0.20 ± 0.09) and balloon angioplasty (0.41 ± 0.10 vs. 0.19 ± 0.08) in concentric plaques. Coronary stenting also induced a greater luminal gain index than directional atherectomy in calcific plaques (0.30 ± 0.11 vs. 0.18 ± 0.09). In conclusion, these data show that plaque morphology assessed by preprocedure intracoronary ultrasound influences the acute luminal enlargement achieved by different coronary interventions. The knowledge of plaque composition may be useful in guiding the choice of the device to be used to obtain a larger acute luminal gain.

Coronary Stenting

Rodriguez and colleagues[145] in Buenos Aires, Argentina; Boston, Massachusetts; and Birmingham, Alabama, studied 66 patients with >0.3 mm early loss of minimal luminal diameter after successful PTCA as shown by 24-hour later quantitative coronary arteriography. The patients were randomly assigned to two groups: group 1 received a Gianturco-Roubin stent (n=33) and group 2 served as controls and received medical therapy only (n=33). All lesions were suitable for stenting. Baseline demographic, clinical, and angiographic characteristics were similar in the two groups. Restenosis (≥50% stenosis) for the overall group occurred in 32 of 66 patients (48%) at 4 ± 1 months follow-up angiography. Restenosis was significantly greater in group 2 than in group 1 patients (75% vs. 21%). Vascular complications and length of hospital stay were higher for the stent group. Although at follow-up, there were no differences in mortality or incidence of AMI between the 2 groups, patients in the control group had a higher incidence of repeat revascularization procedures (73% vs. 21%). Thus, in patients with successful PTCA but reduced luminal diameter demonstrated by repeat angiography at 24 hours, the Gianturco-Roubin stent appears to reduce angiographic restenosis at follow-up.

Colombo and colleagues[146] in Bari, Italy, tested the hypothesis that systemic anticoagulation is not necessary when adequate coronary artery stent expansion is achieved. From March 1993 to January 1994, 359 patients underwent Palmaz-Schatz coronary stent insertion. After an initial successful angiographic result with <20% stenosis by visual estimation, intravascular ultrasound imaging was performed. Further balloon dilatation of the stent was guided by observation of the intravascular ultrasound images. All patients with adequate stent expansion confirmed by ultrasound were treated only with antiplatelet therapy (either ticlopidine for 1 month with short-term aspirin for 5 days or only aspirin). Clinical success at 2 months was achieved in 338 patients or 94%. With an inflation pressure of 15±3 atmospheres and a balloon-to-vessel ratio of 1.2 ± 0.2, optimal stent expansion was achieved in 321 of 334 patients (96%) who underwent intravascular ultrasound evaluation. Despite the absence of anticoagulation, there were only two acute stent thromboses (0.6%) and one subacute stent thrombosis (0.3%) at the 2-month clinical follow-up. Follow-up angiography at 3–6 months documented two additional occlusions at the stent site. At the 6-month clinical follow-up, angiographically documented stent occlusion had occurred in 5 patients (2%), and there was a 6% incidence of AMI, a 6% rate of CABG, and a 2% incidence of death. Emergency intervention, including emergency PTCA or bailout stent for a stent thrombotic event, was performed in three patients (0.8%). The overall event rate was relatively high because of intraprocedural complications that occurred in 16 patients (5%).

The Strecker stent is a balloon-expandable, flexible endoprosthesis constructed of knitted tantalum wire and has been implanted successfully in peripheral arteries. This study by Hamm and associates[147] from Hamburg, Rotenburg, and Frankfurt am Main, Germany, presents the first multicenter experience with implantation of this radiopaque device in the coronary arteries in 64 patients of 6591 consecutive PTCA procedures complicated by abrupt closure. In all except 1 patient, the stents (n = 72) were correctly placed, and flow could be reestablished immediately. During hospitalization 12 (19%) patients had stent closures; 5 (8%) patients had Q wave myocardial infarctions; and 13 (20%) patients underwent CABG (4 on emergency basis). The in-hospital mortality was 9%: 2 patients died after thrombotic stent occlusions, 2 had fatal bleeding complications, and 2 died after CABG. Major bleeding complications at the puncture site were observed in 8 (13%) patients. Angiograms (n = 45) after 17 ± 5 weeks revealed a stent patency rate of 89%. Thus, the Strecker coronary stent proved to be helpful in the management of acute vessel closure during PTCA. However, in this first series a high incidence of early thrombotic occlusions and bleeding complications warrants close anticoagulation monitoring and limits broader indications.

To assess the risk of late side branch occlusion after Palmaz-Schatz stent deployment, Pan and associates[148] from Cordoba and Las Palmas de Gran Canaria, Spain, analyzed the angiographic evolution of 62 patients treated by successful stent implantation who had a total of 85 side branches starting from the stented segment. Side branches were considered minor (n = 39) when the diameter was <1 mm and intermediate (n = 46) when the vessel had ≥1 mm diameter. One angiographic follow-up study was available in all patients at 8 ± 5 months. Eight minor branches presented some degree of stenosis at origin before stent deployment (4 totally occluded). After stent deployment, 32 (82%) of 39 remained unchanged and 3 became occluded. Late progression at origin occurred in 4 of 34 (3 occluded). Before stent deployment, 48% of the intermediate branches had some compromise degree at their starting point (1 totally occluded). Eight of 45 intermediate branches became occluded after stent implantation. Late progression at origin happened in four of 32 branches (2 occluded). Some degree of follow-up stenosis regression at the origin was observed in 22 (26%) of 85 arteries. Neither clinical nor angiographic factors could be identified as predictors of late side branch occlusion or stenosis progression at its origin. Later occlusion or progression at origin of a side branch covered by a Palmaz-Schatz stent seems to be an uncommon occurrence (7% and 12%, respectively) that cannot be predicted by angiographic or clinical factors. On the contrary, regression at follow-up of a side branch-origin stenosis can also come about.

Aorto-ostial location is an important predictor of early and late failure of conventional balloon angioplasty in both native arteries and saphenous vein grafts. Rechavia and associates[149] from Los Angeles, California, deployed Palmaz or Palmaz-Schatz stents in 29 patients with complex vein graft aorto-ostial lesion morphology. All patients had angina at rest. Thirty-two stents were deployed in 25 new and 4 restenotic aorto-ostial stents. Stent implantation was successful in all patients. There was no death, Q wave myocardial infarction, CABG or stent thrombosis in the first 30 days. Stenting improved minimal lumen diameter from 0.7 to 3.3 mm. CABG and PTCA were required in one and two patients, respectively. These authors concluded that Palmaz or Palmaz-Schatz stent implantation for saphenous vein graft aorto-ostial stenosis has a high likelihood of immediate success and is associated with a large immediate gain in lumen diameter. Thirty-day and long-term adverse event rates are low. These data suggest that stenting saphenous vein graft aorto-ostial lesions is an acceptable therapeutic option in selected elderly patients with unstable angina and large diameter vessels.

The stent delivery system is a sheath-covered Palmaz-Schatz stent mounted on a 3.0-, 3.5- or 4.0-mm compliant polyethylene balloon catheter; the balloon resists maximal inflation pressures of 5.7, 6.2, or 6.0 atm, respectively. It is postulated that these pressures are too low to obtain optimal stent deployment. Because optimal stent deployment is a prerequisite for optimal short- and long-term outcome, Kiemeneij and associates[150] from Amsterdam, the Netherlands, performed an intravascular ultrasound study of the mode of stent deployment after delivery with the stent delivery system and after high-pressure dilatations with low-compliant, oversized balloon catheters. In 23 patients an intravascular ultrasound study (30 MHz, 4.3F transducer) was performed to the geometry of 29 stents immediately after delivery with the stent delivery system and after successive high-pressure inflations with low-compliant balloons. After delivery with the stent delivery system (3.3 ± 0.4 mm), stent diameter was 3.0 ± 0.4 mm. After high-pressure dilatations (12.4 ± 1.4 atm) with low-compliant balloons (3.9 ± 0.5 mm), stent diameter increased to 3.4 ± 0.4 mm. Only 8 (28%) stents were completely and symmetrically expanded to the corresponding reference diameter with good apposition after delivery with the stent delivery system. Diameter of incompletely deployed stents (n = 16) was 2.8 ± 0.3 mm. After high-pressure dilatations with low-compliant balloons (3.9 ± 0.5 mm), diameter increased to 3.4 ± 0.4 mm. Twenty (69%) stents became completely and symmetrically expanded to a diameter corresponding to the reference diameter. In conclusion, most stents are suboptimally deployed after delivery with the stent delivery system. Stent expansion and geometry can be improved by dilatations with low-compliant, high-pressure, oversized balloons.

Between July 1992 and February 1994, Urban and associates[151] from Geneva, Switzerland, attempted bailout Palmaz-Schatz stent implantation through a 6F guiding catheter after 52 failed PTCA procedures to reverse (14 [27%] cases) or prevent (38 [73%] cases) abrupt vessel closure. The stents or half-stents were manually crimped onto a monorail balloon catheter for delivery. Thirty-nine (75%) procedures involved a single stent, and 13 (25%) involved 2 or 3 stents. Technical success was achieved in 50 (96%) procedures, and clinical success without major complications was obtained in 45 (87%) cases. Target vessel occlusion was documented angiographically or suggested clinically in 2 (4%) cases. Two (4%) patients underwent semielective CABG, and in 4 (8%) patients a non–Q wave and in one (2%) a Q wave AMI developed. There were no deaths. Major bleeding occurred in 2 patients: 1 had an important groin hematoma that was treated with local surgery followed by CABG, and 1 had macroscopic hematuria that required interruption of anticoagulation therapy on day 4. Three (6%) femoral pseudoaneurysms were diagnosed by ultrasound and could be obliterated by external compression alone. Bailout coronary stent implantation through 6F guiding catheters after failed PTCA is technically reliable, safe, and cost efficient. As a consequence, use of 6F guiding catheters is a good option for a large majority of routine balloon angioplasty procedures.

Liu and associates[152] from Birmingham, Alabama, and West Lafayette, Indiana, carried out a study to stratify the risk of stent thrombosis by using 3 predictors: stent size, poststenting residual dissection, and residual filling defect. In the multicenter clinical trial, 1318 patients had successful deployment of Gianturco-Roubin coronary stents for threatened and acute closure. The 714 (54%) patients having none of these risk factors were designated a low-risk group; 484 (37%) had 1 factor and were designated an intermediate-risk group; 120 (9%) had 2 or all three factors and were designated a high-risk group. The incidence of stent thrombosis was 5.6%, 9.4%, and 17% in the low-, intermediate-, and high-risk groups; the difference among the 3 groups was highly significant. With these 3 predictors, the risk of stent thrombosis can be stratified. Avoiding the use of small stents (<3.00 mm) and achieving optimal angiographic results after stenting for acute or threatened closure are useful strategies in reducing stent thrombosis.

Kiemeneij and Laarman[153] from Amsterdam, the Netherlands, evaluated the feasibility and safety of implantation of unsheathed Palmaz-Schatz coronary stents introduced via the radial artery. Anticoagulation after coronary stenting carries the risk of vascular complications if large-bore guiding catheters are introduced via the femoral artery. These complications have serious local sequelae and lead to suboptimal anticoagulation and prolonged hospitalization. By combining 6F guiding catheters and low-profile dilatation catheters mounted with Palmaz-Schatz stents, smaller vessels such as the radial artery can be selected as the entry site. It is hypothesized that with this technique, major puncture site-related complications rarely occur because hemostasis is easily achieved and because no veins and nerves are near this artery. With the double blood supply to the hand, radial artery occlusion is well tolerated. In 100 consecutive patients, stent implantation was attempted for 122 lesions in 104 vessels. Immediately after stent implantation and final angiography, the introducer sheath was withdrawn and intense anticoagulation and mobilization initiated. The radial artery puncture site was studied by two-dimensional and Doppler ultrasound. Successful stent implantation via the radial artery was achieved in 96 patients. In 2 patients, arterial puncture failed but was followed by successful stenting via another entry site. In 1 patient, stent implantation was achieved with a stent delivery system via the femoral artery after a failed attempt to cross the lesion with a bare stent via the radial approach, complicated by groin bleeding requiring transfusions and vascular surgery. One patient was referred for CABG because the stent could not reach a dissection in a tortuous LAD coronary artery. Lesions were of type A (n = 43 [35%]), B (n = 30 [25%]), and C (n = 49 [40%]). The reference diameter of the stented segments was 3.3 ± 0.5 mm (1.2 to 5.0 mm). Minimal luminal diameter increased from 1.1 ± 0.4 mm (0 to 2.1 mm) to 3.1 ± 0.5 mm (1.0 to 4.2 mm). Diameter stenosis was reduced from 67 ± 11% (37% to 100%) to 13 ± 10% (0% to 68%). Procedural success and an uncomplicated clinical course were achieved in 93 (93%) patients. One (1%) patient had subacute stent thrombosis, which was followed by successful PTCA and CABG. Another patient died 2 days after stenting for unstable angina and poor LV function, without signs of stent occlusion. In 1 patient radial artery bleeding developed and required surgical repair. None of the 4 patients with postprocedure radial artery occlusion showed signs of ischemia of the hand. Hospital stay was 5.2 ± 4.1 days. Patients (n = 64) receiving coumadin at the time of admission were hospitalized for 4.1 ± 4.2 days; of this group 22 (34%) patients were discharged <24 hours after stenting. It is concluded that transradial artery Palmaz-Schatz coronary stenting is feasible and safe. With intense anticoagulation, early major entry site-related complications were rarely encountered.

To evaluate the impact of a more liberal use of endoluminal stenting on the incidence of emergency CABG, Stauffer and associates[154] from Lausanne, Switzerland, analyzed the attitude toward abrupt or threatened closure after PTCA from 1986 through 1993. In 3083 procedures performed, 204 (6.6%) patients had abrupt or threatened closure. The incidence of closure or threatened closure remained stable during the 8 years, ranging between 5% (1986) and 8% (1987). Endoluminal stent implantation was attempted in 92 patients and successfully achieved in 90 (98%), and emergency CABG had to be performed in 41 patients. The proportion without adverse end point (death or AMI) was higher in the patients treated by endoluminal stenting than in patients treated with CABG (71/90 [79%] patients vs. 17/41 [40%] patients, respectively). The use of bailout stenting gradually increased from 0.4% (1986) to 5.6% (1993) of all procedures, whereas the incidence of emergency CABG decreased from 2.7% (1986) to 0.7% (1993). Meanwhile, the incidence of AMI remained stable between 5.6% (1988) and 1.8% (1992) and death rates decreased from 1.4% (1988) to 0.2% (1993). It is concluded that "stent-by" is a highly effective therapeutic approach (79% in the present study) toward closure after PTCA and that, although surgical "stand-by" is certainly mandatory for selected cases, routine CABG stand-by is questionable.

Bartorelli and associates[155] from Milan, Italy, reported the safety and efficacy of sealing the femoral puncture site with percutaneously applied collagen after Palmaz-Schatz stent implantation in 100 consecutive patients. Patients were anticoagulated with continuous heparin infusion, overlapping oral anticoagulants, and antiplatelet therapy by dextran, aspirin, and dipyridamole. At the time of sheath removal and collagen application, the mean activated partial thromboplastin time and prothrombin time values expressed as international normalized ratio were 3.2 ± 2.1 and 1.6 ± 0.7, respectively. The hemostasis time ranged from 1 to 8 minutes (mean, 2.18 ± 2.08 minutes). Only 2 (2%) patients had major puncture-site bleeding (not seal related in one case) that required surgery and blood transfusions. Small (<6 cm) and medium (6 to 10 cm) hematomas observed in 12 (12%) and 2 (2%) patients, respectively, resolved spontaneously without sequelae. Local infection developed in 2 (2%) patients, who were successfully treated with antibiotics without clinical consequences. Subacute stent thrombosis was observed in only 1 (1%) patient. Repeat catheterization through the same femoral artery was performed at 6-month follow-up in 55 patients without difficulty or vascular complications. These findings suggest that percutaneous collagen application after coronary stenting is a secure method of achieving prompt and effective femoral hemostasis with a low incidence of major vascular bleeding complications despite intense anticoagulation. Stable hemostasis may allow continued full-dose anticoagulation, reducing the risk of stent subacute thrombosis.

To determine the feasibility and safety of deployment of this new stent, Ozaki and coworkers[156] in Rotterdam, the Netherlands deployed 28 AVE Micro stents in 23 native coronary artery lesions in 20 patients who developed acute or threatened closure after balloon PTCA. Ten stents were deployed in the LAD, 10 in the LC, and 8 in the right circumflex coronary artery. Luminal dimensions were measured using a computer-based quantitative coronary angiographic analysis system. Stent deployment was successful in 27 of 28 attempts (96%). In 1 patient with a threatened closure of the LAD associated with proximal vessel tortuosity, attempted stent deployment was unsuccessful. The clinical course of the other 19 patients in whom stent deployment was successful was free of coronary reintervention, CABG, and death. AMI was observed in 2 patients (10%): in 1 the stent was implanted within 24 hours after the onset of AMI, and in the other acute vessel occlusion was present for 58 minutes before stent implantation. No subacute occlusion was observed. Event-free survival at 30 days after stent implantation was 85%. Minimal luminal diameter was 0.85 mm before and 1.19 mm after balloon PTCA, 2.61 mm during balloon inflation, 3.26 mm during and 2.74 mm after stenting, 3.43 mm during balloon inflation after high-pressure intrastent balloon inflation, and 2.85 mm after high-pressure intrastent balloon inflation. Average percent diameter stenosis was reduced from 69% before to 56% after balloon PTCA and 17% after stenting. During the initial stent implantation, stent recoil was 0.52 mm. A high-pressure intrastent balloon inflation was performed in 14 stents with an average pressure of 14 atm, and residual stenosis was reduced from 2.55 mm to 2.85 mm in these lesions. Angiographic success (<30% residual diameter stenosis) was achieved in all stented lesions. The results of this early experience would indicate that the new AVE Micro stent may be deployed with a high procedural success rate and a minimal learning curve. Implantation of the stent for the bailout management of failed balloon PTCA can be achieved with a low incidence of adverse cardiac events and a high angiographic success rate.

Saphenous vein graft angioplasty is associated with frequent periprocedural complications and a high frequency of restenosis. Stent implantation has been shown to reduce restenosis with improved long-term outcomes in the treatment of native CAD. Twenty US investigators enrolled a total 589 symptomatic patients for the treatment of focal vein graft stenoses between January 1990 and April 1992. This study[157] reported the multicenter registry experience evaluating the safety and efficacy of the Palmaz-Schatz stent in the treatment of saphenous vein graft disease. Stent delivery was successful in 98.8% of cases and procedural success rate was 97.1%. Major in-hospital complications occurred in 2.9%, with stent thrombosis in 1.4% and major vascular or bleeding complications in 14.3%. Six-month angiographic follow-up revealed an overall restenosis rate of 30%. The 12-month actuarial event-free survival was 76%. These authors concluded that stent implantation in patients with focal saphenous vein graft lesions can be achieved with a high rate of procedural success, acceptable major complications, reduced angiographic restenosis, and favorable late clinical outcome. The rigorous anticoagulation regimen after stent placement results in more frequent vascular and other bleeding complications. Future randomized studies comparing standard balloon angioplasty with stent implan-

TABLE 2-13. Overall 1-Year Medical Care Costs

	PTCA Group (n = 105)	Stent Group (n = 102)	Δ	P
Initial hospitalization	$7505 ± 5015	$9738 ± 3248	+30%	<0.001
Repeat hospitalization	$3359 ± 7100	$1918 ± 4841	−43%	0.21
Total 1-year cost	$10 865 ± 9073	$11 656 ± 5674	+7%	<0.001

PTCA indicates percutaneous transluminal coronary angioplasty; Δ, cost difference compared with PTCA.
Reproduced with permission of Cohen et al.[158]

tation are required to properly assess the full impact of stent placement in the treatment of saphenous vein graft lesions.

Cohen and colleagues[158] in Boston, Massachusetts, determined the impact of coronary stenting on long-term medical care costs in the interval between January 1991 and June 1993 in 207 consecutive patients with symptomatic CAD requiring revascularization of a single coronary lesion. These patients were randomly assigned to receive initial treatment by either PTCA (n = 105) or a Palmaz-Schatz coronary stent (n = 102) in the multicenter STRESS trial. Detailed resource utilization and cost data were collected for each patient's initial hospitalization and any subsequent hospital visit for 1 year after randomization. Compared with conventional PTCA, coronary stenting resulted in additional catheterization laboratory costs, increased vascular complications, and longer length of stay. Initial hospital costs were approximately $2200 higher for stenting than for PTCA (Table 2-13). Over the first year of follow-up, however, patients assigned to initial stenting were less likely to require rehospitalization for a cardiac condition and underwent fewer subsequent revascularization procedures. Follow-up medical care costs thus tended to be lower for stenting than for conventional PTCA. Cumulative 1-year medical care costs remained higher for patients undergoing initial stenting, even after adjustment for the higher incidence of vascular complications in the stent group (Figure 2-28). Thus, elective coronary stenting, as performed in the randomized STRESS trial, increased total 1-year medical care costs by approximately $800 per patient compared with conventional PTCA.

This observational single-center trial by Eeckhout and colleagues[159] from Lausanne, Switzerland, examine the safety and efficacy of unplanned endoluminal stenting for the treatment of a suboptimal angiographic result (defined as a residual stenosis after PTCA of 40% to 50% without delayed runoff as estimated by visual assessment) after conventional PTCA in native, new-onset CAD. Between October 1991 and April 1994, 101 patients with suboptimal results after PTCA in new-onset lesions were treated by endoluminal Wiktor (41 patients) and Palmaz-Schatz (60 patients) stent implantation. Stenting was a technical and angiographic success in all cases. In-hospital complications were subacute closure (2%) and vascular complications at puncture site necessitating surgery (12%) or blood transfusion (3%). No AMI occurred, nor was any urgent CABG performed. At follow-up, restenosis was detected in 16 (20%; 80% angiographic follow-up rate) patients requiring repeat angioplasty (8%) and elective CABG (4%). AMI was not documented. However, 1 patient died suddenly at 5 months of follow-up. The unplanned use of intracoronary stents

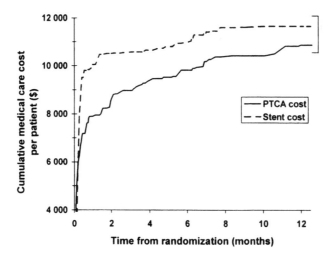

FIGURE 2-28. Plot of cumulative medical care costs in patients randomly assigned to initial percutaneous transluminal coronary angioplasty (PTCA) (n = 105) or coronary stenting (n = 102). The initial higher cost of stenting was partly offset by $1400 in follow-up cost savings, but 1-year costs remained significantly higher with stenting ($11 656 ± 5674 vs. $10 865 ± 9073, $P < 0.001$). Of note, the difference in long-term treatment costs continued to narrow between 6 and 12 months after randomization because of additional hospital admissions for percutaneous revascularization and bypass surgery, mainly in the PTCA group. Bracket indicates $P < 0.001$. Reproduced by permission of Cohen et al.[158]

is a safe and effective therapeutic option for the treatment of a suboptimal angiographic result after conventional angioplasty in new-onset lesions. This approach guarantees a high immediate angiographic success but implies a considerable incidence of vascular complications at puncture site.

Coronary Artery Bypass Grafting

Review

Nwasokwa[160] from New Hyde Park, New York, did a MEDLINE search of articles published on saphenous veins and arterial bypass grafts from 1968–1994. This review covers a number of different topics on this subject and the number of references alone numbers 148. Thus, it is a good source of information on CABG. The author concluded that by 10 years after CABG that 50% of the conduits had closed. The best way to prevent vein graft disease is to use the internal mammary artery as the graft.

Society of Thoracic Surgeons National Cardiac Database

Clark[161] for the Committee for the National Database for Thoracic Surgery, summarized some recently collected data of the Society of Thoracic Surgeons (STS) National Cardiac Database which started in 1990. More than 1500 surgeons working in 706 hospitals have contributed more than one-half million patient records. Geographic distribution of those participating is proportional to the number of centers performing heart surgery. The STS system is in use in all 49 states where centers are operating. There has been a significant decrease

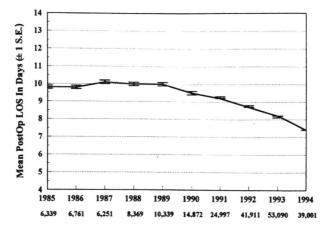

FIGURE 2-29. Annual postoperative length of stay (LOS) for first operation, elective coronary artery bypass grafting. There has been an approximate 25% decline in 5 years. (Data for 1994 are first half of the year only. Patients missing dates are censored.) (SE indicates standard error of the mean.) Reproduced with permission of Clark et al.[161]

in length of stay (Figure 2-29) for most patients having heart operations and a modest fall in CABG operative mortality from 3.7% to 3.3% over the past 3 years (Figure 2-30). CABG case mix also is changing nationally as evidenced by a decline of 17% in the best-risk cases and concomitant increases in those with predicted risks of 5% to 10% and greater. New uses for local data in addition to self assessment and quality assurance include development of critical clinical pathways, support for managed-care group applications, and regional use.

Relation of Volume to Outcome

To examine the evidence for a relation between volume of CABG and hospital death rates, and to assess the degree to which this could be due to

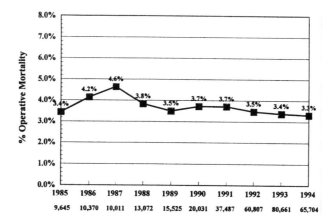

FIGURE 2-30. Annual average mortality for patients (n = 325 / 438) undergoing coronary artery bypass grafting, including all reoperations and elective, urgent, emergent, and salvage categories. A gradual decline is noted for the past 5 years and reached 3.3% in 1994. (Data for 1994 are first half of the year only.) Reproduced with permission of Clark et al.[161]

confounding because of differences in case mix, Sowden and associates[162] from York, UK, identified 15 studies using observational data from the USA from 1972–1992 and after review included 6 of the studies in their analysis. One was included in a sensitivity analysis and 8 were excluded because of duplicate analyses in data sources and methods of reporting results. The seven studies analyzed reported a reduced mortality when the volume was above 200 procedures per year, which was considered their definition of high volume. Studies with better adjustment for case mix, however, indicated less reduction in mortality with increased volume. The apparent advantages of high volume also decreased over time. The authors concluded that the evidence for reduced mortality in hospitals with a high volume of CABG is based entirely on observational studies. The authors believed that these studies may have over-estimated the benefit of increased volume because of the poor adjustment for case mix.

Regionalization of Bypass Surgery

To determine how regionalization of facilities for CABG effects geographic access to CABG and surgical outcomes, Grumbach and associates[163] from several US and Canadian medical centers used computerized hospital discharge records to measure hospital CABG volume and in-hospital post-CABG mortality rates. Included in the study were all nonfederal hospitals in New York, California, Ontario, Manitoba, and British Columbia. Included in the study were all adult residents of these five jurisdictions who underwent CABG in a hospital in their jurisdiction from 1987–1989. In New York and Canada, approximately 60% of all CABG operations took place in hospitals performing 500 or more CABG operations per year, compared with only 26% in California. The highest mortality rates were found among California hospitals performing fewer than 100 CABG operations per year (adjusted 14-day in-hospital mortality was 4.7% compared with 2.4% in high-volume California hospitals). The percentage of the population residing within 25 miles of a CABG hospital was 91% in California, 82% in New York, and less than 60% in Canada. Eliminating very low-volume (<100 cases per year) CABG hospitals in California would increase travel distances to a CABG hospital only slightly for a small number of residents. The Canadian degree of regionalization was not associated with lower CABG rates within provinces for populations living at more remote distances from the nearest CABG hospital. Regionalization of CABG facilities in New York and Canada largely avoids the problem of low-volume outlier hospitals with high postoperative mortality rates found in California. New York has avoided the redundancy of facilities that exists in California while still providing residents a geographically convenient selection of CABG hospitals. Stricter regionalization in Canada may leave residents with a more narrow choice of facilities, but does not disproportionately affect access to surgery for populations living at remote distances from CABG facilities.

Wait Before Bypass

Deaths and delays in patients waiting for CABG in Canada have been highlighted by groups in other countries opposed to "socialized medicine." Since 1991, all 9 cardiac surgery centers in Ontario, Canada, register and follow patients after acceptance for CABG. Naylor and associates[164] for the Steering

Committee of the Adult Cardiac Care Network of Ontario examined the experience in 8517 consecutive patients leaving the registry from October 1991 to July 1993. Individual acuity scores were determined based on symptoms, angiographic findings, LV function, and, where available, noninvasive tests of ischemic jeopardy. Planned CABG was declined or deferred for 3.2% of registrants. While in the queue, 31 (0.4%) patients died and 3 had CABG indefinitely deferred after a nonfatal AMI. Among 8213 patients receiving CABG, the median wait was 17 days (range, 4–51), ranging from 1 day (0:4) for patients needing very urgent CABG (acuity score, 2–3) to 42 days (range, 18–77) for those rated low priority (acuity score, 6–7). In a multivariate analysis, the most important determinant of waiting time was symptom status, followed by anatomy. Age did not alter waiting time; depending on statistical methods, female sex was either not significant or independently associated with approximately 11% relative delay. Whether controlling for significant clinical factors or the multifactorial acuity scores, waiting times clearly varied among hospitals. The authors concluded that, during 1991–1993, patients queuing for CABG in Ontario rarely suffered critical events or extreme delays, and individual variation in waiting times primarily reflected clinical acuity. Nonetheless, symptoms provoked by very modest exertion were commonplace in the queue, and waiting times did vary inequitably among hospitals.

In Octogenarians

Cane and associates[165] from Browns Mills and New Brunswick, New Jersey, described results of CABG in 121 consecutive octogenarians operated on from January 1982 through April 1991. There were 67 men (55%) and 54 women (45%). The age range was 80–89 years (mean, 82). Sixty-nine percent of the patients were having class III or IV symptoms. There were 12 hospital deaths (9%); risk factors included longer cardiopulmonary bypass time, higher preoperative LV end-diastolic pressure, advanced age, history of renal disease, and AMI. Late death occurred in 34 patients (31%) at a mean of 27 months postoperatively; univariate risk factors included chronic obstructive pulmonary disease, higher LV end-diastolic pressure, and AMI. Actuarial survival, including hospital death, was 33% at 80 months, compared with 38% for an age-, sex-, and race-matched population. Most late survivors (84%) were in New York Heart Association class I or II. The authors concluded that CABG can be performed in octogenarians with an acceptable, although increased, risk. Hospital survivors have a good late functional status but are at risk for pulmonary and other atherosclerosis-related events, which impair overall survival.

Williams and associates[166] from Miami Beach, Florida, reviewed their results of CABG in 300 consecutive patients 80 years of age and older having CABG at their institution. There were 176 men (59%) and 124 women (41%). The mean age was 81 years. Preoperatively, 274 patients (91%) had disabling angina, 76 (25%) had left main coronary stenosis >50%, and 293 patients (98%) were in New York Heart Association class III or IV. The overall hospital mortality was 11% (33 of 300) with an elective mortality of 10% (23 of 240), urgent mortality of 11% (5 of 45), and emergent mortality of 33% (5 of 15). Significant independent predictors of operative mortality were preoperative renal dysfunction, postoperative pulmonary insufficiency, postoperative renal dysfunction, use of intra-aortic balloon pumping, and sternal wound infection. The actuarial survival for patients discharged from the hospital was 75 ± 6% (SEM) at 54 months. A favorable outcome may be expected when CABG is performed in patients 80 years of age or older with severe angina.

In Chronic Obstructive Pulmonary Disease

Cohen and associates[167] from Holon and Tel Aviv, Israel, evaluated the effect of chronic obstructive pulmonary disease on the results of patients undergoing CABG. Between June 1991 and June 1993, 651 patients underwent CABG; 37 patients (group 1) had significant chronic obstructive pulmonary disease. These patients were compared with 37 matched control subjects (group 2). Comparison of the groups was made with regard to postoperative morbidity and mortality. Quality of life of survivors was compared at the last follow-up. More patients in group 1 had preoperative arrhythmias (8 vs. 1). Group 1 patients had lower values of forced expiratory volume in 1 second (1.366 ± 0.032 L vs. 2.335 ± 0.49 L), lower oxygen tension (63.5 ± 8.2 vs. 79.1 ± 13.4 mm Hg), and higher carbon dioxide tension (44.8 ± 6.5 vs. 39.7 ± 3.6 mm Hg). After operation patients in group 1 had a longer hospital stay (8.1 ± 3.6 days vs. 6.6 ± 1.7 days) and longer intensive care unit stay (2.64 ± 0.9 days vs. 1.23 ± 0.49 days). More patients in group 1 required prolonged intubation (7 vs. 1) and reintubation (5 vs. 1). More patients in group 1 had significant arrhythmias (27 vs. 9). During a 16-month follow-up period, 5 patients in group 1 died, whereas none in group 2 died. Four deaths were related to arrhythmias. More group 1 patients were not functionally improved by the operation (17 vs. 3). The results of CABG in patients with significant chronic obstructive pulmonary disease were not favorable in midterm follow-up. A major cause for morbidity and mortality was postoperative arrhythmias.

After Successful Angioplasty

Johnson and associates[168] from Boston, Massachusetts, sought characteristics predictive of the need for operative revascularization subsequent to successful PTCA. Through June 1993, 128 patients who had successful PTCAs between January 1982 and March 1989 required subsequent CABG at their hospitals. These cases were matched with 128 control subjects who had a successful PTCA but did not require subsequent CABG. Control subjects were matched to cases by the date of their initial PTCA. Before initial PTCA there were no differences between the patients and control subjects in terms of age, sex, prior AMI, EF, duration of anginal symptoms, hypertension, hyperlipidemia, family history, or obesity. A greater number of cases had diabetes. Angiography before initial PTCA revealed that cases had a greater mean number of total lesions (4.1 vs. 3.3) and a higher incidence of LAD and LC stenoses of ≥70%. The mean number of narrowings successfully dilated was greater in the cases (2.4 versus 1.7). The cases had CABG at a mean interval of 16.7 ± 23 months. There were 17 late deaths among cases and 9 among the controls at a mean of 38.6 ± 30 months. Initial revascularization by PTCA is followed by CABG at a brief interval in a subset of patients who have markers of early CABG. Patients treated with PTCA and CABG have a poorer long-term survival.

After Failed Angioplasty

Boylan and associates[169] from Cleveland, Ohio, described outcomes and findings in 253 patients who had emergent CABG within 24 hours after failed PTCA among 9145 patients having PTCA from 1980–1990. The patients were divided into 2 cohorts based on the date of PTCA: 1980–1985 (n = 109) and 1986–1990 (n = 144). The incidence of PTCA failure was 3.8% during 1980–1985 (109 of 2903) and decreased to 2.3% (144 of 6242) for 1986–1990. Comparison of pre-PTCA patient characteristics between the 2 periods showed that only a history of a previous PTCA and class III or class IV symptoms were more common in the recent years. In-hospital mortality after emergency operation was 4.6% (5 of 109) during 1980–1985 and 7.6% (11 of 144) from 1985–1990. This trend toward increased mortality appeared to be related to an increased number of patients who underwent operation in a state of severe hemodynamic compromise in the more recent period. The in-hospital mortality rate for patients in shock or undergoing cardiopulmonary resuscitation was 28.3% (13 of 46) compared with 1.4% (3 of 207) for patients with less severe hemodynamic derangement. Use of the intra-aortic balloon pump preoperatively increased from 12.8% to 32.6%. Late survival was 92% at 2 and 87% at 5 postoperative years. Although the incidence of PTCA failure necessitating emergent surgical intervention has decreased over time, there has been a trend toward an increased in-hospital mortality rate for those patients that does not appear to be related to more severe pre-PTCA characteristics. This trend does correlate with an increased prevalence of severe hemodynamic compromise in patients needing emergent operation and has occurred despite increased use of intra-aortic balloon pump support.

A databank search was performed by Berger and associates[170] in Rochester, Minnesota, and 148 consecutive patients were identified who underwent emergency CABG at the Mayo Clinic between November 20, 1979, and February 12, 1992, immediately after unsuccessful PTCA. At the end of the PTCA procedure, there was no anterograde coronary blood flow in the treated artery in 54%, ongoing chest pain in 78%, and hemodynamic compromise required intravenous vasopressor therapy in 25% of patients; 127 patients (86%) had at least 1 of these adverse characteristics. After leaving the catheterization laboratory, the median time from arrival in the operating room to initiation of coronary pulmonary bypass was 86 minutes; to administration of cardioplegia, 98 minutes; and to removal of the aortic cross clamp, 135 minutes. In-hospital mortality was 11%, and 18% developed non–fatal Q wave AMI. Thus, significant time is required to achieve surgical reperfusion after unsuccessful PTCA.

After Failed Stenting

Intracoronary stents are being used to treat acute and threatened closure after PTCA and to prevent restenosis. Craver and associates[171] from Atlanta, Georgia, reviewed the outcome of 68 patients having CABG after stent placement. The mean age was 60.5 ± 9.7 years, and 71% were male. Thirty-seven percent had hypertension, 13% had diabetes, 62% had class III or IV angina, 60% had multivessel disease, and 40% had sustained a prior AMI. Fifty-three patients underwent emergency operation, 22 with hemodynamic collapse immediately after PTCA, and seven others required urgent revascularization within 24 hours of angioplasty. Seventeen underwent CABG for acute closure of the stented vessel several days after the angioplasty procedure. There was no correlation between urgency of the procedure, previous infarction, or previous CABG with successful procedure. The in-hospital mortality was 4.4%, 21% had a Q wave AMI, and 1.5% sustained a stroke. EF was the only correlate of long-term mortality. Coronary artery injury for which stents are placed for acute or threatened occlusion or to prevent restenosis but then fail, thus necessitating CABG, can be treated successfully. Although the Q wave AMI is substantial and related to the initial ischemic insult, the long-term survival and event rates are excellent with prompt surgical revascularization.

In Familial Hypercholesterolemia

Familial hypercholesterolemia is an autosomal dominant disorder caused by a mutation of the gene for the LDL cholesterol receptor and is characterized by rapidly progressing coronary atherosclerosis. Kawasuji and associates[172] from Kanazawa, Japan, assessed the long-term results of CABG performed during the past 13 years in 62 patients with heterozygous familial hypercholesterolemia whose mean plasma total and LDL cholesterol level were 327 and 238 mg/dL, respectively. The patients had severe coronary atherosclerosis, with coronary stenosis index of 19.7, and the prevalence of extracoronary atherosclerotic lesions was 27%. Sixty-one patients underwent successful coronary artery by-pass operation, with an average of 2.5 grafts, and the coronary stenosis index decreased to 7.1. After operation, all patients consumed a cholesterol-lowering diet and received drug therapy with pravastatin, probucol, or cholestyramine. Seven patients who were resistant to drug therapy were treated with plasma LDL apheresis. The cholesterol-lowering therapy reduced plasma total cholesterol level by 37%; LDL cholesterol level by 42%, and the LDL/HDL cholesterol ratio by 37%. During the follow-up period (mean, 52 months; range, 10–157 months), there were no deaths from cardiac causes, but three patients died of malignant disease. The actuarial survival rate was 95% at 5 years and 89% at 12 years after operation. Th actuarial freedom from recurrent angina was 90% at 5 years and 53% at 11 years after operation. Four patients underwent reoperation, an average of 8 years postoperatively, because of vein graft atherosclerosis. In spite of severe coronary atherosclerosis, these patients with familial hypercholesterolemia showed good long-term outcome after coronary artery bypass operation. The present findings suggest that aggressive use of arterial grafts, intensive cholesterol-lowering drug therapy, and LDL apheresis may be useful in patients with familial hypercholesterolemia.

With Peripheral Vascular Disease

Rihal and colleagues[173] in Rochester, Minnesota, used prospectively collected data from the CASS registry to conduct a retrospective cohort analysis of 1834 patients (mean age, 56 years), 20% of whom were women with both CAD and peripheral vascular disease, and evaluated their long-term outcomes. Among these patients, 986 received CABG and 848 were treated medically in a nonrandom manner. Perioperative mortality was 4% overall and 2.9% in the absence of peripheral vascular disease. During a mean follow-up of 10 years, 1100 deaths occurred with an estimated 80% due to cardiovascular causes. For the surgical group, 4-, 8-, 12-, and 16-year estimated probabilities of survival were 88%, 72%, 55%, and 41%, respectively, whereas they were 73%, 57%, 44%, and 34%, respectively, for the medical group. These were significant differences in survival. Multivariate analysis demonstrated that the type of therapy received was independently associated with survival. Subgroup analyses suggested that benefits of surgical therapy on survival occurred in patients with 3-vessel CAD and were inversely related to LVEF. Survival free of death or AMI was also significantly better among the surgical group. Therefore, these data suggest that surgical treatment provides long-term benefit for certain subgroups of patients with combined CAD and peripheral vascular disease.

Concomitant Insertion of an Implantable Cardioverter Defibrillator

Previous studies have reported a significant morbidity and mortality associated with CABG in conjunction with the placement of an implantable cardioverter defibrillator with an epicardial lead system. In the absence of a control group, how significantly the component of concomitant placement of the implantable cardioverter defibrillator system contributes to these untoward outcomes remains unknown. The purpose of this study by Daoud and associates[174] from Ann Arbor, Michigan, was to assess the short- and long-term complications in patients undergoing CABG in conjunction with the placement of an implantable cardioverter defibrillator with epicardial leads and to compare these complications with those of patients who had only CABG (control group). The study group (group A) consisted of 56 patients who underwent CABG and placement of an implantable cardioverter defibrillator pulse generator with epicardial leads. A control group (group B) consisted of 56 patients who underwent CABG only during the same period. The two groups were matched for age, sex distribution, LV function, surgical approach, number of bypass grafts per patient, bypass pump time, and length of follow-up period. The early mortality for group A was 7.1% versus 1.8% for group B. The incidence of early morbidity (CHF, infection, or supraventricular and ventricular arrhythmias) for groups A and B was similar (27% vs. 25%). The incidence of late mortality and morbidity (progression of CHF, recurrence of coronary events, chronic AF) for group A and group B were 7.7% vs. 5.5% and 23% vs. 22%, respectively. However, death caused by cardiopulmonary difficulties was more frequent in group A than group B (13% vs. 1.8%). With the availability of the nonthoracotomy lead system and the pulse generator capable of delivering biphasic shock waveform, to place such an implantable cardioverter defibrillator system at a later time after CABG appears to be the preferred approach to treat patients who need both surgical coronary revascularization and implantable cardioverter defibrillator.

Concomitant Carotid Endarterectomy

Controversy exists concerning the best management of patients with concurrent severe carotid and CAD. Akins and associates[175] from Boston, Massachusetts, reviewed the records of 200 consecutive patients having concurrent carotid endarterectomy and CABG from 1979–1993, and follow-up was obtained in 99% of them. Of the group (77% male; mean age, 67 years), 134 (67%) had

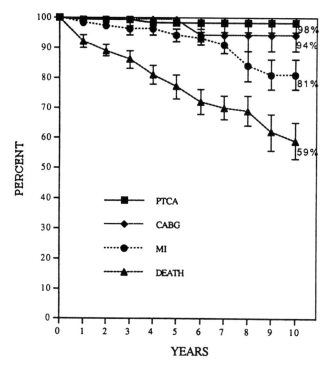

Figure 2-31. Actuarial event-free rates for late cardiac events. CABG indicates coronary artery bypass grafting; MI, myocardial infarction; PTCA, percutaneous transluminal coronary angioplasty. Reproduced with permission of Akins et al.[175]

unstable angina, 130 (65%) had 3-vessel CAD, and 86 (43%) had left main CAD. Preoperative investigation disclosed asymptomatic bruits in 116 (58%), transient ischemia in 65 (32%), strokes in 31 (16%), and bilateral carotid disease in 44 patients (22%). Nonelective operations were required in 66 patients (33%). Hospital death occurred in 7 patients (3.5%), AMI in 5 (2.5%), and permanent stroke in 6 (3%). Ten-year actuarial event-free rates were as follows: death, 58%; AMI, 81%; stroke, 92%; PTCA, 98%; redo CABG, 94%; and all morbidity and mortality, 56% (Figure 2-31). Significant multivariate predictors of hospital death were postoperative stroke, failure to use an internal mammary artery graft, intraoperative intra-aortic balloon, and nonelective operation. Significant predictors of postoperative stroke were peripheral vascular disease and vascular disease and unstable angina. Significant predictors of prolonged hospital stay were postoperative stroke, advanced age, and nonelective operation. Concomitant carotid endarterectomy and CABG can be performed with acceptably low operative risk and good long-term freedom from coronary and neurological events.

Concomitant Abdominal Aortic Aneurysmal Surgery

Mohr and colleagues[176] in Göttingen, Germany, determined whether one-stage surgery, including myocardial revascularization and simultaneous abdominal aneurysm repair are helpful in highly symptomatic patients with severe multivessel CAD. In 25 patients (24 men) with a mean age of 69 years, combined open heart and intra-abdominal aortic surgery were performed. Eighteen patients had severe 3-vessel CAD and impaired LVEFs (mean LVEFs, <35%). In addition, 3 patients had severe aortic valvular stenosis and/or insufficiency. Seven patients had 1- or 2-vessel CAD with low LVEFs (15% to 30%). All patients were in New York Heart Association functional class III or IV. Twenty-one of 25 patients had symptomatic infrarenal abdominal aortic aneurysms, perianeurysm hematomas were present in 9 patients, and 12 patients had signs of beginning aneurysm perforation. Four patients with aortoiliac occlusive disease and limb ischemia were simultaneously operated on. The surgical procedures began with CABG. After completion of myocardial revascularization, aortic aneurysm repair was performed while extracorporeal circulation was continued for mechanical cardiac assist until aortic surgery was completed. An average of 3 coronary bypass grafts were placed, including 17 internal thoracic artery grafts. Three aortic valves were replaced. In the abdominal aortic position, 12 straight tube grafts and 13 bifurcation grafts were placed and 3 renal and 2 carotid arteries were simultaneously repaired. The total time of surgery varied from 2 to 9 hours (mean, 4 hours). One intraoperative AMI occurred despite open grafts. Intensive care unit treatment lasted 1 to 13 days with a mean of 4 days. Three patients died after surgery (12%), 1 from acute renal failure induced by an adverse reaction to heparin, 1 from AMI, and 1 from multiorgan failure. One-year actuarial survival rate was 88%, which compares favorably with survival after isolated abdominal aortic aneurysm surgery in this high-risk patient subgroup. These data indicate that 1-stage surgery is a possible approach to highly symptomatic patients with severe multivessel CAD. Patients with severely impaired LVEF and unstable CAD have a higher risk of CHF and/or AMI during abdominal aortic surgery. The data from this study suggest that extracorporeal circulation protects the heart from hemodynamic changes after aortic clamping or declamping during abdominal aortic surgery. The present study results indicate that 1-stage procedure is a reasonable option for this patient subgroup.

Body Size and Outcome

Although small body size and coronary artery diameter are recognized as major contributors to the increased risk of CABG in women, few studies have established the independent influence of body size and gender on outcome. Christakis and associates[177] from Toronto, Canada, studied 7025 consecutive patients (5694 men and 1331 women) undergoing isolated CABG between 1990 and 1994. Women were older, had higher preoperative prevalences of urgent operation because of unstable angina, diabetes, peripheral vascular disease, hypertension, and single-vessel CAD, and a lower prevalence of LVEF ≤40%. The prevalences of operative mortality (men, 2%; women, 4%), low-output syndrome (men, 7%; women, 15%), and AMI (men, 3%; women, 6%) were higher in women. Patients were divided into quartiles for body surface area, weight, height, and BMI. For both men and women, there was no difference in operative mortality between the highest and lowest quartiles of body size. Women, however, had a higher prevalence of operative mortality than men in the lower quartiles of body surface area, height, and weight and in the higher quartiles of BMI. Among men, the prevalence of low-output syndrome increased with decreasing body surface area, weight, and BMI, suggesting that body size did influence the prevalence of low-output syndrome. However, women had a higher prevalence of low-output syndrome than men in every category and quartile of body size. Multivariable analysis identified gender as a significant determinant of operative mortality and low-output syndrome. When multivariable adjustments were made for body size and preoperative risk factors, gender remained a predictor of both operative mortality and low-output syndrome. Multivariable assessment of risk for men and women separately identified that urgent operation was a predictor of operative mortality and low-output syndrome in women but not men. In conclusion, the increased risk of CABG in women may be explained in part by dramatic differences in preoperative risk factors between men and women. In both men and women, small body size did not increase the risk of operative mortality, but may have contributed to the risk of low-output syndrome. After adjusting for preoperative risk variables and body size, gender remains a significant independent predictor of operative mortality and low-output syndrome.

Predicting Atrial Fibrillation Afterwards

AF occurs commonly after CABG. Despite numerous attempts at prediction, no accurate and generally accepted method exists to predict its occurrence. In this investigation Klein and associates[178] from New York, New York, performed P wave-triggered P wave signal averaging on 54 patients before CABG to evaluate the utility of this method to predict AF after CABG. After excluding six patients with unevaluable P wave signal averages and 3 patients with postoperative arrhythmias other than AF, the P wave signal averages of 45 patients were analyzed. Sixteen patients had postoperative AF and 29 did not. The mean P wave duration of the filtered, signal-averaged P wave was 163 ± 19 msec in the 16 patients with AF and 144 ± 16 msec in the 29 patients without. LA enlargement on the surface electrocardiogram was the only other statistically significant variable that correlated with the onset of postoperative AF. Other clinical variables such as P wave duration in electrocardiographic lead II; LV hypertrophy on electrocardiogram, age, sex, hypertension; and LVEF were not significantly different between the 2 groups. A cut point of 155 msec yielded a sensitivity of 69%, a specificity of 79%, a positive predictive value of 65%, and a negative predictive value of 82%. Signal-averaging of the P wave in patients before CABG provides a good predictor of postoperative AF.

Left Ventricular Function Afterwards

Improvement in LV performance after CABG remains the gold standard in myocardial viability assessment. The time-related changes, however, are not well known. This study by Ghods and associates[179] from Philadelphia, Pennsylvania, examined the LVEF by gated blood pool imaging early (6 ± 4 days) and late (62 ± 24 days) after surgery in patients with normal preoperative EF (group 1, n = 12) and those with LV dysfunction (group 2, n = 15). There were no changes in the critical status between the early and late studies, and all patients had normal sinus rhythm. Group 1 had no significant change in EF (preoperatively, 62%; early postoperatively, 64%; and late postoperatively, 63%). In group 2, EF was 26 ± 8% preoperatively; 30 ± 10% early postoperatively; and

34 ± 8% late postoperatively. Postoperatively, there was a ≥5% improvement in EF in four patients early and 11 patients late. Patients who showed early improvement continued to do so in the late study, but additionally, seven patients showed improvement only in the late study. Thus, the timing of EF measurement after surgery is important in patients with LV dysfunction but not in patients with normal LV function. Early assessment may underestimate the prevalence and degree of recovery.

Recurrence of Angina Afterwards

After bypass surgery, angina occurs in 20–30% of patients during the first year. Cameron and colleagues[180] evaluated the CASS registry to study the predictors and prognosis of postoperative angina in this large sample of 9557 patients who underwent bypass CABG. Angina recurred in the first year in 24% of patients and by the sixth year in 40%. The significant predictors in a multivariate analysis were minimal coronary artery disease, preoperative angina, use of vein grafts only, previous myocardial infarction, incomplete revascularization, female gender, smoking, and younger age. They concluded that these predictors of postoperative angina could be predicted before CABG. Thus, patients with these features could be advised that they would be more likely to experience postoperative angina than those without these features. Postoperative angina was associated with an increased risk of late AMI and reoperation.

Risk Factors Afterwards

The coronary risk factor status of women before and after CABG has not been fully described. Allen and Blumenthal[181] in Baltimore, Maryland, performed a prospective investigation of 136 women who underwent first-time, isolated CABG between February 1992 and October 1993. Major coronary risk factors were measured at the time of surgery and again 6 months later. The sample was 22% black, had a mean age of 64 years, and an average of 11 years of education. Substantial favorable changes in risk factor status occurred in the prevalence of smoking and the number of cigarettes smoked per day among smokers. Although the self-reported dietary intake of fat decreased significantly, the dietary consumption of fat, saturated fat, and cholesterol remained above the recommended levels of the Step-II diet and weights remained essentially the same (Table 2-14). Mean systolic and diastolic BPs significantly increased and a substantial number of patients (59%) continued to exhibit hypertension at 6 months. No significant changes in plasma lipid concentrations were achieved. At 6 months, one third of the women exceeded recommended levels for triglycerides, 85% for total cholesterol, and 92% for LDL. In addition, 34% had HDL levels <40 mg/dL. Health care professionals need to target these women for effective secondary prevention.

Deep Vein Thrombosis Afterwards

Although venous thrombosis may occur often after CABG, prophylaxis with low-dose heparin is rarely used due to the risk of bleeding. Therefore, Goldhaber and colleagues[182] in Boston, Massachusetts, compared the efficacy of two mechanical regimens of prophylaxis against deep vein thrombosis. Con-

TABLE 2-14. Comparison of Risk Factors in Women Before and Six Months After Coronary Artery Bypass Surgery (n = 136)

Risk Factor	Before	After	P Value
Smoking status			
Current smoker (%)	24	12	0.0008
Cigarettes/d for smokers	24 ± 12	9 ± 9	0.0001
Body composition measures			
Weight (kg)	74 ± 16	73 ± 16	NS
Body mass index (kg/m²)	29.1 ± 6	28.6 ± 6	NS
Blood pressure (mm Hg)			
Systolic	130 ± 20	142 ± 22	0.0001
Diastolic	74 ± 10	79 ± 12	0.0004
Dietary assessments			
Calories from fat (%)	39 ± 10	33 ± 9	0.0001
Calories from saturated fat (%)	12.3 ± 3	10.5 ± 3	0.0001
Cholesterol intake (mg/d)	222 ± 172	160 ± 79	0.0002
Fiber intake (g/d)	13.8 ± 7	13.8 ± 7	NS
Lipid profile (mg/dL)			
Triglycerides	189 ± 100	191 ± 100	NS
Total cholesterol	233 ± 50	241 ± 46	NS
LDL cholesterol	144 ± 39	153 ± 45	NS
HDL cholesterol	48 ± 15	46 ± 15	NS
Hypolipidemic drug intervention (%)	22	26	NS

Values are expressed as mean ± SD unless otherwise indicated.

HDL = high-density lipoprotein; LDL = low-density lipoprotein.

Reproduced with permission of Allen and Blumenthal.[181]

secutive patients undergoing CABG without concomitant valve surgery or coronary endarterectomy were randomly assigned to either a more intensive regimen of intermittent pneumatic compression plus graduated compression stockings versus standard compression stockings alone. Of 611 patients screened, 184 were excluded due to peripheral vascular disease, postoperative intra-aortic balloon support, or immediate postoperative anticoagulation. An additional 83 patients refused consent, leaving 172 in each prophylaxis group. The primary study end point was deep venous thrombosis diagnosed by a predischarge leg ultrasound examination performed on postoperative days 4–6. Of 344 patients enrolled 330 (96%) underwent predischarge ultrasonography. Deep vein thrombosis was detected in 19% of patients assigned to intermittent pneumatic compression plus stockings vs. 22% assigned to graduated compression stockings alone. The addition of intermittent pneumatic compression did not add significant incremental benefits to graduated compression stockings alone for deep vein thrombosis prophylaxis among patients undergoing CABG.

Rehabilitation Afterwards

Enrollment in cardiac rehabilitation has been reported to improve exercise capacity, psychological well-being, and survival. However, participation rates are low and the reasons for nonparticipation have not been adequately defined. Harlan and colleagues[183] in Durham, North Carolina evaluated the major correlates of nonparticipation and examined the level of participation of patients who stand to benefit most on the basis of preenrollment functional status and health behaviors. Three hundred ninety-three patients undergoing CABG (1) had baseline functional status and quality-of-life data collected, and (2) were recruited for participation in the Duke Center for Living comprehensive 3-week post-CABG rehabilitation program. Baseline demographic, clinical, catheterization, functional status, psychological status, and health behavior descriptors were analyzed to identify univariate and multivariate correlates of a patient's decision to participate in the program. At baseline, most clinical factors were similar in participants and nonparticipants, but the nonparticipants were more often women (26% vs. 12%). Participants were also more likely to be employed (63% vs. 45%) and had a higher education and income distribution than nonparticipants. On 2 separate scales, nonparticipants had significantly more baseline functional impairment than participants. In multivariate analysis, the independent correlates of higher participation rates were: higher education (college graduates were 71% more likely to participate than high school graduates) and better baseline Duke Activity Status Index (patients with mild functional impairment were at least 42% more likely to participate than patients with moderate impairment). Thus, patients with greater functional impairment and with lower socioeconomic status were disproportionately underrepresented in the cardiac rehabilitation program despite active recruitment and a waiver of direct costs offered to patients who could not afford the program.

Physical and Psychological Function Afterwards

To assess whether physical and psychosocial functioning differs between women and men Ayanian and associates[184] from Boston, Massachusetts, studied 454 consecutive patients who received CABG from June 1989 through March 1990. Before CABG, women were much more likely than men to have had class IV angina (51% vs. 30%), a recent AMI (32% vs. 18%), and CHF (34% vs. 18%). On a range from 0 (severe impairment) to 100 (no impairment), adjusted postoperative functioning was equivalent for women and men in IADLs (87 vs. 89), social activities (95 vs. 95), mental health (73 vs. 76), and vitality (58 vs. 63) (Table 2-15). Women reported similar or greater adjusted improvements than men for IADLs (27 vs. 20), social activities (21 vs. 8), mental health (11 vs. 6), and vitality (22 vs. 13) (Table 2-16). Women were more severely ill than men at the time of CABG, but women and men reported similar physical and psychosocial functioning 6 months after surgery. These findings demonstrate important functional benefits of this procedure among both women and men.

Resternotomy for Bleeding

Over a 2-year period, from January 1, 1992, to December 31, 1993, of 2221 patients undergoing cardiac operations at St. George's Hospital, London, UK, and reported by Unsworth-White and associates,[185] 85 (3.8%) were reopened for the control of bleeding (nine patients more than once). The incidence of resternotomy in coronary cases was 2.3%, but resternotomy was more than three times as likely in valve cases.

Blood Urea Nitrogen as Mortality Determinant

Although information on blood urea nitrogen (BUN) is universally available for patients who undergo CABG, BUN has not often been considered a risk

TABLE 2-15. Functional Status 6 Months After Coronary Artery Bypass Surgery by Sex

Functional Scale	Women (n = 66)	Men (n = 240)	P*
Instrumental activities of daily living, mean (SE)			
Unadjusted	83.9 (2.4)	89.6 (1.1)	0.02
Adjusted	86.7 (2.4)	89.1 (1.2)	0.38
Social activities, mean (SE)			
Unadjusted	94.4 (2.3)	95.7 (1.0)	0.58
Adjusted	95.2 (2.2)	95.3 (1.1)	0.98
Mental health, mean (SE)			
Unadjusted	72.3 (2.5)	76.1 (1.1)	0.18
Adjusted	72.6 (2.4)	76.0 (1.2)	0.23
Vitality, mean (SE)			
Unadjusted	54.8 (3.0)	63.0 (1.4)	0.009
Adjusted	58.1 (3.0)	62.5 (1.5)	0.20

*Unadjusted means were compared with t tests, and adjusted means were compared with analysis of covariance, controlling for age, acute myocardial infarction in the month before admission, New York Heart Association angina class at admission, history of congestive heart failure, the number of coexisting illnesses, education, and marital status.

Reproduced with permission of Ayanian et al.[184]

Table 2-16. Health Status 6 Months After Coronary Artery Bypass Surgery by Sex

Health Status	Women (n = 66)	Men (n = 240)	P*
Overall health, %			
Excellent	11.3	15.5	
Very good	22.6	34.3	
Good	45.2	36.1	0.04
Fair	19.4	11.6	
Poor	1.6	2.6	
Days confined to bed in prior month, %			
0	85.7	93.1	
1–3	7.1	5.1	0.07
>3	7.1	1.8	
Days with heart-related symptoms in prior month, %			
0	61.4	71.9	0.17
1-3	15.9	11.7	
>3	22.7	16.3	

*Wilcoxon rank sum test used to compare the distribution of each variable.

Reproduced with permission of Ayanian et al.[184]

factor for mortality. Hartz and associates[186] from Milwaukee, Wisconsin, evaluated four data sets that differed with respect to the types of patients and available patient information. Each data set was used to examine the relation between BUN and mortality after adjusting for other risks factors. BUN level was strongly associated with mortality in each data set. After adjustment for the available risk factors other than creatinine level, patients with BUN levels >30 mg/dL had a relative odds of mortality ranging between 1.86 and 2.49. Even after adjustment for creatinine level, as well as the other variables, BUN was statistically significant for three of the data sets.

Thyroid Hormone Treatment Afterwards

Thyroid hormone has many effects on the cardiovascular system. During and after cardiopulmonary bypass the serum triiodothyronine concentrations decline transiently, which may contribute to postoperative hemodynamic dysfunction. Klemperer and associates[187] from New York, New York, investigated whether the perioperative administration of triiodothyronine (liothyronine sodium) enhances cardiovascular performance in high-risk patients undergoing CABG. The authors administered triiodothyronine or placebo to 142 patients with CAD and depressed LV function. The hormone was administered as an intravenous bolus of 0.8 µg/kg of body weight when the aortic cross-clamp was removed after the completion of CABG and then as an infusion of 0.113 µg/kg per hour for 6 hours. Clinical and hemodynamic responses were serially recorded, as was any need for inotropic or vasodilator drugs. The patients' preoperative serum triiodothyronine concentrations were normal (mean [±SD] value, 81 ± 22 ng/dL [1.2 ± 0.3 nmol/L]), and they decreased by 40% 30 minutes after the onset of cardiopulmonary bypass. The concentrations in patients given intravenous triiodothyronine became supranormal and were significantly higher than those in patients given placebo. However, the concentrations were once again similar in the 2 groups 24 hours after surgery. The mean postoperative cardiac index was higher in the triiodothyronine group (2.97 ± 0.72 vs. 2.67 ± 0.61 L/min per square meter of body-surface area), and systemic vascular resistance was lower (1073 ± 314 vs. 1235 + 387 dyn/sec.cm^{-5}). The two groups did not differ significantly in the incidence of arrhythmia or the need for therapy with inotropic and vasodilator drugs during the 24 hours after CABG, or in perioperative mortality and morbidity. Raising serum triiodothyronine concentrations in patients undergoing CABG increases cardiac output and lowers systemic vascular resistance but does not change outcome or alter the need for standard postoperative therapy.

Survival After Left Main Narrowing

Caracciolo and colleagues[188] in St. Louis, Missouri; Seattle, Washington; Bethesda, Maryland; Rochester, Minnesota, and Birmingham, Alabama, described results in 1484 patients with left main CAD in the CASS registry, thereby extending the originally published 5-year survival for surgical and medical groups to more than 16 years of follow-up and permitting a further analysis of the left main CAD patient subgroups. The CASS Registry had 1484 patients with ≥50% left main CAD initially treated with either surgery or nonsurgical therapy. The 15-year cumulative survival estimates were 37% for the 1153 patients in the surgical group compared with 27% for the 331 patients in the medical group. Median survival in the surgical group was 13 years compared with only 7 years in the medical group (Figure 2-32). Median survival was also significantly longer in the surgical group stratified by age, sex, anginal class, LV function, coronary anatomy, and the extent of left main CAD. However, CABG did not significantly prolong median survival in patient subgroups with (1) left main CAD of 50% to 59%; (2) normal LV systolic function; (3) normal and mildly abnormal LV systolic function and a right coronary artery stenosis ≥70%; and (4) a nonstenotic right coronary artery. The 15-year cumulative survival for patients with normal LV systolic function in the surgical and medi-

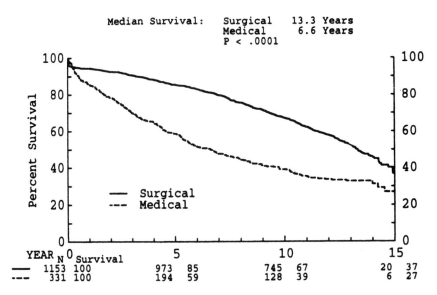

Median Survival: Surgical   13.3 Years
                   Medical   6.6 Years
                   P < .0001

Figure 2-32. Graph showing 15-year cumulative survival estimates in 1484 Coronary Artery Surgery Study Registry patients with ≥50% left main coronary artery stenosis who were initially treated with coronary artery bypass graft surgery (1153 patients) and nonsurgical therapy (331 patients). The number of patients at risk for each follow-up interval is depicted next to the cumulative survival. Reproduced with permission of Caracciolo et al.[188]

cal groups was 42% and 51%, respectively. Median survival was 15 years in the surgical group and >15 years in the medical group. In patients with normal LV systolic function and a right coronary artery stenosis ≥70%, 15-year cumulative survival rates were also similar in the surgical and medical groups. Fifteen-year cumulative survival estimates for all subgroups were affected by convergence of the surgical and medical survival group curves owing to a disproportionate increase in late surgical group mortality. Twenty-five percent of patients in the medical group ultimately had CABG. If medical group patients had survived long enough, approximately 47% would be estimated to have had surgery by 15 years. Thus, these data extend follow-up of more than 16 years in the CASS registry patients with left main CAD and demonstrate that CABG prolongs life in most clinical and angiographic subsets. However, median survival was not prolonged by CABG surgery in patients with normal LV systolic function, even if a significant right coronary artery stenosis was also present.

Graft Patency by Computed Tomography

Thallium-201 single-photon–emission computed tomography is superior to planar imaging for localizing native coronary stenoses, but has not yet been studied for assessing graft patency late after CABG. Accordingly, Lakkis and coworkers[189] in Houston, Texas, studied 50 patients (40 males; average age, 58 years), who presented for evaluation of angina (30 patients), atypical chest pain (20 patients), and other symptoms (9 patients) late after CABG (51 months). Patients with prior AMI were excluded. The mean EF was 58%. All patients underwent coronary angiography within 3 weeks of symptom-limited exercise thallium-201 computed tomography. There were 119 grafts, of which 48 had >50% stenosis by angiograpy. Thallium-201 tomography detected 40 of these

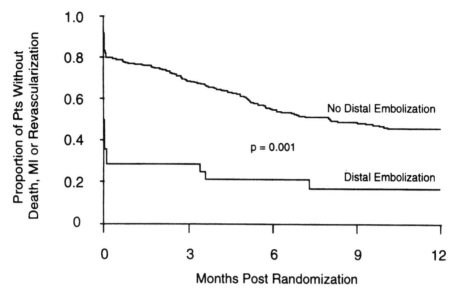

FIGURE 2-33. Kaplan-Meier plots for freedom from the composite clinical end point of death, MI, repeat intervention, or CABG for patients (Pts) with and without distal embolization. Reproduced with permission of Lefkovits et al.[190]

48 (83%) stenosed grafts. The sensitivity of thallium-201 tomography for detecting any graft stenosis was higher than that of the exercise electrocardiogram in patients with typical recurrent angina (84% vs. 24%), as well as in those with atypical symptoms (70% vs. 50%). The sensitivity of thallium-201 tomography for correctly localizing the graft stenosis site was 82% for the LAD, 92% for the right coronary, and 75% for the LC. In conclusion, exercise thallium-201 computed tomography is an excellent method to detect and localize graft stenosis late after CABG; it is far superior to the exercise electrocardiogram alone, both in patients with and without typical recurrent angina.

Venous Graft Angioplasty and Atherectomy

Lefkovits and colleagues[190] and the CAVEAT II investigators identified the predictors and sequelae of distal embolization associated with distal coronary atherectomy (DCA) and PTCA in a multicenter, randomized trial of saphenous vein graft intervention involving 305 patients randomly assigned to DCA (149 patients) or PTCA (156 patients) for lesions with >60% diameter stenosis in vein grafts ≥3 mm in diameter. Distal embolization occurred in 20 patients (13%) assigned to DCA and eight patients (5%) assigned to PTCA. Independent predictors of distal embolization were use of DCA and the presence of thrombus. In-hospital events were more frequent after distal embolization (Figure 2-33). At 12-month follow-up, adverse event rates were also higher in patients with distal embolization. Thus, in this first prospective multicenter trial of saphenous vein graft intervention, distal embolization was more common after DCA than PTCA and in lesions containing thrombus. It also was associated with a poorer in-hospital and 12-month outcome. The concern for distal embolization should be considered when choosing a treatment strategy for saphenous vein graft disease.

Late Survival

The CASS trial was initiated in 1972 by the National Heart, Lung, and Blood Institute to compare CABG with conventional medical therapy for CAD. The study[191] was carried out at 15 participating medical centers in the United States and Canada and was designed as a randomized trial within a larger registry. For the registry, every patient who had coronary angiography for evaluation of suspected CAD during the period of enrollment from 1974 to 1979 was asked to participate. Of these 18 876 men and 6082 women in the CASS registry population, 1250 men and 241 women were excluded from the analysis because they had previous CABG. In the remaining 23 467 patients, 4486 men and 3401 women were excluded because they did not meet the definition of operable CAD. Survival results in this study were based on 6018 men and 1095 women with operable CAD and initial medical management, and 6922 men and 1291 women initially managed surgically. At 15 years, CABG rates (75%) were the same for both men and women. The 15-year survival rate was 50% for men and 49% for women with initial medical treatment and 52% for men and 48% for women with initial surgical treatment. These authors concluded that the rate of bypass surgery and survival did not differ between men and women. In general, both men and women with initial surgical treatment survived longer although benefits were clinically and statistically significant only in those at high risk.

Minimal Access Bypass

The benefits of a minimal-access approach with less surgical trauma have been adopted by an increasing number of surgical specialties. Stanbridge and associates[192] from London, UK, revascularized the LAD coronary artery with the left internal mammary artery without the use of cardiopulmonary bypass and using a minimal-access approach. The authors credited the minimal-access technique to Subramanian at a lecture of the Egyptian Society of Cardiology, Cairo, Egypt, in April 1995, and Subramanian had used an anterior medial sternotomy approach via an 8-cm vertical parasternal incision. Excision of small segments of the third and fourth costal cartilage allowed the left IMA to be mobilized between the second and fifth ribs and then grafted on a beating heart to the LAD having first opened the parietal pericardium. (Figure 2-34). Stanbridge and associates successfully performed this procedure on 4 patients aged 43–67 years including 1 reoperation. The patients required minimal or no intensive care management. There were no intraoperative cardiac arrhythmias and no postoperative hemorrhages. All patients were ready for discharge on the fourth postoperative day and arterial imaging revealed all had patent anastomoses. The authors believe that the minimal-access approach to coronary bypass will have a major impact on the management of patients with single- or double-vessel CAD.

Decline in Mortality

To examine the longitudinal relationship between surgery volume and hospital mortality for CABG in New York State and to explain changes in mortality that occurred over time, Hannan and associates[193] from Albany, New

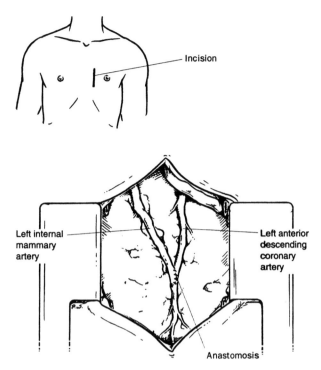

FIGURE 2-34. Site of incision and operative field. Reproduced with permission of Stanbridge et al.[192]

York, examined data produced by the 30 New York State hospitals in which CABG was performed from 1989–1992. Risk-adjusted in-hospital mortality decreased for all categories of surgeons. Low-volume surgeons (≤50 operations per year) experienced a 60% reduction in risk-adjusted mortality in the 4-year period, whereas the highest-volume surgeons (>150 operations per year) experienced a 34% reduction. The percentage of patients undergoing CABG by low-volume surgeons decreased from 7.6% in 1989 to 5.7% in 1992, a 25% decrease. The overall decline in risk-adjusted mortality could not be explained by shifts in patients away from low-volume surgeons to high-volume surgeons. The proportionately larger decrease in risk-adjusted mortality for low-volume surgeons could not be explained by changes in patient case mix or by improvements in the performance of surgeons with persistently low volumes. Part of the decrease was a result of the exodus of low-volume surgeons with high risk-adjusted mortality (in all years studied), the markedly better performance of surgeons who were not consistently low-volume surgeons (especially in 1992).

Without Cardiopulmonary Bypass

Moshkovitz and associates[194] from Tel Hashomer, Israel, reported 220 patients who underwent CABG without cardiopulmonary bypass. Early unfavorable outcome events included operative mortality (seven patients, 3.2%), nonfatal perioperative AMI (6 patients, 2.7%), cerebrovascular accident (1 patient, 0.4%), and sternal infection (3 patients, 1.4%). There were 2 deaths (13%) among 15 patients with calcified aorta and 4 (12%) in 33 patients who underwent emergency operation. Multivariate analysis revealed these 2 risk factors to be the only predictors of early mortality (OR, 8.0 and 9.8, respectively). Preoperative risk factors such as LV dysfunction (EF, ≤35%) (40 patients, 18%), CHF (46 patients, 21%), AMI (59 patients, 27%), cardiogenic shock (seven patients, 3%), age 70 years or older (59 patients, 27%), renal failure (19 patients, 9%), and cerebrovascular accident and carotid artery disease (11 patients, 5%) were not found to be major predictors of early mortality or unfavorable outcome. During 12 months of follow-up (range, 1–21 months), there were 4 cardiac and 3 noncardiac deaths (1-year actuarial survival 93%) and 17 cases (7.7%) of early return of angina. Calcified aorta, nonuse of the internal mammary artery, reoperation, and diabetes mellitus were independent predictors of unfavorable events. The authors conclude that CABG without cardiopulmonary bypass can be done with relatively low operative mortality, although there seems to be an increased risk for early return of angina. This procedure should therefore be considered for patients with appropriate coronary anatomy, in whom cardiopulmonary bypass poses a high risk.

1. The Clinical Quality Improvement Network Investigators: Low incidence of assessment and modification of risk factors in acute care patients at high risk for cardiovascular events, particularly among females and the elderly. Am J Cardiol 1995 (September 15);76:570–573.
2. Mangano DT, Goldman L: Preoperative assessment of patients with known or suspected coronary disease. N Eng J Med 1995 (December 28);333:1750–1756.
3. Mason JJ, Owens DK, Harris RA, Cooke JP, Hlatky MA: The role of coronary angiography and coronary revascularization before noncardiac vascular surgery. JAMA 1995 (June 28);273:24:1919–1925.
4. Lee JG, Krucoff MW, Brazer SR: Periprocedural myocardial ischemia in patients with severe symptomatic coronary artery disease undergoing endoscopy: Prevalence and risk factors. Am J Med 1995 (September);99:270–275.
5. Pilote L, Bourassa MG, Bacon C, Bost J, Ketre K, Mark DB, Pitt B, Reeder G, Rogers WJ, Ryan T, Schwartz L, Smith H, Whitlow P, Wiens R, Hlatky MA: Better functional status in American than Canadian patients with heart disease: An effect of medical care? J Am Coll Cardiol 1995 (November 1);26:1115–1120.
6. Ramanathan KB, El-Zeky F, Zwaag RV, Sullivan JM, Mirvis DM: Long-term survival of patients with coronary artery disease during the 1970s. Chest 1995 (January);107:1:20–27.
7. Carney RM, Saunders RD, Freedland KE, Stein P, Rich MW, Jaffe AS: Association of depression with reduced heart rate variability in coronary artery disease. Am J Cardiol 1995 (September 15);76:562–564.
8. Allison TG, Williams DE, Miller TD, Patten CA, Bailey KR, Squires RW, Gau GT: Medical and economic costs of psychologic distress in patients with coronary artery disease. Mayo Clin Proc 1995 (August);70:734–742.
9. McPherson DD, Sirna S, Collins SM, Ross AF, Moyers JR, Kane BJ, Hiratzka LF, Marcus ML, Kerber RE: Can atherosclerotic coronary arteries vasodilate? An intraoperative high-frequency epicardial echocardiographic study. Am J Cardiol 1995 (July 1);76:21–25.
10. Juillière Y, Berder V, Suty-Selton C, Buffet P, Danchin N, Cherrier F: Isolated myocardial bridges with angiographic milking of the left anterior descending coronary artery: A long-term follow-up study. Am Heart J 1995 (April);129:663–665.
11. Ferrières J, Lambert J, Lussier-Cacan S, Davignon J: Coronary artery disease in heterozygous familial hypercholesterolemia patients with the same LDL receptor gene mutation. Circulation 1995 (August);92:290–295.
12. Hollander JD: The management of cocaine-associated myocardial ischemia. N Engl J Med 1995 (November 9);333:1267–1272.

13. Carroll RJ, Horn SD, Soderfeldt B, James BC, Mahmberg L: International comparison of waiting times for selected cardiovascular procedures. J Am Coll Cardiol 1995 (March 1);25:557–563.

14. Ge J, Liu F, Kearney P, Gorge G, Haude M, Baumgart D, Ashry M, Erbel R: Intravascular ultrasound approach to the diagnosis of coronary artery aneurysms. Am Heart J 1995 (October);130:765–771.

15. Wilke NA, Sheldahl LM, Dougherty SM, Hanna RD, Nickele GA, Tristani FE: Energy expenditure during household tasks in women with coronary artery disease. Am J Cardiol 1995 (April 1);75:670–674.

16. Patterson RE, Eisner RL, Horowitz SF: Comparison of cost-effectiveness and utility of exercise ECG, single photon emission computed tomography, positron emission tomography, and coronary angiography for diagnosis of coronary artery disease. Circulation 1995 (January);91:54–65.

17. Devries S, Wolfkiel C, Fusman B, Bakdash H, Ahmed A, Levy P, Chomka E, Kondos G, Zajac E, Rich S: Influence of age and gender on the presence of coronary calcium detected by ultrafast computed tomography. J Am Coll Cardiol 1995 (January);25:76–82.

18. Rumberger JA, Sheedy PF III, Breen JF, Schwartz RS: Coronary calcium, as determined by electron beam computed tomography, and coronary disease on arteriogram: Effect of patient's sex on diagnosis. Circulation 1995 (March);91:1363–1367.

19. Kaufmann RB, Sheedy PF, Maher JE, Bielak LF, Breen JF, Schwartz RS, Peyser PA: Quantity of coronary artery calcium detected by electron beam computed tomography in asymptomatic subjects and angiographically studied patients. Mayo Clin Proc 1995 (March);70:223–232.

20. Johnston DL, Daley JR, Hodge DO, Hopfenspirger MR, Gibbons RJ: Hemodynamic responses and adverse effects associated with adenosine and dipyridamole pharmacologic stress testing: A comparison in 2,000 patients. Mayo Clin Proc 1995 (April);70:331–336.

21. Dennis CA, Pool PE, Perrins EJ, Mohiuddin SM, Sklar J, Kostuk WJ, Muller DWM, Starling MR: Stress testing with closed-loop arbutamine as an alternative to exercise. J Am Coll Cardiol 1995 (November 1);26:1151–1158.

22. Kiat H, Iskandrian AS, Villegas BJ, Starling MR, Berman DS: Arbutamine stress thallium-201 single-photon emission computed tomography using a computerized closed-loop delivery system: Multicenter trial for evaluation of safety and diagnosis. J Am Coll Cardiol 1995 (November 1);26:1159–1167.

23. Roger VL, Pellikka PA, Oh J, Miller FA, Seward JB, Tajik AJ: Stress echocardiography. Part I. Exercise echocardiography: Techniques, implementation, clinical applications, and correlations. Mayo Clin Proc 1995 (January);70:5–15.

24. Roger VL, Pellikka PA, Oh JK, Miller FA, Seward JB, Tajik AJ: Stress echocardiography. Part II. Dobutamine stress echocardiography: Techniques, implementation, clinical applications, and correlations. Mayo Clin Proc 1995 (January);70:16–27.

25. Frohwein S, Klein JL, Lane A, Taylor WR: Transesophageal dobutamine stress echocardiography in the evaluation of coronary artery disease. J Am Coll Cardiol 1995 (March 15);25:823–829.

26. Sohn DW, Shin GJ, Oh JK, Tajik AJ, Click RL, Miller FA Jr, Seward JB: Role of transesophageal echocardiography in hemodynamically unstable patients. Mayo Clin Proc 1995 (October);70:925–931.

27. Mintz GS, Popma JJ, Pichard AD, Kent KM, Satler LF, Chuang YC, Ditrano CJ, Leon MB: Patterns of calcification in coronary artery disease: A statistical analysis of intravascular ultrasound and coronary angiography in 1155 lesions. Circulation 1995 (April);91:1959–1965.

28. Mintz GS, Painter JA, Pichard AD, Kent KM, Satler LF, Popma JJ, Chuang YC, Bucher TA, Sokolowicz LE, Leon MB: Atherosclerosis in angiographically "normal" coronary artery reference segments: An intravascular ultrasound study with clinical correlations. J Am Coll Cardiol 1995 (June);25:1479–1485.

29. Lee D-Y, Eigler N, Luo H, Nishioka T, Tabaka SW, Forrester JS, Siegel RJ: Effect of intracoronary ultrasound imaging on clinical decision making. Am Heart J 1995 (June);129:1084–1093.

30. Koyama J, Yamagishi M, Tamai J, Kawano S, Daikoku S, Miyatake K: Comparison of vessel wall morphologic appearance at sites of focal and diffuse coronary vasospasm by intravascular ultrasound. Am Heart J 1995 (September);130:440–445.

31. Maheswaran B, Leung CY, Gutfinger DE, Nakamura S, Russo RJ, Hiro T, Tobis JM: Intravascular ultrasound appearance of normal and mildly diseased coronary arteries: Correlation with histologic specimens. Am Heart J 1995 (November);130:976–986.

32. Pétursson MK, Jonmundsson EH, Brekkan A, Hardarson T: Angiographic predictors of new coronary occlusions. Am Heart J 1995 (March) 129;515–520.

33. Alfonso F, Giocolea J, Hernandez R, Segovia J, Silva JC, Perez-Vizcayno MJ, Rollan MJ, Banuelos C, Macaya C: Findings of coronary angioscopy in angiographically normal coronary segments of patients with coronary artery disease. Am Heart J 1995 (November);130:987–993.

34. Caracciolo EA, Davis KB, Sopko G, Kaiser GC, Corley SD, Schaff H, Taylor HA, Chaitman BR, for the CASS Investigators: Comparison of surgical and medical group survival in patients with left main equivalent coronary artery disease: Long-term CASS experience. Circulation 1995 (May);91:2335–2344.

35. Weiner DA, Ryan TJ, Parsons L, Fisher LD, Chaitman BR, Sheffield LT, Tristani FE: Long-term prognostic value of exercise testing in men and women from the coronary artery surgery study (CASS) registry. Am J Cardiol 1995 (May 1);75:865–870.

36. Krittayaphong R, Light KC, Biles PL, Ballenger MN, Sheps DS: Increased heart rate response to laboratory induced mental stress predicts frequency and duration of daily life ambulatory myocardial ischemia in patients with coronary artery disease. Am J Cardiol 1995 (October 1);76:657–660.

37. McCully RB, elZeky F, vanderZwaag R, Ramanathan KB, Sullivan JM: Impact of patency of the left anterior descending coronary artery on long-term survival. Am J Cardiol 1995 (August 1);76:250–254.

38. Schreiber TL, Elkhatib A, Grines CL, O'Neill WW: Cardiologist versus internist management of patients with unstable angina: Treatment patterns and outcomes. J Am Coll Cardiol 1995 (September);26:577–582.

39. Calvin JE, Klein LW, VandenBerg BJ, Meyer P. Condon JV, Snell RJ, Ramirez-Morgen LM, Parrillo JE: Risk stratification in unstable angina: Prospective validation of the Braunwald Classification. JAMA 1995 (January 11);273:2:136–141.

40. Stratmann HG, Younis LT, Wittry MD, Amato M, Miller DD: Exercise technetium-99m myocardial tomography for the risk stratification of men with medically treated unstable angina pectoris. Am J Cardiol 1995 (August 1);76:236–240.

41. Cianflone D, Ciccirillo F, Buffon A, Trani C, Scabbia EV, Finocchiaro ML, Crea F: Comparison of coronary angiographic narrowing in stable angina pectoris, unstable angina pectoris, and in acute myocardial infarction. Am J Cardiol 1995 (August 1);76:215–219.

42. Chen L, Chester MR, Redwood S, Huang J, Leatham E, Kaski JC: Angiographic stenosis progression and coronary events in patients with "stabilized" unstable angina. Circulation 1995 (May);91:2319–2324.

43. Kaski JC, Chester MR, Chen L, Katritsis D: Rapid angiographic progression of coronary artery disease in patients with angina pectoris: The role of complex stenosis morphology. Circulation 1995 (October);92:2058–2065.

44. Ricou FJ, Suilen C, Rothmeier C, Gisselbaek AN, Urban P: Coronary angiography in octogenarians: Results and implications for revascularization. Am J Med 1995 (July);99:16–21.

45. de Feyter PJ, Ozaki Y, Baptista J, Escaned J, Di Mario C, de Jaegere PPT, Serruys PW, Roelandt JRTC: Ischemia-related lesion characteristics in patients with stable or unstable angina: A study with intracoronary angioscopy and ultrasound. Circulation 1995 (September);92:1408–1413.

46. Silva JA, Escobar A, Collins TJ, Ramee SR, White CJ: Unstable angina: A comparison of angioscopic findings between diabetic and nondiabetic patients. Circulation 1995 (October);92:1731–1736.

47. Gurfinkel E, Bozovich G, Cerda M, Mejail I, Oxilia A, Mautner B: Time significance of acute thrombotic reactant markers in patients with and without silent myocardial ischemia and overt unstable angina pectoris. Am J Cardiol (July 15);76:121–124.

48. Figueras J, Lidón RM: Early morning reduction in ischemic threshold in patients with unstable angina and significant coronary disease. Circulation 1995 (October);92:1737–1742.

49. Ikeda H, Takajo Y, Ichiki K, Ueno T, Maki S, Noda T, Sugi K, Imaizumi T: Increased soluble form of P-selectin in patients with unstable angina. Circulation 1995 (October);92:1693–1696.

50. Göbel EJAM, Hautvast RWM, Van Gilst WH, Spanjaard JN, Hillege HL, DeJongste MJL, Molhoek GP, Lie KI: Randomised, double-blind trial of intravenous diltiazem versus glyceryl trinitrate for unstable angina pectoris. Lancet 1995 (December 23/30);346:1653–1657.

51. Serneri GGN, Modesti PA, Gensini GF, Branzi A, Melandri G, Poggesi L, Rostagno C, Tamburini C, Carnovali M, Magnani B for the Studio Epoorine Sottocutanea nell'Angina Instobile (SESAIR) Refrattorie Group: Randomised comparison of subcutaneous heparin, intravenous heparin, and aspirin in unstable angina. Lancet 1995 (May 13);345:1201–1204.

52. Fuchs J, Cannon CP, and the TIMI 7 Investigators: Hirulog in the treatment of unstable angina: Results of the Thrombin Inhibition in Myocardial Ischemia (TIMI) 7 trial. Circulation 1995 (August);92:727–733.

53. Nease RJ Jr, Kneelajd T, O'Connor GT, Sumner W, Lumpkins C, Shaw L, Pryor D, Sox HC, Ischemic Heart Disease Patient Outcomes Research Team: Variation in patient utilities for outcomes of the management of chronic stable angina. JAMA 1995 (April 19);273:15:1185–1190.

54. Thompson SG, Kienasdt J, Pyke SDFM, Haverkate F, Van De Loo JCW, European Concerted Action on Thrombosis and Disabilities Angina Pectoris Study Group: Hemostatic factors and the risk of myocardial infarction or sudden death in patients with angina pectoris. N Engl J Med 1995 (March 9);332:635–641.

55. Chester MR, Chen L, Tousoulis D, Poloniecki J, Kaski JC: Differential progression of complex and smooth stenoses within the same coronary tree in men with stable coronary artery disease. J Am Coll Cardiol 1995 (March 15);25:837–842.

56. Uchida Y, Nakamura F, Tomaru T, Morita T, Oshima T, Sasaki T, Morizuki S, Hirose J: Prediction of acute coronary syndromes by percutaneous coronary angioscopy in patients with stable angina. Am Heart J 1995 (August);130:195–203.

57. El-Tamimi H, Mansour M, Pepine CJ, Wargovich TJ, Chen H: Circadian variation in coronary tone in patients with stable angina: Protective role of the endothelium. Circulation 1995 (December);92:3201–3205.

58. Niebauer J, Hambrecht R, Marburger C, Hauer K, Velich T, vonHodenberg E, Schlierf G, Kubler W, Schuler G: Impact of intensive physical exercise and a low fat diet on collateral vessel formation in stable angina pectoris and angiographically confirmed coronary artery disease. Am J Cardiol 1995 (October 15);76:771–775.

59. Legault SE, Langer A, Armstrong PW, Freeman MR: Usefulness of ischemic response to mental stress in predicting silent myocardial ischemia during ambulatory monitoring. Am J Cardiol 1995 (May 15);75:1007–1011.

60. Jain D, Burg M, Soufer R, Zaret BL: Prognostic implications of mental stress-induced silent left ventricular dysfunction in patients with stable angina pectoris. Am J Cardiol 1995 (July 1);76:31–35.

61. Matsubara K, Yokota M, Miyahara T, Sobue T, Iwase M, Saito H: Left ventricular performance during exercise testing in patients with silent and symptomatic myocardial ischemia. Am Heart J 1995 (March);129:459–464.

62. Weiner DA, Ryan TJ, Parsons L, Fisher LD, Chaitman BR, Sheffield LT, Tristani FE: Significance of silent myocardial ischemia during exercise testing in women: Report from the Coronary Artery Surgery Study. Am Heart J 1995 (March);129:465–470.

63. Nihoyannopoulos P, Marsonis A, Joshi J, Athanassopoulos G, Oakley CM: Magnitude of myocardial dysfunction is greater in painful than in painless myocardial ischemia: An exercise echocardiographic study. J Am Coll Cardiol 1995 (June);25:1507–1512.

64. Rogers WJ, Bourassa MG, Andrews TC, Bertolet BD, Blumenthal RS, Chaitman BR, Forman SA, Geller NL, Goldberg AD, Habib GB, Masters RG, Moisa RB, Mueller H, Pearce DJ, Pepine CJ, Sopko G, Steingart RM, Stone PH, Knatterud GL, Conti CR: Asymptomatic cardiac ischemia pilot (ACIP) study: Outcome at 1 year for patients with asymptomatic cardiac ischemia randomized to medical therapy or revascularization. J Am Coll Cardiol 1995 (September);26:594–605.

65. Kaski JC, Rosano GMC, Collins P, Nihoyannopoulos P, Maseri A, Poole-Wilson PA: Cardiac syndrome X: Clinical characteristics and left ventricular function. J Am Coll Cardiol 1995 (March 15);25:807–814.

66. Lichtlen PR, Bargheer K, Wenzlaff P: Long-term prognosis of patients with anginalike chest pain and normal coronary angiographic findings. J Am Coll Cardiol 1995 (April);25:1013–1018.

67. Kaikita K, Ogawa H, Yasue H, Sakamoto T, Suefuji H, Sumida H, Okumura K: Soluble P-selectin is released into the coronary circulation after coronary spasm. Circulation 1995 (October);92:1726–1730.

68. Shinozaki K, Suzuki M, Ikebuchi M, Takaki H, Hara Y, Tsushima M, Harano Y: Insulin resistance associated with compensatory hyperinsulinemia as an independent risk factor for vasospastic angina. Circulation 1995 (October);92:1749–1757.

69. Ozaki Y, Keane D, Serruys PW: Progression and regression of coronary stenosis in the long-term follow-up of vasospastic angina. Circulation 1995 (November);92:2446–2456.

70. Ozaki Y, Keane D, Serruys PW: Fluctuation of spastic location in patients with vasospastic angina: A quantitative angiographic study. J Am Coll Cardiol 1995 (December);26:1606–1614.

71. Garcia-Dorado D, Théroux P, Tornos P, Sambola A, Oliveras J, Santos M, Soler JS: Previous aspirin use may attenuate the severity of the manifestation of acute ischemic syndromes. Circulation 1995 (October);92:1743–1748.

72. Abrams J: The role of nitrates in coronary heart disease. Arch Intern Med 1995 (February 27);155:357–364.

73. Parker JD, Parker AB, Farrell B, Parker JO: Intermittent transdermal nitroglycerin therapy: Decreased anginal threshold during the nitrate-free interval. Circulation 1995 (February);91:973–978.

74. Freedman SB, Daxini, BV, Noyce D, Kelly DT: Intermittent transdermal nitrates do not improve ischemia in patients taking beta-blockers or calcium antagonists: Potential role of rebound ischemia during the nitrate-free period. J Am Coll Cardiol 1995 (February);25:349–355.

75. Parker JO, Amies MH, Hawkinson RW, Heilman JM, Hougham AJ, Vollmer MC, Wilson RR, and the Minitran Efficacy Study Group: Intermittent transdermal nitroglycerin therapy in angina pectoris: Clinically effective without tolerance or rebound. Circulation 1995 (March);91:1368–1374.

76. Fallen EL, Nahmias C, Scheffel A, Coates G, Beanlands R, Garnett ES: Redistribution of myocardial blood flow with topical nitroglycerin in patients with coronary artery disease. Circulation 1995 (March);91:1381–1388.

77. Khosla S, Coutinho NB, Megellas MM, Mukherjee D, Somberg JC: Can nitroglycerin convert effort-induced angina in man into silent myocardial ischemia? Am J Cardiol 1995 (August 15);76:337–339.

78. Nadeau C, Hilton D, Savard D, Morin Y, Baird M, Alexander M, Langer G, Roth D, Boulet AP, Lariviere L: Three-month efficacy and safety of once-daily diltiazem in chronic stable angina pectoris. Am J Cardiol 1995 (March 15);75:555–558.

79. Brouwer J, Viersma JW, van Veldhuisen DJ, in'tVeld AJM, Sijbring, P, Haaksma J, Dijk WA, Lie KI: Usefulness of heart rate variability in predicting drug efficacy (metoprolol versus diltiazem) in patients with stable angina pectoris. Am J Cardiol 1995 (October 15);76:759–763.

80. Ardissino D, Savonitto S, Egstrup K, Rasmussen K, Bae EA, Omland T, Schjelderup-Mathiesen PM, Marraccini P, Merlini PA, Wahlqvist I, Rehnqvist N: Selection of medical treatment in stable angina pectoris: Results of the Internal Multicenter Angina Exercise (IMAGE) study. J Am Coll Cardiol 1995 (June);25:1516–1521.

81. Wallén NH, Held C, Rehnqvist N, Hjemdahl P: Platelet aggregability in vivo is attenuated by verapamil but not by metoprolol in patients with stable angina pectoris. Am J Cardiol 1995 (January 1);75:1–6.

82. Diodati JG, Cannon RO III, Hussain N, Quyyumi AA: Inhibitory effect of nitroglycerin and sodium nitroprusside on platelet activation across the coronary circulation in stable angina pectoris. Am J Cardiol 1995 (March 1);75:443–448.

83. Davies RF, Habibi H, Klinke WP, Dessain P, Nadeau C, Phaneuf DC, Lepage S, Raman S, Herbert M, Foris K, Linden W, Buttars JA: Effect of amlodipine, atenolol and their combination on myocardial ischemia during treadmill exercise and ambulatory monitoring. J Am Coll Cardiol 1995 (March 1);25:619–625.

84. Gurfinkel EP, Manos EJ, Mejail RI, Cerda MA, Duronto EA, Gardia CN, Daroca AM, Mautner B: Low molecular weight heparin versus regular heparin or aspirin in the treatment of unstable angina and silent ischemia. J Am Coll Cardiol 1995 (August);26:313–318.

85. Treasure CB, Klein JL, Weintraub WS, Talley JD, Stillabower ME, Kosinski AS, Zhang J, Boccuzzi SJ, Cedarholm JC, Aledander RW: Beneficial effects of cholesterol-lowering therapy on the coronary endothelium in patients with coronary artery disease. N Engl J Med 1995 (February 23);332:8:481–487.

86. Waters D, Higginson L, Gladstone P, Boccuzzi SJ, Cook T, Lespérance J, for the CCAIT Study Group: Effects of cholesterol lowering on the progression of coronary atherosclerosis in women: A Canadian coronary atherosclerosis intervention trial (CCAIT) substudy. Circulation 1995 (November);92:2404–2410.

87. Anderson TJ, Meredith IT, Yeung AC, Frei B, Selwyn AP, Ganz P: The effect of cholesterol-lowering and anti-oxidant therapy on endothelium-dependent coronary vasomotion. N Engl J Med 1995 (February 23);332:8:488–493.

88. Jukema JW, Bruschke AVG, van Boven AJ, Reiber JHC, Bal ET, Zwinderman AH, Jansen H, Boerma GJM, van Rappard FM, Lie KI, on behalf of the REGRESS Study Group: Effects of lipid lowering by pravastatin on progression and regression of coronary artery disease in symptomatic men with normal to moderately elevated serum cholesterol levels: The regression growth evaluation statin study (REGRESS). Circulation 1995 (May);91:2528–2540.

89. Byington RP, Jukema JW, Salonen JT, Pitt B, Bruschke AV, Hoen H, Furberg CD, Mancini J: Reduction in cardiovascular events during pravastatin therapy: Pooled analysis of clinical events of the pravastatin atherosclerosis intervention program. Circulation 1995 (November);92:2419–2425.

90. Pitt B, Mancini GBJ, Ellis SG, Rosman HS, Park JS, McGovern ME: Pravastatin limitation of atherosclerosis in the coronary arteries (PLAC I): Reduction in atherosclerosis progression and clinical events. J Am Coll Cardiol 1995 (November 1);26:1133–1139.

91. Lacoste L, Lam JYT, Hung J, Letchacovski G, Solymoss CB, Waters D: Hyperlipidemia and coronary disease: Correction of the increased thrombogenic potential with cholesterol reduction. Circulation 1995 (December);92:3172–3177.

92. Scandinavian Simvastatin Survival Study Group: Baseline serum cholesterol and treatment effect in the Scandinavian Simvastatin Survival Study (4S). Lancet 1995 (May 20);345:1274–1275.

93. Sacks FM, Stone PH, Gibson CM, Silverman DI, Rosner B, Pasternak RC: Controlled trial of fish oil for regression of human coronary atherosclerosis. J Am Coll Cardiol 1995 (June);25:1492–1498.

94. Herrmann W, Biermann J, Kostner GM: Comparison of effects of N-3 to N-6 fatty acids on serum level lipoprotein (a) in patients with coronary disease. Am J Cardiol 1995 (September 1);76:459–462.

95. Collins P, Rosano GMC, Sarrel PM, Ulrich L, Adamopoulos S, Beale CM, McNeill JG, Poole-Wilson PA: 17 β-estradiol attenuates acetylcholine-induced coronary

arterial constriction in women but not men with coronary heart disease. Circulation 1995 (July);92:24–30.

96. Frishman WH, Pepine CJ, Weiss RJ, Baiker WM: Addition of zatebradine, a direct sinus node inhibitor, provides no greater exercise tolerance benefit in patients with angina taking extended-release nifedipine: Results of a multicenter, randomized, double-blind, placebo-controlled, parallel-group study. J Am Coll Cardiol 1995 (August);26:305–312.

97. CABRI Trial Participants: First-year results of CABRI (Coronary Angioplasty versus Bypass Revascularisation Investigation). Lancet 1995 (November 4);346:1179–1184.

98. Pocock SJ, Henderson RA, Rickards AF, Hampton JR, King SB III, Hamm CW, Puel J, Hueb W, Goy JJ, Rodriguez A: Meta-analysis of randomised trials comparing coronary angioplasty with bypass surgery. Lancet 1995 (November 4);346:1184–1189.

99. Sim I, Gupta M, McDonald K, Bourassa MG, Hlatky MA: A meta-analysis of randomized trials comparing coronary artery bypass grafting with percutaneous transluminal coronary angioplasty in multi-vessel coronary artery disease. Am J Cardiol 1995 (November 15);76:1025–1029.

100. Weintraub WS, Mauldin PD, Becker E, Kosinski AS, King SB III: A comparison of the costs of and quality of life after coronary angioplasty or coronary surgery for multivessel coronary artery disease: Results from the Emory Angioplasty versus Surgery Trial (EAST). Circulation 1995 (November);92:2831–2840.

101. Hueb WA, Bellotti G, Almeida de Oliveira S, Arie S, Piva de Albuquerque C, Jatene AD, Pileggi F: The medicine, angioplasty or surgery study (MASS): A prospective, randomized trial of medical therapy, balloon angioplasty or bypass surgery for single proximal left anterior descending artery stenoses. J Am Coll Cardiol 1995 (December);26:1600–1605.

102. Kiemeneij F, Laarman GJ, de Melker E: Transradial artery coronary angioplasty. Am Heart J 1995 (January);129:1–7.

103. Mehan R, Ambrose JA, Bongu RM, Almeida OD, Israel DH, Torre S, Sharma SK, Ratner DE: Angioplasty of complex lesions in ischemic rest angina: Results of the thrombolysis and angioplasty in unstable angina (TAUSA) trial. J Am Coll Cardiol 1995 (October);26:961–966.

104. Holmes DR Jr, Topol EJ, Califf RM, Berdan LG, Leya F, Berger PB, Whitlow PL, Safian RD, Adelman AG, Kellett MA Jr, Talley JD III, Shani J, Gottlieb RS, Pinkerton CA, Lee KL, Keeler GP, Ellis SG; the CAVEAT-II Investigators: A multicenter, randomized trial of coronary angioplasty versus directional atherectomy for patients with saphenous vein bypass graft lesions. Circulation 1995 (April);91:1966–1974.

105. Bell MR, Grill DE, Garratt KN, Berger PB, Gersh BJ, Holmes DR Jr: Long-term outcome of women compared with men after successful coronary angioplasty. Circulation 1995 (June);91:2876–2881.

106. Harris WO, Holmes DR Jr: Treatment of diffuse coronary artery and vein graft disease with a 60-mm-long balloon: Early clinical experience. Mayo Clin Proc 1995 (November);70:1061–1067.

107. Bell MR, Berger PB, Holmes DR, Mullany CJ, Bailey KR, Gersh BJ: Referral for coronary artery revascularization procedures after diagnostic coronary angiography: Evidence for gender bias? J Am Coll Cardiol 1995 (June);25:1650–1655.

108. Abdelmeguid AE, Whitlow PL, Sapp SK, Ellis SG, Topol EJ: Long-term outcome of transient, uncomplicated in-laboratory coronary artery closure. Circulation 1995 (June);91:2733–2741.

109. Holmes DR Jr, Simpson JB, Berdan LG, Gottlieb RS, Leya F, Keeler GP, Califf RM, Topol EJ: Abrupt closure: The CAVEAT I experience. J Am Coll Cardiol 1995 (November 15);26:1494–1500.

110. Danchin N, Daclin V, Juilliere Y, Dibon O, Bischoff N, Pinelli G, Cuilliere M, Cherrier F: Changes in patient treatment after abrupt closure complicating percutaneous transluminal coronary angioplasty: A historic perspective. Am Heart J 1995 (December);130:1158–1163.

111. Moliterno DJ, Califf RM, Aguirre FV, Anderson K, Sigmon KN, Weisman HF, Topol EJ, for the EPIC Study Investigators: Effect of platelet glycoprotein IIb/IIIa integrin blockade on activated clotting time during percutaneous transluminal coronary angioplasty or directional atherectomy (The EPIC Trial). Am J Cardiol 1995 (March 15);75:559–562.

112. Tcheng JE, Harrington RA, Kottke-Marchant K, Kleiman NS, Ellis SG, Kereiakes DJ, Mick MJ, Navetta FI, Smith JE, Worley SJ, Miller JA, Joseph DM, Sigmon KN, Kitt MM, du Mée CP, Califf RM, Topol EJ, for the IMPACT Investigators: Multicenter, randomized, double-blind, placebo-controlled trial of the platelet integrin glycoprotein IIb/IIIa blocker Integrelin in elective coronary intervention. Circulation 1995 (April);91:2151–2157.

113. Aguirre FV, Topol EJ, Ferguson JJ, Anderson K, Blankenship JC, Heuser RR, Sigmon K, Taylor M, Gottlieb R, Hanovich G, Rosenberg M, Donohue TJ, Weisman HF, Califf RM; for the EPIC Investigators: Bleeding complications with the chimeric antibody to platelet gylcoprotein IIb/IIIa integrin in patients undergoing percutaneous coronary intervention. Circulation 1995 (June);91:2882–2890.

114. Bittl JA, Strony J, Brinker JA, Ahmed WH, Meckel CR, Chaitman BR, Maraganore J, Deutsch E, Adelman B, Hirulog Angioplasty Study Investigators: Treatment with bivalirudin (hirulog) as compared with heparin during coronary angioplasty for unstable or postinfarction angina. N Engl J Med 1995;333:764–769.

115. Kussmaul WG, Buchbinder M, Whitlow PL, Aker UT, Heuser RR, King SB, Kent KM, Leon MB, Kolansky DM, Sandza JG: Rapid arterial hemostasis and decreased access site complications after catheterization and angioplasty: Results of a randomized trial of a novel hemostasis device. J Am Coll Cardiol 1995 (June);25:1685–1692.

116. van der Lugt A, Gussenhoven EJ, Stijnen T, van Strijen M, van Driel E, van Egmond FC, van Suylen RJ, van Urk H: Comparison of intravascular ultrasonic findings after coronary balloon angioplasty evaluated in vitro with histology. Am J Cardiol 1995 (October 1);76:661–666.

117. Ellis SG, Miller DP, Brown KJ, Omoigui N, Howell GL, Kutner M, Topol EJ: In-hospital cost of percutaneous coronary revascularization: Critical determinants and implications. Circulation 1995 (August);92:741–747.

118. Wolfe MW, Roubin GS, Schweiger M, Isner JM, Ferguson JJ, Cannon AD, Cleman M, Cabin H, Leya F, Bonan R, Strony J, Adelman B, Bittl JA, on behalf of the Heparin Registry Investigators: Length of hospital stay and complications after percutaneous transluminal coronary angioplasty: Clinical and procedural predictors. Circulation 1995 (August);92:311–319.

119. Kimmel SE, Berlin JA, Laskey WK: The relationship between coronary angioplasty procedure volume and major complications. JAMA 1995 (October 11);274:1137–1142.

120. Strauss WE, Fortin T, Hartigan P, Folland ED, Parisi AF; and the Veterans Affairs Study of Angioplasty Compared to Medical Therapy Investigators: A comparison of quality of life scores in patients with angina pectoris after angioplasty compared with after medical therapy: Outcomes of a randomized clinical trial. Circulation 1995 (October);92:1710–1719.

121. Kitazume H, Kubo I, Iwama T, Ageishi Y: Long-term angiographic follow-up of lesions patent 6 months after percutaneous coronary angioplasty. Am Heart J 1995 (March);129:441–444.

122. Detre K, Yeh W, Kelsey S, Williams D, Desvigne-Nickens P, Holmes D Jr, Bourassa M, King S III, Faxon D, Kent K, for the Investigators of the NHLBI Percutaneous Transluminal Coronary Angioplasty Registry: Has improvement in PTCA intervention affected long-term prognosis? The NHLBI PTCA registry experience. Circulation 1995 (June);91:2868–2875.

123. Stein B, Weintraub WS, Gebhart SSP, Cohen-Bernstein CL, Grosswald R, Liberman HA, Douglas JS, Morris DC, King SB III: Influence of diabetes mellitus on early and late outcome after percutaneous transluminal coronary angioplasty. Circulation 1995 (February);91:979–989.

124. de Groote P, Bauters C, McFadden EP, Lablanche J-M, Leroy F, Bertrand ME: Local lesion-related factors and restenosis after coronary angioplasty: Evidence from a

quantitative angiographic study in patients with unstable angina undergoing double-vessel angioplasty. Circulation 1995 (February);91:968–972.

125. Faxon DP, on behalf of the MARCATOR study group: Effect of high dose angiotensin-converting enzyme inhibition on restenosis: Final results of the MARCATOR study, a multicenter, double-blind, placebo-controlled trial of cilazapril. J Am Coll Cardiol 1995 (February);25:362–369.

126. Desmet W, De Scheerder I, Piessens J: Limited value of exercise testing in detection of silent restenosis after successful coronary angioplasty. Am Heart J 1995 (March);129:452–459.

127. Itoh A, Miyazaki S, Nonogi H, Daikoku S, Haze K: Angioscopic prediction of successful dilatation and of restenosis in percutaneous transluminal coronary angioplasty: Significance of yellow plaque. Circulation 1995 (March);91:1389–1396.

128. Desmarais RL, Sarembock IJ, Ayers CR, Vernon SM, Powers ER, Gimple LW: Elevated serum lipoprotein(a) is a risk factor for clinical recurrence after coronary balloon angioplasty. Circulation 1995 (March);91:1403–1409.

129. Violaris AG, Melkert R, Serruys PW: Long-term luminal renarrowing after successful elective coronary angioplasty of total occlusions: A quantitative angiographic analysis. Circulation 1995 (April);91:2140–2150.

130. Montalescot G, Ankri A, Vicaut E, Drobinski G, Grosgogeat Y, Thomas D: Fibrinogen after coronary angioplasty as a risk factor for restenosis. Circulation 1995 (July);92:31–38.

131. Eriksen UH, Amtorp O, Bagger JP, Emanuelsson H, Foegh M, Henningsen P, Saunamaki K, Schaeffer M, Thayssen P, Orskov H, Kuntz RE, Popma JJ: Randomized double-blind Scandinavian trial of angiopeptin versus placebo for the prevention of clinical events and restenosis after coronary balloon angioplasty. Am Heart J 1995 (July);130:108.

132. Serruys PW, Herrman JPR, Simon R, Rutsch W, Bode C, Laarman GJ, Van Dijk R, Van Den Bos AA, Umans VAWM, Fox KAA, Close P, Deckers JW, Helvetica Investigators: A comparison of hirudin with heparin in the prevention of restenosis after coronary angioplasty. New Engl J Med 1995 (September);333:757–763.

133. Brack MJ, Ray S, Chauhan A, Fox J, Hubner PJB, Schofield P, Harley A, Gershlick AH: The subcutaneous heparin and angioplasty restenosis prevention (SHARP) trial. J Am Coll Cardiol 1995 (October);26:947–954.

134. Bauters C, Lablanche J-M, McFadden EP, Hamon M, Bertrand ME: Relation of coronary angioscopic findings at coronary angioplasty to angiographic restenosis. Circulation 1995 (November);92:2473–2479.

135. Yamamoto H, Imazu M, Yamabe T, Ueda H, Hattori Y, Yamakido M: Risk factors for restenosis after percutaneous transluminal coronary angioplasty: Role of lipoprotein (a). Am Heart J 1995 (December);130:1168–1173.

136. Waksman R, Douglas JS Jr, Scott NA, Ghazzal ZMB, Yee-Peterson J, King SB III: Distal embolization is common after directional atherectomy in coronary arteries and saphenous vein grafts. Am Heart J 1995 (February);129:430–435.

137. Arbustini E, De Servi S, Bramucci E, Porcu E, Costante AM, Grasso M, Diegoli M, Fasani R, Morbini P, Angoli L, Boscarini M, Repetto S, Danzi G, Niccoli L, Campolo L, Lucreziotti S, Specchia G: Comparison of coronary lesions obtained by directional coronary atherectomy in unstable angina, stable angina, and restenosis after either atherectomy or angioplasty. Am J Cardiol 1995 (April 1);75:675–682.

138. Elliott JM, Berdan LG, Holmes DR, Isner JM, King SB, Keeler GP, Kearney M, Califf RM, Topol EJ, for the CAVEAT Study Investigators: One-year follow-up in the coronary angioplasty versus excisional atherectomy trial (CAVEAT I). Circulation 1995 (April);91:2158–2166.

139. Boehrer JD, Ellis SG, Pieper K, Holmes DR, Keeler GP, DeBowey D, Chapekis AT, Leya F, Mooney MR, Gottlieb RS, Serruys PW, Califf RM, Topol EJ: Directional atherectomy versus balloon angioplasty for coronary ostial and nonostial left anterior descending coronary artery lesions: Results from a randomized multicenter trial. J Am Coll Cardiol 1995 (May);25:1380–1386.

140. Nakamura S, Mahon DJ, Leung CY, Maheswaran B, Gutfinger DE, Yang J, Zelman R, Tobis JM: Intracoronary ultrasound imaging before and after directional coronary atherectomy in vitro and clinical observations. Am Heart J 1995 (May);129:841–851.

141. Farb A, Roberts DK, Picard AD, Kent KM, Virmani R: Coronary artery morphologic features after coronary rotational atherectomy: Insights into mechanisms of lumen enlargement and embolization. Am Heart J 1995 (June);129:1058–1067.

142. Umans VA, Baptista J, di Mario C, von Birgelen C, Quaedvlieg P, de Feyter PJ, Serruys PW: Angiographic, ultrasonic, and angioscopic assessment of the coronary artery wall and lumen area configuration after directional atherectomy: The mechanisms revisited. Am Heart J 1995 (August);130:217–227.

143. Haft JI, Christou CP, Goldstein JE, Carnes RE: Correlation of atherectomy specimen histology with coronary arteriographic lesion morphologic appearance in patients with stable and unstable angina. Am Heart J 1995 (September);130:420–424.

144. Marsico F, De Servi S, Ku??ca J, Angoli L, Bramucci E, Valentini P, Klersy C, Specchia G: Influence of plaque composition on luminal gain after balloon angioplasty, directional atherectomy, and coronary stenting. Am Heart J 1995 (November);130:971–975.

145. Rodriguez AE, Santaera O, Larribau M, Fernandez M, Sarmiento R, Perez Baliño N, Newell JB, Roubin GS, Palacios IF: Coronary stenting decreases restenosis in lesions with early loss in luminal diameter 24 hours after successful PTCA. Circulation 1995 (March);91:1397–1402.

146. Colombo A, Hall P, Nakamura S, Almagor Y, Maiello L, Martini G, Gaglione A, Goldberg SL, Tobis JM: Intracoronary stenting without anticoagulation accomplished with intravascular ultrasound guidance. Circulation 1995 (March);91:1676–1688.

147. Hamm CW, Beythien C, Sievert H, Langer A, Utech A, Terres W, Reifart N: Multicenter evaluation of the Strecker tantalum stent for acute coronary occlusion after angioplasty. Am Heart J 1995 (March);129:423–429.

148. Pan M, Medina A, Suarez de Lezo J, Romero M, Melian F, Pavlovic D, Hernandez E, Segura J, Marrero J, Torres F, Gimenez D, Ortega JR: Follow-up patency of side branches covered by intracoronary Palmaz-Schatz stent. Am Heart J 1995 (March);129:436–440.

149. Rechavia E, Litvack F, Macko G, Eigler NL: Stent implantation of saphenous vein graft aorto-ostial lesions in patients with unstable ischemic syndromes: Immediate angiographic results and long-term clinical outcome. J Am Coll Cardiol 1995 (March 15);25:866–870.

150. Kiemeneij F, Laarman G, Slagboom T: Mode of deployment of coronary Palmaz-Schatz stents after implantation with the stent delivery system: An intravascular ultrasound study. Am Heart J 1995 (April);129:638–644.

151. Urban P, Chatelain P, Brzostek T, Jaup T, Verine V, Rutishauser W: Bailout coronary stenting with 6F guiding catheters for failed balloon angioplasty. Am Heart J 1995 (June);129:1078–1083.

152. Liu MW, Voorhees WD III, Agrawal S, Dean LS, Roubin GS: Stratification of the risk of thrombosis after intracoronary stenting for threatened or acute closure complicating coronary balloon angioplasty: A Cook registry study. Am Heart J 1995 (July);130:8–13.

153. Kiemeneij F, Laarman GJ: Transradial artery Palmaz-Schatz coronary stent implantation: Results of a single-center feasibility study. Am Heart J 1995 (July);130:14–21.

154. Stauffer J-C, Eeckhout E, Vogt P, Kappenberger L, Goy J-J: Stand-by versus stent-by during percutaneous transluminal coronary angioplasty. Am Heart J (July);130:21–26.

155. Bartorelli AL, Sganzerla P, Fabbiocchi F, Montorsi P, De Cesare N, Child M, Tavasci E, Passaretti B, Loaldi A: Prompt and safe femoral hemostasis with a collagen device after intracoronary implantation of Palmaz-Schatz stents. Am Heart J 1995 (July);130:26–32.

156. Ozaki Y, Keane D, Ruygrok P, de Feyter P, Stertzer S, Serruys PW: Acute clinical and angiographic results with the new AVE micro coronary stent in bailout management. Am J Cardiol (July 15);76:112–116.

157. Wong SC, Baim DS, Schatz RA, Teirstein PS, King SB, Curry RC Jr, Heuser RR, Ellis SG, Cleman MW, Overlie P, Hirshfeld JW, Walker CM, Litvack F, Fish D, Brinker JA, Buchbinder M, Goldberg S, Chuang YC, Leon MB: Immediate results and late outcomes after stent implantation in saphenous vein graft lesions: The multicenter U.S. Palmaz-Schatz stent experience. J Am Coll Cardiol 1995 (September);26:704–712.

158. Cohen DJ, Krumholz HM, Sukin CA, Ho KKL, Siegrist RB, Cleman M, Heuser RR, Brinker JA, Moses JW, Savage MP, Detre K, Leon MB, Baim DS, for the Stent Restenosis Study Investigators: In-hospital and one-year economic outcomes after coronary stenting or balloon angioplasty: Results from a randomized clinical trial. Circulation 1995 (November);92:2480–2487.

159. Eeckhout E, Stauffer J-C, Vogt P, Debbas N, Kappenberger L, Goy J-J: Unplanned use of intracoronary stents for the treatment of a suboptimal angiographic result after conventional balloon angioplasty. Am Heart J 1995 (December);130:1164–1167.

160. Nwasokwa ON: Coronary artery bypass graft disease. Ann Intern Med 1995 (October 1);123:528–545.

161. Clark RE, Committee for the National Database for Thoracic Surgery: The STS cardiac surgery national database: An update. Ann Thorac Surg 1995 (June);59:1376–1381.

162. Sowden AJ, Deeks JJ, Sheldon TA: Volume and outcome in coronary artery bypass graft surgery: True association or artefact? Br Med J 1995 (July 15);311:151–155.

163. Grumbach K, Anderson GM, Luft HS, Roos LL, Brook R: Regionalization of cardiac surgery in the United States and Canada. JAMA 1995 (October 25);274:1282–1288.

164. Naylor CD, Sykora K, Jaglal SB, Jefferson S, the Steering Committee of the Adult Cardiac Care Network of Ontario: Waiting for coronary artery bypass surgery: Population-based study of 8517 consecutive patients in Ontario, Canada. Lancet 1995 (December 16);346:1605–1609.

165. Cane ME, Chen C, Bailey BM, Fernandez J, Laub GW, Anderson WA, McGrath LB: CABG in octogenarians: Early and late events and actuarial survival in comparison with a matched population. Ann Thorac Surg 1995 (October);90:1033–1037.

166. Williams DB, Carrillo RG, Traad EA. Wyatt CH, Grahowksi R, Wittels SH, Ebra G: Determinants of operative mortality in octogenarians undergoing coronary bypass. Ann Thorac Surg 1995 (October);60:1038–1043.

167. Cohen A, Katz M, Katz R, Hauptman E, Schachner A: Chronic obstructive pulmonary disease in patients undergoing coronary artery bypass grafting. J Thorac Cardiovasc Surg 1995 (March);109:3:574–581.

168. Johnson RG, Sirois G, Watkins JF, Thurere RL, Sellke FW, Cohn WE, Kuntz RE, Weintraub RM: CABG after successful PTCA: A case-control study. Ann Thorac Surg 1995 (June);59:1391–1396.

169. Boylan MJ, Lytle BW, Taylor PC, Loop FD, Proudfit W, Bhorsh JA, Cosgrove DM III: Have PTCA failures requiring emergent bypass operation changed? Ann Thorac Surg 1995 (February);59:2:283–287.

170. Berger PB, Stensrud PE, Daly RC, Grill D, Bell MR, Garratt KN, Holmes DR Jr: Time to reperfusion and other procedural characteristics of emergency coronary artery bypass surgery after unsuccessful coronary angioplasty. Am J Cardiol 1995 (September 15);76:565–569.

171. Craver JM, Justicz AG, Weintraub WS, Shen Y, Guyton RA, Gott JP, Jones EL: Coronary artery bypass grafting in patients after failure of intracoronary stenting. Ann Thorac Surg 1995 (July);60:1:60–66.

172. Kawasuji M, Sakakibara N, Takemura H, Matsumoto Y, Mabuchi HJ, Watanabe Y: Coronary artery bypass grafting in familial hypercholesterolemia. J Thorac Cardiovasc Surg 1995 (February);109:2:364–369.

173. Rihal CS, Eagle KA, Mickel MC, Foster ED, Sopko G, Gersh BJ: Surgical therapy for coronary artery disease among patients with combined coronary artery and peripheral vascular disease. Circulation 1995 (January);91:46–53.

174. Daoud EG, Strickberger SA, Man KC, Bolling SF, Kirsh MM, Morady F, Kou WH: Comparison of early and late complications in patients undergoing coronary artery

bypass graft surgery with and without concomitant placement of an implantable cardioverter defibrillator. Am Heart J 1995 (October);130:780–785.

175. Akins CW, Moncure AC, Daggett WM, Cambria RP, Hilgenberg AD, Torchiana DF, Vlahakes GJ: Safety and efficacy of concomitant carotid and coronary artery operations. Ann Thorac Surg 1995 (August);60(2):311–318.

176. Mohr FW, Falk V, Autschbach R, Diegeler A, Schorn B, Weyland A, Vettelschoss M, Frank B, Gummert J, Dalichau H: One-stage surgery of coronary arteries and abdominal aorta in patients with impaired left ventricular function. Circulation 1995 (January);91:379–385.

177. Christakis GT, Weisel RD, Buth KJ, Fremes SE, Rao V, Panagiotopoulos KP, Vanov J, Goldman BS, David TE: Is body size the cause for poor outcomes of coronary artery bypass operations in women? J Thorac Cardiovasc Surg 1995 (November);110:1344–1358.

178. Klein M, Evans SJL, Blumberg S, Cataldo L, Bodenheimer MM: Use of P-wave-triggered, P-wave signal-averaged electrocardiogram to predict atrial fibrillation after coronary artery bypass surgery. Am Heart J 1995 (May);129:895–901.

179. Ghods M, Pancholy S, Cave V, Cassell D, Heo J, Iskandrian AS: Serial changes in left ventricular function after coronary artery bypass: Implications in viability assessment. Am Heart J 1995 (January);129:20–23.

180. Cameron AAC, David KB, Rogers WJ: Recurrence of angina after coronary bypass surgery: Predictors and prognosis (CASS Registry). J Am Coll Cardiol 1995 (October);26:895–899.

181. Allen JK, Blumenthal RS: Coronary risk factors in women six months after coronary artery bypass grafting. Am J Cardiol (June 1);75:1092–1095.

182. Goldhaber SZ, Hirsch DR, MacDougall RC, Polak JF, Crager MA, Cohn LH: Prevention of venous thrombosis after coronary artery bypass surgery (a randomized trial comparing two mechanical prophylaxis strategies). Am J Cardiol 1995 (November 15);76:993–996.

183. Harlan WR III, Sandler SA, Lee KL, Lam LC, Mark DB: Importance of baseline functional and socioeconomic factors for participation in cardiac rehabilitation. Am J Cardiol 1995 (July 1);76:36–39.

184. Ayanian JZ, Guadagnoli E, Cleary PD: Physical and psychosocial functioning of women and men after coronary artery bypass surgery. JAMA 1995 (December 13);274:1767–1770.

185. Unsworth-White MJ, Herriot A, Valencia O, Poloniecki J, Smith EEJ, Murday AJ, Parker DJ, Treasure T: Resternotomy for bleeding after cardiac operation: A marker for increased morbidity and mortality. Ann Thorac Surg 1995 (March);59:3:664–667.

186. Hartz AJ, Kuhn EM, Kayser KL, Johnson WD: BUN as a risk factor for mortality after coronary artery bypass grafting. Ann Thorac Surg 1995 (August);60(2):398–404.

187. Klemperer JD, Klein I, Gomez M, Helm RE, Ojamaa K, Thomas SJ, Isom OW, Krieger K: Thyroid hormone treatment after coronary-artery bypass surgery. N Engl J Med 1995 (December 7);333:1522–1527.

188. Caracciolo EA, Davis KB, Sopko G, Kaiser GC, Corley SD, Schaff H, Taylor HA, Chaitman BR, for the CASS Investigators: Comparison of surgical and medical group survival in patients with left main coronary artery disease: Long-term CASS experience. Circulation 1995 (May);91:2325–2334.

189. Lakkis NM, Mahmarian JJ, Verani MS: Exercise thallium-201 single photon emission computed tomography for evaluation of coronary artery bypass graft patency. Am J Cardiol 1995 (July 15);76:107–111.

190. Lefkovits J, Holmes DR, Califf RM, Safian RD, Pieper K, Keeler G, Topol EJ, for the CAVEAT-II Investigators: Predictors and sequelae of distal embolization during saphenous vein graft intervention from the CAVEAT-II trial. Circulation 1995 (August);92:734–740.

191. Davis KB, Chaitman B, Ryan T, Bittner V, Kennedy JW: Comparison of 15-year survival for men and women after initial medical or surgical treatment for coronary artery disease: A CASS Registry Study. J Am Coll Cardiol 1995 (April);25:1000–1009.

192. Stanbridge RDL, Symons GV, Banwell PE (Letters to the Editor): Minimal-access surgery for coronary artery revascularization. Lancet 1995 (September 23);346:837.
193. Hannan EL, Siu AL, Kumar D, Kilburn H Jr, Chassdin MR: The decline in coronary artery bypass graft surgery mortality in New York State. JAMA 1995 (January 18);273:3:209–213.
194. Moshkovitz Y, Lusky A, Mohr R: Coronary artery bypass without cardiopulmonary bypass: Analysis of short-term and mid-term outcome in 220 patients. J Thorac Cardiovasc Surg 1995 (October);110:979–987.

3

Acute Myocardial Infarction

General Topics

Variation in Use of Cardiac Procedures

Lower rates of invasive cardiac procedures have been reported for blacks and women than for white men. Few studies have adjusted for differences in the type of hospital admission, insurance status, and disease severity. Utilizing data from the National Hospital Discharge Survey, Giles and associates[1] from Atlanta, Georgia, and Birmingham, Alabama, investigated race and sex differences in rates of cardiac catheterization, PTCA, and CABG among 10 348 persons hospitalized for AMI (Tables 3-1, 3-2, and 3-3). White men consistently had the highest procedure rates, followed by white women, black men, and black women. After matching for the hospital of admission and adjusting for age, in-hospital mortality, health insurance, and hospital transfer rates (with white men as the referent), the ORs for cardiac catheterization were 0.67 for black men, 0.72 for white women, and 0.50 for black women. Similar race-sex differences were noted for PTCA and CABG. Race and sex differentials in the rates of invasive cardiac procedures remained despite matching for the hospital of admission and controlling for other factors that influence procedure rates.

Since the introduction of thrombolytic therapy for patients with AMI, the use of coronary angiography has substantially increased. Behar and associates[2] for the Israeli Thrombolytic Survey Group sought to determine whether the presence of on-site coronary angiographic facilities influenced the utilization of coronary procedures in patients with AMI hospitalized in Israel's coronary care units. A prospective survey was conducted in January and February 1992 in the 25 coronary care units operating in Israel, 15 of which had on-site catheterization facilities. Data on demographics, clinical features, thrombolytic therapy, and the type of coronary diagnostic or therapeutic procedures performed during the current in-hospital stay were recorded. Mortality, both in-hospital and 1 year after discharge, was assessed for all patients in the survey. One thousand fourteen consecutive patients with AMI were hospitalized during the survey, 307 (30%) of whom were admitted to 10 coronary care units without and 707 of whom were treated in hospitals with on-site coronary angiography facilities. Demographic and baseline characteristics were similar in both groups. Thrombolytic therapy was provided equally (46%) to patients admitted to hospital with and without catheterization laboratories. Patients admitted to hospitals with these laboratories underwent coronary angiography (26%) and PTCA and/or CABG (12%) in greater numbers than counterparts admitted to hospitals without such laboratories (10% and 5%, respectively). Hospital and cumulative 1-year mortality rates were 11% and 18%, respectively, in patients admitted to hospitals with on-site catheterization facilities vs. 10% and 17%, respec-

Table 3-1. Age-Adjusted Cardiac Procedure Rates for Patients With Acute Myocardial Infarction, National Hospital Discharge Survey, 1988–1990

	No.	Procedure Rate, %		
		Cardiac Catheterization	Percutaneous Transluminal Coronary Angioplasty	Coronary Artery Bypass Surgery
Age group, y				
35–44	445	55.0	13.7	10.4
45–54	1166	45.3	11.9	11.7
55–64	2189	40.0	11.3	12.7
65–74	3110	36.4	8.8	10.6
≥75	3436	12.8	3.3	4.3
Type of health insurance				
Private or Blue Cross	3139	34.2	10.5	10.1
Medicare	6529	31.0	7.3	9.2
Medicaid or none	680	18.3	4.9	3.0
Size of hospital				
<200 beds	865	4.4	1.2	0.5
200–300 beds	2373	13.6	2.1	1.7
>300 beds	7110	45.3	12.3	14.3
Type of hospital				
Proprietary	912	32.9	6.4	10.2
Government	762	29.4	5.8	7.2
Nonprofit	8674	31.2	8.6	9.2
Region				
Northeast	3854	24.0	5.2	6.4
Midwest	2438	35.1	10.3	10.6
South	2892	31.6	7.4	9.3
West	1164	37.5	11.5	10.9
Hospital transfer*				
Yes	1300	11.3	0.3	0.9
No	9048	34.4	9.4	10.7

*Transferred to another hospital at the time of discharge.
Reproduced with permission from Giles et al.[1]

Table 3-2. Age-Adjusted Cardiac Procedure and In-Hospital Mortality Rates for Patients With Acute Myocardial Infarction, National Hospital Discharge Survey, 1988–1990

	No. of Patients	Procedure Rate, %			In-Hospital Mortality Rate
		Cardiac Catheterization	Percutaneous Transluminal Coronary Angioplasty	Coronary Artery Bypass Surgery	
White men	5503	33.3	8.8	11.2	14.6
Black men	581	28.5	3.3	6.7	12.4
White women	3786	29.0	8.0	6.7	15.7
Black women	478	24.1	4.8	3.6	16.1

Reproduced with permission from Giles et al.[1]

Table 3-3. Age-Adjusted Cardiac Procedure Rates for Patients With Acute Myocardial Infarction Stratified by Type of Health Insurance, National Hospital Discharge Survey, 1988–1990

Types of Health Insurance	No. of Patients	Procedure Rates, %			
		White Men	Black Men	White Women	Black Women
		Cardiac Catheterization			
Private or Blue Cross	3139	36.2	36.0	29.9	28.5
Medicare	6529	33.0	27.0	29.0	25.7
Medicaid or none	680	18.0	11.8	24.2	13.4
		Percutaneous Transluminal Coronary Angioplasty			
Private or Blue Cross	3139	11.9	5.5	8.0	6.5
Medicare	6529	7.2	3.1	7.9	5.5
Medicaid or none	680	8.0	0.1	3.3	0.4
		Coronary Artery Bypass Surgery			
Private or Blue Cross	3139	12.1	11.1	6.2	3.7
Medicare	6529	11.3	5.4	6.9	4.2
Medicaid or none	680	3.9	2.0	5.1	1.5

Reproduced with permission from Giles et al.[1]

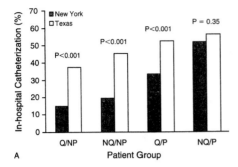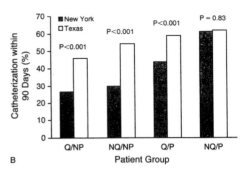

Figure 3-1. Use of cardiac catheterization during the index hospitalization (panel A) and within 90 days of the index hospitalization (panel B), according to state and patient group. Q indicates new or evolving Q-wave infarction; NQ, non–Q-wave infarction; NP, no serious chest pain more than 24 hours after admission; P, serious chest pain more than 24 hours after admission. Reproduced with permission from Guadagnoli et al.[3]

tively, in the patient group admitted to the other hospitals. Patients receiving thrombolytic therapy had similar hospital mortality rates unrelated to the availability of coronary catheterization laboratories. This national survey showed that the availability of invasive coronary facilities led to increased use of diagnostic and therapeutic coronary procedures among patients with AMI. There was no difference in hospital or 1-year mortality rates in patients admitted to hospitals with or without on-site coronary angiographic facilities.

There are large geographic differences in the frequency with which coronary angiography and revascularization are performed. Guadagnoli and associates[3] from Boston, Massachusetts, attempted to assess whether the differences in case mix or in the treatment of specific groups of patients may explain this variability. The authors also assessed the consequences of various patterns of treatment. The authors studied patients covered by Medicare who were 65–79 years of age and were admitted to 478 hospitals with AMI during 1990 in New York (1852 patients), where the rate of use of cardiac procedures is low, and in Texas (1837 patients), where the rate of use of such procedures is high. The authors compared the patterns of treatment of clinically similar groups of patients in the 2 states. They also compared mortality rates and measures of the health-related quality of life. Coronary angiography was performed more often in Texas than in New York (45% vs. 30%). The frequency of use in Texas was significantly higher than that in New York for all the clinical subgroups of patients analyzed except those at greatest risk for reinfarction (Figure 3-1). Over a 2-year period, the adjusted likelihood of death was lower in New York than in Texas. Patients from Texas were 41% more likely to report angina and 62% more likely to say they could not perform activities requiring energy expenditure of 5 or more metabolic equivalents than patients from New York approximately 2 years after infarction. Physicians in Texas were more likely to perform angiography than physicians in New York for patients whose conditions allowed more discretion in the use of cardiac procedures. On average, there appears to be no advantage with respect to mortality or health-related quality of life to performing the procedures at the higher rate used in Texas.

Spertus and associates[4] for the Myocardial Infarction Triage and Intervention Project investigators examined the relation between variables that predict

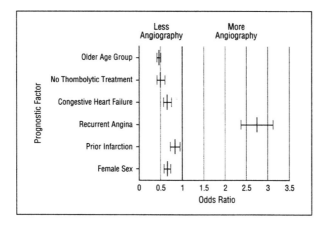

Figure 3-2. Multivariable analysis of the use of angiography after acute myocardial infarction. Odds ratio with 95% confidence intervals are shown for all prognostic factors that were significantly associated with the use of angiography in 4823 survivors of acute myocardial infarction who did not undergo catheterization between 6 hours and 5 days after their infarction. Older age group refers to the odds of going from a younger age group to the next older group; age groups were younger than 45 years, 46 to 59 years, 60 to 74 years, and older than 75 years. Reproduced with permission from Spertus et al.[4]

mortality and the use of angiography and revascularization after AMI. The authors studied 4823 survivors of AMI who underwent angiography between 6 hours and 5 days of admission to determine the relation between factors that predict mortality and the use of angiography (n = 2274), angioplasty (n = 692), and CABG (n = 469). Except for recurrent angina, clinical factors that predict higher mortality were associated with a lower use of angiography (the multivariable adjusted OR was 0.47 for older age, 0.85 for a history of AMI, 0.50 for patients not receiving thrombolytic medications, 0.64 for new heart failure, and 2.75 for recurrent angina (Figure 3-2). A similar relation was observed among patients selected for angioplasty (the odds ratio was 0.51 for an EF of <490%, 0.72 for those patients not receiving thrombolytic medications, 0.74 for a history of AMI, and 1.94 for recurrent angina). In contrast, patients with unfavorable prognostic profiles were much more likely to undergo CABG (the OR was 1.46 for recurrent angina, 1.28 for older age groups, 2.23 for new heart failure, 1.28 for patients not receiving thrombolytic medications, and 1.46 for a history of AMI) (Figure 3-3). These data suggest that aside from symptoms of recurrent angina, the use of angiography and angioplasty is not driven by mortality risk stratification. In contrast, CABG was preferentially performed in patients at increased risk for mortality.

Previous studies have reported conflicting results on gender differences in the management of AMI and have not evaluated hospital length of stay or cost. To determine gender-based differences in presentation, management, length of stay, cost and prognosis after AMI, Paul and colleagues[5] in Boston, Massachusetts, studied 561 patients with AMI. Women were older, had systemic hypertension, diabetes mellitus, and a non–Q-wave AMI more frequently, whereas more men smoked cigarettes. Predictors of coronary angiography were male gender, chest pain at presentation, recurrent angina, admission via the emergency room, and younger age. Gender did not predict mortality. Among pres-

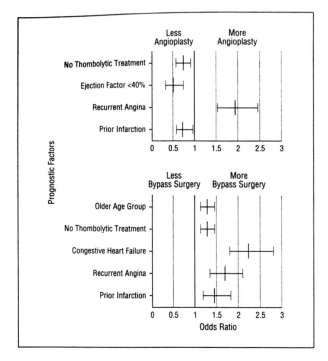

Figure 3-3. Top: Multivariable analyses of the use of revascularization after acute myocardial infarction. Odds ratios with 95% confidence intervals are shown for all prognostic factors that were significantly associated with the use of angioplasty in 1388 survivors of acute myocardial infarction who underwent catheterization between 6 hours and 5 days after infarction and who had an estimation of ejection fraction at the time of angiography. Bottom: Odds ratios with 95% confidence intervals are shown for all prognostic factors that were significantly associated with the use of bypass surgery in 2274 survivors of acute myocardial infarction who underwent catheterization between 6 hours and 5 days after infarction. Older age group refers to the odds of going from a younger age group to the next older group; age groups were younger than 45 years, 46 to 59 years, 60 to 74 years, and older than 75 years. Reproduced with permission from Spertus et al.[4]

enting features, the predictors of length of stay were diabetes, prior CABG, and prior PTCA in men and age alone in women. Pulmonary edema and need for CABG during the hospital course were predictors of length of stay in men alone. Among presenting features, predictors of cost were diabetes in men and CHF in women. Predictors of cost during hospitalization for men were pulmonary edema, coronary angiography, intra-aortic balloon pump use, and CABG; for women, they were peak levels of creatine kinase and CABG. Thus, predictors of length of stay and hospitalization cost differ based on gender.

Effect of Psychosocial Factors

O'Connor and colleagues[6] in Boston, Massachusetts, evaluated the relation between type A personality and suppressed vs. expressed anger and risk of nonfatal AMI in 340 patients and 340 age-, sex-, and community-matched control subjects. Subjects were interviewed at home to assess behavior and medical cardiovascular risk factors and fasting blood samples were obtained. Type A personality was associated with nonfatal AMI in crude matched-pair analyses. Adjusting for known cardiovascular risk factors, including treated hypertension, BMI, treated diabetes, family history of premature AMI, physical activity, smoking, alcohol, total calories per day, and saturated fat did not substantially change the magnitude of the point estimate, although the finding was no longer statistically significant. Further adjustment for lipids, including total cholesterol, HDL, HDL subfractions, and triglycerides attenuated the association, an effect due almost entirely to HDL cholesterol. Suppressed anger was positively associated with increased risk of AMI in crude matched-pair analyses, in analysis adjusted for behavioral and medical cardiovascular risk factors, and after adjustment for lipids. Thus, these data suggest a possible association of type A but not suppressed anger with risk of nonfatal AMI.

Mittleman and colleagues[7] in Boston Massachusetts, interviewed 1623 patients an average of 4 days after AMI. The interview identified the time, place, and quality of AMI pain and other symptoms, the estimated usual frequency of anger during the previous year, and the intensity and timing of anger and other potentially triggering factors during the 26 hours before AMI. Anger was assessed by the onset anger scale, a single-item, seven-level, self-report scale, and the state anger subscale of the State-Trait Personality Inventory. Occurrence of anger in the 2 hours preceding the onset of AMI was compared with its expected frequency using two types of self-matched control data based on the case-crossover study design. The onset anger scale identified 39 patients with episodes of anger in the 2 hours before AMI. The RR of AMI in the 2 hours after an episode of anger was 2.3. The state anger subscale corroborated these findings with a relative risk of 1.9. Regular users of aspirin had a significantly lower RR value than nonusers. Thus, episodes of anger are capable of triggering the onset of AMI, but aspirin may reduce this risk.

Relation to Smoking

To assess the effects of cigarette smoking on the incidence of nonfatal AMI and to compare tar in different types of manufactured cigarettes, Parish and associates[8] for the International Studies of Infarct Survival (ISIS) collaborators obtained responses of questionnaires from 13 926 survivors of AMI recently discharged from hospitals in the United Kingdom and 32 389 of their relatives (control subjects). At ages 30–49 the rates of AMI in smokers were about 5 times those in nonsmokers; at ages 50–59, they were 3 times those of the nonsmokers; and even at ages 60–79, they were twice as great as in nonsmokers (Figure 3-4). The rate of nonfatal AMI was 10% higher in medium tar than in low tar cigarette smokers (Figure 3-5). This study indicates that the imminent change of tar yields to comply with an upper limit of 12 mg per cigarette will not increase and may somewhat decrease the incidence of AMI unless they indirectly help perpetuate tobacco use. Even low tar cigarettes still greatly increase rates of AMI, especially among people aged 30–50, and far more risk is aborted by not smoking than by changing from 1 type of cigarette to another.

Relation to Gray Hair, Baldness, and Facial Wrinkling

To investigate a possible relation between aging signs such as graying of the hair, baldness and facial wrinkling and AMI, Schnohr and colleagues[9] from Copenhagen, Denmark, analyzed data from the Copenhagen City Heart Study.

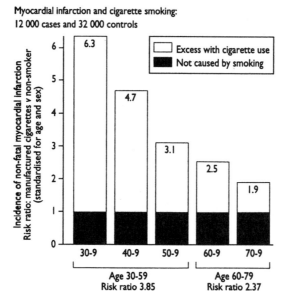

Myocardial infarction and cigarette smoking:
12 000 cases and 32 000 controls

Figure 3-4. Cigarettes and nonfatal myocardial infarction as a first event: risk ratios at various ages. Results in people with no previous history of major neoplastic or vascular disease. Each risk ratio is standardized for sex and quinquennium of age and compares those using manufactured cigarettes only with those who were not currently using any tobacco and had not been regular cigarette smokers at any time in the past 10 years. Risk ratio is given within each column. (As all cases recruited from ISIS-4 were cigarette smokers, this figure involves cases only from ISIS-3). Reproduced with permission from Parish et al.[8]

During the 12-year follow-up, 750 cases of first-time AMI were observed. After statistical adjustment for possible confounders, they found a correlation between graying of the hair, facial wrinkling, and frontoparietal baldness and crown-top baldness and AMI in men. For example, the RR was 1.4 for men with moderately gray hair compared with men with no gray hair and 1.9 for men with completely gray hair. With regard to gray hair, a similar trend was seen in women. It was concluded that, in addition to established coronary risk factors, aging signs like graying of the hair, male baldness, and facial wrinkling indicate an additional risk of AMI.

Effect of Previous Aspirin Therapy

While consumption of aspirin has been shown to decrease the occurrence of nonfatal cardiac events, most studies have not demonstrated any impact of aspirin on cardiovascular mortality. Col and associates[10] from Worcester, Massachusetts, and Tucson, Arizona, asked if aspirin consumption affected the presentation or severity of AMI? The authors monitored the use of aspirin before admission for 2114 patients with a validated diagnosis of AMI in 16 hospitals in the Worcester, Massachusetts, metropolitan area during 1986, 1988, and 1990. The AMIs were characterized as Q-wave vs. non–Q-wave and large (peak creatine kinase levels more than 5 times normal) vs. small (peak creatine kinase levels less than 2 times normal). A total of 332 patients (16%) with validated AMI took aspirin before hospital admission. Nearly 65% of aspirin users had non–Q-wave AMIs, compared 49% of nonaspirin users. Thirty percent of aspirin

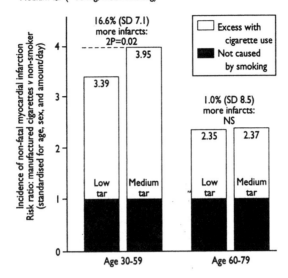

Figure 3-5. Cigarette tar yields and risk of nonfatal myocardial infarction. Standardized for age, sex, and amount smoked, comparisons at ages 30–59 indicate that nonfatal myocardial infarction rates were 1.166 (SD 0.071) times as great among medium tar as among low tar cigarette smokers (2P = 0.02; table III). The same standardized comparisons at ages 60–79 give 1.010 (0.085) (NS). These two estimates (1.166 and 1.010) are combined with the risk ratios of 3.85 and 2.37 for cigarette smokers vs. nonsmokers to yield the cited risk ratios for smokers of low and medium tar cigarettes: 3.39 and 3.95 at ages 30–59 and 2.35 and 2.37 at ages 60–79. Reproduced with permission from Parish et al.[8]

users sustained small infarcts, compared with 22% of nonaspirin users. These findings persisted after stratifying for previous AMI, history of CAD, receipt of thrombolytic therapy, and exclusion of early hospital deaths. Using multivariable regression models to control for age, gender, previous evidence of CAD, and use of other medications, prior aspirin consumption remained independently associated with AMI type (non–Q-wave AMI) and smaller infarct size. Aspirin consumption appears to modify the presentation of AMI, increasing the likelihood that the infarct will be of the small, non–Q-wave variety.

Risk of Serum C3 Levels

Serum complement and IgA levels have been found to be retrospectively associated with the presence of diffuse atherosclerosis. Muscari and associates[11] from Bologna, Italy, assessed whether serum immunoglobulins and complement components were predictive of future myocardial ischemic events. The baseline values of IgG, IgA, IgM, C3, and C4 were measured in the sera from a cohort of 860 inhabitants of the town of Brisighella, Italy. There were 444 men and 416 women (mean age, 53.9 years; SD 12.4; range, 23–84) who had not had any ischemic events (AMI, angina pectoris, stroke, transient ischemic attack, or intermittent claudication) at the time of blood sampling in 1984. Their baseline values for the main recognized risk factors for atherosclerosis were known at baseline and for 4 years of follow-up. Multiple logistic regression analysis was performed for associations between ischemic events and immunologic variables (including serum IgG, IgA, IgM, C3, and C4) and risk factors for atherosclerosis (including age, sex, diastolic BP, cigarette consumption, Quetelet index, total cholesterol, HDL cholesterol, triglycerides, and blood glucose). During follow-up, 57 subjects experienced ischemic events, including 28 cases of CAD (17 AMI and 11 angina pectoris). Of the immunological variables studied, only serum C3 was found to be independently associated with ischemic events. The population was divided into thirds according to C3 values. The cumulative incidence of AMI was 7.1 per 1000 in the low third, 10.6 per 1000 in the middle third, and 40.8 per 1000 in the high third (risk ratio for high vs. middle plus low, 4.2 after adjustment for age and sex). A separate analysis for the sexes showed that serum C3 was a particularly powerful predictor of AMI in men. Men whose C3 levels were in the top third had a 72.6 per 1000 incidence of AMI while the incidence in the rest of the male population was 6.2 per 1000 (risk ratio, 10.7 after adjustment for age). When similar analyses were performed for angina pectoris, stroke, and intermittent claudication, no significant increase in risk was found to be associated with serum C3. C3 levels measured in sera from male subjects without previous ischemic events are independently associated with the risk of AMI.

Quality of Care of Medicare Patients

To develop and test indicators of the quality of care for patients with AMI, Ellerbeck and associates[12] from several USA centers retrospectively reviewed medical records of all acute care hospitals in Alabama, Iowa, and Wisconsin. The patients included all hospitalizations for Medicare patients discharged with the principal diagnosis of AMI between June 1, 1992, and February 28, 1993, and 16 869 patients were identified. The authors subtracted data from 16 124 (96%) of the hospitalizations, representing 14 108 primary hospitalizations and 2016 hospitalizations resulting from transfers. Potential exclusions to the use of standard treatments in AMI care were common with 90% and 70% of patients having potential exclusions for thrombolytics and β-blockers, respectively (Table 3-4 and 3-5). In cohorts of "ideal candidates" for specific interventions, 83% received aspirin, 69% received thrombolytics, and 70% received β-blockers at discharge (Table 3-6). These data demonstrate that many Medicare patients may not be ideal candidates for standard AMI therapies, but these treatments are underused, even in the absence of discernible contraindications. Hospitals and physicians who apply these quality indicators to their practices are likely to find opportunities for improvement.

Characteristics When "Unrecognized"

To evaluate the incidence, prevalence, characteristics, and prognosis associated with clinically unrecognized AMI as diagnosed by electrocardiographic changes, Sigurdsson and associates[13] studied 9141 men residing in Reykjavik, Iceland; all the men were born between 1907 and 1934. Prevalence was strongly influenced by age. Nearly undetectable in the youngest age group, it increased to >5% in the group aged 75–79 years. Incidence was almost zero up to age 40, then increased steeply to more than 300 cases per year per 100 000 persons at age 60, and decreased with age after age 65. Ten- and 15-year survival

Table 3-4. Quality Indicators for an Initial Hospitalization for an Acute Myocardial Infarction (AMI)

Thrombolytics
  Potential candidates: Confirmed AMI and not received in transfer from another emergency department (n = 11371).
  Exclusions: Patients without ST-segment elevation or AMI on their admission electrocardiogram (62%); with chest pain lasting <30 min or with an onset of chest pain >6 h prior to admission or inadequate documentation of the chest pain (55%); chronic liver disease, history of gastrointestinal bleeding, peptic ulcer disease, surgery in the past month, recent head trauma, intracranial neoplasm, recent cardiopulmonary resuscitation, suspected dissecting aneurysm, or coagulopathy (15%); blood in stool on admission or hemorrhagic eye disorder (1%); warfarin on admission (6%); a history of stroke or uncontrolled hypertension (12%); age >80 y (29%); or documentation that thrombolysis was considered but the physician or patient decided against it (9%).
  Criterion: Receive thrombolytics.

Aspirin during the hospitalization
  Potential candidates: Confirmed AMI (n = 12332).
  Exclusions: Patients who died or were transferred on the day of admission (4%); and those with blood in their stools or evidence of bleeding on admission or during the hospitalization (13%); history of gastrointestinal bleeding or a hemorrhagic stroke, chronic liver disease, coagulopathy, platelet count $<100 \times 10^6$/L, recent head trauma, or intracranial neoplasm (6%); a serum creatinine level >265 μmol/L (3 mg/dL) (3%); history of peptic ulcer disease or a discharge diagnosis of an upper gastrointestinal disorder (5%); hemoglobin level <100 g/L or hematocrit <0.30 (5%); allergy to aspirin (4%); treatment with warfarin on admission (6%); or metastatic cancer or other terminal illness (9%).
  Criterion: Receive aspirin during the hospitalization.

Heparin (full or low dose)
  Potential candidates: Confirmed AMI (n = 12332).
  Exclusions: Patients with blood in their stools or evidence of bleeding on admission or during the hospitalization (13%); coagulopathy, platelet count $<100 \times 10^6$/L, prothrombin time > 14 sec on admission, history of a hemorrhagic cerebrovascular accident, head trauma or intracranial neoplasm (15%); hemoglobin level <100 g/L or hematocrit <0.30 (5%); allergy to heparin (0%); or those taking warfarin prior to admission with a prothrombin time of >16 sec (5%).
  Criterion: Receive >4000 U of heparin per 24 h (excludes those just receiving heparin flushes).

Intravenous nitroglycerin for persistent chest pain
  Potential candidates: All patients with confirmed AMI and persistent chest pain (n = 1978).
  Exclusions: Patients with shock or hypotension on admission (11%).
  Criterion: Receive intravenous nitroglycerin.

Timing of thrombolytics
  Potential candidates: All patients with confirmed AMI receiving thrombolytics (n = 2005).
  Exclusions: Inadequate documentation of the time of arrival or the time of administration of the thrombolytic (27%).
  Criterion: The time (in minutes) from arrival at the hospital until the beginning of administration of the thrombolytic.

Timing of aspirin
  Potential candidates: All patients with confirmed AMI receiving aspirin (n = 9272).
  Exclusions: Missing date when aspirin was first begun (10%).
  Criterion: The time (in days) from arrival at the hospital until the beginning of administration of the aspirin.

Reproduced with permission from Ellerbeck et al.[12]

Table 3-5. Quality Indicators at the Time of Discharge for an Acute Myocardial Infarction (AMI), Excluding Patients Who Died or Were Transferred to Another Acute Care Hospital

Aspirin at discharge
Potential candidates: Discharged alive (n = 10015).
Exclusions: Patients with blood in their stools or evidence of bleeding on admission or during the hospitalization (13%); history of gastrointestinal bleeding or a hemorrhagic stroke, chronic liver disease. coagulopathy, platelet count <100 × 10⁹/L, recent head trauma, or intracranial neoplasm (6%); a serum creatinine level >265 μmol/L (3mg/dL) (3%); history of peptic ulcer disease or a discharge diagnosis of an upper gastrointestinal disorder (5%); hemoglobin level <100g/L or hematocrit <0.30 (5%) (5%); allergy to aspirin (4%); treatment with warfarin (15%); metastatic cancer or other terminal illness (7%).
Criterion: Discharged on aspirin.

β-Blockers at discharge
Potential candidates: Discharged alive (n = 10015).
Exclusions: Patients with left ventricular ejection fraction (LVEF) <35% (15%); pulmonary edema or congestive heart failure (unless measured LVEF >50%) (36%); hypotension or shock during the hospitalization or systolic blood pressure at discharge of <100 mm Hg (18%); history of chronic obstructive pulmonary disease (20%); symptomatic bradycardia or pulse at discharge of <50 beats per minute (7%); diagnosis of depression or treatment with antidepressants (5%); treatment with insulin (11%); dementia (4%); conduction disorder including Mobitz type II block, third-degree heart block, or bifascicular block (7%); no significant coronary artery disease (2%); or those at very low risk as determined by the presence of all of the following: no recurrent chest pain; no arrhythmias; no previous AMI; normal stress test; and no LVEF <50% (2%).
Criterion: Discharged on a β-blocker.

Angiotensin-converting enzyme (ACE) inhibitors for low LVEF
Potential candidates: Discharged with an LVEF <40% (n = 2036).
Exclusions: Patients with aortic stenosis (5%); an allergy or intolerance to ACE inhibitor (5%); a serum creatinine level >176 μmol/L (2 mg/dL) (16%); or a systolic blood pressure <100 mm Hg at discharge (8%).
Criterion: Discharged on an ACE inhibitor.

No calcium channel blockers with low LVEF
Potential candidates: Discharged with an LVEF <40% or evidence of shock or pulmonary edema during the hospitalization (n = 2246).
Exclusions: Patients with atrial fibrillation at any time during the hospitalization (33%); recurrent chest pain (27%); or those receiving calcium channel blockers prior to admission (33%).
Criterion: Not discharged on a certain channel blocker.

Smoking cessation advice
Potential candidates: Cigarette smokers discharged alive (n = 1691).
Exclusions: None.
Criterion: Documentation in the chart of advice or counseling on smoking cessation.

Reproduced with permission from Ellerbeck et al.[12]

probabilities were 51% and 45%, respectively, and were similar to those for patients with recognized AMI (Table 3-7). One third of men with unrecognized and 58% of men with recognized AMI had a history of angina pectoris. Angina pectoris had a greater effect on CAD mortality in the former group than in the latter. The risk ratio for unrecognized AMI was 4.6 without angina and 16.9 with angina; the risk ratio for recognized AMI was 6.3 without angina and 8.5 with angina. At least 1/3 of all AMIs were unrecognized. Prognosis and risk factor profiles for patients with recognized and unrecognized AMI were similar.

Table 3-6. Interventions During the Hospitalization and at Discharge in Patients With AMI Who Are Potential Candidates, Ideal Candidates, or Less-Than-Ideal Candidates (Excluded Patients) for These Interventions*

Intervention	Potential Candidates, No.	No. Excluded (%)	Rate of Use of the Intervention, %		
			All Potential Candidates	Excluded Patients	Ideal Candidates
During the initial hospitalization					
Aspirin	12332	4846(39)	75	64	83
Heparin (full or low dose)	12332	2475(20)	68	61	69
Thrombolytics	11371	10266(90)	18	12	70
Intravenous nitroglycerin for persistent pain	1978	224(11)	74	74	74
At the time of or prior to discharge					
Aspirin	10015	4174(42)	66	51	77
β-Blockers	10015	7039(70)	32	27	45
ACE inhibitors for low LVEF	2036	563(28)	60	64	59
Avoidance of calcium channel blockers with low LVEF, shock, or severe CHF	2246	1461(65)	69	64	79
Smoking cessation advice for smokers	1691	0	...	...	28

*AMI indicates acute myocardial infarction; IV, intravenous; ACE, angiotensin-converting enzyme; LVEF, left ventricular ejection fraction; and CHF, congestive heart failure. Ellipses indicated not applicable because there were no exclusions for the smoking cessation indicator.
Reproduced with permission of Ellerbeck et al.[12]

Table 3-7. Clinical Characteristics of Patients with Unrecognized and Recognized Myocardial Infarction*

	Mean Value (95% CI)	
Variable	Patients with Unrecognized Myocardial Infarction (n = 83)	Patients with Recognized Myocardial Infarction (n = 154)
Age, *y*	60 (58 to 62)	59 (58 to 60)
Cholesterol level, *mg/dL*	256 (247 to 265)	254 (248 to 260)
Triglyceride level, *mg/dL*	133 (118 to 148)	147 (133 to 161)
Blood glucose level, *mg/dL*	83 (65 to 101)	83 (80 to 86)
Glucose tolerance (90 min), *mg/dL*	120 (111 to 129)	122 (115 to 129)
Blood pressure, *mm Hg*		
Systolic	141 (136 to 146)	142.0 (139 to 145)
Diastolic	88 (86 to 90)	88.0 (86 to 90)
Body mass index	26.0 (25.2 to 26.8)	26.0 (25.6 to 26.4)
Cardiomegaly, %	18 (10 to 28)	21 (14 to 27)
Smoking habits, %		
Never	10 (4 to 18)	12 (7 to 17)
Former	41 (30 to 52)	45 (37 to 53)
Pipe or cigars	14 (8 to 24)	20 (14 to 26)
1 to 15 cigarettes/d	14 (8 to 24)	12 (7 to 18)
15 to 24 cigarettes/d	12 (6 to 21)	6 (3 to 12)
>25 cigarettes/d	8 (3 to 17)	5 (2 to 9)
Drug therapy, %		
Hypertension	13 (7 to 22)	21 (14 to 27)
Diuretics	11 (5 to 20)	10 (6 to 15)
Digoxin	6 (2 to 14)	16 (10 to 22)
Angina, %	34 (24 to 45)	58 (50 to 66)

*Data pooled from all stages of the study.
Reproduced with permission from Sigurdsson et al.[13]

Although those with unrecognized AMI were less likely than those with recognized AMI to have a history of angina pectoris, angina in these cases was usually associated with ischemic electrocardiographic changes and a poor prognosis, suggesting severe CAD.

Decreasing Mortality

Behar and associates[14] from Tel Hashomer, Israel, compared the outcome of patients with a first AMI among 3 large cohorts of patients hospitalized between 1966 and 1992 in Israel, in view of changes in treatment facilities and investigation methods. Patients with a first AMI constituted 71% of all myocardial infarctions in 1966, 74% in 1981–1983, and 71% in 1992. The male-to-female ratio and the distribution of the site of infarction also remained stable from 1966 to 1992. The mean age of patients increased over time. Thrombolytic therapy was not available in 1966 and 1981–1983, whereas 53% of patients were treated with a thrombolytic agent and 22% examined with coronary angiography in 1992. The 21-day mortality rate decreased markedly, from 22% in 1966 to 14% in 1981–1983 and to 8% in 1992. The decrease was similar in both genders and among 10-year age groups. The 1-year postdischarge mortality rate (not evaluated in 1966) decreased from 7% in 1981–1983 to 6% in 1992. It was concluded that a significant reduction in mortality rate after a first AMI took place over the 25-year period. Changes in treatment modality and management of the acute phase may explain this decrease in mortality rate over time.

Associated With Cocaine Use

The frequency of complications in patients with cocaine-associated AMI is unknown. Hollander and associates[15] for the associated AMI study group determined the short-term mortality and morbidity secondary to cocaine-associated AMI. The authors performed retrospective cohort study at 29 hospital centers throughout the USA. Patients with cocaine-associated AMI that occurred between 1987 and 1993 were identified through record review. The primary outcome measures were in-hospital mortality and the incidence and timing of major cardiovascular complications. Cocaine-associated AMI was identified 136 times in 130 patients. Patients were generally young (mean age, 38 years), nonwhite (72%), tobacco smokers (91%) with a history of cocaine use in the previous 24 hours (88%). The initial electrocardiogram disclosed AMI in 44% and ischemia in an additional 18% of patients. AMI was evenly distributed between anterior (45%) and inferior (44%) walls and was most often non–Q-wave (61%). Complications occurred 64 times in 49 patients (36%); including CHF in 9 patients, VT in 23 patients, SVT in 6 patients, and bradydysrhythmias in 26 patients. Most patients who had complications (90%) had them within 12 hours of presentation. Acute in-hospital mortality was zero. The mortality of patients hospitalized with cocaine-associated AMI was low. Most complications occurred within 12 hours of presentation.

Diagnosis and Early Testing

Creatine Kinase–MB Isoenzyme, Troponin T, Myoglobin, and Leukocyte Differential

To test whether automated measurements of cortisol-induced changes in the leukocyte differential can provide an early marker of AMI, especially when combined with the rapid creatine kinase–MB isoenzyme, Thomson and associates[16] from Rochester, Minnesota, studied 511 consecutive patients presenting to the emergency department with chest pain: 127 patients with infection, trauma, or metastatic cancer or receiving myelosuppressive or glucocorticoid therapy were excluded. Of 69 patients with AMI, only 39% had diagnostic electrocardiographic ST-segment elevation. ST-segment elevation had a specificity of 99% and a positive predictive value of 93%. A relative lymphocytopenia (lymphocyte decrease <20.3%) or elevated rapid creatine kinase–MB level (>4.7 ng/mL) was more sensitive than ST-segment elevation (sensitivities of 58% and 56%, respectively) but less specific (specificities of 91% and 93%, respectively). The presence of both a relative lymphocytopenia and an elevated rapid creatine kinase–MB level had a sensitivity of 44%, a specificity of 99.7%, and a positive predictive value of 97%. Both a relative lymphocytopenia and an elevated rapid creatine kinase–MB level were independent predictors of infarction in patients without ST-segment elevation. If AMI was suspected by the presence of both abnormal markers or ST-segment elevation, the sensitivity for early diagnosis increased from 39% (ST elevation alone) to 65%; the specificity was 99%; and the positive predictive value was 94%. The presence of both a relative lymphocytopenia and an elevated rapid creatine kinase–MB level was an accurate early marker of AMI that appeared to improve the sensitivity of early diagnosis compared with that of ST-segment elevation alone.

A retrospective study of patients with possible AMI was conducted by Dorogy and associates[17] of Aurora, Colorado, over a 2-year period to evaluate the clinical characteristics, angiographic findings, and in-hospital prognosis in patients with normal total creatine kinase activity and increased MB isoenzyme activity. Thirty-nine cases were identified (study group) and compared with cases of Q-wave (n=77) and non–Q-wave (n=60) infarctions. Compared with the Q-wave group, study group patients were older (68±9.0 vs. 61±12 years) and more often had previous diagnoses of CAD (53% vs. 18%) and peripheral vascular disease (29% vs. 10%). Angina (92% vs. 66%) and ST elevation (82% vs. 13%) were more common in the Q-wave group. Nearly identical clinical profiles and electrocardiographic findings were observed in the study and non–Q-wave groups. Angiographic analysis revealed a higher frequency of multivessel disease in the study group (90%) than in the Q-wave group (49%) but no difference between the study group and the non–Q-wave group (80%). LV function and in-hospital complications were similar among groups. It is concluded that patients with normal total creatine kinase activity and increased creatine kinase–MB concentration represent a subgroup of patients with non–Q-wave infarction with a high prevalence of multivessel CAD.

Müller-Bardorff and colleagues[18] in Heidelberg, Germany, developed a whole blood rapid assay device for cardiac troponin T detection that provides a test result within 20 minutes in order to assess patients with chest pain. Monoclonal antibody M7 labeled with gold particles, and antibody 1B10 labeled with biotin were used in the assay. Both antibodies, as well as buffer substances and detergents, were absorbed onto paper fleeces mounted below an application well. Heparinized blood applied to this well solubilizes the dry chemistry reagents. Blood cells were separated from plasma using a glass-fiber fleece. The immunocomplexes formed were concentrated within the reading zone by binding of the biotin-labeled antibody with streptavidin immobilized to the test device. Troponin T bound to the test device served as a control. The detection limit of the assay is 0.18 µg/L with a cross-reactivity with skeletal troponin T of 0.5%. In clinical analyses involving 25 healthy volunteers, 62 patients with chest pain but without myocardial ischemia, 35 patients with AMI, 24 patients with minor myocardial damage due to radiofrequency ablation, and 35 patients with unstable angina, the rapid assay was comparable to the troponin T enzyme immunoassay as regards sensitivity and specificity. Thus, this newly developed assay allows accurate, rapid, and convenient diagnosis of AMI in patients.

de Winter and colleagues[19] in Amsterdam, the Netherlands, studied the value of myoglobin, creatine kinase–MB, and troponin T in excluding AMI in the emergency room in 309 consecutive patients presenting with chest pain. The gold standard for AMI recognition was a combination of history, electrocardiography, and a typical curve of the creatine kinase–MB activity. Myoglobin

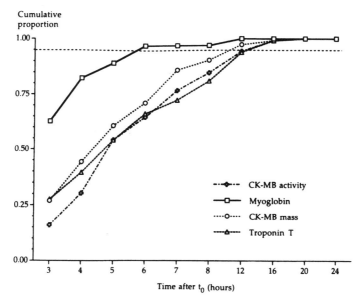

Figure 3-6. Plot showing the cumulative proportion of patients with AMI with a sample above the upper reference limit, comparing CK-MB$_{act}$, CK-MB$_{mass}$, myoglobin, and troponin T. The cumulative proportion of patients with a myoglobin result above the upper reference limit was significantly higher in the early hours than for CK-MB$_{mass}$ and troponin T ($P < 0.0001$). At 6 hours, 97% of patients with AMI had a myoglobin result above the upper reference limit. The cumulative proportion of CK-MB$_{mass}$ was significantly earlier than troponin T ($P < 0.0001$). Differences between the three curves were tested with the Wilcoxon rank-sum test. Reproduced with permission from de Winter.[19]

was the earliest marker, and its negative predictive value was significantly higher than for creatine kinase–MB and troponin T from 3 to 6 hours after the onset of symptoms (Figure 3-6). The negative predictive value of myoglobin reached 89% at 4 hours after symptom onset. The negative predictive value of creatine kinase–MB reached 95% at 7 hours after the onset of symptoms. Troponin T was not an early marker for ruling out AMI and negative predictive value changed over time together with creatine kinase–MB. The early negative predictive value was higher in a subgroup of patients with a low probability of the presence of AMI for the three markers. Cardiac markers rise early in patients with large AMI as indicated in this study by the proportion of patients with a marker substance above the upper reference level at each time point of analysis. These data suggest that for ruling out AMI in the emergency room, myoglobin is a better marker than creatine kinase–MB or troponin T from 3 until 6 hours after symptom onset, but the maximum negative predictive value reaches only 89%. By 7 hours after symptom onset, the negative predictive value of creatine kinase–MB is 95%.

Echocardiography

Res and coworkers[20] in Amsterdam, the Netherlands, combined transesophageal atrial stimulation with 2-dimensional echocardiography in 69 consecutive patients on days 3–5 of their first uncomplicated AMI to determine if inducible remote asynergy (not directly adjacent to the infarcted area and supposedly related to another vascular territory) provided information regarding 1) extent of CAD and 2) future ischemic events. Uncomplicated adequate stress studies were performed in 59 of 69 patients (86%); all of these patients had regional asynergy at rest. Remote asynergy at rest was present in 7 patients and during transesophageal atrial stimulation in 26 patients. Coronary angiography was performed within 2 to 3 weeks after the acute phase. Multivessel CAD was present in 23 of these patients and absent in 3. Of the 33 patients without remote asynergy during transesophageal atrial stimulation, 5 had multivessel CAD. Sensitivity of remote asynergy during esophageal atrial stimulation for detecting multivessel CAD was 82%, specificity 90% and predictive accuracy 86%. New ischemic events defined as recurrent infarction, cardiac death or revascularization within 12 to 18 months occurred in 24 patients (41%); remote asynergy during esophageal atrial simulation was present in 16 of these patients (67%). The investigators concluded that transesophageal atrial stimulation combined with 2-dimensional echocardiography can safely be performed in the early days of AMI; remote asynergy during esophageal atrial stimulation reliably identifies patients with multivessel CAD and future ischemic events.

Heart Rate Variability

Vanoli and colleagues[21] in Oklahoma City, Oklahoma; Milan, Italy; and Montescano, Italy, evaluated heart rate variability during various sleep stages in normal subjects and in patients with AMI. Heart rate variability was measured from 5 minutes of continuous electrocardiographic recordings in 8 individuals with no clinical evidence of CAD (mean age, 47 years) and in 8 patients with a recent AMI (mean age, 51 years) in the awake stage and during non–rapid eye movement (REM) and REM sleep. In normal subjects, the low- to high-frequency ratio derived from power spectral analysis of heart rate variability decreased significantly from the awake state to non-REM sleep. During REM sleep, the low- to high-frequency ratio increased to 3. In patients after AMI, the low-frequency/high-frequency ratio showed an opposite trend toward an increase from 3 to 5. REM sleep produced a further increase in the low-frequency/high-frequency up to 9. Thus, AMI causes a loss in the capability of the vagus to physiologically activate during sleep resulting in a condition of relative sympathetic dominance even during sleep.

Predictors of Non–Q-Wave Infarction

Among patients with acute ischemic syndromes, patients with non–Q-wave AMI are known to be at higher risk for death, reinfarction, and other morbidity than those with unstable angina. The aim of a study by Cannon and coinvestigators[22] in Boston, Massachusetts, was to develop a clinically useful prediction rule to assist in distinguishing, at the time of presentation, patients with non–Q-wave AMI from those with unstable angina. The TIMI IIIB trial enrolled 1473 patients presenting with ischemic pain at rest within 24 hours who had either electrocardiographic changes or documented CAD. Non–Q-wave AMI on presentation was documented by elevation of creatine kinase–MB in 33% of patients. Fifty clinical and electrocardiographic variables were compared between the patients with non–Q-wave AMI and unstable angina. After performing logistic regression, 4 baseline characteristics independently

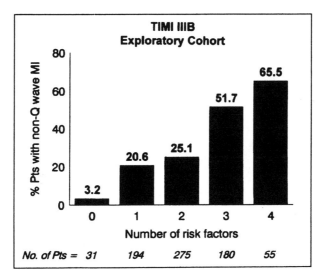

Figure 3-7. Prevalence of non–Q-wave acute myocardial infarction (AMI) based on four baseline characteristics (risk factors) which independently predicted non-Q-wave AMI in the Thrombolysis in Myocardial Infarction (TIMI) IIIB trial exploratory cohort: (1) absence of prior percutaneous transluminal coronary angioplasty; (2) duration of pain ≥60 minutes; (3) ST-segment deviation on the qualifying electrocardiogram; and (4) recent-onset angina. Reproduced by permission from Cannon et al.[22]

predicted non–Q-wave myocardial AMI: the absence of prior PTCA, duration of chest pain ≥60 minutes, ST-segment deviation on the qualifying electrocardiogram, and recent-onset angina (Figure 3-7). Using these four characteristics, a prediction rule for non–Q-wave AMI was developed. For the entire cohort of patients in TIMI III, the percentages of patients with non–Q-wave AMI when 0, 1, 2, 3, and 4 risk factors were present were 7%, 20%, 24%, 50%, and 71%, respectively. Thus, easily identifiable characteristics of presentation can be used to assess the likelihood of non–Q-wave AMI.

Early vs. Late Responders

Burnett and coworkers[23] in Durham, North Carolina, identified factors that distinguish early responders (i.e., requested medical assistance <60 minutes after the onset of AMI symptoms) from late responders (i.e., request ≥60 minutes after symptom onset). A questionnaire developed to assess demographic characteristics, contextual factors, antecedents to symptom onset, and behavioral, affective, and cognitive responses was administered in the hospital to 501 patients with documented AMI. Patients who believed that their symptoms were cardiac in nature were more likely to be early responders, whereas patients who attributed their symptoms to indigestion, muscle pain, fatigue, or another cause responded later. Early responders believed their symptoms to be more serious, felt more comfortable seeking medical assistance, were more anxious or upset when they first noticed symptoms, and perceived that they had less control of their symptoms than late responders. A stepwise multiple regression analysis further suggested that unmarried patients responded significantly later than married patients, and patients who first experienced their symptoms at

Table 3-8. Infarction Pain Duration, Severity and Time Course, and Concomitant Symptoms in Patients With Anterior or Inferior Wall Acute Myocardial Infarction

	Anterior AMI (n = 48)	Inferior AMI (n = 56)
Pain duration (hrs)	6.1 ± 6.4	6.5 ± 5.4
Pain severity (mm)	68 ± 21	61 ± 21
Pre-AMI angina (%)	26 (54)	24 (43)
Continuous pain (%)	34 (71)	42 (75)
Sweating (%)	46 (96)	54 (96)
Nausea (%)	23 (48)	39 (70)*
Vomiting (%)	18 (38)	25 (45)
Hiccups (%)	0 (0)	4 (7)

*$P < 0.05$.
AMI indicates acute myocardial infarction.
Reproduced with permission from Pasceri et al.[24]

work responded significantly later than those who first experienced their symptoms outside of the home but not at work. These results suggest that situational and psychological variables are important determinants of lengthy decision delays in responding to symptoms of AMI.

Relation of Pain Location and Infarct Site

Pasceri and coworkers[24] in Rome, Italy, assessed the location, severity, duration, and time course of pain in 104 consecutive patients with either first or second anterior or inferior Q-wave AMI. Pain severity was assessed using a visual analog scale. Pain location and radiation were similar in 48 patients with anterior and 56 patients with inferior wall AMI. Pain duration and severity were also similar. The pain was continuous in 34 patients with anterior and in 42 with inferior wall AMI. Among the 41 patients who did not receive thrombolytic therapy, 18 patients with continuous pain had a higher creatine kinase peak level than the remaining 23 patients with intermittent pain or preinfarction angina, or both. The incidence of gastrointestinal symptoms was slightly higher in patients with inferior than anterior wall AMI (Table 3-8). Among 32 patients admitted with a second AMI, pain location was similar in 14 who had both infarcts in the same myocardial region but different in 12 of 18 who had a first and second infarct in different regions. Thus, patients with anterior or inferior wall AMI experienced pain in similar body regions. However, in patients who presented with >1 AMI, different locations of the infarction pain were highly predictive of ischemia occurring in different myocardial regions. Finally, patients with preinfarction angina or intermittent pain tended to have smaller infarcts.

Prognostic Indices

Ischemic Time

Hasche and colleagues[25] from Sydney, Australia, performed a prospective study to document the role of ischemia time as a determinant of infarct size in humans. The authors studied 61 patients, including 50 men with a mean age of 57 years admitted with a first AMI (31 anterior and 30 inferior) who had continuous 12-lead electrocardiographic monitoring to document ischemia time. As identified by 32-point QRS score on day 7, changes in regional myocardial blood flow as determined by echocardiography during the following month were related to ischemia time. Among patients with <3 hours of ischemia (n = 16), mean infarct size on day 7 was 21% of potential infarct size. In patients with 3 to 6 hours of ischemia (n = 23), infarct size was 38% of potential and in patients with 6 to 9 hours of ischemia (n = 10), infarct size was 66% of potential. In contrast, the 12 patients with an ischemia time >9 hours had a final infarct size of 77% of potential. Multivariate regression identified size of risk region, duration of ischemia, and duration of initial ST-segment elevation as independent predictors of infarct size. Among these, the most important variable was ischemia time. The regression models developed predicted both individual absolute infarct size and individual infarct/risk ratio. Patients with <6 hours of ischemia had significant recovery of myocardial wall motion by day 7, but patients with 6–9 hours of ischemia had less recovery by 1 month and patients with >9 hours of ischemia had very little recovery of wall motion at 1 month. Thus, measurement of infarct size allows improved prediction of infarct size in humans. The data in this study suggest that significant myocardial salvage and functional recovery may be achieved by reperfusion up to 9 hours after coronary occlusion.

Blood Pressure

Flack and colleagues[26] in Winston-Salem, North Carolina, evaluated the relation between BP and death from CAD and all causes for men with a history of AMI. The study cohort included men ages 35 to 57 years screened for the Multiple Risk Factor Intervention Trial (MRFIT) in 1973 through 1975 and followed for an average of 16 years through 1990. There were 5362 men who reported prior hospitalization for AMI of at least 2 weeks' duration at the initiation of the MRFIT study. There was a J-shaped relation between systolic BP and diastolic BP with CAD and all-cause mortality during the first 2 years of follow-up in the older men (ages 45 to 57 years) only. The risk nadirs for systolic BP were 152 and 145 mm Hg, respectively, for CAD death and all-cause mortality. The diastolic BP risk nadirs were 94 and 90 mm Hg. After the first 2 years, there was a positive association between systolic BP and death from CAD and all causes. At 15 years, cumulative CAD mortality percentages for men with screening systolic BP <120, 120 to 139, 140 to 159, and ≥160 mm Hg were 20%, 21%, 28%, and 32%, respectively (Figure 3-8). When deaths only after year 2 were considered, the quadratic term for diastolic BP was no longer significant. The relation still appeared J-shaped as cumulative mortality for those with diastolic BP <70, 70 to 79, 80 to 89, 90 to 99, and ≥100 mm Hg was 24%, 21%, 21%, 26%, and 30%, respectively (Figure 3-9). When the joint relation of systolic BP and diastolic BP was considered, there were no survival differences among the four cohorts with a systolic BP ≥140 and diastolic BP <80, systolic BP ≥140 and diastolic BP ≤80, systolic BP ≤140 and diastolic BP <80, and systolic BP ≤140 and diastolic BP ≥80 in the first 2 years of evaluation. Following 2 years, both CAD and all-cause mortality rates were approximately 40% higher for participants with systolic BP ≥ 140 mm Hg vs. <140 mm Hg regardless of diastolic BP. Thus, in this large cohort of men with prior AMI,

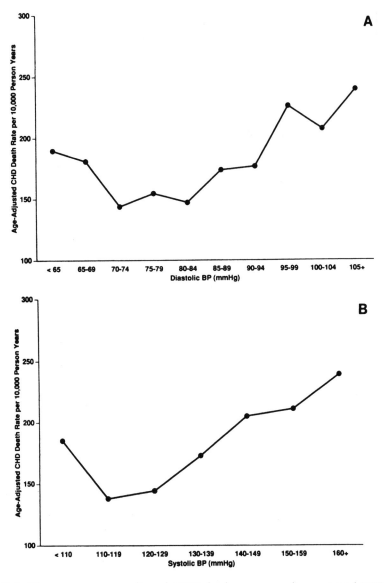

Figure 3-8. Plots represent age-adjusted CHD death rates according to initial DBP (**A**) and SBP (**B**) level, respectively, in the 5362 MRFIT men with prior history of hospitalization of at least 2 weeks' duration for MI. Reproduced with permission from Flack et al.[26]

the association of systolic and diastolic BP with CAD and all-cause mortality varied over a 16-year follow-up period. During early follow-up in older men, only J- or U-shaped relations were evident. However, after 2 years, these same relations had become positive and graded. Given the substantial excess mortality risk in this cohort associated with elevated BP, especially systolic BP, lower BP should receive high priority among hypertensive men with prior AMI.

Previous Angina Pectoris

Experimental studies indicate that brief transient period episodes of ischemia render the heart somewhat resistant to AMI from a subsequent sustained

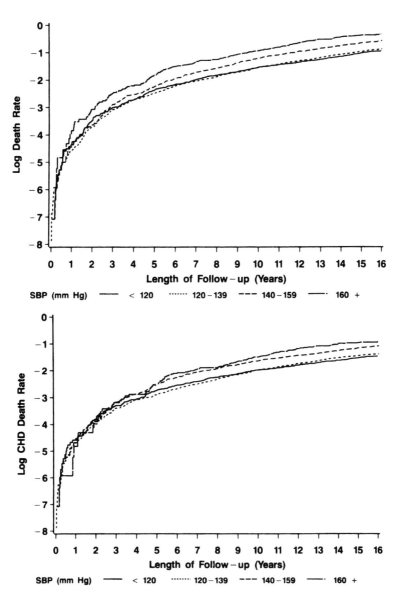

Figure 3-9. Curves of CHD-adjusted mortality by SBP level in MRFIT men with previous MI. Mortality is adjusted for age, cholesterol, and cigarettes smoked per day. Reproduced with permission from Flack et al.[26]

ischemic insult. Nakagawa and colleagues[27] from Osaka, Japan, attempted to determine if this phenomenon might also be operative in patients undergoing AMI. Eight-four patients with an AMI who achieved reflow within 6 hours of onset were classified into 3 groups on the basis of duration of antecedent angina pectoris. Group 1 had no angina, group 2 had new angina occurring within 7 days of the onset of AMI, and group 3 had angina pectoris lasting >7 days before the onset of the infarction. Angiographic collateral flow grade was higher in group 3 than in groups 1 and 2. Although there were no differences in baseline EF and regional wall motion among the 3 groups, the degree of improvement was significantly greater in groups 2 and 3 than in group 1. These authors concluded that episodes of angina pectoris occurring shortly before the onset of AMI may preserve myocardial contractile function in reperfused AMI despite less support from collateral flow channels.

When in Young Adults

There are few data regarding AMI in young adults. Of the 8839 patients with a history of AMI in the CASS study, there were 294 men <35 years of age and 210 women <45 years of age.[28] In reviewing these patients, these authors noted that these young men and women often had angiographically normal coronary arteries, nonobstructive CAD, <70% stenosis, and single vessel CAD more commonly than older patients. Current smoking was more frequent in young patients. Systemic hypertension and diabetes mellitus were more frequent in both older men and women whereas a positive family history of premature CAD was significantly more prevalent only in young women. The survival rate at 7 years was improved for young men compared with that in older men (84% vs. 75%) and for young women compared with older women (90% vs. 77%). These authors concluded that younger patients with AMI have a more favorable prognosis compared with older patients.

ST-Segment Elevation on Holter Monitoring

The correlation between episodes of ST-segment on Holter monitoring, clinical characteristics, LV function, exercise testing, and long-term prognosis was determined by Mickley and coworkers[29] in Odense, Denmark, in 123 consecutive patients (average age, 55 years) with a first AMI. During 36 hours of Holter recording 11 days after AMI, 11 patients (9%) had 91 episodes of ST-segment elevation (group 1), whereas 112 patients had no such episodes (group 2). Most episodes of ST-segment elevation occurred in leads with pathological Q waves or small, indistinct R waves. Large anterior Q-wave AMIs were more prevalent in group 1 than in group 2 and in hospital CHF also occurred more frequently in group 1 patients (82% vs. 23%). Regional and global LV function was reduced in group 1 compared with group 2: EF 33% vs. 50%. All episodes of ST elevation were asymptomatic and did not correlate with different indicators of myocardial ischemia. Indeed, exercise-induced ST-segment depression was more prevalent in group 2 than in group 1: 57% vs. 18%. Over a mean of 5 years of follow-up, an association between episodes of ST-segment elevation on Holter monitoring and 1) cardiac death and 2) cardiac death and nonfatal reinfarction was found. If, however, the symptomatic need for coronary revascularization was included as an end point, no association between episodes of ST-segment elevation and long-term outcome could be demonstrated.

Maximal Exercise Testing

The GISSI-2 database allowed reevaluation of the prognostic role of exercise testing in patients with AMI treated with thrombolysis. Villella and associates[30] on behalf of the GISSI-2 Investigators performed the exercise tests in 6296

Table 3-9. Distribution of Historical and Clinical Variables by Exercise Testing Results

	Maximal negative (n = 2381)	Not diagnostic (n = 2244)	Positive (n = 1626)	Positive for ECG (n = 1089)	Positive for angina (n = 537)
Female sex (%)	17.9	6.0	11.1	9.8	3.8
Age > 70 years (%)	9.7	7.8	9.5	9.0	10.4
Smoking (%)					
Past	21.7	20.1	25.9	24.9	27.9
Present	55.0	68.0	54.9	57.4	49.7
History (%)					
Myocardial infarction	8.5	11.4	14.6	12.2	19.4
Angina	16.1	17.9	24.0	18.4	35.6
Hypertension (treated)	24.7	23.6	28.0	25.4	33.1
Insulin-dependent diabetes	1.5	1.6	1.2	0.9	1.7
Hospital course (%)					
tPA administration	50.4	50.8	49.1	47.5	52.3
Heparin administration	51.2	48.8	48.7	49.8	46.6
Early LV failure	9.2	7.6	7.7	7.5	8.0
Late LV failure	3.9	3.8	4.1	4.3	3.5
Postinfarction angina	6.1	7.4	10.3	7.4	16.0
Electrocardiogram (%)					
Anterior site	37.0	33.2	18.8	14.1	28.1
QRS score > 10	16.1	13.4	10.7	10.1	11.9
Special tests (%)					
Electrical instability (Holter)	27.7	26.3	30.6	29.8	32.2
Recovery-phase LV dysfunction (Echo)	11.0	9.9	9.6	8.9	11.0
6-month follow-up (%)					
Angina	9.4	12.7	22.5	15.6	36.5
CABG	1.2	2.0	7.4	4.7	13.0
PTCA	1.3	1.5	4.1	3.6	5.2

Reproduced with permission from Villella et al.[30]

patients, on average 28 days after randomization (Table 3-9 and Figure 3-10). The test was performed in 2923 patients because of contraindications. The test was judged positive for residual ischemia in 26% of the patients, negative in 38%, and nondiagnostic in 36%. Among the patients with positive stress test results, 33% had symptoms, whereas 67% had silent myocardial ischemia. The mortality rate was 7.1% among patients who did not have an exercise test and 7.1% for those with a positive test, 0.9% for those who had a negative test, and 1.3% for those who did not have a diagnostic test. In the adjusted analysis, symptomatic induced ischemia, submaximal positive result, low work capacity, and abnormal systolic BP were independent predictors of 6-month mortality. However, when these factors were tested simultaneously, only symptomatic induced ischemia and low work capacity were confirmed as independent predictors of mortality. Patients with a normal exercise response have an excellent medium-term prognosis and do not need further investigation. However, more

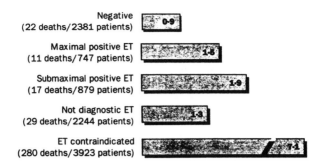

Negative
(22 deaths/2381 patients) 0-9

Maximal positive ET
(11 deaths/747 patients) 1.5

Submaximal positive ET
(17 deaths/879 patients) 1.9

Not diagnostic ET
(29 deaths/2244 patients) 1.3

ET contraindicated
(280 deaths/3923 patients) 7.1

Figure 3-10. 6-Month total mortality by exercise test results. Reproduced with permission from Villella et al.[30]

evaluation should be devoted to the patients who cannot undergo exercise testing, because the potential to influence outcome appears to be much greater.

Older Age

Seventy patients ≥70 years of age admitted to the coronary care unit with non–Q-wave AMI were followed prospectively by Chung and associates[31] in St. Louis, Missouri, for 1 year, and the clinical course in these patients was compared with that in 61 patients <70 years with non–Q-wave AMI and 56 patients ≥70 years with Q-wave AMI. Compared with the younger patients with non–Q-wave AMI, older patients were more likely to develop AF (23% vs. 8%) and CHF (53% vs. 30%), and less likely to receive thrombolytic therapy (9% vs. 28%), cardiac catheterization (41% vs. 72%), and coronary angioplasty (20% vs. 39%). Hospital mortality did not differ significantly between older and younger non–Q-wave AMI patients (10% vs. 3%), but 1-year mortality was higher in the elderly (36% vs. 16%) (Table 3-10), Elderly patients with Q-wave AMI had more in-hospital complications, including death (25 vs. 10%), than elderly patients with non–Q-wave AMI. In contrast, postdischarge mortality

Table 3-10. Predictors of One-Year Mortality Among Hospital Survivors Aged ≥70 Years with Non–Q-Wave Acute Myocardial Infarction.

	Alive (n = 45)	Died (n = 18)	P
Age (years)	77 ± 5	82 ± 6	0.001
Men (%)	24 (53)	6 (33)	NS
Systemic hypertension (%)	30 (67)	14 (78)	NS
Diabetes mellitus (%)	15 (33)	6 (33)	NS
Prior myocardial infarction (%)	15 (33)	10 (56)	NS
New York Heart Association class	1.4 ± 0.7	2.1 ± 0.8	0.003
Jugular venous distention (%)	7 (16)	10 (56)	0.008
Killip class	1.3 ± 0.5	1.8 ± 1.0	0.02
Peak creatine kinase (U)	692 ± 807	358 ± 249	0.02
Anterior infarction (%)	14 (31)	4 (22)	NS
Left ventricular ejection fraction (%)	55 ± 14	41 ± 18	0.007
Cardiac catheterization (%)	22 (49)	2 (11)	0.005
Revascularization (%)	18 (40)	2 (11)	0.02

Reproduced with permission from Chung et al.[31]

was higher in elderly patients with non–Q-wave AMI, so that total mortality at 1 year was similar in the 2 groups. Overall, elderly patients with non–Q-wave AMI accounted for 62% of all deaths occurring during the first year after discharge. Thus, elderly patients with non–Q-wave AMI have a significantly increased mortality risk during the year after hospital discharge compared with other patients with AMI, suggesting that an aggressive diagnostic and therapeutic approach may be of particular benefit in these patients.

Despite the advancements in reperfusion therapy, elderly patients with AMI continue to have higher mortality and complication rates than younger patients. To evaluate this group, Devlin and colleagues[32] in Royal Oak, Michigan, reviewed 994 consecutive patients with AMI at their hospital during a 24-month period. There were 307 patients aged >75 years and 687 younger patients. Demographic analysis of the 2 groups showed that the elderly had a higher proportion of women (56% vs. 31%), more previous AMI (32% vs. 23%), and a higher incidence of BBB (18% vs. 8%). Only 8% of the elderly and 36% of the younger patients were considered eligible for thrombolysis. In the elderly, risk of bleeding and late presentation were the most common reasons for exclusion from treatment with thrombolytic therapy. Despite a higher proportion of non–Q-wave AMI (56% vs. 44%) in the elderly, the incidence of CHF (47% vs. 23%) and death (28% vs. 11%) was greater. Causes of death were not significantly different. Increased mortality in the elderly was not due to multisystem failure but to impaired myocardial reserve, suggesting that more aggressive reperfusion strategies may improve prognosis.

Sex

Bueno and colleagues[33] in Madrid, Spain, determined the differences between sexes and the outcome of AMI in the elderly by comparing the clinical history and evolution of 204 consecutive patients ≥75 years of age admitted with a first AMI. Women had a higher prevalence of hypertension and diabetes, and men were more frequently smokers. These factors were associated with higher rates of CHF. Women showed a lower LVEF and a higher rate of CHF and shock (Figure 3-11). Mortality rate was higher in women; however, sex was excluded as an independent predictor of in-hospital mortality in every regression model tested. Thus, after a first AMI, elderly women have a more complicated hospital course than men, and the increase in mortality appears to be related to extensive cardiovascular risk factors and their influence on LVEF more than to gender itself.

Depression

Over 18 months, Frasure-Smith and colleagues[34] in Montreal, Canada, examined the impact of depression on prognosis in patients after AMI by studying 222 patients who responded to a modified version of the National Institute of Mental Health Diagnostic Interview Schedule for a major depressive episode approximately 7 days after AMI. The Beck Depression Inventory was also completed by 218 of the patients. All patients and/or families were contacted at 18 months to determine survival status. Thirty-five patients met the modified Mental Health Diagnostic Interview Schedule criteria for major in-hospital depression after AMI. Sixty-eight had scores indicative of mild to moderate depres-

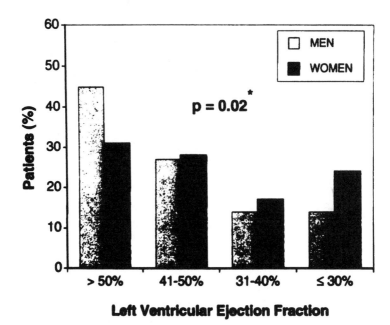

Figure 3-11. Bar graph comparing left ventricular ejection fraction determined by 2-dimensional echocardiography in both groups. *Mantel-Haenszel test. Reproduced with permission from Bueno et al.[33]

sion. There were 21 deaths during the follow-up period, including 19 from cardiac causes. Seven of these deaths occurred among patients who met criteria for depression and 12 occurred among patients with elevated scores. Multiple logistic regression analyses showed that both the test and elevated scores were significantly related to 18-month cardiac mortality. After controlling for other significant multivariate predictors of mortality, the impact of the score remained significant. The interaction of VPCs and the depression score marginally improved the model. Deaths were concentrated among depressed patients with VPCs of ≥10 per hour. Thus, depression while in the hospital after AMI is a significant predictor of 18-month after AMI cardiac mortality.

Neurohumoral Factors

Omland and colleagues[35] in Boston, Massachusetts, evaluated the prognostic accuracy and usefulness of neurohumoral determination as a risk stratification tool after AMI by comparing the long-term prognostic value of subacute neurohumoral measurements with other established indicators of adverse outcome. The study included 145 patients with documented AMI. During a median follow-up of 3.7 years, 30 cardiovascular and six noncardiovascular deaths occurred. By univariate analysis, plasma atrial natriuretic factor and endothelin levels were strongly related to long-term cardiovascular mortality. In multivariate models, both peptides added prognostic information to that obtained from clinical evaluation but not to that obtained from LVEF. Estimation of the area under the receiver-operating characteristic curve showed comparable prognostic accuracy for LVEF, plasma atrial natriuretic factor, plasma endothelin, and Killip classification, meaning that for all these prognostic indicators, a randomly selected patient from the group of patients dying will have a test value larger than that of a randomly selected patient from the group of surviving patients 75% to 82% of the time. The clinical usefulness of neurohumoral determination in routine risk stratification after AMI appears to be limited, because no additional prognostic information to that provided by objective evaluation of LV systolic function is obtained. However, in patients for whom objective assessment of LV performance is not readily available, measurement of plasma atrial natriuretic factor and endothelin may be helpful in identifying asymptomatic patients at risk for cardiac death.

Infarct Size

Two hundred seventy-four consecutive patients with AMI had technitium-99m sestamibi imaging on arrival at the hospital to determine myocardium at risk before reperfusion therapy and at hospital discharge to measure the amount of salvage myocardium and final infarct size in a study by Miller and colleagues[36] in Washington, DC. Defect size on the sestamibi imaging was quantified using a threshold value of 60% of peak counts from the circumferential count profile curves generated for five representative slices of the LV. Patients were followed after hospital discharge to evaluate the association between final infarct size and subsequent mortality. The median infarct size measured was 27% of the LV at presentation to the hospital and was 12% of the LV at hospital discharge. Almost one half of the patients had a final infarct size of ≤10%. The median amount of myocardium salvaged was 9%. During a median duration of follow-up at 12 months, there were 10 deaths and 1 resuscitated out-of-hospital cardiac arrest. There was a significant association between infarct size and overall mortality and cardiac mortality. Two-year mortality was 7% for patients whose infarct size was ≥12% compared with 0% for patients whose infarct size was <12%. There was also a significant association between myocardium at risk and cardiac mortality (Figure 3-12). There was no association between myocardium at risk and overall mortality or myocardium salvaged and either overall mortality or cardiac mortality. These data indicate that larger infarct size measured by technitium-99m sestamibi imaging after AMI was associated with increased mortality risk during short-term follow-up.

Signal-Averaged Electrocardiography

Mercando and colleagues[37] in Tuckahoe, New York, performed signal-average electrocardiography and 24-hour ambulatory electrocardiographic monitoring in 121 elderly patients >6 months after AMI. All patients had asymptomatic complex ventricular arrhythmias and a LVEF >40%. Rates of sudden, cardiac, and total death were compared between groups with and without sustained VT and between normal and abnormal signal-average cardiographic studies. The prevalence of an abnormal signal-averaged electrocardiographic study was 36%. Thirty-seven percent of the patients had nonsustained VT, and the remaining patients had complex ventricular arrhythmias other than VT. There were 27 sudden and 48 total cardiac deaths and 66 deaths from all causes during a mean follow-up of 30 months. Kaplan-Meier survival analysis showed a lower rate of sudden and cardiac death in the group without sustained VT. Although there was a trend toward a lower rate of sudden death in patients with

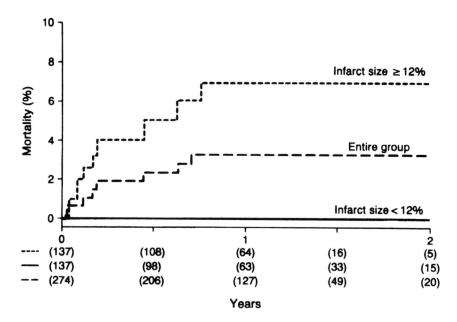

Figure 3-12. Plot of mortality curves for the entire study population and for the population divided into two groups on the basis of median infarct size. Numbers in parentheses at the bottom of the figure indicate the patients from each group available for analysis at the given points in time. Reproduced with permission from Miller et al.[36]

a normal signal-average electrocardiogram, there was no statistical difference in the ranges of sudden, total cardiac, or total death between patients with normal or abnormal studies. The negative predictive value of having neither an abnormal signal-averaged electrocardiogram nor sustained VT was 94% with sudden death. In elderly patients with complex ventricular arrhythmias and EF greater than 40% at least 6 months after an AMI, presence of nonsustained VT predicted a higher rate of sudden and cardiac death. Signal-averaged electrocardiography alone was not predictive.

Pharmacological Echocardiography

To determine the prognostic value of the high-dose (0.84 mg/kg over a 10-minute period) dipyridamole echocardiography test after a first AMI in comparison with clinical, electrocardiographic, echocardiographic, and angiographic variables, follow-up data over an average period of 16 months were obtained in 93 consecutive patients in this study by Nešković and associates[38] from Belgrade, Yugoslavia. There were 41 total cardiac events: 1 death, 2 reinfarctions, 13 cases of postinfarction angina, 5 PTCA procedures, and 20 CABG procedures. Total cardiac events without revascularization procedures were considered adverse cardiac events. The dipyridamole echocardiography tests results were positive in 28 of 41 patients with total cardiac events and in only 4 of 52 patients without total cardiac events. The sensitivity, specificity, and accuracy of positive dipyridamole echocardiography tests in predicting total cardiac events were 68%, 92%, and 82%, respectively. The best predictor of total cardiac events was positivity of dipyridamole echocardiography test, followed by multivessel CAD and patent infarct–related artery. Dipyridamole echocardiography test was positive in 12 of 16 patients with adverse cardiac events and 20 of 77 patients without adverse cardiac events. The sensitivity, specificity, and accuracy of dipyridamole echocardiography test in predicting adverse cardiac events were 75%, 74%, and 74%, respectively. Significant predictors of adverse cardiac events were positivity of dipyridamole echocardiography test and EF ≤40% at the time of dipyridamole echocardiography test. These data indicate that the positivity of dipyridamole echocardiography test is an excellent predictor of cardiac events after AMI and is more powerful as a predictor than the extent of CAD, suggesting its ability to identify functionally critical stenosis. A positive dipyridamole echocardiography test result can identify high-risk revascularization procedures.

Picano and colleagues[39] from Pisa, Italy, assessed the value of dipyridamole echocardiography in predicting reinfarction in 1080 patients evaluated early after uncomplicated AMI and followed for 14 months. Dipyridamole echocardiography was positive in 475 patients (44%). During follow-up, there were 50 reinfarctions: 45 nonfatal and 5 fatal. Reinfarction occurred in 30 patients with positive and 20 with negative results. Reinfarction was fatal in 5 of 30 patients with positive and in none of 20 with negative results. The RR value of reinfarction was 1.9. These authors concluded that dipyridamole echocardiography was helpful in identifying patients evaluated early after uncomplicated acute myocardial infarction, especially for fatal reinfarction.

Exercise Capacity

An inverse association between mortality and exercise capacity has been demonstrated previously in patients with CAD. Physical training generally increases exercise capacity. Only one study investigated the prognostic value of exercise capacity after training but only in a limited number of patients. No data are available on the relation between mortality and the change in peak exercise performance with training. Therefore, Vanhees and coworkers[40] in Pellenberg, Belgium, measured peak oxygen uptake before and after a 3-month, predominantly dynamic training period in 407 patients with CAD. Apart from peak oxygen uptake, several patient characteristics, risk factors for cardiovascular disease, and exercise data were considered in a Cox proportional-hazards model. Peak oxygen uptake had increased by 33% after the training period. During the total follow-up of 2583 patient-years, 37 patients died. Cause of death was cardiovascular in 21. The prognostic value of peak oxygen uptake was higher after training than before training, even after adjustment for age and other significant covariates. Cardiovascular mortality decreased more with greater increases in peak oxygen uptake after training. Relative hazard rate of 0.98 indicates that a 1% greater increase in peak oxygen uptake after training would be associated with a decrease in cardiovascular mortality of 2%. No differences in prognostic values in training effects were observed between patients with myocardial infarcts and patients after CABG. Peak oxygen uptake, evaluated after a physical training program, and its change in response to training are independent predictors for cardiovascular mortality in patients with CAD.

Complications

Angina Pectoris Afterwards

Using coronary angioscopy and angiography, Tabata and colleagues[41] from Saitama and Chiba, Japan, determined the prevalence of intracoronary thrombus and associated anatomic abnormalities in patients with postinfarction angina. Fifty-one consecutive patients with a diagnosis of AMI underwent coronary catheterization. Coronary angioscopy was performed in 17 patients with and 34 patients without postinfarction angina during the same period. The frequency of thrombus as observed by angiography was significantly higher in patients with than without postinfarction angina (all 17 vs. 5 of 34). There were no significant differences between groups with respect to degree of stenosis in the infarct-related artery, number of vessels with significant stenosis, presence of collateral flow, type of therapy, and risk factors. These authors concluded that infarct-related artery thrombus is present in postinfarction angina and may be the primary pathogenic factor. Angioscopy is more sensitive than coronary angiography for detection of coronary thrombus.

Right Ventricular Infarction

To test the hypothesis that flow characteristics from pulmonary regurgitation can predict RV involvement in patients with inferior wall AMI, Cohen and coinvestigators[42] in Paris, France, prospectively recorded continuous-wave Doppler tracings and right-sided cardiac hemodynamics in 48 consecutive patients with inferior wall AMI and pulmonary regurgitation. Right heart hemodynamics enabled the identification of 29 patients with (group 1) and 19 without (group 2) RV involvement. In patients with RV involvement, the pulmonary regurgitant flow pattern was characterized by a rapid rise in flow velocity to a peak level followed by an abrupt deceleration in mid-diastole, whereas in patients without RV involvement, the deceleration in mid-diastole was gradual (Figure 3-13). The pressure half-time of pulmonary regurgitation and the lowest mid-diastolic to peak early diastolic velocity ratio were significantly lower in group 1 than in group 2. The best diagnostic accuracy (95%) was obtained with cutoff values of pressure half-time of pulmonary regurgitation ≤ 150 msec and the lowest mid-diastolic to peak early diastolic velocity ratio ≤ 0.5: sensitivity 100%, specificity 89%, positive predictive value 94%, and negative predictive value 100%. Using multiple logistic regression analysis, the investigators found that the pressure half-time of pulmonary regurgitation was the strongest predictor of RV involvement. Thus, these parameters, derived from pulmonary regurgitant tracings, are useful in the noninvasive bedside diagnosis of RV infarction.

Congestive Heart Failure

Lystash and coworkers[43] in Charlottesville, Virginia, determined the incidence and clinical, noninvasive, and angiographic variables contributing to postdischarge early (≤ 3 months) and late (>3 months) CHF after anterior wall AMI. The patient cohort consisted of 94 consecutive patients <65 years of age who underwent predischarge exercise thallium-201 planar scintigraphy, rest

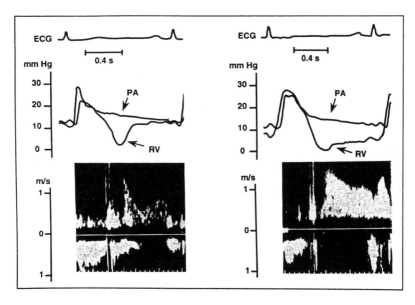

Figure 3-13. Hemodynamic tracings (upper panels) and Doppler pulmonary regurgitation tracings (lower panels) from a patient with (left panels) and in another patient without (right panels) right ventricular (RV) involvement. ECG indicates electrocardiogram; PA, pulmonary artery. Reproduced with permission from Cohen et al.[42]

radionuclide angiography, and coronary arteriography. At a mean of 49 months of follow-up, 10 of the 68 medically managed patients developed early CHF and 10 had late CHF. The 10 patients with early CHF had significantly higher peak creatine kinase values (2494 vs. 1032 IU/L), and at discharge, a lower LVEF (28% vs. 41%), more persistent thallium-201 defects (3.4 vs. 2.1), and fewer stress-induced redistribution defects (1.4 vs. 0.4) than those with late CHF. The early group had less multivessel disease (40% vs. 90%). Fifty percent (5 of 10) of patients who developed late CHF did so after a recurrent infarction compared with 10% (1 of 10) in the early CHF group and 8% in the group without CHF. The 26 patients who underwent CABG within 3 months had an LVEF and extent of ischemia and extent of angiographic stenoses comparable to patients with late CHF. None required hospitalization for CHF or had sustained a recurrent infarction. These data suggest that risk variables for developing CHF early after discharge after an uncomplicated anterior infarction are related to infarct size and early LV dysfunction, whereas late-onset CHF is related to extent of CAD and recurrent ischemic events. Early revascularization in patients with residual ischemia and multivessel disease may reduce incidence of CHF by diminishing risk of future ischemic events.

Cardiogenic Shock

Cardiogenic shock remains a frequently lethal complication of AMI. Early revascularization of the infarct-related artery by coronary angioplasty has been suggested to significantly improve patient survival. In this study by Eltchaninoff and associates[44] from Cleveland, Ohio, in-hospital and 1-year survival was assessed in 50 patients hospitalized for AMI complicated by cardiogenic shock. All patients received medical treatment and intra-aortic balloon pump support.

Thirty-three patients underwent PTCA, whereas 17 patients remained on conventional therapy (no-PTCA group). The 2 groups were comparable for all baseline characteristics. Survival was significantly better in the PTCA group than in the no-PTCA group: 64% vs. 24% in-hospital survival and 52% vs. 12% at 1 year. When angioplasty was successful in achieving reperfusion, survival was further enhanced: in-hospital survival rate was 76% vs. 25% in patients with unsuccessful angioplasty and 60% vs. 25% at 1 year.

Despite advances in the treatment of acute ischemic syndromes, cardiogenic shock is associated with significant morbidity and mortality. Holmes and colleagues[45] for the Global Utilization of Streptokinase and Tissue Plasminogen Activator for Occluded Coronary Arteries (GUSTO) trial reviewed the management of shock in patients who presented within 6 hours of symptom onset according to four treatment strategies: 1) streptokinase plus subcutaneous heparin, 2) streptokinase plus intravenous heparin, 3) accelerated rt-PA plus intravenous heparin, or 4) streptokinase and rt-PA plus intravenous heparin. The primary end point was 30-day all-cause mortality. Shock occurred in 7.2% (2972 patients) in the GUSTO trial. Of this group, 11% had shock on arrival and 89% developed shock after hospital admission. Reinfarction occurred in 11% of patients who developed shock compared with 3% of patients without shock. The shock developed significantly less frequently in patients receiving rt-PA. Patients who developed shock had a significantly lower 30-day mortality rate if angioplasty was performed. These authors concluded that because cardiogenic shock occurred most often after admission and with recurring ischemia and reinfarction, recognizing the signs of incipient shock may improve outcome. Only angioplasty was associated with a significantly lower mortality rate.

Cardiac Rupture

Acute or subacute myocardial rupture is a serious and often lethal complication of AMI. The role of an occluded or open culprit coronary artery on the occurrence of this complication is not clear. Therefore, Cheriex and associates[46] from Maastricht, the Netherlands, reviewed the perfusion status of the infarct-related coronary artery retrospectively in 57 patients who had an initially nonfatal rupture (group A) and 28 patients (including 9 patients from group A) with a postmortem diagnosis of myocardial rupture (group B). In 35 of the 57 patients in group A, a coronary angiogram was available. Complete occlusion or ineffective reperfusion was present in 30 (89%) of 35 patients. The remaining 22 patients of group A showed no clinical signs of reperfusion. All 28 patients of group B had inadequate reperfusion of the infarcted area on postmortem angiography and macroscopic examination of the coronary artery. These observations suggest that myocardial rupture typically occurs in an infarcted area without reperfusion.

The Late Assessment of Thrombolytic Efficacy (LATE) study,[47] a randomized, double-blind trial of 5711 patients with symptoms and electrocardiographic criteria consistent with AMI, demonstrated a 25% mortality reduction in favor of treatment with rt-PA activator and suggested that some patients may benefit even when treated >12 hours after symptom onset. This ancillary study was conducted to determine the association between the time from symptom onset to treatment, and cardiac rupture in patients with AMI. Of the 5711 patients who were prospectively randomized to receive either rt-PA or placebo within 6 and 24 hours from symptom onset, 177 patients had died by day 35. There was cardiac rupture in 53 patients, electromechanical dissociation in 42 patients and asystole in 82 patients. In patients treated after 12 hours, there was no evidence of an increased incidence of rupture with rt-PA and the proportion of deaths due to rupture in this group was lower than that of patients given placebo. However, there was evidence of a difference between rt-PA and placebo with respect to the time that the rupture became clinically manifest. Coronary thrombolysis appears to accelerate rupture events, typically to within 24 hours of treatment.

Figueras and coworkers[48] in Barcelona, Spain, compared clinical and electrocardiographic features of 227 patients who died of an AMI with those of 150 survivors of a first AMI. Of these 227 patients, LV free wall rupture was found in 93, who were older than 50 years. The incidence of healed infarct, CHF, and BBB was lower in patients with than without LV rupture. In patients with anterior AMI and early rupture (1 day), admission ST-segment elevation was higher than in those with LV rupture later than 1 day. However, lateral wall AMI had minimal ST elevation and accounted for 10% of ruptures. On day 2, the decrease in ST-segment in patients with late LV rupture was less than in survivors. Admission systolic BP in patients who had early rupture was higher than in survivors and in those with late rupture. Late rupture was associated with infarct thinning triggered by a physical strain in 18 of 45 patients (40%); infarct thinning, however, was present only in 4 of 48 patients (8%) with early rupture. The investigators concluded that 1) patients with LV rupture are among those greater than 50 years of age with a first transmural AMI without conduction abnormalities or heart failure; and 2) patients with anterior AMI, hypertension on admission, and high ST elevation, are at risk for early rupture, whereas those without initial hypertension or high ST segment that remains elevated may have late rupture in an expanded AMI, often after an undue strain.

General Treatment

Regional Differences in Management

Differences in the management of patients with AMI have been reported among countries, but few studies have investigated the issue in the USA. Pilote and associates[49] from multiple centers for the GUSTO-1 investigators compared the management for AMI among census regions across the USA, using data from GUSTO-1 comprising 21 772 patients and from the American Hospital Association. The authors found substantial regional variation in the management of AMI in the USA (Figure 3-14). B-Blockers (prescribed for a range of 55–81% of patients in the various regions), nitrates (prescribed for 61–77%), and ACE inhibitors (prescribed for 18–23%) were used most often in New England, whereas calcium antagonists (31–42%) and lidocaine (14–43%) were used least often there. Similarly, the proportion of patients undergoing various cardiac procedures differed among regions (range for angiography, 52–81% of patients; angioplasty, 22–35%; and CABG, 9–17%) and was lowest in New England. The regional use of cardiac procedures was closely related to their availability, except in New England. After the analysis was adjusted for clinical and hospital variables, patients in New England were found to be less likely to undergo angiography than patients in other

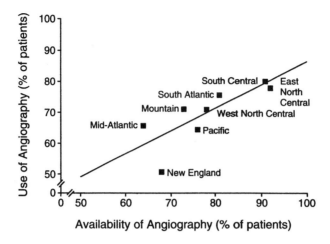

Figure 3-14. Positive association between the use and the availability of coronary angiography in regions of the United States. The outlier status of New England in this analysis is supported by the studentized-residual statistic, which is the distance of the observed value from the regression line, adjusted for the model's variability. The studentized residual for New England was greater than 4, whereas the remaining seven residuals were well within the expected bounds of –2 to 2. Reproduced with permission from Pilote et al.[49]

regions. There was no apparent relation between the use of cardiac procedures and rates of recurrent infarction or death at 30 days or 1 year (Table 3-11). There is substantial regional variation in the use of cardiac medications and procedures to manage AMI in the USA. The use and availability of cardiac procedures are closely related. The management of AMI in New England is atypical in that the relatively limited availability of cardiac procedures does not account for their relatively low use in that region.

Aspirin

Fitch and associates[50] from Minneapolis, Minnesota, and Boston, Massachusetts, examined the effects of aspirin use on mortality and morbidity rates in a subset of the control group of the Program on the Surgical Control of the Hyperlipidemias (POSCH) that was stratified by cigarette-smoking status at the time of randomization. The clinical impact of aspirin intake in cigarette smokers and former cigarette smokers has not been well studied. POSCH was a randomized, controlled, clinical trial designed to ascertain the effects of lipid modification by the partial ileal bypass operation on clinical end points and arteriographic changes in postmyocardial infarction individuals with hypercholesterolemia. Cohorts of cigarette smokers in the diet-control group were evaluated for overall and atherosclerotic CAD mortality rates and recurrent confirmed nonfatal myocardial infarction rates. In current cigarette smokers at baseline (n=90) with a mean follow-up of 8.3 years, the overall mortality rate was 45% in patients with no aspirin use and 10% in patients who reported even infrequent aspirin use. For CAD mortality in this cohort, the RR was 17.1; for the combined end point of CAD mortality and nonfatal AMI, the RR was 2.4. In former cigarette smokers with no aspirin use at baseline (n=92) with a mean follow-up of 8.8 years, the RR of overall mortality was 3.1; CAD mortality, 3.4; and combined atherosclerotic CAD mortal-

Table 3-11. Clinical Outcomes of the Study Patients, According to Region of the United States.

Variable*	New England (n = 2318)	Mid-Atlantic (n = 3758)	South Atlantic (n = 5296)	East North Central (n = 3616)	South Central (n = 1333)	West North Central (n = 1551)	Mountain (n = 1839)	Pacific (n = 2061)
Events in the hospital								
Reinfarction								
% of Patients	4.1	4.1	3.8	3.7	3.9	4.5	3.3	3.1
95% CI	3.3–4.9	3.5–4.7	3.3–4.3	3.1–4.3	2.9–4.9	3.5–5.5	2.5–4.1	2.4–3.8
Stroke								
% of Patients	1.5	1.4	1.6	1.6	1.6	1.8	1.2	1.5
95 % CI	1.0–2.0	1.0–1.8	1.2–2.0	1.2–2.0	0.9–2.3	1.1–2.5	0.7–1.7	1.0–2.0
Death								
% of Patients	6.7	7.1	7.0	6.9	5.4	7.2	6.0	5.8
95% CI	5.7–7.7	6.3–7.9	6.3–7.7	6.1–7.7	4.2–6.6	5.9–8.5	4.9–7.1	4.8–6.8
Death within 30 days								
% of Patients	6.7	7.3	7.3	7.2	5.8	7.7	6.8	6.2
95% CI	5.7–7.7	6.5–8.1	6.6–8.0	6.4–8.0	4.5–7.1	6.4–9.0	5.6–8.0	5.2–7.2
Death by 1 year								
% of Patients	10.1	10.0	10.2	10.3	8.6	9.6	8.9	8.7
95% CI	8.9–11.3	9.0–11.0	9.4–11.0	9.3–11.3	7.1–10.1	8.1–11.1	7.6–10.2	7.5–9.9
Functional status at 1 yr†								
Duke activity status index‡	32 (23,50)	37 (24,51)	32 (19,46)	36 (23,50)	37 (22,51)	35 (24,46)	37 (23,51)	35 (20,50)
Any exertional chest pain (% of patients)	19	20	26	23	19	18	21	16
Any exertional dyspnea (% of patients)	29	23	33	28	27	28	29	30

*CI denotes confidence interval.

†Functional status and symptoms were measured in the following numbers of patients: New England, 227; Mid-Atlantic, 383; South Atlantic, 544; East North Central, 389; South Central, 160; West North Central, 187; Mountain, 214; and Pacific, 172. Chest pain and dyspnea were assessed by interviewing the patients with the Rose questionnaires.

‡Values shown are median scores, followed in parentheses by the 25th and 75th percentiles. Scores are expressed on a scale ranging from 0 (worst) to 52 (best). Reproduced with permission from Pilote et al.[49]

ity and confirmed nonfatal AMI, 1.1. After adjustment for age, gender, LDL cholesterol, HDL cholesterol, EF, extent of CAD at baseline, and length of follow-up, none of these values changed appreciably. The risk of overall mortality, CAD mortality, and combined CAD mortality and recurrent confirmed nonfatal AMI may be significantly reduced by aspirin use in post-AMI cigarette smokers. However, the individuals included in this analysis were highly selected and may not be totally representative of post-AMI patients. Nonetheless, when extensive counseling regarding the negative consequences of continued cigarette smoking fails to cause smoking cessation in post-AMI patients, it may be exceedingly prudent to recommend aspirin usage.

Krumholz and colleagues[51] in New Haven, Connecticut, determined the current pattern of aspirin use and assessed its effectiveness in a large, population-based sample of elderly patients hospitalized with AMI as part of the Cooperative Cardiovascular Project Pilot, a Health Care Financing Administration initiative to improve quality of care for Medicare beneficiaries. Krumholz and colleagues abstracted hospital medical records of Medicare beneficiaries hospitalized in Alabama, Connecticut, Iowa, or Wisconsin from June 1992 through February 1993. Among the 10 018 patients ≥65 years of age who had no contraindication to aspirin, 6140 (61%) received aspirin within the first 2 days after AMI. Patients who were older, had more comorbid medical conditions, presented without chest pain, and had high-risk characteristics, including CHF and shock, were less likely to receive aspirin. The use of aspirin, however, was associated with a lower mortality after adjustment for potential confounders (Figure 3-15). Approximately one third of elderly patients with AMI who had no contraindication to receiving aspirin did not receive it within the first 48 hours after their AMI. The elderly patients with the highest risk of death were, therefore, least likely to receive aspirin. After adjustment for differences between the treatment groups, the use of aspirin was associated with a 22% lower odds of 30-day mortality. Thus, the increased use of aspirin for patients with AMI, especially elderly patients, is an excellent opportunity to improve medical care in these patient groups.

Oral Anticoagulant

To investigate the costs and effects of long-term oral anticoagulant treatment after AMI, Van Bergen and associates[52] from Rotterdam, the Netherlands, performed a cost-effectiveness analysis, based on a randomized, double-blind, placebo-controlled trial involving 60 Dutch hospitals and 3404 hospital survivors of AMI who were randomly assigned within a median period of 4 days after discharge to either oral anticoagulant treatment or placebo. The mean follow-up was 37 months. The oral anticoagulant treatment was aimed at a target international normalized ratio of 2.8–4.8. The costs of oral anticoagulant treatment were estimated at 394 Dutch guilders (Dfl) per patient-year (Dfl1 = $0.58 US). Placebo patients stayed 18 830 days in the hospital compared with 15 083 days for anticoagulation patients (Figure 3-16). Average costs per patient of medical care during follow-up were estimated at Dfl 10 784 for placebo patients and Dfl 9 878 for anticoagulation patients. Thus, costs of long-term anticoagulant treatment are outweighed by the costs of prevented clinical events.

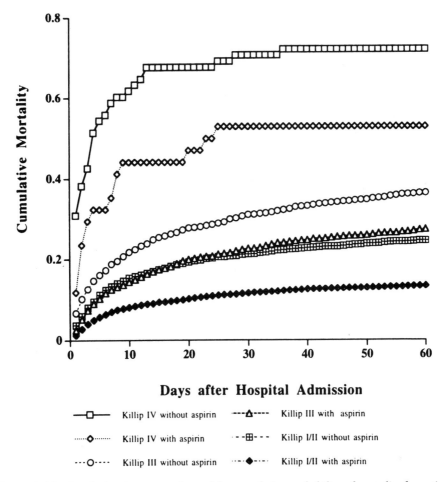

Figure 3-15. Graph showing comparison of the cumulative probability of mortality for patients who received aspirin with those who did not receive aspirin, by Killip class. Reproduced with permission from Krumholz et al.[51]

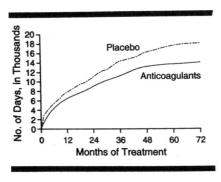

Figure 3-16. Cumulative number of days spent in the hospital by patients of each treatment group during participation in the trial. Reproduced with permission from Van Bergen et al.[52]

β-Blocker

In prospective randomized trials, β-blockers have improved survival after AMI using relatively high doses. In a retrospective analysis of clinical data from 606 consecutive survivors of AMI at 4 university hospitals in 3 countries, Viskin and colleagues[53] from Tel Aviv, Israel; Syracuse, New York; and Mexico City, Mexico, assessed the number of infarct survivors receiving prospectively defined "effective dosages" of β-blockers. Only 58% of infarct survivors with no contraindications to β-blockers received these drugs at the time of hospital discharge and only 11% received dosages equivalent to >50% of the effective dosage. These authors concluded that failure to prescribe β-blockers after AMI is common. Many patients not receiving β-blockers belong to subgroups that would derive the greatest benefit from such treatment. Even when β-blockers were prescribed, the dosages used were considerably lower than those which proved to be effective in preventing death after AMI.

A number of large trials have shown that β-blocker therapy can reduce the incidence of reinfarction and associated mortality after AMI. To evaluate the cardiologists' use of this therapy after hospital discharge, Brand and colleagues[54] from Minneapolis, Minnesota, analyzed insurance claims from 17 network model health plans throughout the United States. The study group included 150 cardiologists who had contacts with one of the health plans and their 280 patients who were plan members. Relative to the American College of Cardiology guidelines, 43% of the cases were apparent deviation from the guidelines. Of the 185 patients who were eligible for therapy with β-blockers, only 48% were treated. These authors concluded that cardiologists currently exhibit a low level of compliance with their specialty's guidelines for postinfarction β-blockade.

Aspirin, β-Blocker, Angiotensin-Converting Enzyme Inhibitor, Calcium Antagonist, and Anticoagulant

Mortality from AMI is reduced after treatment in the recovery period by the selective use of aspirin, β-blockers, warfarin, and ACE inhibitors. Despite evidence from trials, the use of β-blockers has not been translated into clinical practice. Most patients with AMI are managed by general physicians and general practitioners, but immediate coronary care is increasingly complex and the choice of drug for secondary prevention has increased. Smith and Channer[55] from Sheffield, United Kingdom, audited the use of drugs for secondary prevention before and after an intervention aimed at increasing their use. Their study shows that widely accepted and proved treatments for preventing reinfarction and death after recovery from AMI are still underused despite evidence from clinical trials and expert advice. The use of a simple method of marking the case numbers resulted in an increase in prescription for β-blockers so that only 10% of eligible patients were discharged without this treatment. The trials of ACE inhibitors after AMI were published in 1992 and 1993, and their use in clinical practice was facilitated by the intervention. Thus, a simple method of flagging the medical records to highlight a therapeutic decision appears to be beneficial.

Table 3-12. Clinical Outcome of 194 Patients with Acute Myocardial Infarction

	Placebo (n = 98)	Magnesium (n = 96)
Arrhythmias*	39†	26†
Conduction disturbances	15	10
Heart failure	22	18
Hospital mortality	17‡	4‡

Values are expressed as number of patients.
*Arrhythmias were ventricular tachycardia, ventricular fibrillation, and ventricular premature beats (Lown grades 2 to 5).
†p = 0.04; ‡p = 0.01.
Reproduced with permission from Shechter et al.[56]

Magnesium Sulfate

Thrombolytic therapy reduces in-hospital mortality. However, 70% to 80% of patients do not receive thrombolysis and their in-hospital mortality is high. During the last decade some clinical trials demonstrated that magnesium sulfate reduced in-hospital mortality. The aim of a study by Shechter and colleagues[56] in Tel-Hashomer, Israel, was to evaluate the effects of magnesium sulfate in patients with AMI who were considered unsuitable for thrombolytic therapy. Intravenous magnesium sulfate was evaluated in 194 patients with AMI ineligible for thrombolytic therapy in a randomized, double-blind, placebo-controlled study. Group I consisted of 96 patients who received 48-hour intravenous magnesium. Group II consisted of 98 patients who received isotonic glucose as a placebo. Magnesium reduced the incidence of arrhythmias, CHF, and conduction disturbances compared with placebo (Table 3-12). LVEF 72 hours and 1 to 2 months after admission was higher in patients who received magnesium sulfate than in those taking placebo (49% vs. 43% and 52% vs. 45%, respectively). In-hospital mortality was significantly reduced in patients receiving magnesium sulfate than in those receiving placebo (4% vs. 17%), and also in the subgroup of elderly patients (>70 years) (9% vs. 23%). In conclusion, magnesium sulfate should be considered an alternative therapy to thrombolysis in patients with AMI.

Antiarrhythmic Drug

Recent clinical trials have shown increased rather than decreased mortality in patients treated with antiarrhythmic drugs after AMI. To determine whether these findings had an impact on prescription of antiarrhythmic drugs after AMI, Avanzini and associates[57] on behalf of the GISSI investigators from Milan, Italy, retrospectively analyzed the class I and III antiarrhythmic prescription data of 38 072 patients with AMI enrolled in 3 large randomized clinical trials endorsed by a highly representative sample (about 75%) of Italian coronary care units during the last 10 years. The first study was conducted from 1984–1985; the second, from 1988–1989; the pilot for the third, in 1991; and the third, from 1991–1994. Total class I and III antiarrhythmic prescriptions after AMI was halved during the last decade, from 11.9% at discharge and 14.4% at follow-up in the 1984–1985 study to 5.8% and 5.8%, respectively, in 1991–1994. The trend was independent of the different distributions in the 3 studies of the patients' characteristics associated with antiarrhythmic use (i.e., age ≥70 years, anterior AMI, VF during hospitalization, and Killip class ≥ at randomization). The same decreasing trend was observed for each antiarrhythmic drug. The drug most widely used was amiodarone, accounting for about half of the antiarrhythmic prescriptions, followed by mexiletine hydrochloride and propafenone hydrochloride; flecainide acetate was dropped from the prescription last after the publication of the CAST results. The negative results of the recent clinical trials on class I antiarrhythmic drug use after AMI have been rapidly transferred into routine clinical practice in Italy, since the proportion of patients who received class I and III antiarrhythmic drugs after AMI was halved from the early 1980s to the 1990s.

Theophylline

To show that second- or third-degree AV block occurring as an early complication of inferior wall AMI is mediated by adenosine, Bertolet and associates[58] from Gainesville, Florida, studied 8 men who had inferior wall AMI who developed clinically significant AV block. Three had third-degree block, and 5 had high-grade second-degree block. In all patients 1:1 AV nodal conduction was restored and normal sinus rhythm reappeared within 3 minutes of the administration of theophylline. All patients remained free of the arrhythmia for at least 24 hours. Theophylline was administered as 100 mg/min intravenously beginning to a maximum of 250 mg. Thus, adenosine produced by the ischemic myocardium may induce AV nodal block. The AV block in the 8 patients studied was resistant to conventional therapies such as atropine but responded to the adenosine antagonist theophylline.

Captopril

The Chinese Cardiac Study Collaborative Group[59] randomly assigned 13 634 patients entering 650 Chinese hospitals up to 36 hours after the onset of suspected AMI 1 month of oral captopril (6.25 mg initial dose, 12.5 mg 2 hours later, and then 12.5 mg 3 times daily) or matching placebo. Captopril was associated with a nonsignificant reduction in 4-week mortality (617 [9.05%] captopril-allocated vs. 65 [9.59%] placebo-allocated deaths). There was a significant excess of hypotension, mostly early after the start of treatment, but no evidence of any adverse effect on early mortality (even among patients who were hypotensive at entry). Taken together with the other trials of converting enzyme inhibitors started early in AMI, these results indicate that such therapy is generally safe and typically prevents about 5 deaths per 1000 patients treated for the first month.

Lamas and the Survival and Ventricular Enlargement (SAVE) investigators[60] assessed the effect of infarct-related artery patency on outcomes of patients after AMI with LV dysfunction while controlling for differences in LVEF and the extent of CAD. They also determined the effect of ACE inhibitor therapy on patients with patent as well as occluded infarct arteries. The SAVE study consisted of 2231 patients with a documented AMI and an LVEF ≤40%. They were randomly assigned to the ACE inhibitor captopril (50 mg three times a day) or placebo 3 to 16 days after AMI and were followed for an average of 3.5 years. LVEF measured with radionuclide left ventriculography was repeated at the end of the follow-up period. The 946 patients in whom the patency of the infarct-related artery was established before randomization formed the basis of this study. At cardiac catheterization averaging 4 days after AMI, 31% of patients had an initially occluded infarct-related artery. After revascularization an occluded infarct-related artery remained in 162 of the 946 patients (17%) at the time of randomization. One hundred sixty-two patients with persistently occluded infarct-related arteries and 784 with patent infarct-related arteries had similar clinical baseline characteristics, but those with occluded arteries had a slightly lower LVEF than the 784 patients with patent infarct arteries. Cox proportional hazard analyses showed that the independent predictors of all-cause mortality were number of diseased coronary arteries, hypertension, occluded infarct-related artery, LVEF, age, and the use of β-blockers (Figure 3-17). Independent predictors of a composite end point consisting of cardiovascular mortality, morbidity, or reduction of LVEF were occluded infarct-related artery, hypertension, number of diseased vessels, LVEF, use of β-blockers, and randomization to the ACE inhibitor captopril. Thus, infarct-related artery patency within 16 days of AMI predicts a favorable clinical outcome independent of the number of obstructed arteries or LVEF. Beneficial effect of captopril was independent of patency status of the infarct-related artery.

Previous studies after AMI have reported conflicting results on the effect of ACE inhibition on physical working capacity. In an effort to provide more insight into this subject, Hartley and coworkers[61] in Boston, Massachusetts, examined the effects of captopril on working capacity of patients who had low EF but no CHF after AMI. One hundred sixty-six participants were recruited from five centers after randomization to either captopril or placebo for the survival and ventricular enlargement study. Upright cycle ergometer tests were performed with continuous measurements of respiratory gases at 4, 12, and 24 months after AMI. The study concurred with two of three previous post-AMI studies and supported the conclusion that working capacity is not affected by ACE inhibition at 4 or 12 months after AMI in patients without CHF. In addition, no significant effect of captopril was noted at 24 months after AMI. Peak oxygen uptake tended to decrease between 12 and 24 months in the placebo group by an average of –22 mL/min, but to increase in the captopril group +62 mL/min. This post hoc observation suggests that a late beneficial effect may have been masked by inadequate study duration. Known benefits of captopril appear not to include an increase in working capacity within the first 24 months after AMI.

Captopril + Mononitrate + Magnesium Sulfate

The ISIS-4 collaborative group[62] described results from a study of 58 050 patients entering 1086 hospitals up to 24 hours (median, 8 hours) after the onset of suspected AMI with no clear contraindications to study treatments (no cardiogenic shock or persistent, severe hypotension) and the patients were randomly assigned into a 2 × 2 × 2 factorial study. The treatment comparisons were as follows: 1) 1 month of oral captopril (6.25 mg initial dose titrated up to 50 mg twice daily) vs. matching placebo; 2) 1 month of oral, controlled-release mononitrate (30 mg initial dose titrated up to 60 mg once daily) vs. matching placebo; and 3) 24 hours of intravenous magnesium sulfate (8 mmol initial bolus followed by 72 mmol) vs. open control. There were no significant

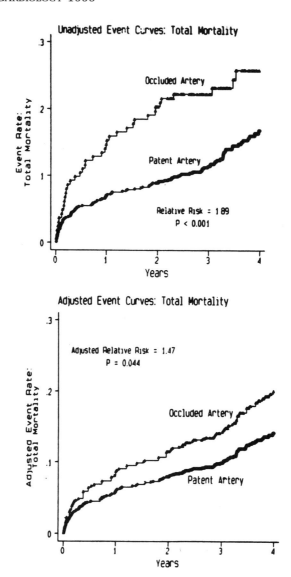

Figure 3-17. Univariate survival curves for (top) total mortality by infarct artery patency and (bottom) cardiovascular mortality by infarct artery patency. Reproduced with permission from Lamas et al.[60]

"interactions" between the effects of these 3 treatments, and the results for each are based on the random comparison of about 29 000 active vs. 29 000 control-allocated patients. There was a significant 7% (SD 3) proportional reduction in 5-week mortality (2088 [7.19%] captopril-allocated deaths vs. 2231 [7.69%] placebo), which corresponds to an absolute difference of 4.9 (SD 2.2) fewer deaths per 1000 patients treated for 1 month (Figure 3-18). The absolute benefits appeared to be larger (perhaps about 10 fewer deaths per 1000) in certain higher-risk groups, such as those presenting with a history of previous AMI or with heart failure. The survival advantage appeared to be maintained in the longer term (5.4 [SD 2.8] fewer deaths per 1000 at 12 months). Captopril

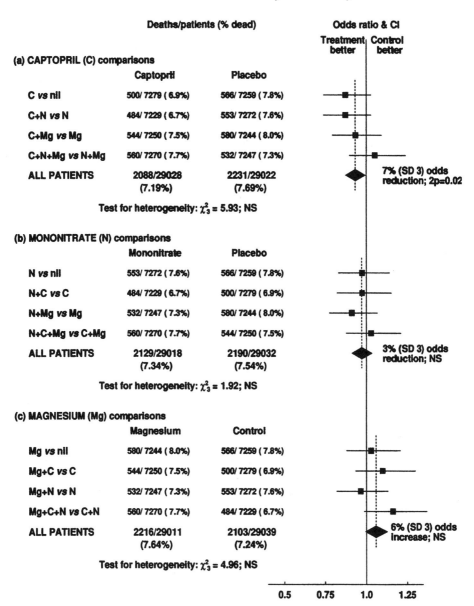

Figure 3-18. Mortality in days 0–35 subdivided by other randomly allocated study treatments. C indicates captopril; N, mononitrate, Mg, magnesium. For example, the subgroup assessment of captopril in the presence of mononitrate is denoted C+N vs. N. Odds ratios (ORs: black squares with areas proportional to the amount of "statistical information" in each subdivision) comparing the mortality among patients allocated the study treatment to that among patients allocated the relevant control are plotted for each of the treatment comparisons, subdivided by the other randomly allocated study treatments, along with their 99% confidence intervals (CIs: horizontal lines). For each of the three study treatment comparisons, the overall result and its 95% CI is represented by a diamond, with the overall proportional reduction (or increase) and statistical significance given alongside. Squares or diamonds to the left of the solid vertical line indicate benefit (significant at 2p < 0.01 when the entire horizontal line is to the left of the vertical line and at 2P < 0.05 when the diamond does not overlap the vertical line). χ^2 tests for evidence of heterogeneity of the sizes of the ORs in the subdivisions are also given. Reproduced with permission from ISIS-4 Collaborative Group.[62]

was associated with an increase of 52 (SD 2) patients per 1000 in hypotension considered severe enough to require termination of study treatment, of 5 (SD 2) per 1000 in reported cardiogenic shock, and of 5 (SD 1) per 1000 in some degree of renal dysfunction. It produced no excess of deaths on days 0 through 1, even among patients with low BP at entry. There was no significant reduction in 5-week mortality, either overall (2129 [7.3%] mononitrate-allocated deaths vs. 2190 [7.54%] placebo) or in any subgroup examined (including those not receiving short-term nonstudy intravenous or oral nitrates at entry). Further follow-up did not indicate any later survival advantage. The only significant side effect of the mononitrate regimen studied was an increase of 15 (SD 2) per 1000 in hypotension. Those assigned to active treatment had somewhat fewer deaths on days 0 through 1, which is reassuring information about the safety of using nitrates early in acute AMI. There was no significant reduction in 5-week mortality, either overall (2216 [7.64%] magnesium-allocated deaths vs. 2103 [7.24%] control) or in any subgroup examined (including those treated early or late after symptom onset or in the presence or absence of fibrinolytic or antiplatelet therapies, or those at high risk of death). Further follow-up did not indicate any later survival advantage. In contrast with some previous small trials, there was a significant excess with magnesium of 12 (SD 3) per 1000 in CHF and of 5 (SD 2) per 12 000 in reported cardiogenic shock during or just after the infusion period. Magnesium was also associated with an increase of 11 (SD 2) per 1000 in hypotension considered severe enough to require termination of study treatment, of 3 (SD 0.6) per 1000 in bradycardia, and of 3 (SD 0.4) per 1000 in a cutaneous flushing or burning sensation (but assessment of magnesium involved open control). There was no evidence of a net adverse effect on mortality on days 0 through 1. Because of its size, ISIS-4 provides reliable evidence about the effects of adding each of these 3 treatments to established treatments for AMI. Intravenous magnesium was ineffective, and although oral nitrate therapy appeared safe, it did not produce a clear reduction in 1-month mortality. Other trials have shown that starting long-term converting enzyme inhibitor therapy in the weeks or months after AMI in patients with impaired ventricular function avoids about 2 deaths per 1000 patients per month of treatment. ISIS-4, GISSI-3, and smaller studies now collectively demonstrate that, for a wide range of patients without clear contraindications, captopril started early in AMI prevents about 5 deaths per 1000 in the first month, with somewhat greater benefits in higher-risk patients. This benefit from 1 month of early treatment seems to persist for at least the first year.

Enalapril

ACE inhibitor therapy can preserve LV function and geometric features and improve survival in subsets of patients with AMI. Carstensen and associates[63] from Copenhagen, Denmark; Stavanger, Norway; and Stockholm and Gothenburg, Sweden, investigated the effect of enalapril treatment initiated <24 hours after AMI on global and regional echocardiographic wall motion indexes obtained at 2 to 5 days and at 1 and 6 months in 428 consecutive patients enrolled in the randomized, placebo-controlled Cooperative New Scandinavian Enalapril Survival Study II. In anterior AMI, the non–infarct-zone index deteriorated in the placebo group but remained unchanged in the enalapril-treated group, an effect related to attenuated LV volume expansion. No treatment effects were observed in nonanterior AMIs or in the entire unselected population. Thus in an unselected population with AMI, early enalapril treatment had no effect on LV function; yet in patients with anterior infarcts, LV function was maintained through the preservation of function in the noninfarcted myocardium.

Infarct expansion starts within hours to days after transmural myocardial injury. Previous echocardiographic and left ventricographic studies demonstrated that ACE inhibitor therapy limits LV dilatation, particularly in patients with anterior wall AMI or impaired LV function. Schulman and coworkers[64] in Baltimore, Maryland, randomly assigned 43 patients with an acute Q-wave AMI within 24 hours of symptom onset to intravenous enalaprilat (1 mg) or a placebo. Patients were then given corresponding oral therapy and follow-up in 1 month. Pretreatment and 1-month gaited blood pool scans were obtained in 32 patients to evaluate changes in cardiac volumes and EF. Twenty-three patients underwent magnetic resonance imaging at 1 month to evaluate LV infarct expansion. BP decreased at 6 hours but returned to baseline in both groups after 1 month of therapy. The change in cardiac volumes from baseline from 1 month differed between the placebo (end-diastolic volume, +16 mL; end-systolic volume, +8 mL), and enalapril (end-diastolic volume, −8 mL; end-systolic volume, −14 mL) groups. Global and infarct zone EF improved significantly at 1 month in the enalapril group (+16% and +19%) but did not change over 1 month in the placebo group. Infarct segment length and infarct expansion index by magnetic resonance imaging were significantly less than those treated with enalapril, suggesting less infarct expansion in this group. Thus, earlier administration of enalapril to patients presenting with the first Q-wave AMI prevents cardiac dilatation and infarct expansion.

Trandolapril

In mortality studies of patients after AMI, exclusion of patients during selection from the screened population may be important for evaluating the impact of trials, but data on patients excluded from studies are rarely presented. In the Trandolapril Cardiac Evaluation (TRACE) trial of the ACE inhibitor trandolapril vs. placebo in patients with LV systolic dysfunction shortly after AMI, Køber and colleagues[65] in Copenhagen, Denmark, accounted for medical history, infarct complication, and survival in all patients screened for entry. A total of 7001 consecutive enzyme-confirmed AMIs were screened for entry in 27 Danish coronary care units. The 1-year mortality of all screened AMI cases was 23%. The target population of the trial were patients with LV systolic dysfunction (echocardiographically determined wall motion index ≤1.2) within 6 days of AMI. The 1-year mortality of this group was 34%. Patients with wall motion index >1.2 had a 1-year mortality of 12%. Of those with wall motion index ≤1.2, 859 (33%) were excluded. A total of 1749 were included in the study. The excluded and included groups had a 1-year mortality of 54% and 24%, respectively. The result of the study will be applicable to two thirds of the patients with LV systolic dysfunction; however, even with this high figure, care should be taken in extrapolating the result to the general population with reduced LV function after AMI since the group excluded from the study had a higher mortality than those who were included.

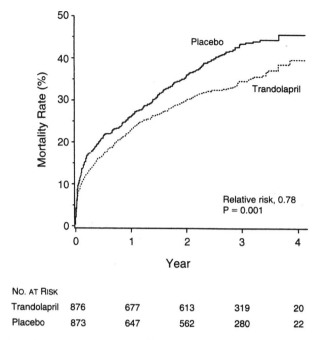

No. at Risk

Trandolapril	876	677	613	319	20
Placebo	873	647	562	280	22

Figure 3-19. Cumulative mortality from all causes among patients receiving trandolapril or placebo. Reproduced with permission from Køber et al.[66]

Treatment with ACE inhibitors reduces mortality among survivors of AMI, but whether to use ACE inhibitors in all patients or only in selected patients is uncertain. Køber and associates[66] for the TRACE study group screened 6676 consecutive patients with 7001 AMIs confirmed by enzyme studies. A total of 2606 patients had echocardiographic evidence of LV systolic dysfunction (EF ≤35%). On days 3–7 after AMI 1749 patients were randomly assigned to receive oral trandolapril (876 patients) or placebo (873 patients). The duration of follow-up was 24–50 months. During the study period, 304 patients (34.7%) in the trandolapril group died compared with 369 (42.3%) in the placebo group (Figure 3-19). The RR of death in the trandolapril group compared with the placebo group was 0.78. Trandolapril also reduced the risk of death from cardiovascular causes (RR, 0.75) and sudden death (RR, 0.71). In contrast, the risk of recurrent AMI (fatal or nonfatal) was not significantly reduced (RR, 0.86). Long-term treatment with trandolapril in patients with reduced LV function soon after AMI significantly reduced the risk of overall mortality, mortality from cardiovascular causes, sudden death, and the development of severe heart failure.

Zofenopril

LV dilatation and neuroendocrine activation are common after AMI. Long-term treatment with an ACE inhibitor may improve outcome by attenuating these processes. Ambrosioni and associates[67] from Bologna, Italy, for the Survival of Myocardial Infarction Long-Term Evaluation (SMILE) study investigators investigated whether zofenopril administered for 6 weeks after the anterior wall AMI could improve both short- and long-term outcome. A total of 1556 patients were enrolled within 24 hours after the onset of symptoms of anterior

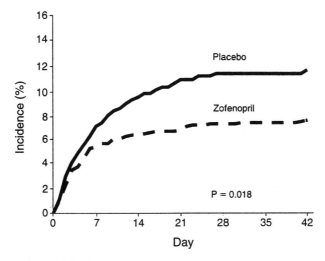

Figure 3-20. Incidence of death or severe congestive heart failure during 6 weeks of treatment with zofenopril or placebo in patients with acute myocardial infarction. Reproduced with permission from Ambrosioni et al.[67]

wall AMI, and they were randomly assigned in a double-blind fashion to receive either placebo (784 patients) or zofenopril (772 patients) for 6 weeks. At this time the incidence of death or severe CHF was assessed. The patients were reexamined after 1 year to assess survival. The incidence of death or severe CHF at 6 weeks was significantly reduced in the zofenopril group (55 patients, 7.1%) compared with the placebo group (83 patients, 10.6%); the cumulative reduction in the risk of death or severe CHF was 34% (Figure 3-20). The reduction in risk was 46% for severe CHF and 25% for death. After 1 year of observation, the mortality rate was significantly lower in the zofenopril group than in the placebo group; the reduction in risk was 29%. Treatment with zofenopril significantly improved both short- and long-term outcome when this drug was started within 24 hours after the onset of anterior wall AMI and continued for 6 weeks.

Insulin-Glucose Infusion

Diabetes mellitus increases the short- and long-term mortality rate after AMI. Marlmberg and colleagues[68] from Stockholm, Sweden, tested the hypothesis that insulin-glucose infusion followed by multidose insulin treatment in diabetic patients with AMI could beneficially affect mortality during the subsequent year. Six hundred twenty patients with AMI were randomly assigned to conventional therapy and to treatment with insulin-glucose infusion followed by multidose subcutaneous insulin for more than 3 months. There was a beneficial reduction in mortality from 26.1% in the control group to 18.6% in the infusion group at 1 year. The mortality reduction was especially evident in patients with a low cardiovascular risk profile and no previous insulin treatment: 8.6% in the infusion group vs. 18% in the control group. These authors concluded that insulin-glucose infusion followed by a multidose insulin regimen improved long-term prognosis in diabetic patients with AMI.

L-Carnitine

L-Carnitine is a physiological compound that appears to perform an essential role in myocardial energy production at the mitochondrial level. The CEDIM trial[69] was a randomized, double-blind placebo-controlled multicenter trial in which 472 patients with a first AMI and high-quality 2-dimensional echocardiograms received either placebo (239 patients) or L-carnitine (233 patients) within 24 hours of onset of chest pain. A significant attenuation of LV dilation occurred in the first year after AMI in the patients treated with L-carnitine compared to those treated with placebo. The combined incidence of death and CHF after discharge was 6% in the L-carnitine treatment group vs. 9.6% in the placebo group. These authors concluded that L-carnitine treatment initiated early after AMI and continued for 12 months can attenuate LV dilation during the first year after an AMI, resulting in smaller LV volumes at 3, 6, and 12 months. Since ACE inhibitors were not used in this trial, however, it is unclear whether L-carnitine would have been additive to ACE inhibitive therapy.

Partial Ileal Bypass

The POSCH[70] trial utilized partial ileal bypass to reduce hypercholesterolemia. In this randomized, secondary lipid/atherosclerosis intervention trial there was evidence for reduction in atherosclerosis progression as demonstrated by clinical and arteriographic end points. A total of 838 patients received American Heart Association step-2 diet instruction and half were also randomly assigned to partial ileal bypass treatment. An overall mortality rate of 10% occurred at 6.7 years in the control group and 9.4 years in the intervention group for a gain in disease-free interval of 2.7 years in the intervention group. A CAD mortality rate of 8% occurred at 7.2 years in the control group and 11 years in the intervention group, for a gain of 3.8 years. Twenty-five percent of patients underwent either revascularization or heart transplantation at 5.4 years in the control group and 12.4 years in the intervention group for a gain of 7 years. The authors concluded that the marked lipid modification achieved by partial ileal bypass in the POSCH trial led to statistically significant increases in the disease-free intervals for overall mortality, CAD mortality, confirmed nonfatal AMI, and coronary intervention procedures (Figure 3-21).

Thrombolysis

Review

Rogers[71] from Birmingham, Alabama, provided an excellent review on contemporary management of AMI. The author pointed out that only 20% of patients with AMI are treated with intravenous thrombolytic agents. The types of thrombolytic agents are summarized in Table 3-13 and the results of using the thrombolytic agents in large trials are summarized in Table 3-14. The author also provided a treatment algorithm for typical patient with AMI (Table 3-15).

Variation in Use

To examine differences in outcomes and patient management in the USA and outside the USA undergoing thrombolysis for AMI, Van de Werf and associ-

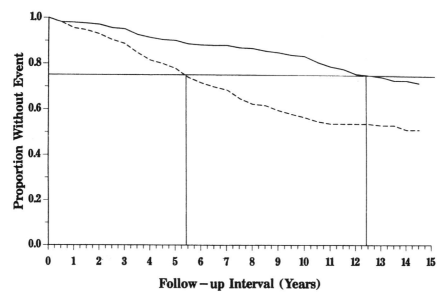

Figure 3-21. Live table analysis for all CABG, PTCA, and heart transplantation procedures. Control group indicated by dashed line (n = 417) and intervention group, solid line (n = 421). Reproduced with permission from Buchwald et al.[70]

ates[72] for the GUSTO investigators randomly assigned patients in the USA (n = 23 105) and 14 other countries (n = 17 916) to receive streptokinase plus either subcutaneous or intravenous heparin, accelerated rt-PA plus intravenous heparin, or combined streptokinase and rt-PA plus intravenous heparin. Differences in 30-day mortality and patient management were compared among treatments and between US and non–US patients. Treatment-by-country interactions were assessed by logistic regression analyses. Expected mortality of US and non–US patients was estimated using a predictive model and was compared with observed mortality. Mortality reduction with accelerated rt-PA vs. streptokinase was greater in the USA (1.2% absolute decrease vs. 0.7% elsewhere), but the test for treatment-by-country interaction against streptokinase was not significant. Benefits of accelerated rt-PA over combination therapy were observed in the USA, but not in other countries (Figure 3-22). Despite differences in baseline characteristics and patient management, 30-day mortality was not significantly different: 6.8% in the USA vs. 7.2% elsewhere. After adjustment for baseline differences, observed versus predicted outcomes were slightly better in the USA (6.8% vs. 7.0%) than elsewhere (7.2% vs. 7.0%), indicating that enrollment in the United States was a marginally significant predictor of better survival. No significant evidence for a differentially greater benefit of accelerated rt-PA over streptokinase was found in US vs. non–US patients. However, increased procedure and treatment use in the United States was associated with only a small decrease in 30-day mortality.

In Men vs. Women

At 12 centers, 395 patients, including 288 men (73%) and 107 women (27%) with AMI, were prospectively randomized by Stone and coworkers[73] in

Table 3-13. Thrombolytic Agents Approved for Intravenous Use in the United States

	Streptokinase	Alteplase (rt-PA)	Anistreplase (APSAC)
Source	Group C β-Hemolytic Streptococcus Bacillus	Human protein produced by recombinant DNA technology	Acylated Complex of Streptokinase and Human Lys-Plasminogen
Circulating half-life (min)	23	5	90
Fibrin specific	No	Yes	No
Antigenic	Yes	No	Yes
Dose (IV)	1.5 million IU over 1 h	100 mg over 3 h or 100 mg over 90 min*	30 IU over 2–5 min
Bolus dosing possible	No	Not	Yes
Cost per dose (to pharmacy)‡	$285	$2,200	$1,649
Concomitant medications recommended	Aspirin, Heparin (controversial) (IV or SQ)	Aspirin, IV Heparin	Aspirin
Mortality benefit proved versus randomized controls	Yes	Yes	Yes

*Alteplase may be given as 1 of 2 IV regimens: (1) 3-hour regimen—give 60 mg over first hour, including a 6–10-mg initial bolus, then give 20 mg over each of the next 2 hours (for patients <65 kg, total dose should be adjusted downward and not exceed 1.25 mg/kg); (2) 90-minute regimen—give 15-mg initial bolus, 0.75 mg/kg (up to 50 mg) over first 30 minutes, and 0.5 mg/kg (up to 35 mg) over next hour.
†Bolus dosing currently under investigation; not yet approved.
‡Source: University of Alabama Hospital Pharmacy, January 1995.
SQ = subcutaneous.
Reproduced with permission from Rogers.[71]

Table 3-14 International Megatrials Comparing Intravenous Thrombolytic Regimens

	International Study	ISIS-3	GUSTO
Number of patients	20,891	41,299	41,021
Types of patients	Suspected AMI	Suspected AMI with ST elevation	Suspected AMI with ST elevation
Upper age limit	No	No	No
Interval from symptom onset to randomization	0–6 h	0–24 h	0–6 h
Thrombolytic regimens compared	(1) SK 1.5 MU over 30–60 min (2) tPA (Alteplase) 100 mg over 3 h	(1) SK 1.5 MU over 1 h (2) tPA (Duteplase) 0.6 MU/kg over 4 h (3) APSAC 30 U over 3 min	(1) SK 1.5 MU over 1 h plus SQ heparin (SK/SQ) (2) SK 1.5MU over 1 h plus IV heparin (SK/IV) (3) Accelerated: tPA (Alteplase) up to 100 mg over 90 min plus IV heparin (4) Combination: tPA (up to 90 mg over 1 h) and SK (1.0 MU over 1 h) plus IV heparin
Double blind	No	Partially	No
Concomitant aspirin	300–325 mg/d	162 mg/d	160–325 mg/d
Concomitant heparin	Randomized to either no heparin or to SQ heparin 12,500 IU q 12 h starting 12 h after thrombolytics	Randomized to either no heparin or to SQ heparin 12,500 IU q 12 h starting 4 h after thrombolytics	SQ regimen: 12,500 IU BID starting 4 h after thrombolytic IV regimen: 5,000-IU bolus plus 1,000 IU/h titrated to aPTT of 60–85s
Primary end point	In-hospital mortality	Mortality at 35 days	Mortality at 30 days
Mortality	SK: 8.5% tPA: 8.9% *P* = NS	SK: 10.6% tPA: 10.3% APSAC: 10.5% *P* = NS for pairwise comparisons	SK/SQ: 7.2% SK/IV: 7.4% tPA: 6.3% Combination: 7.0% *P* < 0.001 for tPA vs SK
Stroke	SK: 0.9% tPA: 1.3%	SK: 1.0% tPA: 1.4% APSAC: 1.3%	SK/SQ: 1.2% SK/IV: 1.4% tPA: 1.55% Combination: 1.6%
Combination of death or nonfatal stroke	Not reported	Not reported	SK/SQ: 7.7% SK/IV: 7.9% tPA: 6.9%

AMI indicates acute myocardial infarction; SK, streptokinase; MU, million units; SQ, subcutaneous; IV, intravenous; APSAC, anistreplase; aPTT, activated partial thromboplastin time.
Reproduced with permission from Rogers.[71]

Table 3-15 Treatment Algorithm for Typical Patient With Acute Myocardial Infarction

Initial stabilization
- Obtain vital signs, IV access, ECG
- Begin continuous rhythm monitoring, supplemental oxygen
- Analgesia for chest pain

Acute reperfusion therapy
- Options include IV thrombolytic therapy or primary PTCA, depending upon patient's eligibility for thrombolytic therapy and local availability of primary PTCA
- If IV thrombolysis employed, favored choices include
  —Accelerated tPA; 15-mg bolus, 50 mg over 30 minutes, 35 mg over 60 minutes
  —Streptokinase: 1.5 MU over 60 minutes

Acute antithrombin and antiplatelet therapy
- Aspirin: 160–325 mg chewed in emergency department, then daily per os
- Heparin (if tPA used): 5,000-IU bolus, 1,000 IU/h initially, keep aPTT 60–85 seconds (Table V)

Other immediate pharmacologic therapy
- IV β-blocker (if no evidence of bradycardia, hypotension, heart failure, heart block or, asthma), for example, metoprolol 5 mg IV × 3, atenolol 5 mg IV × 2, then oral agent
- IV nitroglycerin (especially for continued chest pain, LV dysfunction, hypertension)
- IV magnesium (if serum levels low, ventricular arrhythmias), for example, 2 g over 5 minutes, followed by 8 g over 24 hours
- ACE inhibitor (especially for large, anterior infarcts without hypotension), for example, captopril, beginning at 6.25 mg po TID and titrated to 50 mg po TID over several days
- Avoid: routine lidocaine, calcium channel blockers

Predischarge management
- Noninvasive assessment
  —Ejection fraction
  —Provocative test for ischemia (limited exercise test, dipyridamole thallium, dobutamine echocardiogram, etc.), unless there has been spontaneous recurrence of ischemia
- Coronary arteriography and revascularization, if anatomy feasible, for those with ejection fraction <50% and/or evidence of spontaneous or provocable recurrent ischemia
- Discharge medications
  —Aspirin: 160–325 mg/d or every other day, indefinitely
  —ACE inhibitor (if ejection fraction <40%): eg, captopril 50 mg TID, enalapril 10 mg BID, ramipril 5 mg BID
  —β-blocker (if no contraindication): eg, metoprolol 100 mg BID, atenolol 100 mg qd, timolol 10 mg BID
  —Avoid: routine antiarrhythmic agents, calcium channel blockers

Postdischarge management
- Risk factor modification: especially smoking cessation, treatment of lipid abnormalities
- Cardiac rehabilitation program

ECG indicates electrocardiogram; PTCA, percutaneous transluminal coronary angioplasty; aPTT, activated partial thromboplastin time; LV, left ventricular; ACE, angiotensin-converting enzyme. Reproduced with permission from Rogers.[71]

Royal Oak, Michigan, to treatment with t-PA or primary PTCA. Compared with men, women were older (66 vs. 58 years); more often had diabetes mellitus (19% vs. 10%), systemic hypertension (54% vs. 39%), or prior CHF (5% vs. 0%); and presented later after symptom onset (229 vs. 174 minutes). The in-hospital mortality in women was 3.3-fold higher than men (9.3% vs. 2.8%). After adjustment for comorbid baseline characteristics, however, only advanced age independently correlated with mortality. Among thrombolysis-treated patients, mortality was significantly higher in women than in men (14% vs. 4%) (Figure 3-23). Intracranial hemorrhage after thrombolysis was also more common in women than in men (5.3% vs. 0.7%). In contrast, women and men

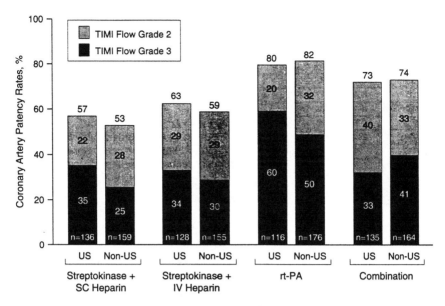

Figure 3-22. Coronary artery patency rates in US and non-US patients per treatment strategy. Percentage of patients with Thrombolysis in Myocardial Infarction (TIMI) flow grade 2 or 3 are shown above the bars, with the percentages with flow grade 2 and grade 3 shown separately within the bars. SC indicates subcutaneous; IV, intravenous; rt-PA, accelerated recombinant tissue-type plasminogen activator; and Combination, rt-PA and streptokinase plus IV heparin. Reproduced with permission from Van de Werf et al.[72]

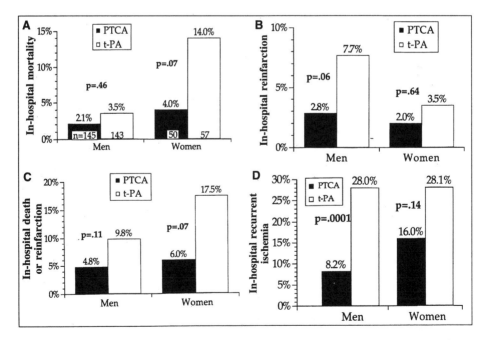

Figure 3-23. Effect of treatment modality on in-hospital outcome stratified by gender: A, mortality; B, nonfatal reinfarction; C, death or reinfarction; D, recurrent ischemia. PTCA indicates percutaneous transluminal coronary angioplasty; t-PA, tissue plasminogen activator. Reproduced with permission from Stone et al.[73]

had similar in-hospital mortality after primary PTCA (4% vs. 2%, respectively). No intracranial bleeding occurred in PTCA-treated patients. A univariate trend was present for reduced in-hospital mortality in women treated with PTCA rather than thrombolysis (4% vs. 14%). By multiple logistic regression analysis of 15 clinical variables, treatment with PTCA rather than thrombolysis, as well as younger age, were independently predictive of in-hospital survival in women. In men in-hospital mortality was similar with both thrombolysis and PTCA (3.5% vs. 2.1%, respectively); only advanced age independently correlated with mortality in men. Compared with men, women with AMI are at increased risk for early mortality and life-threatening hemorrhagic complications after thrombolytic therapy. Primary PTCA reduces the risk of intracranial bleeding and results in improved survival in women, such that the prognosis of men and women is equally favorable.

Gender-related differences in outcome after AMI may relate to biased treatment allocation. To address this concern Vacek and coworkers[74] in Kansas City, Missouri, analyzed 573 patients presenting with ST-segment elevation AMI and treated within 6 hours with reperfusion therapy. Two hundred eighty (49%) patients received direct PTCA, whereas 293 (51%) received thrombolytics followed by PTCA. Seventy-four percent were men and 26% were women, and there were no differences in sex distribution between the two treatment groups. Women were older in both groups. Inferior AMI was seen more often in women (64% of those receiving direct PTCA, 71% of those treated with lytic first) than in men (51% and 59%, respectively). There was no gender-related difference in presence of multivessel CAD, prior AMI, prior CABG, baseline EF, percentage of patients with EF ≤40%, number of narrowings dilated, or PTCA success. Patients who underwent direct PTCA had more multivessel disease and prior CABG. After a mean follow-up of 129 weeks, no gender-related differences were seen in the need for cardiac catheterization, documented restenosis, AMI, CABG, clinical ischemia, or death. Patients treated with direct PTCA were more likely to undergo CABG or to die. Thus, women undergoing reperfusion therapy for ST-segment elevation were older than men, with a higher frequency of inferior wall AMI. No specific gender-related bias in treatment allocation was evident.

In Menstruating Women

Anectodal case reports have suggested that thrombolytic therapy is safe during menstruation. Karnash and colleagues[75] for the GUSTO-I trial identified menstruating women who received thrombolytic therapy while soliciting information on all North American women enrolled in the GUSTO-I trial. Twelve menstruating women were identified with an average age of 46; 75% were cigarette smokers. No woman died or had a stroke or severe bleeding. Three patients had moderate bleeding and required transfusion (25%) compared with 11% of all GUSTO-I patients. These authors concluded that although there was no statistically significant increase in bleeding risk during menstruation, this may have been due to the small number of menstruating women in the study. The results do suggest that there may be a clinically significant increase in the risk of moderate bleeding. Nevertheless the GUSTO-I experience is consistent with the concept that life-saving thrombolytic therapy for acute infarction should generally not be withheld because of active menstruation.

In Smokers vs. Nonsmokers

Grines and colleagues[76] evaluated 1619 patients treated with t-PA, urokinase, or both in six consecutive myocardial infarction trials of whom 878 (54%) were smoking at the time. Patients underwent 90-minute and predischarge cardiac catheterizations. The evaluators were blinded to the patients' smoking status. Baseline fibrinogens and hematocrits were greater in smokers. Although there were no differences between smokers and nonsmokers with regard to 90-minute patency of the infarct-related artery (73% and 74%, respectively), smokers were more likely to have TIMI grade 3 flow (41% vs. 35%) with a larger minimum lumen diameter of the infarct stenosis both acutely and at follow-up. Smokers tended to have reduced in-hospital mortality compared with nonsmokers after adjustment for baseline differences between smokers and nonsmokers in age, inferior AMI, three-vessel CAD, and baseline LVEF. Thus, in this study, smokers had a relatively hypercoagulable state, documented by increased hematocrit and fibrinogen, but the results suggest that the mechanism of AMI in smokers may be more often thrombosis of a less critical atherosclerotic lesion.

Despite the epidemiological studies that show that cigarette smoking is associated with higher rates of AMI and death from CAD, several large clinical trials have demonstrated that smokers who have an AMI have a better prognosis than nonsmokers. Barbash and colleagues[77] evaluated this "smoker's paradox" in the GUSTO-I trial. They analyzed outcomes of baseline characteristics of approximately 12 000 nonsmokers, 11 000 exsmokers, and 17 000 current smokers in the GUSTO-I trial. Smokers were significantly younger by a mean of 11 years. Nonsmokers had significantly higher hospital and 30-day mortality rates (9.9% and 10.3%) compared with smokers (3.7% and 4.0%). Thus, although smokers receiving thrombolysis for AMI had a reduced mortality, they presented 11 years earlier. Furthermore, when other differences in clinical and angiographic baseline factors and therapeutic responses were evaluated, no significant difference in mortality was seen between smokers and nonsmokers.

Effect of Previous Angina on Outcome

Kloner and colleagues[78] in the TIMI-4 study analyzed the effect of a history of previous angina on in-hospital outcomes for patients with AMI. Patients eligible for thrombolytic therapy were enrolled in the study and data were collected from case report forms regarding previous history of angina, in-hospital outcome and 6-week follow-up. Two hundred eighteen patients had a history of previous angina at any time before AMI and 198 patients did not have previous angina. Patients with a previous history of angina were less likely than those without angina to experience in-hospital death (3% vs. 8%), severe CHF or shock (1% vs. 7%) or the combined end points of in-hospital death, severe CHF, or shock (4% vs. 12%). Patients with a history of angina were more likely to have a smaller serum creatine kinase-determined infarct size and less likely to have Q waves on their electrocardiograms. In the subset of patients who had angina within the 48 hours before AMI compared with those who did not, there was a trend toward less likely in-hospital death (3% vs. 6%), a lower incidence of severe CHF or shock (1% vs. 6%), a lower combined end point of death, CHF, or shock (3% vs. 10%), smaller infarct size assessed by serum creatine kinase, and a trend toward fewer Q-wave infarcts. Patients with a history of previous angina tended to have more recurrent ischemic pain. The beneficial in-hospital effects of previous angina were not dependent on angiographically visible coronary collateral vessels. Thus, these data indicate that previous angina provides a beneficial effect on in-hospital outcome after AMI.

Tissue Plasminogen Activator

Kurnik[79] in Camden, New Jersey, evaluated the hypothesis that t-PA has greater efficacy when administered between noon and midnight as measured by coronary patency 90 minutes after initiation of treatment. Seven hundred twenty-eight patients were enrolled in either of two studies in which t-PA was administered under a uniform protocol for the treatment of AMI. Six hundred ninety-two patients had qualifying arteriograms that allowed standardized assessment by a core angiographic laboratory of the primary end point of 90-minute patency. t-PA had a circadian pattern of efficacy with greater TIMI grade 3 patency when administered between noon and midnight (Figure 3-24). When t-PA was given within 2 hours of symptoms, the total patency was highest and there was a trend toward the greatest magnitude difference occurring between AM and PM patency. The onset of AMI was confirmed to have circadian variation with peak incidence about 10:00 AM. The peak efficacy of t-PA was about 8:00 PM, demonstrating a phase difference of about 10 hours after peak AMI incidence. Thus, there is a circadian variation in the ability of t-PA to rapidly open coronary arteries with the highest efficacy between noon and midnight. This finding has implications for understanding the circadian pathophysiology of AMI and for its therapy.

Ottani and colleagues[80] in Forli, Italy, determined whether new-onset prodromal angina, defined as chest pain episodes limited to the 24 hours before AMI, is a clinical correlate of the ischemic preconditioning phenomenon. Twenty-five patients with their first AMI treated with thrombolysis (rt-PA given as 100 mg/3 hours) were included in the study when they met the following criteria: 1) <120 minutes from onset of symptoms to reperfusion therapy; 2) <90 minutes from the beginning of thrombolytic therapy to reperfusion; 3) a patent infarct-related coronary artery with TIMI 3 flow and absence of visible collateral circulation to the infarct related artery; and 4) the presence of new-onset prodromal angina, typical chest pain occurring at rest within 24 hours of AMI. Patients were divided into two groups: group 1 included 13 patients without prodromal angina, and group 2, 12 patients with prodromal angina. Despite no difference in time to treatment and time to reperfusion, the peak of creatine kinase–MB release was markedly lower in group 2 than in group 1 patients. Both groups were comparable in terms of area at risk defined as amount of myocardium beyond the infarct-related stenosis and hypokinetic segments in groups 1 and 2, but the final infarct size was smaller in group 2 patients. There was an additional 33% reduction infarct size in the group of patients with prodromal angina. Therefore, despite a similar area at risk, patients with new-onset prodromal angina showed a significantly smaller infarct size compared with patients without prodromal symptoms. This might be explained by their having ischemic preconditioning.

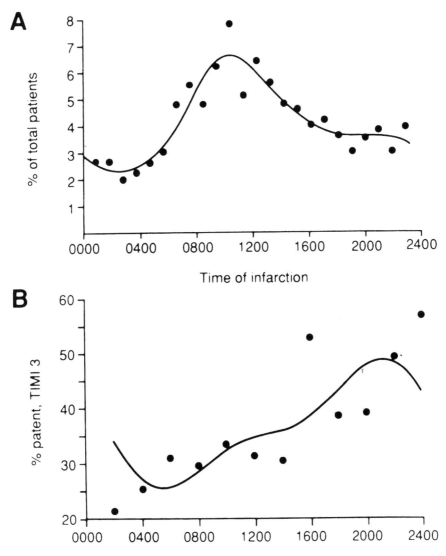

Figure 3-24. Plots of circadian patterns of infarction incidence and of tissue-type plasminogen activator (t-PA) efficacy. **A,** circadian pattern of the frequency distribution of an event (onset of infarction); **B,** circadian pattern of efficacy of an intervention (patency 90 minutes after t-PA). There is a phase lag of about 10 hours from peak incidence of infarction (about 10:00 AM) to peak efficacy of t-PA (about 8:00 PM). The second-order harmonic regression models are superimposed on the measured data. A given patient will be represented at a later time on B than on A because of the time lapse between onset of infarction and initiation of thrombolytic therapy. Reproduced with permission from Kurnik et al.[79]

Of a total of 3339 patients enrolled in TIMI II, 1681 were randomly assigned to an invasive strategy and 1658 to a conservative strategy.[81] One hundred forty-two patients died before 14 days but the remaining 3197 patients had a radionuclide ventriculographic study. As seen in Figure 3-25, there was a hyperbolic relationship between 1-year all cause mortality and rest LVEF obtained at about 2 weeks. The highest mortality rate (9.9%) was noted in patients with an EF <30%. Patients unable to exercise were those not having a rest

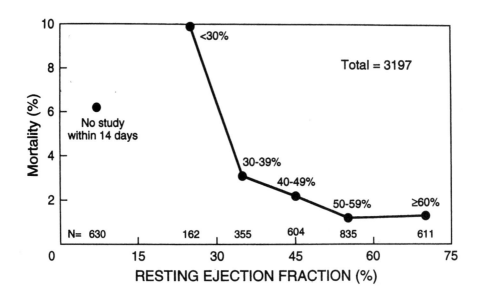

Figure 3-25. Relation of rest ejection fraction to all cause mortality in the TIMI II study. Also note the mortality rate for patients who did not undergo radionuclide ventriculography within 14 days. Reproduced with permission from Zaret et al.[81]

study; they had a 1-year mortality of 6.2%. Peak exercise EF provided prognostic information similar to that of rest EF. These authors concluded that rest EF provides important prognostic information about patients with AMI. Data also suggested that mortality rate was lower in TIMI II patients than in patients in the prethrombolytic era.

Lenderink and colleagues[82] in Rotterdam, the Netherlands, evaluated 5-year survival in patients who received placebo, rt-PA, or rt-PA with additional immediate PTCA in two European Cooperative Study Group trials. Determinants for long-term survival were assessed in 1043 patients discharged alive. Five-year follow-up information on mortality was collected. Hospital mortality was lower after t-PA than placebo (3% vs. 6%) and higher after t-PA with immediate PTCA compared with t-PA without additional intervention (6% vs. 2%). Of the 1043 hospital survivors, data were available for 923 patients of whom 109 died. In the placebo group, mortality after hospital discharge was 11% vs. 11% in the comparative t-PA group. The patients treated with t-PA and immediate PTCA had a mortality rate of 11% vs. 9% in the t-PA group without PTCA. Significant determinants of mortality in multivariate proportional hazards analysis were enzymatic infarct size, indicators of residual LV function, number of diseased vessels, and TIMI perfusion grade at discharge. Patients with TIMI grade 2 flow had mortality rates similar to those with TIMI flow grade 0 and 1, whereas prognosis was better in patients with TIMI flow grade 3 (Figure 3-26). Thus, the initial in-hospital benefit of thrombolysis with intravenous t-PA is maintained throughout 5 years with no early or late beneficial effect of systematic immediate PTCA. Enzymatic infarct size, LVEF, and

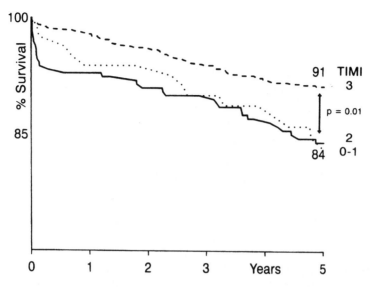

Figure 3-26. Survival curves after hospital discharge with stratification for different TIMI perfusion grades obtained at discharge. Patients with TIMI grades 0 and 1 are combined (solid line). The difference between patients with complete perfusion (TIMI 3; 5-year survival, 95%) and those with TIMI grades 0 to 2 (survival, 84%) was significant (*P* = 0.01). Reproduced with permission from Lenderink et al.[82]

extent of CAD are predictors for long-term survival. TIMI perfusion grade 2 at discharge should be considered an inadequate result of therapy.

Fourteen hundred seventy-three patients were enrolled in the TIMI IIIB trial and were randomly assigned to therapy with either t-PA or placebo, and also to an early invasive management strategy with coronary arteriography at 18 to 48 hours followed by revascularization as soon as possible.[83] Alternatively, an early conservative strategy was used which reserved arteriography and revascularization for failure of initial therapy to prevent recurrent ischemia. At 1 year, the incidence of death or nonfatal infarction for the t-PA and placebo treated groups was similar (12.4% vs. 10.6%). The incidence of death and nonfatal infarction was also similar after 1 year for the early invasive and early consecutive strategies (10.8% vs. 12.2%). Revascularization by 1 year was slightly more common with the early invasive than the early conservative strategy (64% vs. 58%), and was entirely related to a small difference in the PTCA rates. These authors concluded that in this large study of unstable angina and non–Q-wave AMI, the incidence of death and nonfatal reinfarction was low but not trivial after 1 year (4.3% mortality; 8.8% nonfatal infarction). The incidence of death and nonfatal AMI or both did not differ after 1 year by strategy assignment, but fewer patients in the early invasive strategy group underwent later repeat hospital admission (26% vs. 33%). Either strategy was felt to be appropriate for patient management; differences in hospital admissions and revascularization procedures with their attendant costs are likely to be minimal.

Very early administration of thrombolytic therapy for AMI has significantly reduced mortality in eligible patients. The purpose of a study by Maynard and coworkers[84] in Seattle, Washington, was to evaluate factors that influence the time from symptom onset to hospital admission and the time from hospital presentation to the onset of thrombolytic therapy in a large population of patients with AMI. The study included 212 990 patients from 904 hospitals that participated in the National Registry of Myocardial Infarction. The median time from symptom onset to hospital presentation for those treated was 1.5 hours vs. 2.7 hours for those not receiving thrombolytic therapy. The delay was greater for older patients and women as well as for those who arrived at the hospital during daylight hours. Of the 59 802 (28%) patients who received thrombolytic therapy, 23% were treated <30 minutes from admission; 63% <60 minutes, and 83% <90 minutes. Time to treatment increased with age and was longer for women and patients arriving between midnight and early morning. The most important factor associated with shorter time to treatment was initiation of thrombolytic treatment in the emergency department rather than in the coronary care unit (47 vs. 73 minutes). Hospital treatment times are much too long, given that quick identification and treatment of eligible patients are of primary importance in reducing mortality from AMI. To shorten these times, thrombolytic treatment should be initiated in the emergency department, and the effectiveness of hospital programs aimed at reducing time to treatment should be subject to continuing quality improvement surveillance.

Tissue Plasminogen Activator vs. Streptokinase

Patients with AMI who were treated with accelerated t-PA given over a period of 90 minutes rather than the conventional 180 minutes, and with two thirds of the dose given in the first 30 minutes, had a 30-day mortality that was 15% lower than that of patients treated with streptokinase in the GUSTO study. This was equivalent to an absolute decrease of 1% in 30-day mortality. Mark and associates[85] from multiple worldwide medical centers sought to assess whether the use of t-PA, compared with streptokinase, is cost effective. Their primary, or base case, analysis of cost-effectiveness, used data from the GUSTO study and life expectancy projected on the basis of the records of survivors of AMI in the Duke Cardiovascular Disease Database. In the primary analysis, we assumed that there were no additional treatment costs caused by the use of t-PA after the first year and that the comparative survival benefit of t-PA was still evident 1 year after enrollment. One year after enrollment, patients who received t-PA had both higher costs ($2845) and a higher survival rate (an increase of 1.1%, or 11 per 1000 patients treated) than streptokinase-treated patients. On the basis of the projected life expectancy of each treatment group, the incremental cost-effectiveness ratio—with both future costs and benefits discounted at 5% per year—was $32 678 per year of life saved. The use of t-PA was least cost effective in older patients. At all ages, the use of t-PA in patients with anterior infarctions yielded more favorable cost-effectiveness values. In their secondary analyses, the cost-effectiveness values were most sensitive to a lowering of the projected long-term survival benefits of t-PA and to moderate or greater increases in the projected medical costs for patients in the t-PA group after the first year. In contrast, their results were not sensitive to even very unfavorable assumptions about the additional costs associated with the higher rate of disabling stroke that was noted in patients treated with t-PA in the GUSTO study. The cost-effectiveness of treatment with accelerated t-PA rather than streptokinase compares favorably with that of other therapies whose added medical benefit for dollars spent is judged by society to be worthwhile.

Anistreplase

The outcome of patients with TIMI grade 2 flow is worse than that of patients with grade III flow after thrombolytic therapy for AMI. It is unclear whether myocardial infarction grade 2 flow represents incomplete recanalization of the culprit lesion or poor distal runoff. The Thrombolytic Trial of Eminase (anistreplase) in AMI (TEAM) 2 and TEAM 3 were randomized trials comparing anistreplase with streptokinase (TEAM 2, n = 370) or with alteplase (t-PA) (TEAM 3, n = 325). Zahger and coinvestigators[86] in Los Angeles, California, compared the minimal luminal diameter of the culprit lesion in patients with TIMI grade 2 flow with that in patients with TIMI grade 3 flow both 90 minutes (TEAM 2) and 1 day (TEAM 3) after thrombolysis. Patients with TIMI grade 2 flow had a lower residual luminal diameter in the culprit lesion than patients with TIMI grade 3 flow. Residual percent stenosis was correspondingly higher in patients with TIMI grade 2 flow. At the early angiogram, 66% of patients with grade 2 flow, but only 35% of those with grade 3 flow, had a minimal luminal diameter of 0.6 mm. Incomplete recanalization of the culprit lesion may thus be an important determinant of TIMI grade 2 flow after thrombolysis.

Within 1 year, Ozbek and colleagues[87] in Homburg/Saar, Germany, evaluated 434 patients with AMI who were admitted to 14 hospitals less than 4 hours after the onset of symptoms. Group A consisted of 171 patients (39%) treated with thrombolysis, and group B consisted of 263 patients (61%) with contraindications. Patients in group A more likely had a definite AMI (91%) than patients in group B (67%). Group B had 277 contraindications (1.6 per patient), with increased risk for life-threatening bleeding being the most frequently recorded at admission. The in-hospital mortality in group A was 7% (11 of 158) and in group B 27% (47 of 177). Age and type of therapy (thrombolysis or no thrombolysis) were identified as independent predictors of increased mortality. Thus, although most patients with an AMI are excluded from thrombolytic therapy because of contraindications, these data suggest that in-hospital mortality is unexpectedly high. Furthermore, evaluation of this group of patients is warranted to define the impact of contraindications as an independent factor for mortality.

Reteplase vs. Streptokinase

Streptokinase and alteplase are established therapies in AMI. Reteplase is a new thrombolytic agent that can be given as a double bolus. The International Joint Efficacy Comparison of Thrombolytics (INJECT) trial was designed to determine whether the effect of reteplase on survival was at least equivalent (within 1% fatality rate) to that of a standard streptokinase regimen.[88] Patients from 208 centers in nine countries (n = 6010) with symptoms and electrocardiographic criteria consistent with AMI were randomly assigned to receive in a double-blind manner either streptokinase 1.5 MU intravenously over 60 minutes or reteplase 2 boluses of 10 MU given 30 minutes apart. Treatment could be started up to 12 hours from onset of symptoms. All patients received intravenous heparin for at least 24 hours. The primary end point was a 35-day outcome. There were 270

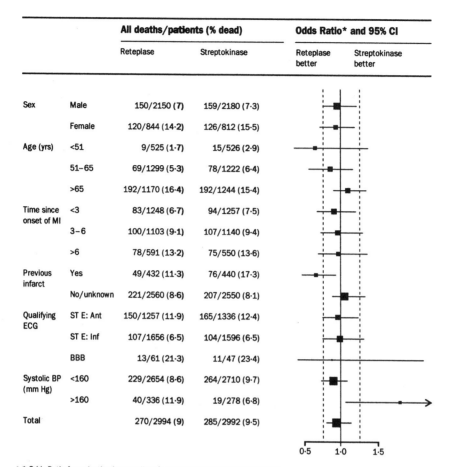

		All deaths/patients (% dead)		Odds Ratio* and 95% CI	
		Reteplase	Streptokinase	Reteplase better	Streptokinase better
Sex	Male	150/2150 (7)	159/2180 (7·3)		
	Female	120/844 (14·2)	126/812 (15·5)		
Age (yrs)	<51	9/525 (1·7)	15/526 (2·9)		
	51–65	69/1299 (5·3)	78/1222 (6·4)		
	>65	192/1170 (16·4)	192/1244 (15·4)		
Time since onset of MI	<3	83/1248 (6·7)	94/1257 (7·5)		
	3–6	100/1103 (9·1)	107/1140 (9·4)		
	>6	78/591 (13·2)	75/550 (13·6)		
Previous infarct	Yes	49/432 (11·3)	76/440 (17·3)		
	No/unknown	221/2560 (8·6)	207/2550 (8·1)		
Qualifying ECG	ST E: Ant	150/1257 (11·9)	165/1336 (12·4)		
	ST E: Inf	107/1656 (6·5)	104/1596 (6·5)		
	BBB	13/61 (21·3)	11/47 (23·4)		
Systolic BP (mm Hg)	<160	229/2654 (8·6)	264/2710 (9·7)		
	>160	40/336 (11·9)	19/278 (6·8)		
Total		270/2994 (9)	285/2992 (9·5)		

0·5   1·0   1·5

* Odds Ratio for reduction in mortality of reteplase relative to streptokinase

Figure 3-27. 35-day mortality by subgroups. Reproduced with permission from International Joint Efficacy Comparison of Thrombolytics et al.[88]

deaths (9.02%) in the reteplase and 285 deaths (9.53%) in the streptokinase group, a nonsignificant difference (Figure 3-27). Among patients who received treatment (99%) there were 263 deaths (9.43%) in the streptokinase group (a difference of −0.53%). Because the upper limit of the 90% CI for this difference was 0.71%, this result shows that reteplase is at least as effective as streptokinase. In-hospital stroke rates were 1.23% for reteplase and 1.00% for streptokinase. Bleeding events were similar in the 2 treatment groups (0.7% reteplase and 1.0% streptokinase). The incidence of recurrent AMI was similar, but there were significantly fewer cases of AF, asystole, cardiac shock, CHF, and hypotension in the reteplase group. The authors concluded that reteplase is an effective drug in the treatment of AMI. It is clinically safe, its administration is simple, and it will be a useful addition to the range of thrombolytic agents available.

Reteplase vs. Alteplase

Smalling and colleagues[89] for the RAPID Investigators tested the hypothesis that bolus administration of one or more dosage regimens of a mutant r-PA (reteplase) a nonglycosylated deletion mutant of the wild-type t-PA is superior to standard-dose t-PA (alteplase) in leading to infarct-related artery patency 90 minutes after initiation of therapy. Six hundred six patients with AMI were randomly assigned 1 of 4 treatment arms: 1) t-PA 100 mg intravenously over 3 hours; 2) r-PA as a 15-MU single bolus; 3) r-PA as a 10-MU bolus followed by 5 MU 30 minutes later; or 4) r-PA as a 10-MU bolus followed by 10 MU 30 minutes later. Coronary arteriography was performed at 30, 60, and 90 minutes after initiation of treatment and at hospital discharge. In this study, the 10 + 10 MU r-PA group had the best 90-minute and 5- to 14-day TIMI grade III flow. The TIMI grade 3 flow in the 10 + 10 MU r-PA group at 60 minutes was equivalent to that in the t-PA group at 90 minutes (51% vs. 49%). Global LVEF and regional wall motion in the 10 + 10 MU r-PA were superior to those of the t-PA at hospital discharge. The 15 MU and 10 + 5 MU r-PA patency and LVEF were similar to those of t-PA and inferior to those of the 10 + 10 MU r-PA group. Bleeding complications appeared to be similar among the different groups of patients. Thus, these data suggest that this mutant t-PA given as a double bolus of 10 + 10 MU achieves more rapid, complete, and sustained thrombolysis of the infarct-related artery than standard dose t-PA without an apparent increased risk of complications. The improvement in thrombolysis is associated with improved global and regional LV function at hospital discharge.

Streptokinase + Hirulog + Heparin

Théroux and colleagues[90] in Montreal, Canada, studied the potential protective effect of hirulog, a direct thrombin inhibitor, to improve early patency rates obtained with streptokinase and aspirin in patients with AMI. Angiographic patency of the culprit coronary artery lesion was assessed at 90 and 120 minutes after the initiation of streptokinase and aspirin and again after 4 days in 68 patients with AMI. Patients were randomly assigned to hirulog 0.5 mg/kg per hour for 12 hours followed by 0.1 mg/kg per hour infusion (low dose), 1.0 mg/kg per hour for 12 hours followed by placebo (high dose), or to heparin 5000 U bolus followed by 1000 U per hour titrated to an activated partial thromboplastin time 2 to 2.5 times greater than control after 12 hours. After 90 minutes, TIMI flow grade 2 or 3 was observed in 96% of patients treated with the low dose of hirulog, in 79% with the high dose, and in 46% with heparin and TIMI flow grade 3 was observed in 85%, 61%, and 31% of these patients, respectively. After 120 minutes, these figures were 100%, 82%, and 62% for TIMI flow grades 2 and 3 and 92%, 68%, and 46% for TIMI flow grade 3. At 90 minutes, the RR value for restoring TIMI flow grade 3 was 2.77 with hirulog at 0.5 mg/kg per hour compared with heparin and 1.4 compared with hirulog 1.0 mg/kg per minute. Patients who received a placebo infusion after 12 hours had more clinical events and reocclusion during the following 4 days than patients in the other 2 groups. These data suggest that hirulog, a direct thrombin inhibitor, yields higher early patency rates in the culprit coronary artery than heparin when used as adjunctive therapy to streptokinase and aspirin in the early phases of AMI. High doses are not required and may be less effective than lower doses suggesting that too much thrombin inhibition may be harmful.

Recombinant Staphylokinase vs. Alteplase

Vanderschueren and colleagues[91] in Leuven, Belgium, assessed the thrombolytic efficacy, safety, and fibrin specificity of a recombinant staphylokinase, which previously has been shown to offer promise for coronary artery thrombolysis in patients with AMI. One hundred patients with evolving AMI of <6 hours' duration and with ST-segment elevation were allocated to accelerated and weight-adjusted rt-PA or recombinant staphylokinase. All patients received aspirin and intravenous heparin. The primary end points of the study were coronary artery patency and plasma fibrinogen levels at 90 minutes after therapy. TIMI perfusion grade 3 at 90 minutes was achieved in 62% of the staphylokinase-treated patients and 58% of the t-PA–treated patients. TIMI perfusion grade 3 patency was present in 50% of patients treated with staphylokinase given a 10-mg dose and 74% of patients receiving a 20-mg dose. Residual fibrinogen levels at 90 minutes were 118% of baseline with staphylokinase and 68% with t-PA. Staphylokinase therapy was not associated with an excess mortality or hemorrhagic, mechanical, or allergic complications. However, patients developed antibody-mediated staphylokinase-neutralizing activity from the second week after staphylokinase treatment. These data suggest staphylokinase is at least as effective for early coronary recanalization and significantly more fibrin-specific than accelerated t-PA in patients with evolving AMI. The limitation of administering staphylokinase may be its antigenic potential.

Recombinant Urokinase Type Plasminogen Activator (Saruplase)

The LIMITS study was instituted to evaluate and characterize the effect of a prethrombolytic heparin bolus (5,000 IU) on the efficacy and safety of saruplase in patients with AMI. The study[92] was designed as a randomized, parallel-group, double-blind, multicenter trial. Fifty-six patients were treated within 6 hours of onset with either a bolus of 5000 IU of heparin or placebo before thrombolytic treatment with saruplase was given as a 20-mg bolus followed by an infusion of 60 mg over 60 minutes. Thirty minutes after completion of thrombolysis, intravenous heparin infusion was administered for 5 days. In the heparin pretreatment group, 78.6% of patients had an open infarct-related vessel (TIMI flow grade 2 or 3) compared with 56.5% in the placebo group. Twelve patients died during the hospital stay, including 3 in the initial heparin group compared with 9 in the control group. These authors concluded that in AMI, the administration of a heparin bolus before thrombolytic therapy with saruplase is associated with a significantly higher patency rate at angiography 6 to 12 hours after the start of thrombolysis without any appreciable increase in the risk of bleeding.

Patency Afterwards

To determine whether pharmacological reperfusion to TIMI grade 2 flow (delayed inflow or outflow of contrast throughout the infarct vessel) during AMI confers the same clinical benefit as restoration of grade 3 flow (brisk and complete filling), Lincoff and co workers[93] in Cleveland, Ohio, analyzed in-hospital clinical and angiographic outcomes in 1229 patients prospectively enrolled in the Thrombolysis and Angioplasty in Myocardial Infarction trials.

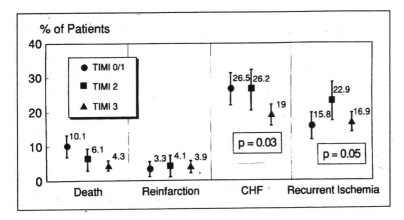

Figure 3-28. In-hospital clinical outcome in patient groups defined by 90-minute Thrombolysis in Myocardial Infarction (TIMI) trial flow. Values are displayed as percentage of patients with 95% confidence intervals; p values are for the difference between TIMI 2 and 3 groups. CHF indicates congestive heart failure. Reproduced with permission from Lincoff et al.[93]

Patients were treated with intravenous tissue plasminogen activator or urokinase, or both. Angiography of the infarct-related artery 90 minutes after initiation of thrombolytic therapy demonstrated TIMI grades 0, 1, 2, or 3 flow in 20%, 7%, 17%, and 55% of vessels, respectively. Rescue or adjunctive PTCA was performed in 80%, 27%, and 16% of patients with TIMI 0/1, 2, or 3 flow, respectively. Predischarge angiography was performed in 963 patients. A significant gradient of increasing mortality was seen in patients with lower TIMI flow grades (Figure 3-28). The incidence of CHF and recurrent ischemia was significantly higher in patients with TIMI flow grade 2 than with flow grade 3 perfusion. Acute LVEF and infarct zone regional wall motion were also significantly improved in patients with TIMI flow grade 3 compared with grade 2 flow, with trends toward better improvement in global and regional function in the TIMI flow grade 3 group. These findings were not affected by the use of acute PTCA. Thus, TIMI 2 and 3 flow grades are not equivalent with regard to clinical outcome, and flow grade 2 after thrombolysis for AMI should not be regarded as patency in the sense of predicting a good clinical outcome.

Effect of Nitroglycerin

Romeo and associates[94] from Rome, Catania, and Vibo Valentia, Italy, and Gainesville, Florida, evaluated the impact of concurrent nitroglycerin administration on the thrombolytic efficacy of rt-PA in patients with anterior AMI. Sixty patients (53 men and 7 women; mean age, 54±7 years) with anterior AMI entered the study. Thirty-three patients were randomly assigned to receive rt-PA alone (100 mg in 3 hours) (group A) and 27 to receive rt-PA plus nitroglycerin (100 μg/min) (group B). Time from the onset of chest pain and delivery of rt-PA was similar in the 2 groups of patients. Patients in group A had signs of reperfusion more often than the patients in group B (25 of 33 or 76% vs. 15 of 27 or 56%). Time to reperfusion was also shorter in group A than in group B (20±9.4 vs. 38±5.9 minutes). Group B had a greater incidence of in-hospital adverse events (9 of 27 vs. 5 of 33) and a higher incidence of coronary artery reocclusion (8 of 15, or 53%, vs. 6 of 25, or 24%). Peak plasma levels of rt-PA antigen were higher in group A compared with group B (1427±679 vs. 512±312 ng/mL). In conclusion, concurrent nitroglycerin administration reduces the thrombolytic efficacy of rt-PA in patients with anterior AMI probably by lowering the plasma levels of rt-PA antigen. The diminished efficacy of rt-PA is associated with an adverse outcome.

Elevated ST Segment Augmentation and Resolution

To investigate the significance of abrupt augmentation of ST segment elevation immediately after reperfusion, 36 patients with an initial AMI successfully treated with thrombolysis were studied by Yokoshiki and associates[95] from Sapporo and Asahikawa, Japan. Immediately after reperfusion was performed, 17 (47%) patients showed abrupt augmentation of ST segment elevation of anterior area (E group), and 19 (53%) patients did not (N group). The time to reperfusion was not significantly different between the 2 groups. In the E group the peak level of creatine kinase–MB isozyme was higher than in the N group. The LVEF did not increase in the E group from acute to chronic phase. However, in the N group EF increased significantly. The difference in EF in the chronic phase was significant between the 2 groups. The infarcted regional wall motion did not increase in the E group, whereas in the N group it increased markedly. In addition, the infarcted regional wall motion in the chronic phase was worse in the E group than in the N group. Abrupt augmentation of ST segment elevation associated with successful reperfusion appears to reflect diminished myocardial salvage.

Some studies have shown that the use of cut-off points for ST segment resolution within 3 hours after the start of thrombolysis is effective in predicting outcome. Schroder and colleagues[96] for the INJECT trial compared mortality in 6010 patients randomized to receive either rateplase or streptokinase. The 1909 German patients form the basis of this sub-study. In 1398 who presented less than 6 hours from the onset of AMI, the 35-day mortality rate for complete, partial, and no ST segment resolution was 2.5%, 4.3%, and 17.5%, respectively. When baseline characteristics were included, ST segment resolution was the most powerful independent predictor of 35-day mortality. These authors concluded that no ST segment resolution indicated failed thrombolysis and predicted a very high early mortality. On the other hand, complete resolution was associated with a small infarct area and low mortality. Partial ST segment resolution also predicted larger infarct areas, but early mortality was relatively low. These data suggest that the different extents of ST segment resolution may serve as a surrogate end point in clinical trials.

Biochemical Markers of Reperfusion

Laperche and colleagues[97] in Paris, France, evaluated biochemical methods for the early diagnosis of patency after thrombolysis in patients with AMI to establish the optimal diagnostic criteria. In 97 patients with AMI treated with thrombolytic agents ≤6 hours after symptom onset, myoglobin, troponin T, and creatine kinase and its MB isoenzyme and MM isoforms were measured just before thrombolysis began and 90 minutes later. Thrombolytic agents used in this study included streptokinase, rt-PA, urokinase, and combinations of these agents in individual patients. Infarct-related artery patency was assessed by a 90-minute coronary angiogram. For each marker, expected sensitivity and specificity based on published thresholds for the diagnosis of patency were compared with observed values. With receiver-operator characteristic curve analysis of the slopes of increase and relative increases in each marker over 90 minutes, the best diagnostic performance was achieved by demonstrating a relative increase in myoglobin, troponin T, and the creatine kinase–MM isoforms MM3/MM1 in patients treated >3 hours after onset of symptoms. These data indicate that effective early noninvasive diagnosis of patency after thrombolysis is possible in patients treated >3 hours after symptom onset using relative increase over 90 minutes in selected plasma markers, especially myoglobin, troponin T, and creatine kinase isoforms MM3/MM1.

Q-Wave Regression Afterwards

Iwasaki and colleagues[98] in Okayama, Japan, examined the relation of Q-wave regression to LV indexes in anterior AMI in relation to reperfusion therapy. A total of 94 patients with their first anterior wall AMI (segment 6 or 7 occlusion according to the American Heart Association classification) were classified. The follow-up period with 12-lead electrocardiograms ranged from 6 to 60 months. An abnormal Q wave was defined as >40 msec and >25% of the R-wave amplitude. Q-wave regression was defined as Q-wave disappearance and r-wave regression >0.1 mV in ≥1 leads. Contingency tables with the χ-square test and analysis of variance were used for assessment of the relation between Q-wave regression and angiographic and clinical indexes. Q-wave regression in one or more leads was found in 77% of the patients. The incidence of Q-wave regression in patients with patent infarct-related artery (81%) was not significantly different from that in those with an occluded lesion (67%). Q-wave regression appeared within 1 month in 60% of patients with a patent infarct-related artery but in 25% of those with an occluded lesion. No difference in the incidence of Q-wave regression was seen between patients with lesions at segments 6 (81%) and 7 (70%) or between those with (75%) and without (77%) collateral circulation. Q-wave regression did not correlate with LVEF, LV end-diastolic or end-systolic volumes, or regional wall motion. In conclusion, Q-wave regression in patients with anterior wall AMI does not reflect improvement in LV function and its prognostic significance is poor.

Impaired Tissue Reperfusion

Maes and colleagues[99] in Leuven, Belgium, used PET to determine whether there is impaired tissue reperfusion after successful thrombolytic therapy in selected patients with AMI. Thirty patients with an AMI and TIMI flow grade 3 of the infarct-related vessel at 90 minutes after thrombolytic therapy were evaluated. Within 24 hours after thrombolysis, at 5 days, and at 3 months, myocardial blood flow was measured with $^{13}NH_3$. Fluorodeoxyglucose uptake as an estimate of myocardial viability was measured at 5 days. Radionuclide LV angiograms were acquired at 5 days and 3 months after thrombolytic therapy. In 11 patients (37%), regional myocardial flow was severely impaired and was <50% of the normally perfused myocardium despite successful thrombolysis. No recovery of segmental LV function occurred in any of these patients at 3 months. In 12 patients (40%), intermediate flows (50% to 75% of normal) were found with functional improvement after PTCA only in regions with a PET mismatch between perfusion and viability, i.e., reduced perfusion but continued viability as evidenced by fluorodeoxyglucose uptake. Seven patients (23%) had high flow values early after successful thrombolysis (>75% of normal) and showed preserved regional contractile function at 3 months. Thus, these data demonstrate impaired myocardial tissue perfusion in some patients after successful thrombolysis with AMI. Functional recovery of the reperfused myocardium is observed only when adequate tissue flow is restored.

Recurrent Myocardial Ischemia or Infarction Afterwards

PTCA has become increasingly common as a therapeutic measure for patients with AMI. In the Primary Angioplasty and Myocardial Infarction (PAMI) trial Stone and colleagues[100] evaluated the rates and effects of recurrent ischemia after different reperfusion strategies in AMI. At 12 centers, 395 patients presenting within 12 hours of the onset of AMI were prospectively randomized to receive rt-PA or primary PTCA. Recurrent ischemia developed in 19.2% of patients before hospital discharge, resulting in reinfarction in 4.6% of patients and death in 2.6%. Recurrent ischemia occurred in 28% after rt-PA but in only 10.3% after PTCA. After hospital day 2, recurrent ischemia occurred in only 1.1% of patients who received primary PTCA vs. 13.5% of patients who received rt-PA. These authors concluded that the much lower rate of recurrent ischemia after primary PTCA than after rt-PA resulted in improved survival without reinfarction and allowed a shorter, less complicated hospital stay. They also concluded that safe, early discharge on day 3 after primary PTCA should be feasible in selected patients with AMI.

Mueller and colleagues[101] evaluated the event rate of nonfatal reinfarction over a 3-year follow-up in patients entered into the TIMI II trial. During this 3-year follow-up, 349 of 3339 patients had a nonfatal reinfarction. Univariate predictors were history of angina, hypertension, multivessel disease, and not a current smoker. The RR value of death in patients with a nonfatal reinfarction compared to those without a nonfatal reinfarction was 1.9 if reinfarction occurred within 42 days. The RR was 6.2 if reinfarction occurred between 43 and 365 days, and 2.9 for reinfarction between 1 and 3 years. Cumulative 3-year death rate was 14% in patients with a nonfatal reinfarction compared with 7.9% in a matched control group. These authors concluded that nonfatal reinfarction is a strong and independent predictor for sudden death. It represents a powerful component for a composite end point in patients receiving thrombolytic therapy after AMI.

Early postinfarction angina implies an unfavorable prognosis. Most published information on this outcome represents data collected in the prethrombolytic era in which definitions and populations differ considerably. The purpose of a study by Barbagelata and colleagues[102] in Durham, North Carolina, was to evaluate the incidence and importance of recurrent ischemia after administration of thrombolytic therapy. The investigators studied patients enrolled in the TIMI studies. Patients were enrolled in 3 studies with similar entry criteria; 552 patients were treated with t-PA, 293 were treated with urokinase, and 385 received both thrombolytic agents. Recurrent ischemia was defined as symptoms in association with electrocardiographic changes; reinfarction was defined as a reevaluation of creatinine kinase–MB isoenzyme in an appropriate clinical setting. Both recurrent ischemia and infarction occurred in 42 patients (3%), recurrent ischemia alone occurred in 226 (18%), and neither occurred in 964 (78%). Although baseline characteristics were similar among the 3 groups, in-hospital cardiac events (73 deaths and 253 CHF episodes) were not: in-hospital mortality in patients with reinfarction was 21%; with recurrent ischemia, 11%; and with neither event, 4%. The in-hospital CHF rate of patients with reinfarction was 50%; with recurrent ischemia alone, 31%; and with neither event, 17%. As expected, median in-hospital costs were highest in patients with reinfarction ($26 802), intermediate for those with recurrent ischemia alone ($18 422), and lowest in patients with neither event ($15 623). Recurrent myocardial ischemia after thrombolytic therapy is a frequent, important, and expensive adverse clinical outcome, making it a critical target for therapeutic intervention.

Early and Late Mortality

Lee and colleagues[103] representing the GUSTO-I trial used data from the 41 021 patients enrolled in GUSTO-I, a randomized trial of four thrombolytic strategies, to obtain a comprehensive analysis of relations between baseline clinical data and 30-day mortality and developed a multivariable statistical model for risk assessment in candidates for thrombolytic therapy. The relation between clinical descriptors collected at initial presentation and death within 30 days, which occurred in 7% of the population, was examined with both univariable and multivariable analyses. Variables studied included demographics, history and risk factors, presenting characteristics, and treatment assignment. Risk modeling was performed with logistic multiple regression and validated with bootstrapping techniques. Multivariable analysis identified age as the most significant factor influencing 30-day mortality with a rate of 1% in the youngest decile (<45 years) and 21% in patients >75 years of age. Other variables associated with increased mortality included lower systolic BP, higher Killip class, and an anterior wall AMI. These 5 characteristics contained 90% of the prognostic information in the baseline clinical data. Other significant though less important factors included previous AMI, height, time to treatment, diabetes, weight, smoking status, type of thrombolytic agent used, previous CABG, hypertension, and previous cerebrovascular disease. Clinical determinants of mortality in patients treated with thrombolytic therapy within 6 hours of symptom onset are multifactorial and the relations are complex. It is necessary to consider multiple characteristics, including age, medical history, physiological significance of the AMI, and medical treatment to predict prognosis for individual patients.

Simes and colleagues[104] in Sydney, Australia; Rochester, Minnesota; Auckland, New Zealand; Berlin, Germany; Rotterdam, the Netherlands; Atlanta, Georgia; Barcelona, Spain; Durham, North Carolina; Cleveland, Ohio; and Washington, DC, tested what thrombolytic strategies achieve more complete, early, sustained coronary artery patency and whether this correlates with further reductions in mortality in patients with AMI. The GUSTO-I trial was used to make these determinations. An angiographic substudy within GUSTO-I provided a unique opportunity to examine the relation between mortality and degree of coronary artery patency among the various regimens. Four thrombolytic strategies were compared in 41 021 patients in GUSTO-I. Streptokinase with subcutaneous or intravenous heparin, accelerated t-PA with intravenous heparin, and combined streptokinase plus t-PA with intravenous heparin were used. Accelerated t-PA was associated with a lower 30-day mortality (6%) than the other strategies (7%, 7%, and 7%, respectively). Among the 1210 patients in the angiographic substudy randomly assigned to angiography 90 minutes after starting treatment, there was improved patency as evidenced by the TIMI grade 3 flow with accelerated t-PA having more patients with TIMI grade 3 flow than the other regimens (Table 3-16). To evaluate whether differences in mortality among the four strategies matched differences in 90-minute patency, a model was developed for predicting mortality differences in the main trial from the angiographic substudy. The model assumed that differences in treatment effects on 30-day mortality were mediated through differences in 90-minute patency for the four treatments. The predicted rates were compared with observed mortality rates in the remaining patients in the main trial for each treatment group. The predicted and observed 30-day mortality rates for the four treatments were streptokinase with subcutaneous heparin, 7% compared with 7%; streptokinase with intravenous heparin, 7% vs. 7%; accelerated t-PA 6% vs. 6%; and streptokinase plus t-PA, 7% vs. 7%. The correlation between predicted and observed results was 0.97. Thus, the close relation between the predicted and observed 30-day mortality rates supports the hypothesis that an important mechanism for improved survival with thrombolytic therapy is achievement of early and relatively normal perfusion. These data provide a biological explanation for the mortality differences seen in the GUSTO-I trial.

Aguirre and colleagues[105] for the TIMI II study group evaluated clinical outcomes and potential indications for routine postmyocardial infarction cardiac catheterization and revascularization of patients who have a non–Q-wave vs. Q-wave infarct after thrombolytic therapy. A secondary analysis of 2634 patients enrolled in the TIMI II trial with a first AMI was performed to determine 6-week and 1-year cardiac event rates and identify clinical and angiographic differences between the 1867 patients (71%) who developed a Q-wave AMI and the 767 patients (29%) who sustained a non–Q-wave AMI after intravenous thrombolytic therapy. Male sex and anterior wall AMIs were more frequent in the Q-wave vs. the non–Q-wave groups. During rt-PA infusion, a greater percentage of non–Q-wave AMI patients had normalization of initial ST segment elevation. Infarct-related artery patency as judged by TIMI flow grade 2 or 3, complete infarct-related artery reperfusion, and the percentage of patients with a predischarge resting LVEF >55% were greater in the non–Q-wave group. New CHF during hospitalization developed more frequently in Q-wave patients. After 42 days, the occurrence of reinfarction, death, and combined death or reinfarction were similar in patients assigned to the invasive or conservative postthrombolytic management strategy, regardless of infarct type. One-year mortality was 3% vs. 3% for non–Q-wave and 4% for Q-wave infarcts. Thus, angiographic and clinical differences were observed between patients who present with initial ST segment elevation and develop early non–Q-wave vs. Q-wave AMIs after treatment with t-PA, heparin, and aspirin. Early mortality and adverse clinical events in these patients were not different after a conserva-

Table 3-16 Coronary Artery Patency at 90 Minutes by Thrombolytic Therapy and 30-Day Mortality*

TIMI Grade	Total	SK-SQ n = 296	SK-IV n = 286	TPA n = 292	TPA + SK n = 302	30-Day Mortality, %
0	285	97 (33)	83 (29)	41 (14)	64 (21)	8.4
1	98	38 (13)	29 (10)	14 (5)	17 (6)	9.2
2	341	75 (25)	80 (28)	79 (27)	107 (35)	7.9
3	452	86 (29)	94 (33)	158 (54)	114 (38)	4.0
Unknown	34	7	6	11	10	18.2
Total	1210	303	292	303	312	

TIMI indicates Thrombolysis in Myocardial Infarction; SK-SQ, streptokinase with subcutaneous heparin; SK-IV, streptokinase with intravenous heparin; TPA, accelerated tissue-type plasminogen activator with IV heparin; and TPA + SK, tissue-type plasminogen activator plus streptokinase with intravenous heparin. Values are numbers (percentages) of patients receiving each treatment at each TIMI grade who also had angiographic results.
*For the 1210 patients randomized to the 90-minute angiographic substudy. Results are of the first angiogram irrespective of time done. Those without any angiogram are given as unknown.
Reproduced with permission from Simes et al.[104]

tive compared with invasive treatment strategy, regardless of whether the infarct type is non–Q-wave or Q-wave.

Coronary Angioplasty

The PAMI trial randomized 395 patients presenting within 12 hours of the onset of acute transmural myocardial infarction to receive either t-PA or undergo primary PTCA. Stone and associates in this 12-center study examined the predictors of in-hospital and 6-month outcome after these 2 different reperfusion strategies.[106] Only advanced age and treatment by t-PA vs. PTCA correlated with increased in-hospital mortality. Reduction of in-hospital death or reinfarction with PTCA vs. t-PA was particularly marked in patients >65 years (8.6% vs. 20%). Management with primary PTCA vs. t-PA was the most powerful multivariate correlate of freedom from recurrent ischemic events (10.3% vs. 28%). The independent beneficial effect of angioplasty on freedom from death or reinfarction was maintained at the 6-month follow-up examination (8.2% vs. 17%). These authors concluded that primary PTCA is a preferred alternative for reperfusion following AMI.

Bauters and colleagues[107] in Lille Cedex, France, studied 300 consecutive patients who after thrombolysis for AMI underwent delayed PTCA of the infarct-related lesion at an average of 11 days after their infarct. Procedural success was obtained in 253 patients (84%) and angiographic follow-up was performed in 205 of this group (81%) at a mean of 7 months. Restenosis defined as >50% stenosis was present in 105 patients (51%). Only 34 of the 105 patients with angiographic restenosis were symptomatic; the others had clinically silent restenosis. Among these 105 patients, 27 had reocclusion at the dilated site at follow-up. The severity of the stenosis at follow-up and the late loss in minimal lumen diameter followed a nearly Gaussian distribution if the lesions that were totally occluded at follow-up were excluded. By multivariate analysis, two independent predictors of reocclusion were identified: a small reference diameter and the presence of collateral vessels before the procedure. Only one factor was associated with restenosis in 178 patients who did not have reocclusion at follow-up: a TIMI flow grade ≤2 before the procedure. There was a significantly higher LVEF in patients without restenosis (56%) and in patients without total occlusion than in patients with reocclusion (46%). Thus, despite a satisfactory clinical outcome, delayed PTCA of an infarct-related lesion is associated with a high rate of angiographic recurrence.

Harrington et al[108] in a multicenter trial examined the results of the CAVEAT trial to determine the characteristics and consequences of creatine kinase and creatine kinase–MB myocardial isoenzyme fraction elevations after percutaneous coronary intervention. Patients with new native lesions undergoing coronary intervention at 35 clinical sites were randomly assigned to undergo PTCA (n = 500) or directional coronary atherectomy (n = 512). Cardiac enzyme levels were measured 12 and 24 hours after the interventional procedure and when clinically indicated for recurrent myocardial ischemia. There were 78 AMIs in the atherectomy group and 34 in the PTCA group. Hospital length of stay was increased among patients with an infarction. Postprocedural myocardial infarction was highly predictive of mortality, CABG or repeat intervention within 30 days. These authors concluded that AMI occurred commonly after coronary intervention in CAVEAT and was associated with a worse clinical outcome. Although the incidence of AMI was higher with atherectomy than with PTCA, the baseline characteristics and consequences of the infarctions were similar between the treatments with regard to 30-day outcome. Myocardial enzyme elevations after an otherwise successful interventional procedure may identify a population at risk for a future cardiac event.

Morishima and associates[109] from Ogaki, Japan, evaluated the clinical significance of the angiographic no-reflow phenomenon in 93 patients with AMI treated by PTCA. On the basis of the post-PTCA angiograms, patients were divided into 3 groups: normal angiogram (group 1, n = 65), slight no-reflow (group 2, n = 13), and severe no-reflow (group 3, n = 15). Regional wall motion in the chronic phase was depressed in groups 2 and 3 compared with group 1. The proportion of the area of the transmural infarction to that of the total infarction determined by scintigraphy was higher in groups 2 and 3 than in group 1. A significantly higher incidence of myocardial rupture and of death resulting from cardiac causes was observed in group 3 compared with group 1. The severity of this phenomenon immediately after an emergency PTCA correlated well with the severity of myocardial damage, with patients having severe no-reflow showing the poorest prognosis.

Predictions of increased risk or recurrent cardiac events and death after AMI include ischemia, anterior location of the infarct, and non–Q-wave vs. Q-wave AMI. Although PTCA is performed in patients with ischemia after AMI to alleviate apparent symptoms, the outcome, according to location and type of AMI and their effect on the prevention of subsequent infarction and death is not known. To determine if location and type of AMI provide prognostic information in patients with postinfarction ischemia, Welty and coinvestigators[110] in Boston, Massachusetts, analyzed morbidity and mortality during and after PTCA according to the location (anterior vs. inferior) and type (Q-wave vs. non–Q-wave) AMI in 505 consecutive patients. The incidence of recurrent angina, repeat PTCA, CABG, reinfarction, and death during long-term follow-up after hospital discharge with 440 patients with an initial successful angioplasty was also compared. During the procedure there was no difference in the primary success rate or mortality of the different groups; however, more patients with anterior non–Q-wave AMI underwent emergent CABG after successful PTCA. Multivariate Cox proportional hazards analyses controlling for age, gender, number of narrowed coronary arteries, location, type of AMI, and year of angioplasty, revealed that more patients with anterior wall AMI had more than one cardiac event (repeat PTCA, CABG, reinfarction, or death) than did those with inferior wall AMI. The rate of reinfarction or death was 1.9 times higher in patients with anterior than inferior AMI. There was no difference in these cardiac events for Q-wave vs. non–Q-wave AMI. These results suggest that anterior location, but not type of AMI was associated with the greater likelihood of a cardiac event at follow-up.

Rescue PTCA has been advocated as a mechanical method to achieve reperfusion in instances where a myocardial infarct–affected artery remains occluded after thrombolytic therapy. Most prior reports of rescue PTCA have been observational, and analyses of value have been inconclusive. To evaluate the benefit of rescue PTCA, McKendall and coinvestigators[111] in Providence, Rhode Island, studied 133 patients enrolled in the thrombolysis and myocardial infarction phase I open label and phase II trials who had an occluded infarct-related artery after thrombolytic therapy. According to protocol, 100 consecutive patients had no rescue PTCA performed (no-rescue group) and 33 consecutive patients underwent protocol-directed rescue PTCA (rescue group). The 2 cohorts were compared for clinical and angiographic outcome. Baseline characteristics of the two groups were similar. Rescue PTCA was attempted in each rescue group patient and was successful in 82%. In 21 days, the mortality rate was 12% in the rescue group and 7% in the no-rescue group. Failed rescue PTCA was associated with a mortality of 33%. Reinfarction occurred in 6% of patients in the rescue group and 5% of those in the no-rescue group. At 21 days, a mean LVEF was 51% in the rescue group and 41% in the no-rescue group. Investigators concluded that the routine use of rescue PTCA does not appear to offer significant benefit beyond that of contemporary medical therapy after thrombolytic failure.

Coronary Bypass

The TIMI II trial evaluated different therapeutic approaches, including coronary revascularization by CABG or PTCA for appropriate clinical indications. Gersh and associates[112] in this multicenter trial examined the results of CABG after thrombolytic therapy. Of 3339 patients enrolled in the TIMI II trial, CABG was performed on 390 patients (11.7%). Fifty-four (14%) were within 24 hours after entry into the trial or within 24 hours of PTCA and 336 (86%) between 24 hours and 42 days after entry. Perioperative mortality rates were, respectively, 16.7% and 3.9%, and perioperative myocardial infarction rates were 5.6% and 6.2%. On multivariate analysis, the only independent predictor of perioperative mortality was CABG within 24 hours after entry or after PTCA. These authors concluded that the increased mortality rate with CABG after thrombolytic therapy, particularly in patients undergoing the operation within 24 hours of PTCA or during the evolving phase of infarction, must be balanced against the excellent 1-year prognosis.

Creswell and associates[113] from St. Louis, Missouri, examined retrospectively 3942 patients who underwent CABG between 1986 and 1993 and found that 2296 patients had CABG after AMI. The interval between onset and AMI and the CABG varied from <6 hours in 11 patients to >6 weeks in 1023 patients. Of the total 3942 patients, 1646 at no time had an AMI. The operative mortality associated with increasing time intervals between AMI and CABG were 9.1%, 8.3%, 5.2%, 6.5%, and 2.9% for <6 hours, 6 hours to 2 days, 2–14 days, 2–6 weeks, and more than 6 weeks, respectively. For patients undergoing CABG within 14 days of AMI, the operative mortality was 5.3% for those receiving an intra-aortic balloon pump preoperatively for postinfarction angina, but 11.8% for those who underwent urgent/emergent operation without intra-aortic balloon pump support. Elective CABG can be accomplished with acceptable morbidity and mortality early after acute AMI if an elective operation is possible. In addition, the intra-aortic balloon pump should be used aggressively in patients with postinfarction angina to allow for elective rather than urgent/emergent surgery.

Rehabilitation

Despite the known benefits of cardiac rehabilitation, limited data are available on the outcome of this treatment in women, and this secondary prevention strategy may be underutilized. To assess the gender differences in baseline exercise capacity, indexes of obesity, lipid profiles, behavior characteristics, and components of quality of life, as well as the improvements in these components after a secondary prevention program, Lavie and Milani[114] in New Orleans, Louisiana, retrospectively reviewed data from 458 patients (83 women and 375 men) enrolled in a phase II cardiac rehabilitation and exercise program after a major cardiac event. At baseline (6 weeks after the cardiac event and before rehabilitation), exercise capacity and ratio of LDL to HDL cholesterol were lower, but total cholesterol, HDL cholesterol, LDL cholesterol, and percent body fat were higher in women than in men with CAD. In addition, with regard to quality of life, women had lower scores for energy, function, and total quality of life than men. After cardiac rehabilitation and exercise training, women had significant improvements in exercise capacity (+33%) and percent body fat (−7%), which compared favorably with the improvements seen in men, but improvements in BMI and lipids were not statistically significant. Although most behavioral traits and measures of quality of life significantly improved in women, depression, hostility, and measures of mental health were not significantly reduced. However, improvements in all these risk factors, behavioral traits, and components of quality of life were statistically similar in men and women. Because women have a lower exercise capacity, energy, function score, and total quality-of-life score at baseline, these improvements after cardiac rehabilitation may be of greater clinical benefit to women than to men. These data reaffirm that women should be routinely referred to and vigorously encouraged to participate in outpatient cardiac rehabilitation and exercise training after major cardiac events.

A rehabilitation program that relied totally upon the primary health care system was created by Bondestam and colleagues[115] in Göteborg, Sweden, for patients ≥65 years old with AMI. Patients from one primary health care district were assigned to a rehabilitation program (n = 91), whereas patients from a neighboring district constituted a control group (n = 99). The rehabilitation measures were initiated very early after the infarction with individual counseling in the home of the patient and later in the local health center, where 21% of the patients also joined a low-intensity exercise group. The control group was somewhat older and contained a greater number of women compared with the rehabilitation group, but size and course of infarction, complications, and previous morbidity were similar. To control for differences in age, a matching procedure was performed and 71 pairs of the same sex and age were found. During the first 3 months there was a significantly lower incidence of rehospitalization in the intervention group, regarding both percentage of patients and days of rehospitalization. Visits to the emergency department without rehospitalization were also significantly lower in the intervention group. After 12 months the differences still remained, with the exception of days of rehospitalization. In the matched groups the same result was seen. While readmissions and emergency department visits generally were well justified in the intervention group, vague symptoms dominated among the control group. The factor that was most strongly related to readmissions in the intervention group was previous AMI, while in the control group no special factor

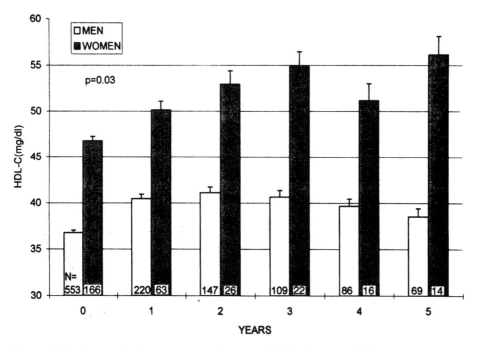

Figure 3-29. Bar graph showing yearly changes in HDL cholesterol (HDL-C) for men and women over 5 years. Values are mean ± SEM. Reproduced with permission from Warner et al.[117]

influencing readmissions could be found. Thus, an uncomplicated rehabilitation model characterized by very early intervention and performed within the primary health care system can significantly reduce the consumption of health care 1 year after AMI in patients ≥65 years old.

CAD is the leading cause of death among black women in the USA. Black women also demonstrate a greater prevalence of coronary risk factors and a higher mortality after AMI than white women. To evaluate the clinical profile and outcome of black women in an urban-based cardiac rehabilitation program, Cannistra and coworkers[116] in Boston, Massachusetts, studied prospectively 35 black women (mean age, 54 years) and 47 white women (mean age, 57 years). Black women had similar admitting diagnoses as white women, with recent AMI being the most common (37%). Coronary risk factors were more prevalent in black women than white women in the program: hypertension (71% vs. 53%), diabetes mellitus (46% vs. 26%), and obesity (74% vs. 49%). Cholesterol and HDL lipoprotein levels were similarly elevated in black (251 mg/dL) and in white (248 mg/dL) women, whereas 34% of black and 21% of white women were active smokers. There was no significant difference in initial exercise capacity at program entry. Fewer black women (51%) completed the 12-week program than white women (64%). Comparison of initial and follow-up exercise tests after 12 weeks of moderate to high-intensity dynamic exercise demonstrated significant and similar improvements in functional capacity in both black and white women. Among obese patients, only the white women lost weight. The cholesterol profile did not change in either group, and most of the smokers (74%) did not complete the pro-

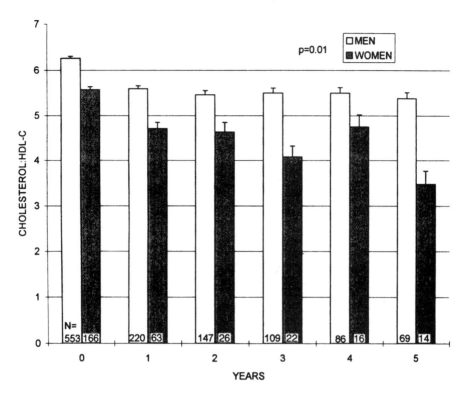

Figure 3-30. Bar graph showing yearly changes in ratio of total cholesterol to HDL cholesterol (HDL-C) for men and women over 5 years. Values are mean ± SEM. Reproduced with permission from Warner et al.[117]

gram. In conclusion, black women in this program demonstrated a high coronary risk profile and low initial functional capacity, which improved after exercise training.

Warner and colleagues[117] in Winston-Salem, North Carolina, determined whether the benefits of a cardiac rehabilitation program were similar in men and women as regards changes in HDL cholesterol. They compared changes in HDL cholesterol and other lipids in 553 men and 166 women participating in a cardiac rehabilitation program for up to 5 years. Patients exercised 3 days a week at 70% to 85% of their maximum heart rate predetermined by symptom-limited treadmill test. Aerobic capacity was estimated in metabolic equivalents and percent body fat was determined by skin-fold measurements. Baseline HDL cholesterol, LDL cholesterol, and total cholesterol were higher in women, whereas a ratio of total cholesterol to HDL cholesterol was lower than in men. Both men and women showed an increase in HDL cholesterol after 1 year, but only the women's level continued to increase over 5 years (Figure 3-29). Sex difference in change for HDL cholesterol remained after adjustment for age and smoking. A nonsignificant trend toward a greater change in HDL cholesterol in women existed after adjustment for baseline percent body fat and estimated metabolic equivalents expended in exercise. Change in the ratio of total cholesterol to HDL cholesterol was also more favorable in women (Figure 3-30). Total cholesterol decreased by 20% in women and 8% in men, whereas LDL cholesterol decreased by 34% in women and 15% in men. There was no sex difference in changes in triglycerides. Thus, women with heart disease who participate in a cardiac rehabilitation program achieve greater lipid benefits over longer periods of time than previously shown to be true for men.

1. Giles WH, Anda RF, Casper ML, Escobedo LG, Taylor HA: Race and sex differences in rates of invasive cardiac procedures in US hospitals. Arch Inter Med 1995 (February 13);155:318–324.
2. Behar S, Hod H, Benari B, Narinsky R, Pauzner H, Rechavia E, Faibel HE, Kat AM, Roth A, Goldhammer E, Freedberg NA, Rougin N, Kracoff O, Shapira C, Jafari J, Lotan C, Daka F, Gottlieb S, Weiss T, Kanetti M, Klutstein M, Rudnik L, Barasch E, Mahul N, Blondheim D, Gelvan A, Barbash G, Israeli Thrombolytic Survey Group: On-site catheterization laboratory and prognosis after acute myocardial infarction. Arch Intern Med 1995 (April 24);155:813–817.
3. Guadagnoli E, Hauptman PJ, Ayanian JZ, Pashos CL, McNeil BJ, Clearly PD: Variation in the use of cardiac procedures after acute myocardial infarction. N Engl J Med 1995 (August 31);333:573–578.
4. Spertus JA, Weiss NS, Every NR, Weaver WD, for the Myocardial Infarction Triage and Intervention Project Investigators: The influence of clinical risk factors on the use of angiography and revascularization after acute myocardial infarction. Arch Intern Med 1995(November 27);155:2309–2316.
5. Paul SD, Eagle KA, Guidry U, DiSalvo TG, Villarreal-Levy G, Smith AJC, O'Donnell CJ, Mahjoub ZA, Muluk V, Newell JB, O'Gara PT: Do gender-based differences in presentation and management influence predictors of hospitalization cost and length of stay after acute myocardial infarction? Am J Cardiol 1995 (December 1);76:1122–1125.
6. O'Connor NJ, Manson JE, O'Connor GT, Buring JE: Psychosocial risk factors and nonfatal myocardial infarction. Circulation 1995 (September);92:1458–1464.
7. Mittleman MA, Maclure M, Sherwood JB, Mulry RP, Tofler GH, Jacobs SC, Friedman R, Benson H, Muller JE, for the Determinants of Myocardial Infarction Onset Study Investigators: Triggering of acute myocardial infarction onset by episodes of anger. Circulation 1995 (October);92:1720–1725.
8. Parish S, Collins R, Peto R, Youngman L, Barton J, Jayne K, Clarke R, Appleby P, Lyon V, Cederholm-Williams S, Marshall J, Sleight P, for the International Studies of Infarct Survival (ISIS) Collaborators: Cigarette smoking, tar yields, and non-fatal myocardial infarction: 14,000 cases and 32,000 controls in the United Kingdom. Br Med J 1995 (August 1);311:471–477.
9. Schnohr P, Lange P, Nyboe J, Appleyard M, Jensen G: Gray hair, baldness, and wrinkles in relation to myocardial infarction: The Copenhagen City Heart Study. Am Heart J 1995 (November);130:1003–1010.
10. Col NF, Yarzebski J, Gore JM, Alpert JS, Goldberg RJ: Does aspirin consumption affect the presentation or severity of acute myocardial infarction? Arch Intern Med 1995 (July 10);155:1386–1389.
11. Muscari A, Bozzoli C, Puddu GM, Sangiorgi Z, Dormi A, Rovinetti C, Descovich GC, Puddu P: Association of serum C3 levels with the risk of myocardial infarction. Am J Med 1995 (April);98:357–364.
12. Ellerbeck EF, Jencks SF, Radford MJ Kresowik TF, Craig AS, Gold JA, Krumholz HM, Vogel RA: Quality of care for Medicare patients with acute myocardial infarction. JAMA 1995 (May 17);273:19:1509–1514.
13. Sigurdsson E, Thorgeirsson G, Sigvaldason H, Sigfusso N: Unrecognized myocardial infarction: Epidemiology, clinical characteristics, and the prognosis role of angina pectoris. Ann Intern Med 1995 (January);122:96–102.
14. Behar S, Goldbourt U, Barbash G, Modan B: Twenty-five year mortality rate decrease in patients in Israel with a first episode of acute myocardial infarction. Am Heart J 1995 (September);130:453–458.
15. Hollander JE, Hoffman RS, Burstein JL, Shih RD, Thode HC Jr, the Cocaine-Associated Myocardial Infarction Study Group: Cocaine-associated myocardial infarction. Arch Intern Med 1995 (May 22);155:1081–1086.

16. Thomson SP, Gibbons RJ, Smars PA, Suman VJ, Pierre RV, Santrach PJ, Jiang NS: Incremental value of the leukocyte differential and the rapid creatine kinase—MB isoenzyme for the early diagnosis of myocardial infarction. Ann Intern Med 1995 (March 1);122:335–341.

17. Dorogy ME, Hooks GS, Cameron RW, Davis RC: Clinical and angiographic correlates of normal creatine kinase with increased MB isoenzymes in possible acute myocardial infarction. Am Heart J 1995 (August);130:211–217.

18. Müller-Bardorff M, Freitag H, Scheffold T, Remppis A, Kübler W, Katus HA: Development and characterization of a rapid assay for bedside determinations of cardiac troponin T. Circulation 1995 (November);92:2869–2875.

19. de Winter RJ, Koster RW, Sturk A, Sanders GT: Value of myoglobin, troponin T, and CK-MB$_{mass}$ in ruling out an acute myocardial infarction in the emergency room. Circulation 1995 (December);92:3401–3407.

20. Res JCJ, Kamp O, Delemarre BJ, Visser CA: Usefulness of combined two dimensional echocardiography and transesophageal atrial stimulation early after acute myocardial infarction. Am J Cardiol 1995 (December 1);76:1112–1114.

21. Vanoli E, Adamson PB, Lin B, Pinna GD, Lazzara R, Orr WC: Heart rate variability during specific sleep stages: A comparison of healthy subjects with patients after myocardial infarction. Circulation 1995 (April);91:1918–1922.

22. Cannon CP, Thompson B, McCabe CH, Mueller HS, Kirshenbaum JM, Herson S, Nasmith JB, Chaitman BR, Braunwald E, for the TIMI III Investigators: Predictors of non-Q-wave acute myocardial infarction in patients with acute ischemic syndromes: An analysis from the Thrombolysis in Myocardial Ischemia (TIMI) III trials. Am J Cardiol (May 15);75:977–981.

23. Burnett RE, Blumenthal JA, Mark DB, Leimberger JD, Califf RM: Distinguishing between early and late responders to symptoms of acute myocardial infarction. Am J Cardiol (May 15);75:1019–1022.

24. Pasceri V, Cianflone D, Finocchiaro ML, Crea F, Maseri A: Relation between myocardial infarction site and pain location in Q-wave acute myocardial infarction. Am J Cardiol 1995 (February 1);75:224–227.

25. Hasche ET, Fernandes C, Freedman SB, Jeremy RW: Relation between ischemia time, infarct size, and left ventricular function in humans. Circulation 1995 (August);92:710–719.

26. Flack JM, Neaton J, Grimm R Jr., Shih J, Cutler J, Ensrud K, MacMahon S, for the Multiple Risk Factor Intervention Trial Research Group: Blood pressure and mortality among men with prior myocardial infarction. Circulation 1995 (November);92:2437–2445.

27. Nakagawa Y, Ito H, Kitakaze M, Kusuoka H, Hori M, Kuzuya T, Higashino Y, Fujii K, Minamino T: Effect of angina pectoris on myocardial protection in patients with reperfused anterior wall myocardial infarction: Retrospective clinical evidence of "preconditioning." J Am Coll Cardiol 1995 (April);25:1076–1083.

28. Zimmerman FH, Cameron A, Fisher LD, Ng G: Myocardial infarction in young adults: Angiographic characterization, risk factors and prognosis (Coronary Artery Surgery Study registry). J Am Coll Cardiol 1995 (September);26:654–661.

29. Mickley H, Nielsen JR, Berning J, Junker A, Moller M: Characteristics and prognostic importance of ST segment elevation on Holter monitoring early after acute myocardial infarction. Am J Cardiol 1995 (September 15);76:537–542.

30. Villella A, Maggioni AP, Villella M, Giordano A, Turazza FM, Santoro E, Franzosi MG, on behalf of the GISSI-2 Investigators: Prognostic significance of maximal exercise testing after myocardial infarction treated with thrombolytic agents: The GISSI-2 database. Lancet 1995 (August 26);346:523–529.

31. Chung MK, Bosner MS, McKenzie JP, Shen J, Rich MW: Prognosis of patients ≥70 years of age with non-Q-wave acute myocardial infarction compared with younger patients with similar infarcts and with patients ≥ 70 years of age with Q-wave acute myocardial infarction. Am J Cardiol 1995 (January 1);75:18–22.

32. Devlin W, Cragg D, Jacks M, Friedman H, O'Neill W, Grines C: Comparison of outcome in patients with acute myocardial infarction aged >75 years with that in younger patients. Am J Cardiol 1995 (March 15);75:573–576.

33. Bueno H, Vidán T, Almazán A, López-Sendón JL, Delcán JL: Influence of sex on the short-term outcome of elderly patients with a first acute myocardial infarction. Circulation 1995 (September);92:1133–1140.

34. Frasure-Smith N, Lespérance F, Talajic M: Depression and 18-month prognosis after myocardial infarction. Circulation 1995 (February);91:999–1005.

35. Omland T, Bonarjee VVS, Lie RT, Caidahl K: Neurohumoral measurements as indicators of long-term prognosis after acute myocardial infarction. Am J Cardiol 1995 (August 1);76:230–235.

36. Miller TD, Christian TF, Hopfenspirger MR, Hodge DO, Gersh BJ, Gibbons RJ: Infarct size after acute myocardial infarction measured by quantitative tomographic ^{99m}Tc sestamibi imaging predicts subsequent mortality. Circulation 1995 (August);92:334–341.

37. Mercando AD, Aronow WS, Epstein S, Fishbach S, Fishbach M: Signal-averaged electrocardiography and ventricular tachycardia as predictors of mortality after acute myocardial infarction in elderly patients. Am J Cardiol 1995 (September 1);76:436–440.

38. Nešković AN, Popovic AD, Babic R, Marinkovic J, Obradovic V: Positive high-dose dipyridamole echocardiography test after acute myocardial infarction is an excellent predictor of cardiac events. Am Heart J 1995 (January);129:31–39.

39. Picano E, Pingitore A, Sicari R, Minardi G, Gandolfo N, Seveso G, Chiarella F, Bolognese L, Chiaranda G, Sclavo MG, Previtali M, Margaria F, Magaia O, Bianchi Pirelli S, Severi S, Raciti M, Landi P, Vassalle C, Bento de Sousa MJ, Felipe L, Duarte M: Stress echocardiographic results predict risk of reinfarction early after uncomplicated acute myocardial infarction: Large-scale multicenter study. J Am Coll Cardiol 1995 (October);26:908–913.

40. Vanhees L, Fagard R, Thijs L, Amery A: Prognostic value of training-induced change in peak exercise capacity in patients with myocardial infarcts and patients with coronary artery bypass surgery. Am J Cardiol 1995 (November 15);76:1014–1019.

41. Tabata H, Mizuno K, Arakawa K, Satomura K, Shibuya T, Kurita A, Nakamura H: Angioscopic identification of coronary thrombus in patients with postinfarction angina. J Am Coll Cardiol 1995 (May);25:1282–1285.

42. Cohen A, Guyon P, Chauvel C, Abergel E, Costagliola D, Raffoul H, Valty J, Diebold B: Relations between Doppler tracings of pulmonary regurgitation and invasive hemodynamics in acute right ventricular infarction complicating inferior wall left ventricular infarction. Am J Cardiol 1995 (March 1);75:425–430.

43. Lystash JC, Gibson RS, Watson DD, Beller GA: Early versus late congestive heart failure after initially uncomplicated anterior wall acute myocardial infarction. Am J Cardiol 1995 (April 1);75:653–658.

44. Eltchaninoff H, Simpfendorfer C, Franco I, Raymond RE, Casale PN, Whitlow PL: Early and 1-year survival rates in acute myocardial infarction complicated by cardiogenic shock: A retrospective study comparing coronary angioplasty with medical treatment. Am Heart J 1995 (September);130:459–464.

45. Holmes DR, Bates ER, Kleiman NS, Sadowski Z, Horgan JHS, Morris DC, Califf RM, Berger PB, Topol EJ: Contemporary reperfusion therapy for cardiogenic shock: The GUSTO-I trial experience. J Am Coll Cardiol 1995 (September);26:668–674.

46. Cheriex EC, de Swart H, Dijkman LW, Havenith MG, Maessen JG, Engelen DJM, Wellens HJJ: Myocardial rupture after myocardial infarction is related to the perfusion status of the infarct-related coronary artery. Am Heart J 1995 (April);129:644–650.

47. Becker RC, Charlesworth A, Wilcox RG, Hampton J, Skene A, Gore JM, Topol EJ: Cardiac rupture associated with thrombolytic therapy: Impact of time to treatment in the last assessment of thrombolytic efficacy (LATE) study. J Am Coll Cardiol 1995 (April);25:1063–1068.

48. Figueras J, Curos A, Cortadellas J, Sans M, Soler-Soler J: Relevance of electrocardiographic findings, heart failure, and infarct site in assessing risk and timing of left ventricular free wall rupture during acute myocardial infarction. Am J Cardiol 1995 (September 15);76:543–547.

49. Pilote L, Califf RM, Sapp SH, Miller DP, Mark DB, Weaver WD, Gore JM, Armstrong PW, Ohman EM, Topol EJ: Regional variation across the United States in the

management of acute myocardial infarction. N Engl J Med 1995 (August 31);333:565–572.

50. Fitch LL, Buchwald H, Matts JP, Johnson JW, Campos CT, Long JM: Effect of aspirin use on death and recurrent myocardial infarction in current and former cigarette smokers. Am Heart J 1995 (April);129:656–662.

51. Krumholz HM, Radford MJ, Ellerbeck EF, Hennen J, Meehan TP, Petrillo M, Wang Y, Kresowik TF, Jencks SF: Aspirin in the treatment of acute myocardial infarction in elderly Medicare beneficiaries: Patterns of use and outcomes. Circulation 1995 (November);92:2841–2847.

52. Van Bergen PFMM, Jonker JJC, Van Hout BA, Van Domburg RT, Deckers JW, Azar AJ, Holman A: Costs and effects of long-term oral anticoagulant treatment after myocardial infarction. JAMA 1995 (March 22/29);273:12:925–928.

53. Viskin S, Kitzis I, Lev E, Zak Z, Heller K, Villa Y, Zajaria A, Laniado S, Belhassen B: Treatment with beta-adrenergic blocking agents after myocardial infarction: From randomized trials to clinical practice. J Am Coll Cardiol 1995 (May);25:1327–1332.

54. Brand DA, Newcomer LN, Freiburger A, Tian H: Cardiologists' practices compared with practice guidelines: Use of beta-blockade after acute myocardial infarction. J Am Coll Cardiol 1995 (November 15);26:1432–1436.

55. Smith J, Channer KS: Increasing prescription of drugs for secondary prevention after myocardial infarction. Br Med J 1995 (October 7);311:917–918.

56. Shechter M, Hod Hanoch, Chouraqui P, Kaplinsky E, Rabinowitz B: Magnesium therapy in acute myocardial infarction when patients are not candidates for thrombolytic therapy. Am J Cardiol 1995 (February 15);75:321–323.

57. Avanzini F, Latini R, Maggioni A, Colombo F, Santoro E, Franzosi MG, Tognoni G, and the GISSI Investigators: Antiarrhythmic drug prescription in patients after myocardial infarction in the last decade. Arch Intern Med 1955 (May 22);155:1041–1045.

58. Bertolet BD, McMurtrie EB, Hill JA, Belardinelli L: Theophylline for the treatment of atrioventricular block after myocardial infarction. Ann Intern Med 1995 (October 1);123:509–511.

59. Chinese Cardiac Study Collaborative Group: Oral captopril versus placebo among 13,634 patients with suspected acute myocardial infarction: Interim report from the Chinese Cardiac Study (CCS-1). Lancet 1995 (March 18);345:686–687.

60. Lamas GA, Flaker GC, Mitchell G, Smith SC Jr., Gersh BJ, Wun C-C, Moyé L, Rouleau JL, Rutherford JD, Pfeffer MA, Braunwald E, for the Survival and Ventricular Enlargement Investigators: Effect of infarct artery patency on prognosis after acute myocardial infarction. Circulation 1995 (September);92:1101–1109.

61. Hartley LH, Flaker G, Basta L, Menapace F, Goldman S, Davis B, Hamm P, Lamas G, Moye L, Wun C-C, Pfeffer M: Physical working capacity after acute myocardial infarction in patients with low ejection fraction and effect of captopril. Am J Cardiol 1995 (November 1);76:857–860.

62. ISIS-4(Fourth International Study of Infarct Survival) Collaborative Group: A randomised factorial trial assessing early oral captopril, oral mononitrate, and intravenous magnesium sulphate in 58,050 patients with suspected acute myocardial infarction. Lancet 1995 (March 18);345:669–685.

63. Carstensen S, Bonarjee VVS, Berning J, Edner M, Nilsen DWT, Caidahl K: Effects of early enalapril treatment on global and regional wall motion in acute myocardial infarction. Am Heart J 1995 (June);129:1101–1108.

64. Schulman SP, Weiss JL, Becker LC, Guerci AD, Shapiro EP, Charndra NC, Siu C, Flaherty JT, Coombs V, Taube JC, Bahr R, McVeigh ER, Weisman HF, Weisfeldt ML, Gerstenblith G: Effect of early enalapril therapy on left ventricular function and structure in acute myocardial infarction. Am J Cardiol 1995 (October 15); 76:764–770.

65. Køber L, Torp-Pedersen C, on behalf of the TRACE Study Group: Clinical characteristics and mortality of patients screened for entry into the Trandolapril Cardiac Evaluation (TRACE) Study. Am J Cardiol 1995 (July 1);76:1–5.

66. Køber L, Torp-Pedersen C, Carlsen JE, Bagger H, Eliasen P, Lyngborg K, Videbek J, Cole DS, Auclert L, Pauly NC, Aliot E, Persson S, Camm AJ, for the Trandolapril Cardiac Evaluation (TRACE) study group: A clinical trial of the angiotensin-con-

verting—enzyme inhibitor Trandolapril in patients with left ventricular dysfunction after myocardial infarction. N Engl J Med 1995 (December 21);333:1670–1676.

67. Ambrosioni E, Borghi C, Magnani B, and The Survival of Myocardial Infarction Long-Term Evaluation (SMILE) Study Investigators: The effect of the angiotensin-converting-enzyme inhibitor zofenopril on mortality and morbidity after anterior myocardial infarction. N Engl J Med 1995 (January 12);80–85.

68. Marlmberg K, Ryden L, Efendic S, Herlitz J, Nicol P, Waldenstrom A, Wedel H, Welin: Randomized trial of insulin-glucose infusion followed by subcutaneous insulin treatment in diabetic patients with acute myocardial infarction (DIGAMI Study): Effects on mortality at 1 year. J Am Coll Cardiol 1995 (July);26:57–65.

69. Iliceto S, Scrutinio D, Bruzzi P, D'Ambrosio G, Boni L, DiBiase M, Biasco G, Hugenholtz PG, Rizzon P: Effects of L-carnitine administration on left ventricular remodeling after acute anterior myocardial infarction: The L-carnitine ecocardiografia digitalizzata infarto miocardico (CEDIM) trial. J Am Coll Cardiol 1995 (August);26:380–387.

70. Buchwald H, Campos CT, Boen JR, Nguyen PA, Williams SE: Disease-free intervals after partial ileal bypass in patients with coronary heart disease and hypercholesterolemia: Report from the program on the surgical control of the hyperlipidemias (POSCH). J Am Coll Cardiol 1995 (August);26:351–357.

71. Rogers WJ: Contemporary management of acute myocardial infarction. Am J Med 1995 (August);99:195–206.

72. Van de Werf F, Topol EJ, Lee KL, Woodlief LH, Granger CB, Armstrong PW, Barbash GI, Hampton JR, Guerci A, Simes RJ, Ross AM, Califf RM, GUSTO Investigators: Variations in patient management and outcomes for acute myocardial infarction in the United States and other countries. JAMA 1995 (May 24/31);273:20:1586–1591.

73. Stone GW, Grines CL, Browne KF, Marco J, Rothbaum D, O'Keefe J, Hartzler GO, Overlie P, Donohue B, Chelliah N, Vliestra R, Puchrowicz-Ochocki S, O'Neill WW: Comparison of in-hospital outcome in men versus women treated by either thrombolytic therapy or primary coronary angioplasty for acute myocardial infarction. Am J Cardiol (May 15);75:987–992.

74. Vacek JL, Handlin LR, Rosamond TL, Beauchamp G: Gender-related differences in reperfusion treatment allocation and outcome for acute myocardial infarction. Am J Cardiol 1995 (August 1);76:226–229.

75. Karnash SL, Granger CB, White HD, Woodlief LH, Topol EJ, Califf RM: Treating menstruating women with thrombolytic therapy: Insights from the global utilization of streptokinase and tissue plasminogen activator for occluded coronary arteries (GUSTO-I) trial. J Am Coll Cardiol 1995 (December);26:1651–1656.

76. Grines CL, Topol EJ, O'Neill WW, George BS, Kereiakes D, Phillips HR, Leimberger JD, Woodlief LH, Califf RM: Effect of cigarette smoking on outcome after thrombolytic therapy for myocardial infarction. Circulation 1995 (January);91:298–303.

77. Barbash GI, Reiner J, White HD, Wilcox RG, Armstrong PW, Sadowski Z, Morris D, Aylward P, Woodlief LH, Topol EJ, Califf RM, Ross AM: Evaluation of paradoxic beneficial effects of smoking in patients receiving thrombolytic therapy for acute myocardial infarction: Mechanism of the "smoker's paradox" from the GUSTO-I trial, with angiography. J Am Coll Cardiol 1995 (November 1);26:1222–1229.

78. Kloner RA, Shook T, Przyklenk K, Davis VG, Junio L, Matthews RV, Burstein S, Gibson CM, Poole WK, Cannon CP, McCabe CH, Braunwald E, for the TIMI 4 Investigators: Previous angina alters in-hospital outcome in TIMI 4: A clinical correlate to preconditioning? Circulation 1995 (January);91:37–47.

79. Kurnik PB: Circadian variation in the efficacy of tissue-type plasminogen activator. Circulation 1995 (March);91:1341–1346.

80. Ottani F, Galvani M, Ferrini D, Sorbello F, Limonetti P, Pantoli D, Rusticali F: Prodromal angina limits infarct size: A role for ischemic preconditioning. Circulation 1995 (January);91:291–297.

81. Zaret BL, Wackers FJ, Terrin ML, Forman SA, Williams DO, Knatterud GL, Braunwald E: Value of radionuclide rest and exercise left ventricular ejection fraction in assessing survival of patients after thrombolytic therapy for acute myocardial infarction: Results of thrombolysis in myocardial infarction (TIMI) phase II study. J Am Coll Cardiol 1995 (July);26:73–79.

82. Lenderink T, Simoons ML, Van Es G-A, Van de Werf F, Verstraete M, Arnold AER, for the European Cooperative Study Group: Benefit of thrombolytic therapy is sustained throughout five years and is related to TIMI perfusion grade 3 but not grade 2 flow at discharge. Circulation 1995 (September);92:1110–1116.

83. Anderson HV, Cannon CP, Stone PH, Williams DO, McCabe CH, Knatterud GL, Thompson B, Willerson JT, Braunwald E: One-year results of the thrombolysis in myocardial infarction (TIMI) IIIB clinical trial. J Am Coll Cardiol 1995 (December);26:1643–1650.

84. Maynard C, Weaver WD, Lambreu C, Bowlby LJ, Rogers WJ, Rubison M for the participants in the National Registry of Myocardial Infarction: Factors influencing in the time to administration of thrombolytic therapy with recombinant tissue plasminogen activator (Data from the National Registry of Myocardial Infarction). Am J Cardiol 1995 (September 15);76:548–552.

85. Mark DB, Hlatky MA, Califf RM, Naylor CD, Lee KL, Armstrong PW, Barbash G, White H, Simoons ML, Nelson CL, Clapp-Channing N, Knight JD, Harrell FE Jr, Simes J, Topol EJ: Cost effectiveness of thrombolytic therapy with tissue plasminogen activator as compared with streptokinase for acute myocardial infarction. N Engl J Med 1995 (May 25);332:1418–1424.

86. Zahger D, Karagounis LA, Cercek B, Anderson JL, Sorensen S, Moreno F, Shah PK for the TEAM Investigators: Incomplete recanalization as an important determinant of thrombolysis in myocardial infarction (TIMI) Grade II flow after thrombolytic therapy for acute myocardial infarction. Am J Cardiol 1995 (October 15);76:749–752.

87. Ozbek C, Heisel A, Krause M, Berg G, Hammer B, Bay W, Sen S, Schieffer H: Comparison of mortality from acute myocardial infarction in patients receiving anistreplase with those not receiving thrombolysis. Am J Cardiol 1995 (December 1);76:1103–1107.

88. International Joint Efficacy Comparison of Thrombolytics: Randomized, double-blind comparison of reteplase double-bolus administration with streptokinase in acute myocardial infarction (INJECT) trial to investigate equivalence. Lancet 1995 (August 5);346:329–336.

89. Smalling RW, Bode C, Kalbfleisch J, Sen S, Limbourg P, Forycki F, Habib G, Feldman R, Hohnloser S, Seals A, and the RAPID Investigators: More rapid, complete, and stable coronary thrombolysis with bolus administration of reteplase compared with alteplase infusion in acute myocardial infarction. Circulation 1995 (June);91:2725–2732.

90. Théroux P, Pérez-Villa F, Waters D, Lespérance J, Shabani F, Bonan R: Randomized double-blind comparison of two doses of hirulog with heparin as adjunctive therapy to streptokinase to promote early patency of the infarct-related artery in acute myocardial infarction. Circulation 1995 (April);91:2132–2139.

91. Vanderschueren S, Barrios L, Kerdsinchai P, Van den Heuvel P, Hermans L, Vrolix M, De Man F, Benit E, Muyldermans L, Collen D, Van de Werf F, for the STAR Trial Group: A randomized trial of recombinant staphylokinase versus alteplase for coronary artery patency in acute myocardial infarction. Circulation 1995 (October);92:2044–2049.

92. Tebbe U, Windeler J, Boesl I, Hoffmann H, Wojcik J, Ashmawy M, Schwarz ER, von Loewis of Menar P, Rosemyeer P, Hopkins G, Barth H: Thrombolysis with recombinant unglycosylated single-chain urokinase-type plasminogen activator (saruplase) in acute myocardial infarction: Influence of heparin on early patency rate (LIMITS study). J Am Coll Cardiol 1995 (August);26:365–373.

93. Lincoff AM, Topol EJ, Califf RM, Sigmon KN, Lee KL, Ohman EM, Rosenschein U, Ellis SG, for the Thrombolysis and Angioplasty in Myocardial Infarction Study Group: Significance of a coronary artery with Thrombolysis in Myocardial Infarction grade 2 flow "patency" (outcome in the Thrombolysis and Angioplasty in Myocardial Infarction trials). Am J Cardiol (May 1);75:871–876.

94. Romeo F, Rosano GMC, Martuscelli E, De Luca F, Bianco C, Colistra C, Comito M, Cardona N, Miceli F, Rosano V, Mehta JL: Concurrent nitroglycerin administration reduces the efficacy of recombinant tissue-type plasminogen activator in patients with acute anterior wall myocardial infarction. Am Heart J 1995 (October);130:692–697.

95. Yokoshiki H, Kohya T, Tateda K, Shishido T, Hirasawa K, Kitabatake A: Abrupt augmentation of ST segment elevation associated with successful reperfusion: A sign of diminished myocardial salvage. Am Heart J 1995 (October);130:698–704.

96. Schroder R, Wegscheider K, Schroder K, Dissmann R, Meyer-Sabellek W: Extent of early ST segment elevation resolution: A strong predictor of outcome in patients with acute myocardial infarction and a sensitive measure to compare thrombolytic regimens. J Am Coll Cardiol 1995 (December);26:1657–1664.

97. Laperche T, Steg PG, Dehoux M, Benessiano J, Grollier G, Aliot E, Mossard J-M, Aubry P, Coisne D, Hanssen M, Iliou M-C, for the PERM Study Group: A study of biochemical markers of reperfusion early after thrombolysis for acute myocardial infarction. Circulation 1995 (October);92:2079–2086.

98. Iwasaki K, Kusachi S, Hina K, Yamasaki S, Kita T, Endo C, Tsuji T: Q-wave regression unrelated to patency of infarct-related artery or left ventricular ejection fraction or volume after anterior wall acute myocardial infarction treated with or without reperfusion therapy. Am J Cardiol 1995 (July 1);76:14–20.

99. Maes A, Van de Werf F, Nuyts J, Bormans G, Desmet W, Mortelmans L: Impaired myocardial tissue perfusion early after successful thrombolysis: Impact on myocardial flow, metabolism, and function at late follow-up. Circulation 1995 (October);92:2072–2078.

100. Stone GW, Grines CL, Browne KF, Marco J, Rothbaum D, O'Keefe J, Hartzler GO, Overlie P, Donohue B, Chelliah N, Timmis GC, Vlietstra R, Puchrowicz-Ochocki S, O'Neill WW: Implications of recurrent ischemia after reperfusion therapy in acute myocardial infarction: A comparison of thrombolytic therapy and primary angioplasty. J Am Coll Cardiol 1995 (July);26:66–72.

101. Mueller HS, Forman SA, Menegus MA, Cohen LS, Knatterud GL, Braunwald E: Prognostic significance of nonfatal reinfarction during 3-year follow-up: Results of the thrombolysis in myocardial infarction (TIMI) Phase II Clinical Trial. J Am Coll Cardiol 1995 (October);26:900–907.

102. Barbagelata A, Granger CB, Topol EJ, Worley SJ, Kereiakes DJ, George VS, Ohman EM, Leimberger J, Mark DB, Califf RM: Frequency, significance, and cost of recurrent ischemia after thrombolytic therapy for acute myocardial infarction. Am J Cardiol 1995 (November 15);76:1007–1013.

103. Lee KL, Woodlief LH, Topol EJ, Weaver WD, Betriu A, Col J, Simoons M, Aylward P, Van de Werf F, Califf RM, for the GUSTO-I Investigators: Predictors of 30-day mortality in the era of reperfusion for acute myocardial infarction: Results from an international trial of 41021 patients. Circulation 1995 (March);91:1659–1668.

104. Simes RJ, Topol EJ, Holmes DR Jr., White HD, Rutsch WR, Vahanian A, Simoons ML, Morris D, Betriu A, Califf RM, Ross AM, for the GUSTO-1 Investigators: Link between the angiographic substudy and mortality outcomes in a large randomized trial of myocardial reperfusion: Importance of early and complete infarct artery reperfusion. Circulation 1995 (April);91:1923–1928.

105. Aguirre FV, Younis LT, Chaitman BR, Ross AM, McMahon RP, Kern MJ, Berger PB, Sopko G, Rogers WJ, Shaw L, Knatterud G, Braunwald E, for the TIMI II Investigators: Early and 1-year clinical outcome of patients' evolving non-Q-wave versus Q-wave myocardial infarction after thrombolysis: Results from the TIMI II study. Circulation 1995 (May);91:2541–2548.

106. Stone GE, Grines, CL, Browne KF, Marco J, Rothbaum D, O'Keefe J, Hartzler GO, Overlie P, Donohue B, Chelliah N, Timmis GC, Vlietstra R, Strzelecki M, Purchrow-ixz-Ochocki S, O'Neill WW: Predictors of in-hospital and 6-month outcome after acute myocardial infarction in the reperfusion era: The primary angioplasty in myocardial infarction (PAMI) trial. J Am Coll Cardiol 1995 (February);25:370–377.

107. Bauters C, Khanoyan P, Mc Fadden EP, Quandalle P, Lablanche J-M, Bertrand ME: Restenosis after delayed coronary angioplasty of the culprit vessel in patients with a recent myocardial infarction treated by thrombolysis. Circulation 1995 (March);91:1410–1418.

108. Harrington RA, Lincoff AM, Califf RM, Holmes DR, Berdan LG, O'Hanesian MA, Keeler GP, Garratt KN, Ohman EM, Mark DB, Jacobs AK, Topol EJ: Characteristics and consequences of myocardial infarction after percutaneous coronary intervention: Insights from the Coronary Angioplasty Versus Excisional Atherectomy Trial (CAVEAT). J Am Coll Cardiol 1995 (June);25:1693–1699.

109. Morishima I, Sone T, Mokuno S, Taga S, Shimauchi A, Oki Y, Kondo J, Tsuboi H, Sassa H: Clinical significance of no-reflow phenomenon observed on angiography after successful treatment of acute myocardial infarction with percutaneous transluminal coronary angioplasty. Am Heart J 1995 (August);130:239–243.

110. Welty FK, Mittleman, MA, Lewis SM, Healy RW, Shubrooks SJ, Muller JE: Significance of location (anterior versus inferior) and type (Q-wave versus non-Q-wave) of acute myocardial infarction in patients undergoing percutaneous transluminal coronary angioplasty for postinfarction ischemia. Am J Cardiol 1995 (September 1);76:431–435.

111. McKendall GR, Forman S, Sopko G, Braunwald E, Williams DO, and the Thrombolysis in Myocardial Infarction Investigators: Value of rescue percutaneous transluminal coronary angioplasty following unsuccessful thrombolytic therapy in patients with acute myocardial infarction. Am J Cardiol 1995 (December 1);76:1108–1111.

112. Gersh BJ, Bhesebro JH, Braunwald E, Lambrew C, Passamani E, Solomon RE, Ross AM, Ross R, Terrin ML, Knatterud GL: Coronary artery bypass graft surgery after thrombolytic therapy in the Thrombolysis In Myocardial Infarction trial, phase II (TIMI II). J Am Coll Cardiol 1995 (February);25:395–402.

113. Creswell LL, Moulton MJ, Cox JL, Rosenbloom M: Revascularization after acute myocardial infarction. Ann Thorac Surg 1995 (July);60:1:19–26.

114. Lavie CJ and Milani RV: Effects of cardiac rehabilitation and exercise training on exercise capacity, coronary risk factors, behavioral characteristics, and quality of life in women. Am J Cardiol 1995 (February 15);75:340–343.

115. Bondestam E, Breikss A, Hartford M: Effects of early rehabilitation on consumption of medical care during the first year after acute myocardial infarction in patients ≥65 years of age. Am J Cardiol (April 15);75:767–771.

116. Cannistra LB, O'Malley CJ, Balady GJ: Comparison of outcome of cardiac rehabilitation in black women and white women. Am J Cardiol (May 1);75:890–893.

117. Warner JG Jr., Brubaker PH, Zhu Y, Morgan TM, Ribisl PM, Miller HS, Herrington DM: Long-term (5-year) changes in HDL cholesterol in cardiac rehabilitation patients: Do sex differences exist? Circulation 1995 (August);92:773–777.

4

Arrhythmias, Conduction Disturbances, Syncope, and Cardiac Arrest

Atrial Fibrillation/Flutter

Historical Development

Flegel[1] from Montreal, Canada, provided an excellent article on the history of atrial fibrillation. He pointed out that the electrical stimulation of animals' hearts made known the existence of AF in 1874, but AF was not associated with its clinical counterpart, arrhythmia perpetua, until 1909. By this time, simultaneous recordings of the human heart beat, the venous and arterial pulses, and electrocardiographic activity had revealed the common origin of these events. After the electrical basis of AF was found and AF was clearly distinguished from VF, investigation into its mechanism ensued. Two contrasting theories, that of circus movement and that of tachysystole from a single focus, led to 30 years of research and debate. Pivotal to the argument was the notion of blocked conduction. Although the theory of circus movement prevailed for a long time, it appeared to be demolished by electrophysiological experiments done between 1948 and 1950. The realization that blocked conduction could later reenter led to more recent research in animals and humans that revived the notion of circular conduction, although in a much more sophisticated form.

Risk Factors for Development

AF recurs in many patients who are treated with antiarrhythmic therapy to maintain sinus rhythm. In a report by Reimold and associates[2] from Boston, Massachusetts, from March 1985 to August 1991, 214 patients with recurrent symptomatic chronic or paroxysmal AF for which conventional antiarrhythmic agents had failed were treated with propafenone or sotalol. Baseline demographic data including the presence of pacing therapy were collected. Life-table estimates of the duration of freedom from AF were constructed on the basis of pacemaker status. Of 214 patients, 26 (12%) had pacing therapy. Patients with dual-chamber pacing were more likely to remain in sinus rhythm at 6 months (80%) than were patients with ventricular pacing (40%) or patients without pacing therapy (55%). A Cox univariate regression analysis demonstrated that dual-chamber pacing, in contrast to ventricular pacing or no pacing, was associated with a lower risk of recurrent AF. Clinical parameters such as age, gender, LA size, fibrillation pattern, drug assignment, EF, and underlying cardiac disease did not alter the risk of recurrent AF. Dual-chamber pacing was associated with a decreased likelihood of recurrent AF even after adjustment for other clinical covariates in a multivariate model. In patients with recurrent AF treated with propafenone or sotalol, dual-chamber pacing improved maintenance of sinus rhythm.

In addition to antithrombotic therapy, 2 treatment strategies for intermittent AF are evolving: suppression of AF or control of the ventricular response during AF. Clinical and echocardiographic features that predict recurrent AF may influence the choice of management. In a study by Flaker and coworkers[3] in Columbia, Missouri, clinical, echocardiographic, and electrocardiographic data from 486 patients with intermittent AF enrolled in the Stroke Prevention in Atrial Fibrillation studies were analyzed. Patients with intermittent AF were younger, had fewer incidences of systemic hypertension and heart failure, and had more recent-onset AF than patients with constant AF. They also had a smaller mean LA diameter, a lower prevalence of a large LA, better LV performance by echo, and less MR. After a mean follow-up of 26 months, 51% of patients remained in sinus rhythm and 49% of patients developed recurrent AF, including 12% who had AF, as seen on all follow-up electrocardiograms. Clinical factors predicting recurrent AF were age, heart failure, and AMI. An enlarged LA was associated with recurrent intermittent AF; an enlarged LV predicted conversion to constant AF. Thus, clinical and echocardiographic parameters predict recurrent AF in patients with intermittent nonvalvular AF.

Prevalence, Ages, and Gender

Feinberg and associates[4] from 5 United States and Canadian medical centers, reviewed the available epidemiological data to define the age and sex distribution of persons with AF. From 4 large recent population-based surveys, the authors estimated the overall age and gender-specific prevalence of AF (Figure 4-1). The estimates were applied to the recent US census data to calculate the number of men and women with AF in each age group (Figure 4-2). There are an estimated 2.2 million people in the US with AF, with a median age of about 75 years. The prevalence of AF is 2.3% in people older than 40 years and 5.9% in those older than 65 years. Approximately 70% of individuals with AF are between 65 and 85 years of age. The absolute number of men and women with AF is about equal. After age 75 years, about 60% of the people with AF are women. In contrast to people with AF in the general population, patients with AF in recent anticoagulation trials had a mean age of 69 years, and only 20% were older than 75 years. The risks and benefits of antithrombotic therapy in older individuals are important considerations in stroke prevention in AF.

Natural History

Krahn and associates[5] from Winnipeg, Canada, undertook a study to identify the natural history of AF, including risk factors for its development and outcome. The incidence of AF among 3983 male air crew recruits observed continuously for 44 years was calculated based on person-years of observation (Figure 4-3). Age and 23 variables were examined to identify risk factors for AF (Table 4-1). Controlling for age and 9 prognostic variables, the effect of AF on 8 outcomes was examined. Analysis of risk factors for AF and outcome after fibrillation was based on a Cox proportional hazard model using time-dependent covariates. Of the 3983 study members, 299 (7.5%) developed AF

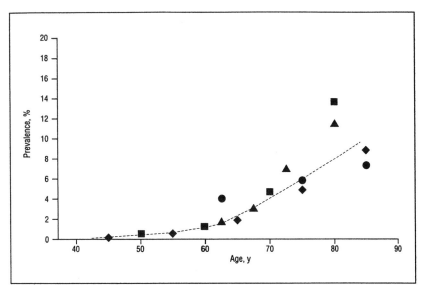

Figure 4-1. Prevalence of atrial fibrillation at various ages. The values are plotted at the midpoint of the age range, i.e., the prevalence of atrial fibrillation from ages 60 to 69 years is plotted at 65 years. Prevalence for "over age 75 years" is plotted at 80 years. Prevalence for "over age 80 years" is plotted at 85 years. The dotted line represents the estimated prevalence values used to calculate absolute numbers of people with atrial fibrillation. Diamonds indicate the Framingham Study; circles, Cardiovascular Health Study; squares, Mayo Clinic Study, Rochester, Minn.; and triangles, Busselton, Western Australia. Reproduced with permission from Feinberg et al.[4]

during 154 131 person-years of observation. The incidence rose with age from less than 0.5 per 1000 person-years before age 50 to 9.7 per 1000 person-years after age 70. Risk for AF was increased with AMI, angina, and ST-T wave abnormalities in the absence of ischemic heart disease. The RR for AF was strongest at the onset of ischemic heart disease and diminished over time. The rate of AF was 1.42 times greater in men with a history of hypertension. CHF, valvular heart disease, and cardiomyopathy were important but uncommon risk factors. AF independently increased the risk for stroke and CHF. Total mortality rate was increased 1.31 times; cardiovascular mortality including and excluding fatal stroke were also increased. The incidence of AF in men increases with advancing age. Clinical cardiac abnormalities, particularly recent CAD and hypertension, are strongly associated with increased risk for AF. AF increases morbidity and mortality, but the magnitude of the increase may be less than previously reported.

Cerebral Infarction

Ezekowitz and colleagues[6] in the Veterans Affairs Cooperative Study used computed tomography scans of the head performed at entry, at the time of any subsequent stroke, and at termination of follow-up to determine the frequency of cerebral infarction in patients with nonrheumatic AF. This study was a double-blind controlled trial designed to determine the efficacy of warfarin for the prevention of stroke in neurologically normal patients with nonrheumatic AF. Patients were followed for 3 years or until the termination of the study.

Age, y	US Population[21] (Thousands)	Estimated Atrial Fibrillation Prevalence, %	Estimated Population With Atrial Fibrillation (Thousands)
40-44	18 754	0.1	19
45-49	14 094	0.3	42
50-54	11 645	0.5	58
55-59	10 442	0.8	83
60-64	10 582	1.5	159
65-69	10 037	3.0	301
70-74	8242	5.0	412
75-79	6279	7.0	440
80-84	4035	10.0	404
85-89	2090	10.0	209
90-94	812	10.0	81
95+	258	10.0	26
US population older than 40 y	97 270	2.3	2234
Total US population	252 177	0.89	2234

*See text for assumptions and derivation of estimated prevalence values for atrial fibrillation.

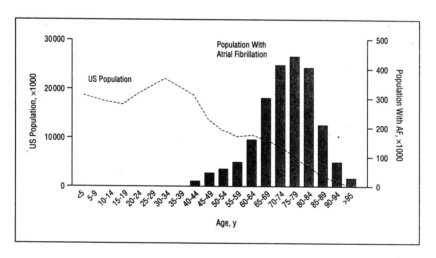

Figure 4-2. Estimated numbers of people with atrial fibrillation (AF) compared with US general population. Bars indicate numbers of people (×10³) with AF per 5-year age group (right axis). Dotted line indicates US population (×10³) per 5-year age group (left axis, 1991 census data). See text for derivation of estimated numbers of people with AF. Reproduced with permission from Feinberg et al.[4]

Of the 516 evaluable scans performed at entry, 76 had evidence of one or more silent cerebral infarcts. Age, history of hypertension, active angina, and elevated mean systolic BP were associated with cerebral infarcts in these patients. Silent cerebral infarction occurred during the study at rates of 1% and 1.6% per year for the placebo and warfarin treatment groups, respectively. Silent cerebral infarction at entry was not an independent predictor of symptomatic stroke, but active angina was a significant predictor; 15% of the placebo-assigned patients with angina had a stroke compared with 5% of placebo-assigned patients without angina. Thus, silent cerebral infarction is frequently seen in asymptomatic patients with AF. Active angina was the only significant indepen-

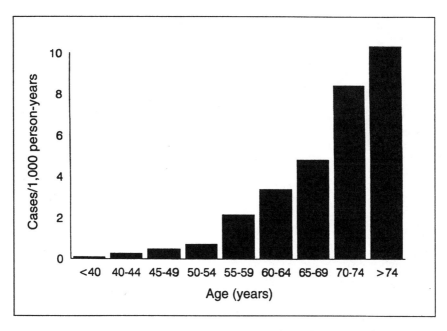

Figure 4-3. Incidence of atrial fibrillation in the Manitoba Follow-Up Study, 1948 to 1992. Reproduced with permission from Krahn et al.[5]

dent predictor associated with silent infarction. The small sample size precluded determining whether warfarin was protective in these patients.

Anticoagulant Therapy

Collins and colleagues[7] performed serial transesophageal echocardiography in 14 patients with nonrheumatic AF after identification of atrial thrombi on the initial transesophageal study. The authors wished to determine the mechanism of benefit of warfarin anticoagulation when given for several weeks before cardioversion. This benefit has previously been ascribed to organization and adherence of atrial thrombi, a finding observed among pathological studies of patients with rheumatic valvular heart disease. All patients received warfarin anticoagulation and were followed clinically for signs of thromboembolism. Eighteen atrial thrombi were identified on the initial study and included 14 thrombi in the left atrial appendage, 2 in the body of the left atrium, 1 in the RA appendage, and 1 in the body of the right atrium. Thrombus size varied from 5 to 20 mm, and 6 appeared to be mobile. After a median period of 4 weeks of warfarin, 16 of 18 atrial thrombi had completely resolved on transesophageal echocardiographic study (Figure 4-4). No new thrombi were identified on follow-up study, and no patient had a clinical thromboembolic event between studies. These data support the hypothesis that among patients with nonrheumatic AF, the mechanism of clinical benefit with 3 to 4 weeks of warfarin before cardioversion is related to thrombus resolution and prevention of new thrombus formation.

A number of studies have demonstrated the efficacy of oral anticoagulant therapy in reducing the risk of stroke and systemic embolism in patients with nonrheumatic AF. Both the targeted and actual levels of anticoagulation differed

Table 4-1. Age-Adjusted Relative Risk for Atrial Fibrillation

Variable	Frequency Among Cases n (%)	Relative Risk
Cardiac		
Ischemic heart disease	109 (36.3)	3.48
Myocardial infarction	67 (22.3)	3.75
Angina	42 (14.0)	3.13
Valvular disease	25 (8.3)	6.95
Congestive heart failure	44 (14.7)	9.93
Cardiomyopathy	5 (1.7)	14.02
Miscellaneous cardiovascular conditions	7 (2.3)	3.01
Hypertension	159 (53.0)	2.32
Palpitations	23 (7.7)	2.77
Murmur	87 (29.0)	2.02
Noncardiac		
Diabetes	35 (11.7)	1.82
Pulmonary embolus	9 (3.0)	3.67
Cerebrovascular disease	26 (8.7)	1.89
Thyroid	9 (3.0)	1.26
Alcohol	26 (8.7)	2.07
Smoking	222 (74.2)	1.37
Obesity	163 (54.3)	1.42
Electrocardiogram		
ST or T wave changes	150 (50.0)	3.11
ST or T wave changes without ischemic heart disease	67 (22.3)	2.57
Left ventricular hypertrophy	16 (5.3)	2.39
Supraventricular rhythm disturbance	78 (26.0)	3.06
Ventricular rhythm disturbance	84 (28.0)	2.18
Heart rate >100	70 (23.3)	1.81
Atrioventricular conduction disturbance	48 (16.0)	2.04
Intraventricular conduction disturbance	74 (24.7)	1.25
Left axis deviation	59 (19.7)	1.27

Reproduced with permission from Krahn et al.[5]

widely among the studies, however, and a number of studies failed to report standardized prothrombin-time ratios as international normalized ratios (INRs). The European Atrial Fibrillation Trial study group, in a report prepared by J.C. Latum, MD, and P.J. Koudstaal, MD,[8] reported an analysis determining the intensity of oral anticoagulant therapy and nonrheumatic AF that provides the best balance between the prevention of thromboembolism and the occurrence of bleeding complications. The investigators calculated INR-specific incidence rates for both ischemic and major events occurring in 214 patients who received anticoagulant therapy in the European Atrial Fibrillation Trial, a secondary-prevention trial in patients with nonrheumatic AF and a recent episode of minor cerebral ischemia. The optimal intensity of anticoagulation was between an INR of 2.0 and 3.9. No treatment effect was apparent with anticoagulation below an INR of 2.0. The rate of thromboembolic events was lowest at INRs from 2.0 to 3.9, and most major bleeding complications occurred with treatment at intensities with INRs of 5.0 or above. To achieve optimal levels of anticoagulation with the lowest risk in patients with AF and a recent episode of cerebral ischemia, the target value for the INR should be set at 3.0, and values below 2.0 and above 5.0 should be avoided.

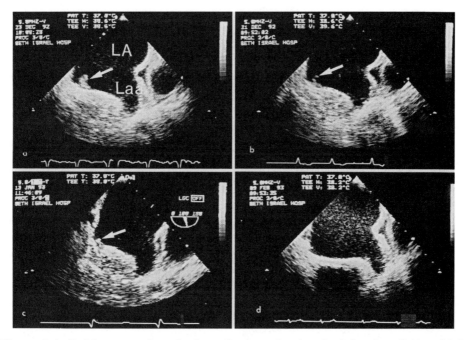

Figure 4-4. Serial transesophageal echocardiograms showing the left atrium (LA) and left atrial appendage (Laa) viewed in the vertical plane with a 5-MHz biplane transesophageal probe. The thrombus (arrow) is in the body of the left atrium, closely associated with the mitral annulus in the posterior portion of the left atrium. a, Initial study demonstrating a mobile 12-mm thrombus. b, Thrombus persists (arrow) but is smaller after 1 week of warfarin therapy. c, After 3 weeks of warfarin, the thrombus continues to be seen (arrow). d, Complete thrombus resolution after 5.5 weeks of warfarin. Reproduced with permission from Collins et al.[7]

Warfarin and Aspirin

To examine the cost-effectiveness of prescribing warfarin sodium in patients who have nonvalvular AF with or without additional stroke risk factors (a prior stroke or transient ischemic attack, diabetes mellitus, systemic hypertension, or heart disease), Gage and associates[9] from Stanford, California, estimated from literature review, phone survey of 75 patients with AF, and Medicare reimbursement. All patients were age 65 and good candidates for warfarin therapy. For patients with nonvalvular AF and additional risk factors for stroke, warfarin therapy led to a greater quality-adjusted survival and cost savings. For patients with nonvalvular AF and 1 additional risk factor, warfarin therapy cost $8000/quality-adjusted life-year saved. For 65-year-old patients with nonvalvular AF alone, warfarin cost about $370 000/quality-adjusted life-year saved, compared with aspirin therapy. However, for 75-year-old patients with nonvalvular AF alone, prescribing warfarin cost $110 000/quality-adjusted life-year saved. For patients who were not prescribed warfarin, aspirin was preferred to no therapy on the basis of both quality-adjusted survival and cost in all patients, regardless of the number of risk factors present. Treatment with warfarin is cost-effective in patients with nonvalvular AF and 1 or more additional risk factors for stroke. In 65-year-old patients with nonvalvular AF but no other risk factors for stroke, prescribing warfarin instead of aspirin would affect quality-adjusted survival minimally but increase costs significantly.

Warfarin vs. Quinidine or Amiodarone

A search was conducted by Middlekauff and associates[10] from Los Angeles, California; and Boston, Massachusetts, of the English-language MEDLINE databases of the National Library of Medicine dated 1966 through December 1992. The search was conducted by intersecting "quinidine," "warfarin," or "amiodarone" with "AF." Six of 249 articles concerning quinidine and 5 of 20 articles concerning warfarin were judged by multiple reviewers to meet predetermined inclusion and exclusion criteria. To the authors' knowledge, no randomized, placebo-controlled trials of amiodarone therapy for AF have been published. Five of 112 identified articles concerning amiodarone involved nonrandomized trials that met the remaining selection criteria and were included in this analysis. Thromboembolic events and fatal nonthromboembolic adverse events during the course of therapy (defined as fatal proarrhythmia, fatal hemorrhage, and fatal noncardiac toxic effects) were considered to have equivalent weight. The total risk during therapy, defined as thromboembolic and fatal nonthromboembolic adverse events during the course of therapy, was evaluated over a range of baseline thromboembolism risks, from 1% to 20% per patient-year. Quinidine therapy compared with no therapy was associated with increased total risk, unless baseline thromboembolism risk exceeded 11% per patient-year. Total risk during warfarin therapy was less than total risk during quinidine therapy for the entire range of baseline thromboembolism risks, from 1% to 20% per patient-year. Total risk during warfarin or amiodarone therapy was similar and less than that with no therapy for the entire range of baseline risks. Based on data from randomized, controlled trials of quinidine and warfarin, warfarin therapy appears to be the safest strategy for thromboembolism prevention in the patient with AF.

Diltiazem

Ellenbogen and coworkers[11] in Richmond, Virginia, examined the efficacy of various doses of intravenous diltiazem to control the ventricular response during AF or atrial flutter. Control of the ventricular response of patients with AF and a rapid ventricular response can provide patients with relief of symptoms and improve hemodynamics. Eighty-four consecutive patients with AF or atrial flutter, or both, received an intravenous bolus dose of diltiazem followed by a continuous infusion of diltiazem at 5, 10, and 15 mg/hr. The mean ventricular response and BP were monitored. Overall, 94% of patients responded to the bolus dose with a >20% reduction in heart rate from baseline, a conversion to sinus rhythm, or a heart rate <100 beats per minute. Seventy-eight patients received the continuous infusion. After 10 hours of infusion, 47% of patients had maintained response with the 5-mg/hr infusion, 68% maintained response after the infusion was titrated to 10 mg/hr, and 76% after titration from the 5- and 10-mg/hr infusion to the 15-mg/hr dose. For the three diltiazem infusions studied, mean heart rate was reduced from a baseline value of 144 beats per minute to 98, 107, 107, 101, 91, and 88 beats per minute at infusion times 0, 1, 2, 4, 8, and 10 hours, respectively. By the end of the infusion, 18% of patients (14 of 78) had conversion to sinus rhythm. Hypotension was the most common side effect, occurring in 13% of patients. Symptomatic hypotension was present in 4% of patients and responded to normal saline solution in all cases. The investigators conclude that a bolus dose of 20 or 25 mg followed by titration of a continuous infusion of 5, 10, and 15 mg/hr of intravenous diltiazem is a safe and effective regimen to rapidly lower heart rate in patients with AF and atrial flutter.

Cardioversion

Murgatroyd and colleagues[12] from London, United Kingdom, evaluated the efficacy and tolerability of low energy shocks for termination of AF in patients using an endocardial electroconfiguration that embraced both atria. Twenty-two consecutive patients with stable AF were studied during electrophysiological testing. A step-up voltage protocol was used starting at 10 or 20 V and increasing to a maximum of 400 V. Patients were conscious at the start of the study and were asked to report symptoms, but were sedated if shocks were not tolerated. Cardioversion was achieved in all 19 patients who completed the study, with a mean leading edge voltage of 237 V. The mean maximal shock delivered without sedation was 116 V. These authors concluded that the delivery of biphasic R-wave synchronous shocks between the right atrium and coronary sinus can terminate AF with very low energies. General anesthesia is not required, but few fully conscious patients are able to tolerate this method of cardioversion.

Because atrial thrombi are poorly seen by conventional imaging techniques, several weeks of prophylactic anticoagulation are routinely prescribed before cardioversion. Transesophageal echo is a superior test for identifying atrial thrombi. Manning and colleagues[13] from Boston, Massachusetts, and Farmington, Connecticut, evaluated the safety of transesophageal echocardiographically guided early cardioversion in conjunction with short-term anticoagulation as a strategy for guiding early cardioversion in hospitalized patients with AF. Over a 4.5-year period, 233 patients agreed to participate, and 230 underwent transesophageal echocardiography. Fifteen percent of patients had identifiable LA or RA thrombi. Ninety-five percent of patients without thrombi had successful cardioversion to sinus rhythm, all without prolonged anticoagulation, and none experienced a clinical thromboembolic event. Eighteen patients with atrial thrombi underwent uneventful cardioversion after prolonged anticoagulation. These authors concluded from this large prospective and consecutive study of patients undergoing transesophageal echo that this treatment algorithm has a safety profile similar to conventional therapy and minimizes both the period of anticoagulation and the overall duration of AF.

The role of transesophageal echocardiography in the guidance of cardioversion of AF was studied in this report by Stoddard and associates[14] from Louisville, Kentucky. Thirty-seven (18%) of 206 patients had LA thrombus. Cardioversion was attempted in 153 patients receiving no (n=107) or <7 days (n=46) of anticoagulation prophylaxis, in 27 patients after ≥3 weeks of anticoagulation, and was canceled in 26 patients, primarily on the basis of transesophageal echocardiography findings. LA thrombus was observed in 37 (18%) of 206 patients. No embolic complications occurred over a 4-week follow-up period. In 7 (41%) of 17 patients new LA appendage spontaneous echocardiographic contrast developed immediately after electric cardioversion. In this group, significant decreases occurred in the LA appendage maximal emptying shear rate, maximal filling shear rate, and peak emptying velocity. In one patient an LA appendage thrombus formed after electric cardioversion. LA thrombus resolved in 1 (5%) of 21 patients, became immobile in 0 (0%) of 16 patients after 3 to 5 weeks of anticoagulation but resolved (n=9) or became immobile (n=6) in 15 (71%) of 21 patients after >5 weeks of anticoagulation. Transesophageal echocardiography–guided cardioversion was safely done without or with <7 days of anticoagulation prophylaxis in selected patients, but the potential for LA thrombus to form after electric cardioversion makes anticoagulation advisable in all patients. The conventional recommendation of 3 to 4 weeks of anticoagulation prophylaxis before cardioversion is usually inadequate for LA thrombus to resolve or to become immobile.

Radiofrequency Catheter Ablation

Patients with drug-refractory AF or flutter may be considered candidates for transvenous ablation of the His bundle with placement of a pacemaker. Della Bella and associates[15] from Milan, Italy, used radiofrequency ablation on the slow AV node pathway in 14 such patients. Radiofrequency current was delivered when patients were in sinus rhythm, atrial flutter, or AF. Permanent complete AV block was induced in one patient who required a pacemaker. During a follow-up of 6 months, 11 patients experienced a recurrence of AF at a rate of 60–95 beats/min. In sinus rhythm the effective refractory period of the AV node was prolonged from 270 to 390 msec and the Wenckebach cycle from 346 to 458 msec. Thus, they concluded that ablation of the slow AV node pathway allows reduction of ventricular rate during AF or flutter while maintaining intact AV conduction during sinus rhythm.

Studies have suggested that radiofrequency current application in the low right atrial region may prevent recurrences of common atrial flutter. Fischer and colleagues[16] from Bordeaux, France, and Tucson, Arizona, evaluated 2 different approaches to target the ablation site in 80 consecutive patients with atrial flutter. Overall, atrial flutter was interrupted and rendered noninducible after a single session in 72 patients (90%) and could not be interrupted in 8 (10%). Three anatomic landmarks were used: area 1, between the tricuspid valve and inferior vena cava orifice; area 2, between the tricuspid valve and coronary sinus ostium; area 3, between the inferior vena cava and coronary sinus. The location of the final successful site in the first group of 50 patients was 39% in area 1, 36% in area 2, and 25% in area 3. In the next 30 patients radiofrequency lesions were placed at several sites and produced success rates of 70%, 40% and 10% at areas 1, 2 and 3, respectively. These authors concluded that radiofrequency catheter ablation of atrial flutter can be performed with a high success rate and is safe. The highest success rate was achieved with radiofrequency energy applied in the isthmus between inferior vena cava orifice and tricuspid valve.

Steinberg and associates[17] from New York, New York, described the procedural success and clinical recurrences after radiofrequency catheter ablation of atrial flutter. A deflectable catheter with a 4- or 5-mm tip was positioned in the posterior right atrium. Radiofrequency energy was delivered sequentially from the tricuspid annulus to the inferior vena cava. Catheter ablation during 18 sessions for 16 patients resulted in abrupt atrial flutter termination and noninducibility in all patients. Successful sites were near the os of the coronary sinus but had no distinguishing electrographic features. During a follow-up period of 8 ± 5 months, 4 (25%) patients had recurrence of atrial flutter; 3 of these patients underwent successful repeat ablation. According to actuarial analysis, 87% of patients remained in normal sinus rhythm 6 months after the initial procedure. The only distinguishing feature of those with recurrence compared with those whose sinus rhythm was maintained was the induction of nonclinical atrial arrhythmia (50% vs. 0%, respectively). One patient had resolution of presumed tachycardia-related cardiomyopathy. Catheter ablation by an anatomic approach was highly successful in terminating type 1 atrial flutter and was associated with good long-term response. This technique represents a meaningful alternative for restoration and maintenance of normal sinus rhythm.

Poty and colleagues[18] in Rouen, France, evaluated 12 patients referred for catheter ablation of atrial flutter. Duodecapolar and decapolar catheters were used for detailed mapping of the tricuspid ring, inferior vena cava/tricuspid annulus isthmus, and the coronary sinus ostium area. Additional multipolar catheters were used for recording activation of the coronary sinus and the coronary sinus/tricuspid annulus isthmus. Atrial flutter was present at baseline in 9 patients and was induced by proximal coronary sinus pacing in 3. Counterclockwise RA activation was recorded in all patients. Primary ablation was considered successful when atrial flutter was no longer inducible even during isoproterenol infusion. Atrial flutter was successfully ablated in all 12 patients with a mean of 4 pulses delivered at the inferior vena cava/tricuspid annulus isthmus. In the 3 patients in whom atrial flutter was induced, during proximal coronary sinus pacing and in sinus rhythm before ablation, a collision of descending and ascending wave fronts was observed in the middle lateral right atrium. This activation pattern of the lateral right atrium was also noted after unsuccessful radiofrequency applications. Noninducibility of atrial flutter after radiofrequency applications was associated with a change of activation pattern at the mid-lateral right atrium and with an inversion of the activation sequence of the inferior vena cava/tricuspid annulus isthmus in 9 patients when pacing from the proximal coronary sinus. In 2 of 3 patients, despite noninducibility of atrial flutter, ablation was pursued to obtain evidence of permanent block of conduction at the inferior vena cava/tricuspid annulus isthmus. A completely descending middle lateral right atrium wave front was observed when pacing from the proximal coronary sinus in all patients except one. Low lateral RA pacing was performed in 4 patients and showed evidence for block in the counterclockwise direction at the isthmus. During a follow-up of 9 months, atrial flutter recurred in 1 patient, the only one who showed no conduction block at the isthmus after the procedure. These data suggest that direction of impulse propagation at mid-lateral right atrium and block of propagation at the inferior vena cava/tricuspid annulus isthmus during proximal coronary sinus and low RA pacing may be useful in predicting success of atrial flutter ablation by radiofrequency energy.

Treatment of Resistant Type

Zarembski and associates[19] from Tucson, Arizona, compared amiodarone to flecainide in maintaining normal sinus rhythm in patients with resistant chronic AF. The authors identified previously reported studies using amiodarone or flecainide in the treatment of patients with chronic AF refractory to class I antiarrhythmic drugs or sotalol. The results of 6 trials of amiodarone (200–400 mg/d; 315 patients) and 2 trials of flecainide (200–300 mg/d; 163 patients) were aggregated using meta-analytic techniques. The percentages of patients taking amiodarone or flecainide and remaining in normal sinus rhythm at 3 and 12 months were compared relative to results for quinidine, which were acquired from a meta-analysis of quinidine used as first-line therapy for AF. After 3 and 12 months of treatment with amiodarone, 217 (73%) of 299 patients and 64 (60%) of 107 patients, respectively, remained in normal sinus rhythm. These percentages were significantly greater than those for quinidine (70% and 50%, respectively). For flecainide, the percentage of patients remaining in normal sinus rhythm was significantly lower than for quinidine: 79 (49%) and 56 (34%) of 163 patients, respectively. The aggregated percentages of patients requiring withdrawal of amiodarone and flecainide were similar: 9.5% and 8.6%, respectively. Mortality and proarrhythmia could not be assessed. This analysis suggests that low-dose amiodarone is more efficacious and equally well tolerated when compared with flecainide in the management of chronic, drug-resistant AF.

Atrial Thrombi

Thromboembolism related to AF is a major cause of morbidity and mortality. Patients with acute thromboembolism and AF are at high risk for early recurrent events. To determine the prevalence of LA thrombi in patients who had acute thromboembolism and newly diagnosed AF, Manning and associates[20] from Boston, Massachusetts, and Farmington, Connecticut, screened adult inpatients with AF to identify those with acute (<36 hours) systemic thromboembolism and newly recognized AF. Of 41 qualifying patients, 31 (76%) agreed to undergo transesophageal echocardiographic study, including 24 with acute neurological events and 7 with peripheral thromboembolism. A control population consisted of 88 adults with newly recognized AF without clinical thromboembolism. Transesophageal echocardiography identified left atrial thrombi in 13 (43%) of the 30 study patients who underwent transesophageal echocardiography compared with 9 (10%) of 87 controls. Spontaneous echocardiographic contrast was identified in 27 (87%) of the study population vs. 42 (48%) of the control group. The prevalence of this marked blood stasis did not differ between patients with LA thrombi without thromboembolism. Duration of AF, prevalence of abnormal LF function, LA size, and MR were similar in both groups. LA thrombi were identified in >40% of patients with acute thromboembolism and newly recognized AF. These data suggest that a major source of recurrent thromboembolism in this group may be residual thrombus migration. Among patients with AF and atrial thrombi, clinical thromboembolism seems to occur randomly or is related to an unidentified process.

Supraventricular Tachycardia with or without the Short P-R Interval Syndrome

Review

A splendid review of supraventricular tachycardia was provided in the January 1995 issue of *The New England Journal of Medicine* by Drs. Leonard I. Ganz and Peter L. Friedman[21] from Boston, Massachusetts.

Incidence of Associated Atrial Fibrillation

Clinical experience has suggested that there is a substantial incidence of AF in patients with paroxysmal SVT. To determine the precise incidence of AF and the factors that determine it, Hamer et al[22] from Durham, North Carolina, followed up 169 patients with paroxysmal SVT during a mean follow-up period of 31 months. Nineteen percent of the patients had an episode of AF, including 6% within 1 month, 9% within 4 months, and 12% within 1 year. The mechanism of paroxysmal SVT was not associated with the time to recurrence of AF. Similarly, the heart rate during paroxysmal SVT was not associated with the time to occurrence of AF. These authors concluded that AF will develop in about 12% of patients with paroxysmal SVT during a 1-year follow-up period, and the occurrence is not related to the mechanism or heart rate of the paroxysmal SVT.

Propafenone

The UK Propafenone PSVT Study Group[23] conducted a double-blind, placebo-controlled trial of the efficacy and tolerability of propafenone in 100 patients with proxysmal SVT or AF or flutter who had 2 or more symptomatic arrhythmia recurrences as documented by transtelephonic electrocardiographic monitoring during a 3-month drug-free observation period. Patients were randomly assigned to 2 consecutive crossover periods of propafenone (300 mg twice daily) compared with placebo, followed by 300 mg propafenone three times daily vs. placebo. Analysis was based on the time to treatment failure, defined as the interval from treatment onset to the occurrence of either electrocardiographically-documented arrhythmia or an adverse event. With a proportional-hazards model, the authors determined that the RR values of treatment failure after the achievement of steady-state drug levels for placebo compared with propafenone 300 mg twice daily were 6.8 for proximal SVT and 6.0 for AF. Due to a greater incidence of adverse events on high-dose propafenone, the relative risk of receiving placebo rather than propafenone 300 mg 3 times a day was 2.2 for proximal SVT and 1.9 for AF. If adverse events were excluded in the high-dose comparison, the RR for arrhythmia recurrence was 15.0 for proximal SVT and incalculable for AF. One episode of wide-complex tachycardia was documented during propafenone therapy. Propafenone is of value in the prophylaxis against both proximal SVT and AF, and a dose of 300 mg twice daily is effective and well tolerated.

Sotalol

Sotalol is an antiarrhythmic agent with combined β-blocking and class III antiarrhythmic properties. Sung and associates[24] from San Francisco, California; Salt Lake City, Utah; Princeton, New Jersey, Boston, Massachusetts; Washington, DC; and Fargo, North Dakota, assessed the safety and efficacy of sotalol in terminating SVT, AF, and atrial flutter. Ninety-three patients with spontaneous or induced SVT (n = 45) or AF (n = 48) with a ventricular rate of ≥120 beats/min were studied. In the first phase, the double-blind phase, patients were randomly assigned to receive placebo or intravenous sotalol, 1.0 or 1.5 mg/kg. If SVT or AF did not convert to sinus rhythm or if the ventricular rate did not slow to <100 beats/min within 30 minutes, patients then entered the open-label phase, which also lasted 30 minutes, and were given 1.5 mg/kg intravenous sotalol. In the SVT group, during the double-blind phase, conversion to sinus rhythm occurred in 2 (14%) of 14 patients who received placebo and 10 (67%) of 15 who received 1.5 mg/kg sotalol; during the open-label phase, 1.5 mg/kg intravenous sotalol converted 7 (41%) of 17 patients to sinus rhythm. In the AF group, during the double-blind phase, conversion to sinus rhythm occurred in 2 (14%) of 14 patients who received placebo, 2 (11%) of 18 who received 1.0 mg/kg sotalol, and 2 (13%) of 16 who received 1.5 mg/kg sotalol; in these groups a >20% reduction of ventricular rate without conversion to sinus rhythm occurred in 0 (0%) of 14, 13 (72%) of 18, and 12 (75%) of 16 patients, respectively. During the open-label phase, 1.5 mg/kg intravenous sotalol converted 7 (30%) of 23 patients to normal sinus rhythm. The most common adverse events were hypotension and dyspnea. During the double-blind phase they occurred in 10% of patients who received placebo, 9% of those who received 1.0 mg/kg sotalol, and 10% of those who received 1.5 mg/kg intravenous sotalol. Most of these events were mild to moderate, but all were transient and clinically manageable. In conclusion, intravenous sotalol is safe and effective for acute termination of SVT and for acute slowing of ventricular rate during AF but not for termination of AF at doses of 1.5 mg/kg.

Ventricular Arrhythmias

Prognostic Predictors

Goldstein and colleagues[25] in the CAST evaluated the association between ease of suppression of ventricular arrhythmias and mortality from all causes. The CAST-I study investigated the effect on arrhythmic death of ventricular premature beat suppression achieved by three drugs—encainide, flecainide, and moricizine—at two different dose levels. The CAST-II study investigated the same effect using moricizine alone at three dose levels. If suppression of VPCs was achieved, patients were randomly assigned to the effective active drug or corresponding placebo. To determine the independence of easily suppressed ventricular arrhythmias as a predictor of arrhythmic death, the authors adjusted statistically for other variables related both to ease of suppression and arrhythmic death. Patients with VPCs that were easy to suppress (n=1778) had fewer arrhythmic deaths during follow-up than those with VPCs that were hard to suppress (n=1173). Patients whose VPCs were easily suppressed were older and had a lower frequency of prior history of CHF and AMI. They also had a higher incidence of anterior MI, VPC frequency, and average LVEF. After adjusting for these variables, the authors found that easily suppressed VPCs were still significant predictors of arrhythmic death. Thus, this study shows that the ease of VPC suppression identifies a subgroup of post-AMI patients who have a low risk of arrhythmic death.

The majority of patients with serious ventricular arrhythmias induced by exercise have ischemic heart disease. These arrhythmias, however, develop only in a minority of the patients with CAD. Berntsen and associates[26] from Tromsø, Norway, investigated whether patients with VT or VF produced by exercise-induced ischemia exhibit any premonitory electrocardiographic indicators of arrhythmia propensity and whether arrhythmia suppression by myocardial revascularization abolished these changes. High-quality exercise electrocardiograms (50 mm/sec) from 30 patients with VT and VF produced by exercise-induced ischemia were studied before and after surgical revascularization. These results were compared with those obtained from 30 control patients matched for age, sex, heart disease, and preoperative exercise capacity. The resting and peak exercise electrocardiograms were examined separately in a blinded manner with respect to QRS duration and ST-segment depression. Patients with BBB patterns were excluded. The QRS duration at rest was similar in case and control patients preoperatively and increased significantly with exercise in both groups. However, the QRS prolongation was 11 ± 3 msec in the case group compared with 4 ± 2 msec in the control group. QRS prolongation ≥15 msec predicted ischemia-related ventricular arrhythmias in 73% of the patients. After surgical revascularization, there was no QRS prolongation with exercise in either group. In both groups, the QRS prolongation was associated with significant ST-segment depression, which was larger in the case patients. After revascularization, the ST-segment depressions at peak exercise were smaller in both groups. The current findings confirm that QRS prolongation is a specific characteristic of ischemia. Furthermore, they indicate that the prolongation is greater in patients exhibiting ischemia-related VT and VF and that arrhythmia suppression by surgical revascularization is associated with a normalization of these changes. QRS prolongation ≥15 msec, in the absence of BBB, may be a useful indicator of risk of ischemic VT or VF related to exercise.

Twenty-nine consecutive patients with a prior myocardial infarction, severely reduced LVEF ($26\pm8\%$), and asymptomatic nonsustained VT were enrolled in a prospective trial by Hernández and associates[27] from Wynnewood and Philadelphia, Pennsylvania. After a negative programmed electric stimulation study (3 extrastimuli at 2 sites with 2 drive trains), the 26 men and 3 women (mean age, 71) were monitored for a mean of 13 months without antiarrhythmic drug therapy. Five patients died suddenly or had sustained VT; 3 others had a cardiac, nonarrhythmic death. Events occurred during the first 13 months of surveillance. Clinical factors associated with a poor outcome included CHF and lack of β-blocker therapy. In addition, patients with events tended to have lower EFs than those without. Thus, a negative programmed electric stimulation study does not necessarily imply a benign outcome in patients with a prior AMI and nonsustained VT if they also have severe LV dysfunction and a history of CHF.

Eisenberg and coworkers[28] in San Francisco, California, delineated the clinical spectrum of 15 patients with polymorphic VT and normal QT intervals in the absence of apparent structural heart disease, adverse drug effects, or electrolyte disturbances. Patients presented with either palpitations, presyncope, syncope, no symptoms, or aborted sudden death. Mean age was 41 years, and mean follow-up was 38 months. LV function was normal as determined by either echocardiogram or left ventriculography. Episodes of polymorphic VT were analyzed in terms of the preceding interval, and the relation of the initiating coupling interval to the QT interval (coupling interval/QT interval = polymorphic VT index). The mean QT for the group as a whole was 0.41 second. Patients could be separated into 3 distinct groups. Four patients had polymorphic VT reproducibly induced by exercise and initiated by late-coupled beats. Isoproterenol induced polymorphic VT in 3 of 4 patients, and all 4 responded to chronic β-blockade. Two patients had polymorphic VT during episodes of coronary artery spasm, and both responded to calcium channel blockade. Polymorphic VT unrelated to exertion or coronary vasospasm occurred in 9 patients. Tachycardia onset was initiated by closely coupled beats and was preceded by a pause in 4 patients and no pause in 5. Sudden death occurred in 5 of 9 patients with the shortest polymorphic VT indexes. Drug therapy and chronic pacing were not reliable in preventing episodes of sudden death. Invasive electrophysiological studies, including the use of monophasic action potential recordings, were not useful in the evaluation or management of these patients. Appropriate therapy for patients presenting with either exercise- or coronary vasospasm–induced polymorphic VT is usually associated with a good prognosis. Conversely, patients with spontaneous episodes of short-coupled polymorphic VT have a high incidence of sudden death and should be considered for automatic implantable cardioverter-defibrillator insertion.

To study prognostic factors in patients with sustained VT or VF complicated by LV dysfunction, Szabó and colleagues[29] from Groningen, the Netherlands, evaluated the predictive value of demographic, clinical, and hemodynamic parameters for cardiac mortality and sudden cardiac death in 85 patients with VT or VF and LVEF <0.45 (mean, 0.27±0.10). Patients underwent serial drug testing and received appropriate antiarrhythmic treatment, with amiodarone given as last-resort therapy. During a follow-up of 24±13 months, 23 patients died of cardiac causes, 18 of them suddenly. LVEF ≤0.27 and amiodarone treatment were related to greater cardiac mortality and increased risk of sudden cardiac death, whereas β-blockade was associated with improved survival. In the multivariate model, cardiac mortality was best predicted by a LVEF ≤0.27, and absence of β-blockade and severe LV dysfunction were the strongest predictors of sudden cardiac death. It was concluded that severe LV dysfunction predicts increased cardiac mortality and high risk of sudden cardiac death. Moreover, β-blocking treatment is associated with lower cardiac mortality and a reduced risk of sudden cardiac death in patients with sustained VT or VF and depressed LV function. β-Blocking agents may therefore be an important addition to conventional antiarrhythmic treatment in patients with VT or VF and LV dysfunction.

In patients with CHF, the frequency of ventricular arrhythmias poorly predicts mortality. It is unknown whether the length of VT is a better predictor of mortality in these patients. Reese and associates[30] from Baltimore, Maryland, investigated the prognostic importance of the length of the longest run of VT, the frequency of VT, and the frequency of VPCs with 24-hour ambulatory electrocardiographic recordings in 122 patients with heart failure. They also determined whether the cause of heart failure affects the prognostic importance of these parameters. Each ambulatory electrocardiographic recording was evaluated for the frequency of VPCs and VT and for the length of the longest run of VT. For each electrocardiographic parameter patients were divided into groups based on the median value of that parameter. Mortality among groups was compared in all patients and then separately for nonischemic and ischemic patients. Neither the frequency of VPCs nor the frequency of VT predicted mortality whether or not cause was considered. When all patients were examined, the length of VT did predict an increased risk of death. However, when cause was considered, length of VT predicted mortality only in the nonischemic patients and not in the ischemic patients.

It was concluded that the length of VT may be the best electrocardiographic predictor of mortality in patients with nonischemic CHF.

Localizing the Arrhythmic Origin

Jadonath and associates[31] from Philadelphia, Pennsylvania, developed an algorithm on the basis of the QRS morphology observed on the 12-lead electrocardiogram that would rapidly locate the site of origin of the monomorphic VT arising from the septal portion of the RV outflow tract. Radiofrequency catheter ablation guided by pace-mapping techniques has proven effective in eliminating the VT originating from the RV outflow tract in the absence of structural heart disease. A method that would rapidly identify the portion of the RV outflow tract septum toward which more detailed pace-mapping should be directed before catheter ablation would be useful in decreasing procedure time and radiation exposure and potentially facilitating a successful ablation procedure. The RV outflow tract septum was divided into 9 sites. In 11 patients, bipolar pacing was performed at each of the 9 designated sites to mimic VT. A standard 12-lead surface electrocardiogram was recorded during pacing. The QRS morphology in the limb leads was characterized and the site of the R-wave transition was determined in the precordial leads. A QS in lead aVR and a monophasic R wave in leads II, III, aVF, and V_6 were noted in each patient at all paced sites. In lead I, pacing at the 3 posterior septal sites always resulted in an R wave. Pacing at the 3 anterior sites produced a dominant Q wave (either QS or Qr) at 17 (52%) of 33 sites or a qR complex at 16 (48%) of 33 sites. In lead aVL, a QS complex was noted while pacing at all anterior sites. Although pacing at posterior sites frequently resulted in a QS complex in lead aVL (20 [61%] of 33 sites), an R wave was frequently observed in this lead (13 [39%] of 33 sites). Early precordial R-wave transition (R/S ≥ 1 in V_1, V_2, or V_3) was observed while pacing at the majority (55%) of the posterior and superior sites but infrequently (20%) at the remaining RV outflow tract septal sites. Moving diagonally from the superior-posterior aspect of RV outflow tract septum to the anterior-inferior region resulted in a delay in the precordial R-wave transition. The QRS morphology in leads I and aVL and the precordial R-wave transition pattern appears to be useful in locating the site on the RV outflow tract septum, from which VT originates. Analysis of the QRS pattern of the VT helps to guide catheter positioning necessary for precise localization before application of radiofrequency energy.

Patterns of Coronary Narrowing

Most patients with serious exercise-induced ventricular arrhythmias have extensive CAD. These arrhythmias develop, however, only in a minority of patients with angina pectoris. Berntsen and associates[32] from Tromsø, Norway, investigated whether these arrhythmia patients are characterized by any specific arrhythmogenic pattern of CAD. Among 1100 consecutive patients undergoing CABG, 30 (2.7%) patients had VT or VF during preoperative exercise testing. For each of these patients, 2 matched control subjects with angina pectoris without ventricular arrhythmia were selected. All patients underwent angiocardiography by standard techniques. The recordings were blinded and interpreted in random order by an experienced invasive cardiologist. Significant stenosis (≥50%) of the LM coronary artery was found in 27% of the case patients compared with 12%

of the matched control subjects; proximal LAD artery stenoses were more frequent in the arrhythmia patients. Although stenosis ≥75% was only moderately more frequent in the case patients, the difference was highly significant for stenosis ≥95%, which was seen in 47% of the case patients compared with 22% of the control patients. The difference was even more pronounced for the combination of left main coronary artery stenosis and/or high-grade stenosis (≥95%) of the LAD artery. This pattern was seen in 60% of the case patients compared with 28% of the matched control patients. In addition, concurrent stenosis of the right coronary artery was seen in 14 (47%) of these case patients compared with 12 (20%) in the matched control patients. These results suggest that exercise-induced VT and VF are associated with a specific arrhythmogenic pattern of coronary artery obstruction consisting of the LM coronary artery or the proximal LAD artery. The additional effect of concurrent right coronary artery involvement may be through an impaired collateral supply to the LAD territory.

Amiodarone

Ammar and coworkers[33] in Los Angeles, California, determined the effects of chronic amiodarone treatment on systolic and diastolic function in patients with cardiac disease undergoing treatment for resistant ventricular arrhythmias. Previous studies have shown that chronic amiodarone treatment either has no effect or increases LVEF, but the effects on diastolic properties of the ventricle have not been defined. Twelve male patients were given loading doses of amiodarone followed by a maintenance regimen. Serial measurements of heart rate, BP, and indexes of systolic and diastolic function were measured by Doppler echocardiographic techniques at baseline conditions and at 2, 8, and 12 weeks of drug therapy. Changes in altered thyroid state were excluded by serial determinations of thyroid function. Amiodarone increased LVEF (+16% by 8 weeks), decreased presystolic ejection period/LV ejection time (−12%), and increased velocity of circumferential fiber shortening (+22%). Amiodarone decreased mitral inflow velocity peak E/peak A, and increased deceleration and isovolumic relaxation times incrementally. Chronically administered amiodarone can improve systolic function and exert a negative lusitropic action in patients with heart disease.

To identify whether electrophysiological study results during early-phase amiodarone therapy can be predicted by previous electrophysiological study, Ferrick and associates[34] from Bronx, New York, reviewed the electrophysiological data of 50 patients with inducible sustained ventricular arrhythmias who underwent 4.3±1.3 drug trials before being given amiodarone. Study results during testing with agents of the modified Vaughan-Williams Ia classification were compared with data obtained after 2 weeks of amiodarone therapy. Partial response by electrophysiological study was defined as well-tolerated VT <150 beats/min associated with BP ≥90 mm Hg. Significant slowing in the rate of induced VT was seen during therapy with both Ia agents and amiodarone, although there was a trend toward greater slowing during amiodarone treatment. Two of 3 patients with noninducible VT during amiodarone showed profound VT slowing during Ia therapy. Thirty-eight of 50 patients demonstrated concordance of electrophysiological study results with regard to achieving partial response criteria. Twenty patients died during a mean follow-up period of

37±29 months; 7 of the 10 sudden deaths occurred in patients who did not meet partial response criteria. It was concluded that patients with inducible sustained ventricular arrhythmias failing serial drug testing with Ia agents only rarely have their VT suppressed during amiodarone therapy. Partial response criteria are often concordant between testing on agents of the Ia classification and amiodarone, and there was no significant difference in survival in patients based on their partial response status.

The efficiency of prophylactic antiarrhythmic treatment with amiodarone in reducing 1-year mortality in patients with reduced LVEF (<35%) and asymptomatic ventricular arrhythmias was investigated in a prospective, multicenter, randomized, controlled study by Garguichevich and colleagues[35] from Rosario, Argentina. Among 127 patients who entered the study, 61 were assigned to no antiarrhythmic therapy (control group) and 66 to amiodarone treatment (amiodarone group). Amiodarone was administered at a dosage of 800 mg/d for 2 weeks followed by 400 mg/d thereafter. A 12-month follow-up was completed for 106 patients (57 in the amiodarone group and 49 in the control group). Amiodarone reduced the overall mortality rate, which was 11% in the amiodarone group vs. 29% in the control group, and sudden death rate, which was 7.0% in the amiodarone group vs. 20% in the control group. Side effects were rare, and in only 3 patients did amiodarone treatment have to be discontinued.

Amiodarone vs. Bretylium

Kowey and colleagues[36] in Wynnewood, Pennsylvania, designed a study to compare the safety and efficacy of a high and a low dose of intravenous amiodarone with bretylium, the only approved class III antiarrhythmic agent. A total of 302 patients with refractory, hemodynamically destabilizing VT or VF were enrolled in this double-blind trial at 82 medical centers in the United States. They were randomly assigned to therapy with intravenous bretylium or intravenous amiodarone administered in a high dose (1.8 g) or a low dose (0.2 g). The primary analysis included arrhythmia event rate during the first 48 hours of therapy, and it showed comparable efficacy between the bretylium group and the high-dose amiodarone group that was greater than noted for the low-dose amiodarone group. Overall mortality in the 48-hour double-blind period was 14% and was not significantly different among the three treatment groups. More patients treated with bretylium had hypotension compared with the 2 amiodarone groups. More patients remained on the 1000 mg amiodarone regimen than the other regimens. Thus, these data suggest that bretylium and amiodarone have comparable efficacy for the treatment of malignant ventricular arrhythmias, but bretylium use may be limited by a higher incidence of hypotension.

Sotalol vs. Procainamide

Sotalol is the prototype class III agent that combines β-blocking properties with the propensity to prolong the effective refractory period by lengthening the action potential duration. Its precise effect on the prevention of VT/VF compared to class I agents has not been evaluated in a blinded study. In a double-blind parallel-design multicenter study by Singh and associates[37] from Los Angeles and San Francisco, California; Chicago, Illinois; Washington, DC; and Princeton, New Jersey, the electrophysiological and antiarrhythmic effects of intravenous and oral sotalol (n=55) and procainamide (n=55) were therefore compared in patients with VT/VF inducible by programmed electric stimulation. Sotalol produced a greater effect on lengthening the ventricular effective refractory period. It prevented the inducibility of VT/VF in 30% vs. 20% for procainamide. In an alternate therapy group (n=41) of similar patients previously refractory to or intolerant of procainamide, intravenous sotalol prevented inducibility in 32%. The pooled overall sotalol efficacy rate was 31%. There was a significant relation between the increase in the ventricular effective refractory period and the prevention of inducibility of VT/VF. Ventricular effective refractory period of ≥300 msec was critical for the prevention of VT/VF inducibility. Thirteen sotalol and 6 procainamide responders from the randomly assigned group and 30 from the nonrandomized groups completed 1 year of sotalol therapy follow-up. Life-table analysis of these patients in each group showed a trend in favor of sotalol. Both sotalol and procainamide were well tolerated. In the randomly assigned group there was 1 case of sudden death during treatment with sotalol and 2 cases of nonfatal torsades de pointes in the procainamide group and 2 in the sotalol group; in the nonrandomized alternate therapy group, there were 6 cases of nonfatal torsades de pointes. These data support the emerging role of sotalol in the control of symptomatic VT and VF.

Radiofrequency Catheter Ablation

Ventricular ectopic activity is commonly encountered in practice and is usually relatively benign. However, frequent VPCs can be symptomatic in some patients. Zhu and colleagues[38] examined the role of radiofrequency catheter ablation in these patients. Ten patients with frequent and severely symptomatic monomorphic ventricular ectopic beats were selected from three tertiary care centers. These patients had been unable to tolerate or were unsuccessfully treated with a mean of 5 antiarrhythmic drugs. The site of origin of ectopic activity was mapped, and frequent VPCs were eliminated by catheter ablation in all 10 patients. None had inducible VT. During a mean follow-up of 10 months, no patient had a recurrence of symptomatic ectopic activity. These authors concluded that radiofrequency catheter ablation can successfully eliminate monomorphic ventricular ectopic activity and is therefore a reasonable alternative for the treatment of severely symptomatic, drug-resistant, monomorphic VPCs in patients without significant structural heart disease.

Cardiac Arrest

Cardiopulmonary Resuscitation

To determine the effect of location within the hospital and preexisting electrocardiographic rhythm on the outcome of cardiopulmonary resuscitation, Karetzky and associates[39] from Newark, New Jersey, retrospectively reviewed the cardiopulmonary resuscitation records for a 3-year period in 668 hospitalized patients. Resuscitation was successful in only 12 patients in the intensive care unit (3.3%) and in 43 patients not in the intensive care unit (14%), 20 of whom were on a telemetry unit. Patients who survived to discharge had similar 1-year survival rates regardless of initial hospital location, although intensive care unit

Table 4-2. Cardiopulmonary Resuscitation Survival by Sex and Race (n = 668)

Group	n	No. (%) Survival to Discharge	1-Y Survival
Sex			
F	346 (51.7)	34 (9.8)	28 (8.0)
M	322 (48.2)	21 (6.5)	16 (4.9)
P	. . .	>.05	>.05
Race			
B	426 (63.7)	28 (6.6)	24 (5.6)
W	242 (36.3)	27 (11.2)	20 (8.3)
P	. . .	<.05	>.05

Reproduced with permission from Karetsky et al.[39]

patients had the best 3-year survival rate, and there were no survivors at 3 years in the group that received cardiopulmonary resuscitation in the nonmonitored hospital bed. Survival was best with an initial cardiac rhythm of VT or VF, but all non-VTs were associated with survival (Table 4-2). Age was not an apparent factor, while survival to hospital discharge favored whites over blacks. Futile resuscitative efforts are routinely performed in part because physicians and patients are unaware of outcome results and factors that influence survival. A wide recognition of the limitations of cardiopulmonary resuscitation should lead to advanced directives that reflect this awareness, with substantially more patients choosing not to have cardiopulmonary resuscitation.

Grubb and associates[40] from Edinburgh, United Kingdom, sought to identify factors that predict in-hospital death among patients who initially survived out-of-hospital cardiac arrests. The authors investigated 346 consecutive cases of out-of-hospital cardiac arrests received by a single center in their city (270 patients examined retrospectively, 76 prospectively). Of the retrospective cohort, 246 cases were thought to be of cardiac origin. There were associations between in-hospital mortality and prearrest variables, resuscitation variables, and factors measured during admission. Crew-witnessed arrests were associated with low mortality; arrest rhythm, resuscitation by a health professional, conscious level on admission, and requirement for ventilation independently predicted in-hospital mortality. A weighted prognostic scoring system based on 3 of these variables accurately predicted the likelihood of in-hospital death in the prospective test group. Further assessment of conscious level during admission with the Glasgow coma score predicted mortality rates in the study population, but coma did not predict a hopeless prognosis in individual cases unless it persisted for 72 hours or more. Accurate prognostic assessment of out-of-hospital cardiac arrest survivors can be made from information available on admission. Of factors that independently predicted outcome, the skill of the resuscitator is most readily modified. This suggests that public training in resuscitation may reduce mortality rates.

To determine factors associated with cardiopulmonary resuscitation being attempted after cardiac arrest from AMI, in or outside of a hospital, and estimate short-term and long-term survival rates, Heller and associates[41] from Newcastle, Australia, examined 4924 men and women (age, 25–69) from a community-based register of all suspected heart attacks and sudden cardiac deaths in the

Lower Hunter region of New South Wales, Australia. Cardiopulmonary resuscitation was attempted in 41% of cases of cardiac arrest after AMI outside of a hospital and 63% of cases in hospital. Survival rates at 28 days were 12% and 39%, respectively. Among the survivors, although 41% had another AMI (or coronary death), 81% of both groups were still alive 2 years later. Younger and better educated people were more likely to receive cardiopulmonary resuscitation in either setting, and being married predicted cardiopulmonary resuscitation being attempted outside of a hospital. Younger age predicted better survival rates after attempted resuscitation in hospital. The reasons for better education to predict cardiopulmonary resuscitation being attempted need explanation. The higher survival rate after cardiopulmonary resuscitation in hospital compared with outside of a hospital and the good long-term prognosis for survivors in both settings suggest that attempts to improve success of cardiopulmonary resuscitation outside of a hospital may be worthwhile.

In Morbid Obesity

Patients with morbid obesity have high rates of sudden, unexpected cardiac death. The mechanism of death in these patients is uncertain. Duflou and associates[42] from Sydney, Australia; Washington, DC; and Baltimore, Maryland, compared 28 patients with morbid obesity (22 sudden cardiac deaths and 6 unnatural deaths) with 11 age-matched nonobese patients with traumatic deaths. Heart weight, LV cavity diameter, LV and RV wall thickness, ventricular septal thickness, epicardial fat thickness, and extent of coronary artery atherosclerosis were determined; myocyte size, nuclear size, and degree of interstitial fibrosis were calculated morphometrically. Mean heart weights in the patients with morbid obesity were increased but remained constant as a percentage of body weight. Of the gross parameters, only heart weight and LV cavity size were independent predictors of obesity. Of microscopic parameters, only nuclear area was an independent predictor of obesity. Of 22 patients with morbid obesity, dilated cardiomyopathy was the most frequent cause of sudden cardiac death (10 patients) followed by severe coronary atherosclerosis (6), concentric LV hypertrophy without LV dilatation (4), pulmonary embolism (1), and hypoplastic coronary arteries (1). The cardiomyopathy of morbid obesity is characterized by cardiomegaly, LV dilatation, and myocyte hypertrophy in the absence of interstitial fibrosis. It is the most common cause of sudden cardiac death in these patients.

Effect of Smoking Cessation

Some of the adverse effects of smoking are reduced when people quit smoking. Peters and colleagues[43] used the CAST trial to evaluate the effect of cigarette smoking cessation on overall mortality and the incidence of arrhythmic death. Of 2752 patients randomly assigned to blinded therapy, 1026 were smoking at the time of their baseline examination. Of these, 517 stopped smoking by the time of the 4-month visit and 509 continued to smoke. Over a mean follow-up period of about 16 months, there were 17 arrhythmic deaths and 32 total deaths among the quitters vs. 30 and 45, respectively, among the smokers. Most of the fatal events occurred in a group at high risk of ongoing ischemia. These authors concluded that smoking cessation was accompanied by a marked reduction in arrhythmic death and overall mortality that achieves statistical significance in a high-risk cohort. These data reaffirm reduction of this important risk factor can benefit patients with advanced ischemic disease.

Shen and colleagues[44] in Rochester, Minnesota, evaluated the incidence and correlates of sudden unexpected nontraumatic death among young adults in a well-surveyed population. The incidence and pathogenesis of sudden unexpected nontraumatic death in a young adult population (age, 20–40 years) have not been well defined. All residents 20–40 years old from Olmsted County, Minnesota, who had nontraumatic sudden death between 1960 and 1989 were included. Histological and gross cardiac specimens were examined. The incidence of sudden death was estimated based on the ratio of number of observed events to relative census data for the Olmsted County population from the last 3 decades. Statistical comparisons between age decades were obtained with χ^2 test. Incidence trends were tested using Poisson regression. Of the 54 subjects, 19 were women ($4.1/10^5$ population annually) and 35 were men ($8.7/10^5$ population annually). An increase in incidence of sudden death was evident in men. Causes of death included CAD, noncardiovascular disease, suspected primary arrhythmia, vascular disease, myocarditis, hypertrophic cardiomyopathy, and unknown causes. Gross and histological features suggestive of RV dysplasia were found in 9 subjects (17%), but 6 of these 9 had other established causes of death. Of the 27 sudden deaths between 1980 and 1989, 9 (33%) had a history of cocaine abuse. A trend in increasing incidence of sudden death in young men is noted. A high prevalence of cocaine abuse was observed in young adults who died suddenly. Histological features of RV dysplasia were prevalent but were not necessarily the primary cause of death.

Effect of β-Blockers

Kendall and associates[45] from Oslo, Norway, evaluated more than 400 original and reviewed articles on the usefulness of β-blockers in preventing sudden coronary death and concluded the following: "Of all the therapies currently available for the prevention of sudden cardiac death, none is more established or more effective than β-blockers. Indeed, the evidence that β-blockers have a cardioprotective effect is compelling. They probably reduce the rate of atheroma formation; they reduce the risk for VF in animal models of myocardial ischemia; they appear to reduce cardiac mortality in primary prevention trials; and they reduce mortality, particularly from sudden death, in patients who have had AMI. Moreover, withholding β-blockers because of problems perceived to be associated with them is usually not warranted and may frequently prevent their use in those who will benefit most from them."

Effect of n-3 Polyunsaturated Fatty Acids

To assess whether the dietary intake of long-chain n-3 polyunsaturated fatty acids from seafood, assessed both directly and indirectly through a biomarker, is associated with a reduced risk of primary cardiac arrest, Siscovick and associates,[46] from several medical centers in the United States, assessed a total of 334 case patients with primary cardiac arrest (age, 25–74 years) attended by paramedics from 1988–1994 and 493 population-based control cases and control subjects, matched for age and sex, randomly identified from the community.

All cases and control subjects were free of prior clinical heart disease, major comorbidity, and use of fish oil supplements. Compared with no dietary intake of eicosapentaenoic acid and docosahexaenoic acid, an intake of 5.5 g of n-3 fatty acids per month (the mean of the third quartile and the equivalent of 1 fatty fish meal per week) was associated with a 50% reduction in the risk of primary cardiac arrest (OR, 0.5), after adjustment for potential confounding factors. Compared with a red blood cell membrane, n-3 polyunsaturated fatty acid level of 3.3% of total fatty acid level of 5.0% of total fatty acids (the mean of the third quartile) was associated with a 70% reduction in the risk of primary cardiac arrest (OR, 0.3). Dietary intake of n-3 polyunsaturated fatty acids from seafood is associated with a reduced risk of primary cardiac arrest.

Effect of Heart Rate Variability

Prospective cohort studies suggest that phobic anxiety is a strong risk factor for fatal CAD, in particular, sudden cardiac death. It has also been established that reduced heart rate variability can identify patients at high risk for subsequent sudden cardiac death. Kawachi and coinvestigators[47] in Boston, Massachusetts, therefore hypothesized that persons with symptoms of phobic anxiety may exhibit reduced heart rate variability. The investigators tested their hypothesis in 581 men (age, 47–86 years) enrolled in the Normative Aging Study who were free of CAD and diabetes. Symptoms of anxiety were assessed using the Crown-Crisp index, an instrument that has been demonstrated in previous prospective studies to strongly predict risk of sudden cardiac death. Heart rate variability was measured under standardized conditions, with paced deep breathing (6 breaths each minute). Two measures of heart rate variability were used: the standard deviation of heart rate and the maximal minus minimal heart rate over 1 minute. Men reporting higher levels of phobic anxiety had a higher resting heart rate. After adjusting for age, mean heart rate, and BMI in analyses of covariance, men reporting higher levels of phobic anxiety had lower heart rate variability, whether measured by the standard deviation of heart rate, or maximal minus minimal heart rate. These data suggest that phobic anxiety is associated with altered cardiac autonomic control, and hence increased risk of sudden cardiac death.

Frequency of "Active" Coronary Lesions

Farb and colleagues[48] in Washington, DC, determined the frequency of active and inactive coronary lesions and AMI in individuals with sudden coronary death. The hearts of persons dying as a result of sudden coronary death underwent perfusion-fixation and postmortem angiography. An active coronary lesion was defined as a disrupted plaque, luminal fibrin/platelet thrombus, or both. Inactive lesions were defined as having a cross-sectional luminal stenosis ≥75% with neither plaque disruption nor luminal thrombus. Ninety hearts were examined from 72 men and 18 women with a mean age at the time of death of 51 years. AMI was present in 19, healed AMI in 37, and no AMI in 34. Active coronary lesions were identified in 51: acute thrombi and disrupted plaques were found in 27, acute thrombi only in 21, and disrupted plaques only in 3. In hearts with AMI, active coronary lesions were significantly more prevalent than in hearts with only healed AMI or hearts lacking an acute or healed AMI.

Hearts without acute or healed AMI and without active lesions were similar to hearts with active lesions as regards heart weight and severity of epicardial CAD. Acute changes in coronary plaque morphology, including thrombus, plaque disruption, or both, were found in 57% of patients with sudden coronary events. In hearts with myocardial scars and no AMI, active coronary lesions were found in 46% of cases. Neither AMI nor an active coronary lesion was present in 19% of hearts.

Syncope

Importance of History for Delineation of Types

Calkins and associates[49] from Ann Arbor and Detroit, Michigan, identified and quantitated the symptoms associated with neurocardiogenic syncope, syncope due to VT, and syncope resulting from AV block. They studied 80 patients referred for evaluation of syncope in whom a diagnosis of neurocardiogenic syncope, AV block, or VT was established. Each patient was interviewed using a standard questionnaire. The clinical histories were then compared to identify which variables best differentiated the cause of syncope. The clinical histories of patients with syncope caused by VT and AV block were similar. Only age, the duration of prodromal symptoms, diaphoresis before syncope, and fatigue after syncope differed. In contrast, the clinical history in patients with neurocardiogenic syncope differed greatly from that obtained in patients with syncope caused by AV block or VT. Features of the clinical history that were predictive of syncope caused by AV block or VT were male sex, age >54 years, two or fewer episodes of syncope, and a duration of warning of ≤5 seconds. Features of the clinical history predictive of syncope not caused by VT or AV block were palpitations, blurred vision, nausea, warmth, diaphoresis, or lightheadedness before syncope, and nausea, warmth, diaphoresis, or fatigue after syncope. The results of this study identify and compare the features of the clinical history obtained in patients with syncope due to VT, AV block, and neurocardiogenic syncope and demonstrate that the clinical history is of value in distinguishing patients with these 3 causes of syncope.

Provocation Maneuvers

The prognosis of patients manifesting prolonged asystole during head-up tilt testing is unclear. Dhala and colleagues[50] in Milwaukee, Wisconsin, found that in 209 consecutive patients with a history of syncope and positive head-up tilt tests, 19 had asystole lasting >5 seconds (group 1a). When compared with patients without asystole (group 1b), group 1a patients were younger (32 vs. 47 years), but clinical manifestations were not any more dramatic (the number of episodes of syncope and injury during syncope were similar). During follow-up (mean, 2 years), with the patient taking pharmacological therapy such as β-blockers, ephedrine, theophylline, or disopyramide, the recurrence rate was 11% and 8% in groups 1a and 1b. No patient in the asystole group underwent pacemaker implantation. Additionally, of 75 normal volunteers (group 2) with no history of syncope undergoing tilt tests to define its specificity, 3 had asystole (mean duration, 10 seconds). During >1 year of follow-up, despite no treatment, all 3 are symptom free. Thus, asystole during head-up tilt testing does not predict either a more malignant outcome or a poor response to pharmacological therapy. Moreover, an asystolic response does not enhance the specificity of the head-up tilt test because it may be present in asymptomatic "normal" volunteers.

Morillo and associates[51] from London, Canada, assessed the rate of positive head-up tilt, specificity, and same-day reproducibility of a head-up tilt at 60° combined with a low-dose isoproterenol infusion in the following patients: 120 consecutive patients with recurrent unexplained syncope, 30 healthy patients in a control group, and 30 patients with documented syncope not related to a vasodepressor reaction. Head-up tilt was positive in 61% (73 of 120) of patients with unexplained syncope. The false-positive rate in both the control and documented syncope groups was 6.6%. The mean isoproterenol dose infused was 1.4±0.5, 1.3±0.4, and 1.3±0.5 μg/min, respectively. Head-up tilt was positive during the drug-free stage in 30 (25%) of 120 patients, and isoproterenol infusion was necessary in the remaining 43 (36%) patients. Immediate reproducibility was assessed in 75 patients, and head-up tilt response was reproduced in 37 (82%) of 45 patients with a baseline positive head-up tilt and in 28 (93%) of 30 patients with a baseline negative response. Overall, sensitivity, specificity, and reproducibility were 61%, 93%, and 86%, respectively. Clinical variables that increased the probability of a positive outcome were age ≤50 years and two or more syncopal episodes in the preceding 6 months in the absence of structural heart disease. These data support the use of a head-up tilt protocol with low-dose isoproterenol infusion for the assessment of patients with recurrent syncope.

Natale and colleagues[52] in Milwaukee, Wisconsin, evaluated the specificity of head-up tilt testing using different tilt angles and isoproterenol infusion rates in normal volunteers with no prior history of syncope. One hundred fifty volunteers were randomly assigned to two groups of 75 each. In group 1, subjects were further randomized to have head-up tilt testing at 60°, 70°, or 80° angle at baseline followed by repeat tilt testing during a low-dose isoproterenol infusion that increased heart rate by an average of 20%. In group 2, after having a baseline head-up tilt test at a 70° angle for a maximum of 20 minutes, subjects were randomized to have a repeat tilt table testing at a 70° angle during low-dose (1.5 μg/min), medium-dose (3 μg/min), or higher-dose (5 μg/min) isoproterenol infusion. In group 1, syncope or presyncope with hypotension developed in 2 subjects during the baseline test at 60° and 70° of tilt and in 5 subjects during tilting at 80°. In 6 of 10 subjects with a positive test at an 80° angle, there was an abnormal response after 10 minutes of tilt testing. In group 2, using various isoproterenol doses with tilt testing at a 70° angle, 1.5, 3, and 5 μg/min elicited abnormal responses in 1, 5, and 14 of the subjects. Regression analysis demonstrated that head-up tilt testing at 80° angle or during 3 and 5 μg/min isoproterenol infusion rates are the most significant predictors of an abnormal response. Thus, head-up tilt testing at a 60° or 70° angle with or without low-dose isoproterenol infusion provides adequate specificity for this type of testing. Caution is needed, however, in interpreting results if the head-up tilt test at 80° is extended beyond 10 minutes or if high doses of isoproterenol are used.

Head-up tilt testing has proved to be useful in provocation of neurocardiogenic syncope. The purpose of this study by Hou and colleagues[53] from Taiwan, Republic of China, was to examine whether simply assuming an upright posture by standing can be an alternative to the head-up tilt testing for diagnosis of neurocardiogenic syncope. Eighty-four patients with recurrent unexplained syncope and 22 normal volunteers were recruited into the study. Forty-seven patients with syncope and all normal volunteers received the standing test. Thirty-seven of the patients with syncope received head-up tilt testing (90°). All individuals laid down for 5 minutes and then assumed an upright posture until syncope or presyncope occurred or until a maximum of 10 minutes was reached in each stage of the test. The tests included 4 stages: baseline and infusion of 1, 2, or 3 µg/min isoproterenol in each of the successive stages. Five individuals could not tolerate the procedure, and further testing was terminated. Overall, the standing test was positive in 83% of the patients with syncope, and its specificity was 74%. The head-up tilt testing was positive in 75% of the patients with syncope. The duration of assuming an upright posture before occurrence of syncope or presyncope was significantly longer in the syncope-tilting group in the third and fourth stage compared with the syncope-standing group. However, the curves of the time course for cumulative positive rates were not significantly different in the 2 groups. The standing test can serve as an alternative to head-up tilt testing and can be applied to patients with recurrent unexplained syncope for confirmation of the diagnosis.

In Athletes

Calkins and associates[54] from Ann Arbor, Michigan, and Baltimore, Maryland, reported a series of patients who were referred for evaluation of syncope that occurred during or immediately after exercise and in whom a diagnosis of vasodepressor syncope was established (9 women and 8 men; mean age, 28±17 years). The approach to management was individualized in each patient. All patients were monitored to determine the frequency and type of recurrent symptoms. The mean age at onset of symptoms was 23±16 years. In 10 patients syncope occurred only in association with exercise. Pharmacological therapy was successful in normalizing the patients' response to upright tilt in each of the 10 patients in whom it was attempted. During a mean follow-up period of 35±9 months, none of the patients placed on pharmacological therapy had recurrent syncope. Seventeen (88%) of 19 patients resumed participation in athletics. The results of this study demonstrate that vasodepressor syncope is a cause of syncope in athletes and that patients with exercise-related vasodepressor syncope can safely continue to participate in athletics.

Pindolol

Cohen and associates[55] from Manhasset, New York, evaluated the efficacy, safety, and tolerance of pindolol as initial therapy for vasovagal syncope. Head-up tilt table testing was performed on 192 patients for syncope or near-syncope of unknown cause. Forty-four (23%) patients had a positive head-up tilt table test for vasovagal syncope, and 28 (64%) received oral pindolol as initial therapy. Three patients were lost to follow-up; of the remaining 25 patients (mean age, 60±22 years), 15 were women, 14 had syncope, and 11 had near-syncope. At 14±6 months follow-up, 16 (64%) patients were without recurrence or side effects from pindolol. Of the 9 patients who stopped taking pindolol, 3 were switched to another regimen for recurrent symptoms, 2 stopped because of side

Table 4-3. Vasovagal International Study Classification for Tilt-Induced Cardioneurogenic (Vasovagal) Syncope*

Type 1, mixed
    Heart rate initially increases with head-up tilt and later decreases, but remains above 40 beats/min or is less than 40 beats/min only briefly (<10 s), and without asystole ≥3 s. Blood pressure may increase initially but later decreases before heart rate decreases.
Type 2A, cardioinhibitory
    Heart rate increases with tilting, then decreases to <40 beats/min for >10 s, or has asystole >3 s. Blood pressure may increase initially but decreases before the heart rate decreases.
Type 2B, cardioinhibitory
    Heart rate increases initially, then decreases to <40 beats/min for >10 s, or has asystole >3 s. Blood pressure decreases to hypotensive levels only at or after the time at which heart rate decreases.
Type 3, pure vasodepressor
    Heart rate increases initially and decreases less than 10% from peak value at time of syncope. Blood pressure decreases to account for syncope.

*This table does not include the exceptions catalogued by the Vasovagal International Study investigators.
Reproduced with permission from Benditt et al.[56]

effects, and 4 did not comply with the regimen. In conclusion, pindolol appears to be safe and effective as initial treatment for vasovagal syncope.

Cardiac Pacing

Benditt and associates[56] from Minneapolis, Minnesota, and London, United Kingdom, and Toledo, Ohio, provided an excellent review on cardiac pacing for prevention of recurrent vasovagal syncope. A vasovagal international study classification for tilt-induced cardioneurogenic (vasovagal) syncope was presented in Table 4-3.

Long Q-T Interval Syndrome

Review

Tan and associates[57] from Stanford, California, provided a superb review of electrophysiological mechanisms of the long QT interval syndromes and torsades de pointes. In their article, the authors provided a table showing the modified Vaughan-Williams classification of antiarrhythmic drugs (Table 4-4), and also a summary of short- and long-term treatment for torsades de pointes caused by acquired and hereditary long QT interval syndromes (Table 4-5).

Genetic Abnormality

Schwartz and colleagues[58] tested the hypothesis that the QT interval would shorten more in patients with long QT syndrome genes linked to chromosome 3 than in those genes linked to chromosome 7 in response to mexiletine and also with increases in heart rate. Fifteen patients with a long QT syndrome were evaluated. Six had the long QT syndrome in association with genes linked to chromosome 3 and 7 with genes linked to chromosome 7. These patients were treated with mexiletine and its effects on QT and QT_c were measured. Mexiletine significantly shortened the QT interval among patients with long

Table 4-4. Modified Vaughan-Williams Classification of Antiarrhythmic Drugs

Class	Pharmacological Effect	Antiarrhythmic Drugs
IA	Depresses rapid action potential upstroke and decreases conduction velocity (Na$^+$ channel blockade) and significantly prolongs repolarization (K$^+$ channel blockade)	Quinidine, procainamide, disopyramide
IB	Depresses rapid action potential upstroke in abnormal tissue (little effect in normal tissue) and enhances repolarization	Mexilitene, lidocaine, tocainide, moricizine*
IC	Markedly depresses rapid action potential upstroke and decreases conduction velocity (Na$^+$ channel blockade) but exerts little effect on repolarization (little or no K$^+$ channel blockade)	Propafenone, encainide, flecainide, moricizine*
II	Blocks adrenergic receptors	Propranolol, metoprolol, atenolol, and others
III	Primarily blocks K$^+$ channels and slows repolarization (little or no Na$^+$ channel blockade)	Sotalol, amiodarone, bretylium, N-acetylprocainamide
IV	Blocks Ca^{2+} channels	Verapamil, diltiazem, nifedipine, and others

*Moricizine has been variously classified as a class IB and class IC agent.
Reproduced with permission from Tan et al.[57]

Table 4-5. Summary of Short- and Long-Term Treatments for Torsades de Pointes Caused by the Acquired and Hereditary Long QT Interval Syndromes*

Treatment	Mechanism	Acquired LQTS (Pause-Dependent)	Hereditary LQTS (Adrenergic-Dependent)
Short-term	Remove inciting factors	Withdraw offending agent and correct predisposing conditions, such as hypokalemia, bradycardia, or hypomagnesemia	Correct contributing or predisposing conditions such as hypokalemia, bradycardia, or hypomagnesemia
	Blockade of Na^+ and Ca^{2+} current	Lidocaine, magnesium	Lidocaine, magnesium
	Increase heart rate and activate K^+ currents	β_1-Adrenergic agonists such as isoproterenol; temporary overdrive electrical pacing	β_1-Adrenergic agonists are contraindicated; temporary overdrive electrical pacing
	Inhibit adrenergic and sympathetic activity	Contraindicated because of negative chronotropic effects	β_1-Adrenergic antagonists such as propranolol and esmolol
Long-term	Avoid inciting factors	Withhold offending agent (and all similar agents) and prevent predisposing metabolic or electrolyte disturbances	Prevent contributing or predisposing metabolic or electrolyte disturbances
	Inhibit adrenergic and sympathetic activity	Contraindicated because of negative chronotropic effects	β_1-Adrenergic blockers such as nadolol; Surgical high thoracic left sympathectomy
	Implantable device therapy	Pacemaker implantation for heart block or bradycardia-dependent LQTS; Cardioverter-defibrillator not indicated if offending agent can be identified and reliably withheld	Permanent pacemaker implantation with β_1-adrenergic blockers such as nadolol; Cardioverter-defibrillator implantation

*LQTS indicates long QT interval syndromes.
Reproduced with permission of Tan et al.[57]

QT interval genes linked to chromosome 3, but not among patients with a long QT interval genes linked to chromosome 7. The long QT interval linked to chromosome 3 patients shortened their QT interval in response to increases in heart rate more than patients in whom the long QT interval genes were linked to chromosome 7 and more than 18 healthy control subjects. There was a trend for patients with a long QT interval genes linked to chromosome 7 to have syncope or cardiac arrest under emotional or physical stress and for the patients whose long QT interval genes are linked to chromosome 3 to have cardiac events either at rest or during sleep. Thus, this study demonstrates differential responses of patients with long QT intervals to interventions targeted to their specific genetic defect. The data suggest that patients whose long QT interval genes are linked to chromosome 3 are more likely to benefit from sodium channel blockers, such as mexiletine, and to cardiac pacing and to be at risk for arrhythmias at slower heart rates. On the other hand, patients with a long QT interval genes linked to chromosome 7 may be at higher risk to develop syncope under stressful conditions because of the combined arrhythmic potential of catecholamines with an insufficient adaptation of the QT interval with heart rate increases.

Moss and colleagues[59] investigated electrocardiographic T-wave patterns in members of families linked to 3 genetically distinct forms of the long QT syndrome. Five quantitative electrocardiographic repolarization variables, i.e., 4 Bazett-corrected time intervals ($QT_{onset-c}$, QT_{peak-c}, QT_c, and $T_{duration-c}$, in milliseconds) and the absolute height of the T wave ($T_{amplitude}$, in millivolts), were measured in 153 members of 6 families with a long QT syndrome linked to markers on chromosome 3. Genotypic data were used to define each family member as being affected or unaffected with a long QT syndrome. Affected members of all 6 families had longer QT intervals than unaffected family members. Each of the three long QT syndrome genotypes was associated with somewhat distinctive electrocardiographic repolarization features. Among affected individuals, the QT was unusually prolonged in those individuals with mutations involving the cardiac sodium channel gene *SCN5A* on chromosome 3. This study emphasizes that a considerable variability exists in the quantitative repolarization variables associated with each genotype with overlap in the T-wave patterns among the 3 genotypes. In this study, three separate genetic loci for the long QT syndrome, including mutations in two cardiac ionic channel genes, were associated with different phenotypic T-wave patterns on the electrocardiogram. This study provides insight into the influence of genetic factors on electrocardiographic manifestations of ventricular repolarization.

Bundle Branch Block

Mairesse and coworkers[60] in Brussels, Belgium, compared the efficacy of dobutamine stress testing using 2-dimensional echocardiography and perfusion tomography for the noninvasive identification of CAD in patients with left BBB. Twenty-four patients with permanent, complete left BBB (11 with previous AMI) were studied prospectively with dobutamine echocardiography and perfusion tomography. The presence of >50% luminal diameter coronary stenosis was compared with the presence of dobutamine-induced fixed or reversible perfusion defects, and with resting or dobutamine-induced abnormalities of wall thickening. For each test, the LAD coronary artery territory was compared with the LC and/or right coronary artery. Significant CAD was found in the LAD coronary artery in 12 patients; all were identified by perfusion imaging, and 10 by two-dimensional stress echocardiography. In the 12 patients without LAD CAD, scintigraphy was also positive in all (specificity, 0%), and echocardiography in only 1 (specificity: 92%). The diagnostic accuracy was 50% and 87%, respectively. This low specificity of perfusion tomography was improved by requiring an associated apical defect to indicate LAD CAD and was corrected by restricting the diagnosis of CAD to those patients with partially reversible defects. In the LC and/or right coronary artery territory, sensitivity and specificity were similar using both techniques. The authors concluded that dobutamine-stress echocardiography is a specific and accurate test for the noninvasive identification of CAD, even in the LAD artery territory of patients with left BBB.

Heart Block

Brink and colleagues[61] in Tygerberg, South Africa, have determined by linkage analysis the approximate chromosomal position of the gene causing progressive familial heart block type I. Progressive familial heart block type I is a dominantly inherited cardiac bundle-branch conduction disorder that has been traced through nine generations of a large South African kindred. Eighty-six members of three pedigrees, 39 members of which were affected with progressive familial heart block type I, were genotyped at four linked polymorphic marker loci mapped to chromosome 19, bands q13.2–q13.3. Maximum 2-point logarithm of the odds scores, which represent the logarithm of the OR of detecting linkage compared with nonlinkage, generated were 6.49 for the kallikrein locus, 5.72 for the myotonic dystrophy locus, 3.44 for the creatine kinase muscle-type locus, and 4.51 for the apolipoprotein C2 locus. The maximum multipoint logarithm of the odds score was 11.6 with a 90% support interval positioning the progressive familial heart block type I locus within a 10 cM distance centering on the kallikrein 1 locus. The gene for progressive familial heart block type I maps to an area of approximately 10 cM on chromosome 19q13.2–13.3. These results provide a means of DNA-based diagnosis in the evaluation of families and a basis for cloning studies to identify the causative gene.

Pacemakers

Pacing the RV apex profoundly modifies the sequence of activation and thus the sequence of contraction and relaxation of the left ventricle. To evaluate the relative importance of preserving normal ventricular activation sequence and optimal AV synchrony in permanent pacing, Leclercq and associates[62] from Rennes, France, compared the effects of 3 pacing modes: AAI, preserving both normal AV synchrony and normal activation sequence; DDD, with complete ventricular capture that preserves only AV synchrony; and VVI, disrupting both, at rest and during exercise. Hemodynamic and radionuclide studies were performed in 11 patients who had normal intrinsic conduction and who were implanted on a long-term basis with a DDDR pacemaker for isolated sinus node dysfunction. AAI vs. DDD and VVI significantly increased cardiac output at rest (6.6±1.3 vs. 6±0.9 vs. 5±1 L/min) and during exercise (14±2 vs. 12±2.2 vs. 14±2.1 L/min). Pulmonary capillary wedge pressure was lowest with AAI (15±4.5 mm Hg), with an average reduction of 17% compared with DDD (20±5 mm Hg) and of 30% compared with VVI (26±7 mm Hg) during exercise. Identical benefits were observed for all other hemodynamic parameters: RA pressure, PA pressure, LV stroke work index, and systemic vascular resistances. LVEF was significantly higher in AAI than in DDD at rest (61% vs 58%, respectively) and during exercise (65% vs 60%, respectively). This improvement in LV systolic function resulted principally from the increase in septal ejection fraction. LV filling also was improved in AAI as demonstrated by a significant increase in peak filling rate at rest and during exercise. These data show the importance of preserving, whenever possible, not only normal AV synchrony but also normal ventricular activation sequence in permanent cardiac pacing.

Cardioverters-Defibrillators

Pinski and Trohman[63] provided an excellent review in the *Annals of Internal Medicine* of implantable cardioverter-defibrillators. The currently available cardioverter-defibrillators are listed in Table 4-6. The causes of frequent implantable cardioverter-defibrillators are summarized in Table 4-7.

Brooks and associates[64] from Boston, Massachusetts, analyzed 177 patients in whom a nonthoracotomy approach was initially used to implant a cardioverter-defibrillator system; 11 (6%) patients also received a separately implanted permanent pacemaker. The main problem encountered in these patients were previously implanted unipolar pacemakers (n=3) and ventricular pacing leads positioned at the RV apex, the latter interfering with optimal placement of the tripolar implantable cardioverter-defibrillator lead (n=9). The approaches used to solve these problems were individualized and included placement of the implantable cardioverter-defibrillator sensing lead at the RV outflow tract (n=3), initial placement (n=1) or subsequent repositioning (n=2) of the RV pacing lead at the outflow tract, upgrade from unipolar to bipolar systems (n=2), reprogramming from the DDD to AAI mode (n=2), inactivation of the pacemaker (n=1), and simultaneous placement of a single-chamber atrial pacemaker with the implantable cardioverter-defibrillator lead (n=2). These revisions fulfilled the pacing needs in each patient and prevented unfavorable sensing interaction between the 2 systems.

The exponential increase in cardioverter-defibrillator implantations has resulted in a need for safe implantations that do not require long waiting periods. Trappe and associates[65] from Hannover, Germany, report intraoperative and follow-up results in 48 patients with ventricular tachyarrhythmias who underwent cardioverter-defibrillator implantation (Cardiac Pacemakers Inc. or Ventritex Systems) in the catheterization laboratory. Twenty-six (54%) patients had their first cardioverter-defibrillator implant (group 1), and 22 (46%) patients underwent pulse-generator replacement (group 2). In all patients, cardioverter-defibrillator implant or pulse-generator replacement were performed with the patient under general anesthesia. In 25 (96%) of 26 patients in group 1, cardioverter-defibrillator implantation was possible with a mean defibrillation threshold of 13±8 J. One patient had a defibrillation threshold of >25 J, and therefore cardi-

Table 4-6. Currently Available Implantable Cardioverter-Defibrillators*

Manufacturer	Model	Therapies	Committed Shocks	Magnet Functions
CPI[†]	Ventak P 1600[‡]	LEC, shock	Committed	Inhibition of detection and therapy (<30 s) Deactivation (>30 s)
CPI[†]	Ventak P2 1625	LEC, shock, VVI	Programmable	Inhibition of detection and therapy (<30 s) Deactivation (>30 s)—programmable
CPI[†]	PRx 1705[‡]	ATP, LEC, shock, VVI	Programmable	Inhibition of detection and therapy (<30 s) Deactivation (>30 s)—programmable
Intermedics[§]	Res-Q	ATP, LEC, shock, VVI	Committed	Inhibition of detection and therapy VVI pacing at 100 beats per minute
Medtronic[‖]	PCD 7217B[‡]	ATP, LEC, shock, VVI	Noncommitted for VT Committed for VF	Inhibition of detection and therapy No effect on pacing
Medtronic[‖]	PCD 7219D	ATP, LEC, shock, VVI	Programmable (first shock), then committed	Inhibition of detection and therapy No effect on pacing
Telectronics[¶]	Guardian 4215	ATP, LEC, shock, VVI	Programmable	Inhibition of detection and therapy
Ventritex[**]	Cadence V100[‡]	ATP, LEC, shock, VVI	Noncommitted	Inhibits detection and therapy—programmable No effect on pacing

*ATP indicates antitachycardia pacing; LEC, low-energy cardioversion; shock, defibrillation shocks; VF, ventricular fibrillation; VT, ventricular tachycardia; VVI, ventricular antibradycardia pacing.
[†]Saint Paul, Minnesota.
[‡]Commercially available in the United States.
[§]Angleton, Texas.
[‖]Minneapolis, Minnesota.
[¶]Englewood, Colorado.
[**]Sunnyvale, California.
Reproduced with permission from Pinski and Trohman.[63]

Table 4-7. Causes of Frequent Implantable Cardiac Defibrillator Shocks

Sustained ventricular tachyarrhythmias
   Frequently recurring episodes, each one terminated by 1 shock
   >1 shock needed to terminate each episode of sustained ventricular tachyarrhythmia
Nonsustained ventricular tachyarrhythmias (committed devices)
Supraventricular rhythms satisfying detection criteria
   Atrial fibrillation
   Sinus tachycardia
   Paroxysmal supraventricular tachycardia
Oversensing of signals
   Sensing lead failure
   Double- and triple-counting of pacing artifacts
   T- and P-wave oversensing
   Electromagnetic interference
Random component failure

Reproduced with permission from Pinski and Trohman.[63]

overter-defibrillator implant was not achieved. This patient underwent epicardial device implantation 1 day later. Another patient in group 1 had vessel rupture (vena subclavia) intraoperatively. During a mean follow-up of 2±1 months, 2 patients died from CHF 2 and 4 months after device implantation. An infection occurred in 1 patient in group 2, 3 months after generator replacement. In conclusion, these data show that in the majority of patients cardioverter-defibrillator implantation in the catheterization laboratory is safe and has a low complication rate and therefore can generally be recommended.

Jordaens and associates[66] from Ghent, Belgium, analyzed 24 patients with VF or sustained VT who underwent implantation of a new Medtronic transvenous defibrillator. All patients had the device implanted without thoracotomy. High placement of a shock lead in the anonymous vein and inversion of the shock-wave polarity allowed avoidance of placement of subcutaneous patches. Implantation time decreased from 138 minutes for the first 12 patients to 82 minutes for the last 12 patients, with 4 and 11 subpectoral pockets, respectively. Three patients required a minor reintervention. No bleeding or infection occurred. One episode of pulmonary edema and 1 pulmonary embolism were seen in the postoperative course. No postoperative deaths were observed. During a mean follow-up period of 4.1 months, 58% of the 24 patients had symptomatic arrhythmic episodes, with shocks in 50% of the 24. Inappropriate shocks were delivered in 3 cases (AF and T-wave sensing). One episode was not terminated even with 4 internal shocks. One patient had VF because of a sensing problem. By reprogramming of sensitivity, back-up pacing, and adjustment of drug therapy these arrhythmic complications could be prevented. Pectoral implantation of a cardioverter-defibrillator is easy and can be performed by cardiologists experienced in pacemaker implantation. Careful postoperative observation reprogramming after the first spontaneous event and prehospital discharge induction of VF prevents arrhythmic complications.

Postoperative electrocardiographic changes are frequently present after insertion of implantable cardioverter-defibrillators and may mimic perioperative myocardial infarction. Osswald and coworkers[67] assessed the incidence and clinical significance of postoperative electrocardiographic changes in relation to clinical, laboratory, and implantation data. In 25 (16%) of 156 patients undergoing implantable cardioverter-defibrillator implantation, significant electrocardiographic changes (≥50% reduction in R-wave amplitude in three or more leads or new Q waves in two or more leads) were present 1 to 3 days after the operation and persisted at hospital discharge in 12 (8%). Presence of thoracotomy, the total number of induced VF episodes, and the number of defibrillation shocks required during defibrillation threshold testing correlated with postoperative electrocardiographic changes. Other factors associated with a significant R-wave loss in the lateral precordial leads included left-sided pleural effusion, lung infiltrates or atelectasis, and large defibrillator patch electrodes over the left ventricle or the lateral chest wall. Myocardial necrosis documented by elevated cardiac enzymes occurred in 6 (5%) of 151 patients without significant electrocardiographic changes and in 3 (12%) with such changes. However, postoperative electrocardiographic changes associated with elevated enzymes were indistinguishable from changes unrelated to necrosis. Therefore, the sensitivity and specificity of the surface electrocardiogram for detection of AMI after implantable cardioverter-defibrillator placement is poor. Multiple factors such as thoracotomy, myocardial injury from defibrillation threshold testing, electric insulation, or shielding of the heart may contribute to the development of electrocardiographic pseudo-infarct patterns.

Circadian variability has been described for the occurrence of many pathophysiological cardiac events in patients with heart disease. Wood and associates[68] from Richmond and Norfolk, Virginia, evaluated circadian variation in VT as detected by implantable cardioverter-defibrillators. Forty-three patients with late generation implantable defibrillators were followed for a mean of 226 days. The weighted distribution of 830 episodes of VT peaked between 2:00 and 3:00 P.M. These authors concluded that the distribution of ventricular tachyarrhythmias detected by the cardioverter-defibrillator follows a circadian pattern with a peak tachycardia frequency between noon and 5:00 P.M. This circadian periodicity has implications for patient management.

Raitt and colleagues[69] in Seattle, Washington, evaluated the records of 111 consecutive patients who had undergone transvenous cardioverter-defibrillator implantation for malignant ventricular arrhythmias. In each patient, all device tachyarrhythmia detections were examined and classified as VF, monomorphic VT, rapid polymorphic VT, or other. The number of events, time to first arrhythmia detection, and cycle length of monomorphic ventricular tachycardias were recorded. There were 55 patients with a history of only VF, and 56 with a history that included an episode of monomorphic VT. Over 14 months of follow-up with all patients initially off of antiarrhythmic medications, monophasic VT was detected by only 18% of patients with a history of only VF compared with 54% of those with a history that included monomorphic VT. Among patients who did detect monomorphic VT, those with a history of only VF had fewer episodes (7 vs. 20) and a shorter mean monomorphic ventricular tachycardia cycle length (279 vs. 314 msec) (Figure 4-5) than those without a clinical history of monomorphic VT. Abrupt onset of VF not preceded by monomorphic VT was detected in 11% of patients with VF only. Male sex, age <60 years, and monomorphic

| | Index Arrhythmia | | |
| | History of VF Only (n=55) | Any History of MVT (n=56) | *P* |
Arrhythmia Detection			
MVT	10 (18%)	30 (54%)	.002
Spontaneous VF	6 (11%)	NA	
>5 episodes of MVT	3 (5%)	21 (38%)	<.001
Mean number of MVTs per patient with MVT	6.6±7	20±31	<.001
Mean MVT cycle length	278±39	314±43	.03

Figure 4-5. Ventricular Arrhythmias Detected on Follow-up. VF indicates ventricular fibrillation; MVT, sustained monomorphic ventricular tachycardia; and NA, not available. Reproduced with permission from Raitt et al.[69]

VT inducible on electrophysiological study were all significantly associated with an increased likelihood of monomorphic VT detection. On multivariate analysis, the inducibility of monomorphic VT was the primary independent predictor of monomorphic VT detection but was of minimal incremental predictive value in the subgroup of patients with a history of only VF. When electrophysiological studies were not considered, arrhythmia history was the primary independent predictor of monomorphic VT. Thus, patients with a history of only VF infrequently have monomorphic VT detected by their defibrillators; when these patients detect monomorphic VT, it is faster than that detected in patients with a clinical history of monomorphic VT before implantable cardioverter-defibrillator surgery. A significant percentage of VF survivors had the abrupt onset of VF not preceded by monomorphic VT suggesting that the deterioration of rapid monomorphic VT to VT is not the only clinically important mechanism of VF induction.

Wever and colleagues[70] from the Netherlands analyzed the effectiveness of the implantable cardioverter-defibrillator as first-choice therapy compared with conventional therapeutic strategy beginning with antiarrhythmic drugs in 60 consecutive survivors of cardiac arrest associated with prior AMI. These patients were randomly assigned to early implantable defibrillator (n= 29) or conventional therapy (n=31). Clinical characteristics were similar in the 2 groups. Therapy in each group was guided by electrocardiographic monitoring, exercise testing, and programmed electrical stimulation. Primary end points, including death, recurrent cardiac arrest, and cardiac transplantation, number of invasive procedures, and antiarrhythmic therapy changes and duration of hospitalization were compared. Median follow-up was 24 months. In the group receiving an early implantable defibrillator, 4 patients died (14%) of cardiac causes. In the patients treated with antiarrhythmic agents, 20 patients failed this therapy and subsequently underwent mapping-guided VT surgery (6 patients) or implantable defibrillator implantation (14 patients). Of the 6 VT surgery patients, 1 died, 1 had a cardiac transplantation, and 1 had an implantable defibrillator placed because of persistent inducibility despite the addition of antiarrhythmic drugs. Among the 11 patients who remained on antiarrhythmic drugs as sole therapy, 2 died in the hospital before they could be retested by programmed electrical stimulation, leaving 9 believed to be adequately protected by antiarrhythmic drugs alone. Among those, 5 died and 1 survived recurrent cardiac arrest followed by implantable cardioverter-defibrillator placement. In total, 16 conventionally treated patients ultimately had implantable cardioverter-defibrillator implantation, 3 of whom died. The total mortality in the conventional group was 11 patients (35%) and 4 died suddenly, 5 died of CHF, and 2 died of noncardiac causes. Comparison of main outcome events in both strategies showed a significant difference in favor of early implantable cardioverter-defibrillator placement. The early cardioverter-defibrillator group had fewer invasive procedures, less therapy changes, and fewer days in the hospital. Therefore, these data suggest that the implantable cardioverter-defibrillator implantation as first choice is superior to conventional antiarrhythmic drug therapy in survivors of cardiac arrest associated with prior AMI.

Nunain and colleagues[71] in Boston, Massachusetts, examined the limitations and complex management problems associated with the use of tiered-therapy implantable cardioverter-defibrillators. The study group consisted of 154 patients having implantation of tiered-therapy implantable cardioverter-defibrillators at the Massachusetts General Hospital in Boston, Massachusetts. Pulse generators from three different manufacturers were used. In 39 patients, a complete nonthoracotomy lead system was used. Perioperative mortality was 1%. Among 154 patients, 37% experienced late postoperative problems. Twenty-one patients required system revision within 37 months of surgery. Reasons for revision were spurious shocks due to electrode fractures (3) or electrode adapter malfunction (2), inadequate signal from endocardial rate-sensing electrodes (3), superior vena cava or RV coil migration (5), failure to correct tachyarrhythmias due to a postimplant rise in defibrillation threshold (5), or pulse generator failure (3). One of the patients required system removal for infection after revision of an endocardial lead. A further 32 patients received inappropriate shocks for AF with a rapid ventricular response or sinus tachycardia. Two of these patients also received shocks for VT initiated by antitachycardia pacing triggered by AF. Ventricular pacing for bradycardia was associated with inappropriate shocks due to excessive autogain in 2 patients. Therefore, despite major diagnostic and therapeutic advantages of tiered-therapy implantable cardioverter-defibrillators, a significant proportion of patients experienced device-related complications or received inappropriate shocks.

Long-term outcomes of all patients who underwent nonthoracotomy implantable cardioverter-defibrillator implantation at the Montefiore Medical Center from April 1991 to October 1994 were studied by Kim and coworkers[72] in New York, New York, using the intention-to-treat analysis. Of 94 consecutive patients, 81 underwent nonthoracotomy implantable cardioverter-defibrillator implantation and 13 underwent thoracotomy. Six of 81 patients had a high defibrillation threshold: 4 subsequently underwent thoracotomy, and 2 were treated with amiodarone. There were no surgical mortalities. The duration of follow-up was 20 months, and was >12 months in 74% of 67 living patients. Actuarial survival rates at 1 and 2 years were, respectively, 98% and 94% for sudden death and 91% and 83% for total mortality. Two-year mortality rates were 12% and 25% in patients with EF ≥30% and <30%, respectively. Thus, instances of sudden death and surgical mortality are very few in patients with nonthoracotomy implantable cardioverter-defibrillators. Deaths during long-term follow-up are mostly due to nonsudden cardiac and noncardiac causes. Therefore, implantable cardioverter-defibrillator therapy may have greater impact on survival in patients with lower risks of nonsudden cardiac and cardiac death than in patients with severe cardiac or noncardiac disease. Prospective studies are needed to address this question.

Currently, there is no national consensus on the advisability of patients with implantable cardioverter-defibrillators being allowed to drive automobiles. Curtis and colleagues[73] from Gainesville, Florida, examined the driving safety of patients at risk for sudden death after implantation of a cardioverter-defibrillator. Surveys were sent to all 742 physicians in the United States involved in cardioverter-defibrillator implantation and follow-up. A total of 30 motor vehicle accidents related to shocks from implantable defibrillators were reported by 25 physicians over a 12-year period, from 1980 to 1992. Nine were fatal accidents involving 8 patients with a defibrillator and 1 passenger in a car driven by a patient. No bystanders were fatally injured. There were 21 nonfatal accidents involving 15 patients, 3 passengers, and 3 bystanders. The estimated fatality rate for patients with a defibrillator, 7.5 per 100 000 patient-years, is significantly lower than that of the general population (18.4 per 100 000 patient-years). Only 10.5% of all defibrillator discharges during driving resulted in accidents. Most physicians recommended that their patients wait a mean of 7 months after implantation or shock before driving again. These authors concluded that the motor vehicle accident rate caused by discharge from an implantable cardioverter-defibrillator is low. Although restricting driving for a short period of time after implantation may be appropriate, excessive restrictions or total ban on driving appears to be unwarranted.

Zipes and colleagues[74] in Indianapolis, Indiana, documented clinical experiences associated with the implantation of 2834 epicardial and endocardial cardioverter-defibrillators in 2807 patients followed for almost 1 year and compared the results between the 2 systems. Patients in the 2 groups had similar clinical characteristics. More than half of the patients had a total of almost 50 000 spontaneous ventricular tachyarrhythmias that were terminated with equal success, approximately 98%, by epicardial and endocardial cardioverter-defibrillators. Lead dislodgement and pocket infection occurred more often with the endocardial than with the epicardial cardioverter-defibrillator, but perioperative mortality was higher with the epicardial than with the endocardial placement. Sudden cardiac death with mortality occurred in 1% of the patients in the epicardial implantable cardioverter-defibrillator group and 0.6% in the endocardial group. Overall mortality at 1 year was 12% and 7% for the epicardial and endocardial groups, respectively, demonstrating the higher surgical mortality for the placement of the epicardial system. Thus, the endocardial implantable cardioverter-defibrillator is as effective as the epicardial system but is associated with lower perioperative mortality.

Coronary revascularization has been suggested as sole therapy for secondary prevention of sudden cardiac arrest associated with ischemia. The use of implantable defibrillators in combination with coronary revascularization for this patient population is unclear. In this investigation by Daoud and associates[75] from Ann Arbor, Michigan, among 412 consecutive patients receiving an implantable defibrillator, 23 (6%) were identified as sudden cardiac arrest survivors who were noninducible with programmed stimulation and had unstable angina or ischemia on a functional study; they underwent successful coronary revascularization. During a follow-up of 34±18 months, 10 (43%) of the 23 patients received implantable defibrillator shocks (8±8 per patient; range, 1 to 22 shocks), and 9 of the 10 patients had syncope/presyncope associated with at least one implantable defibrillator discharge. Patients with implantable defibrillator discharges were compared with those without implantable defibrillator discharges, and no clinical characteristics were statistically different between the 2 groups. In conclusion, revascularization alone may be inadequate therapy for survivors of sudden cardiac arrest associated with ischemia who are noninducible with programmed stimulation, and clinical variables cannot predict which patients are likely to have recurrent malignant ventricular arrhythmias.

Sweeney and colleagues[76] in Boston, Massachusetts, evaluated the effect of treatment for spontaneous ventricular arrhythmias of antiarrhythmic drugs in 53 patients, the implantable cardioverter-defibrillator in 59 patients, and no antiarrhythmic treatment in 179 patients on total mortality and the mechanism of cardiac death in 291 consecutive patients evaluated for cardiac transplantation between January 1986 and January 1995. There were 109 deaths (37%): 63 (22%) were sudden, 40 (14%) nonsudden, and 6 (2%) noncardiac during mean follow-up of 15 months. Clinical variables, medical therapies for CHF, and actuarial rates of transplantation were similar among the treatment groups. Kaplan-Meier sudden death rates were lowest in the patients receiving the implantable cardioverter-defibrillator, intermediate in the no antiarrhythmic treatment group, and highest in the drug treatment group throughout follow-up. Total mortality and nonsudden cardiac death rates did not differ. Cox proportional hazards model revealed that antiarrhythmic drug therapy was associated with sudden death and the implantable cardioverter-defibrillator was associated with nonsudden cardiac death. These data demonstrate that sudden death rates are lowest in patients treated with the implantable cardioverter-defibrillator compared with drug therapy or no antiarrhythmic therapy in patients awaiting cardiac transplantation with severe CHF. However, although the implantable cardioverter-defibrillator reduced sudden death in the high-risk patient with severe LV dysfunction, the effect on long-term survival was limited, especially by the relatively high incidence of nonsudden cardiac death.

Miscellaneous

Palpitations

Barsky and associates[77] from Boston, Massachusetts, did a 6-month follow-up examination of 145 consecutive patients who had been studied earlier because of palpitations and who had had ambulatory electrocardiographic monitoring at the time of the initial visit. At 6-months follow-up, 130 of the initial 145 patients with palpitations and 69 of the initial 70 asymptomatic, nonpatient volunteers were reinterviewed. Eighty-four percent of the patients had recurrent palpitations during the 6-month period. At follow-up, patients with palpitations scored significantly higher than the comparison group on measures of cardiac symptoms and role impairment and had made more physician visits in the preceding 6 months. They also had a higher prevalence of panic disorder and more psychopathic symptoms, somatized more, and were more hypochondriacal. Psychiatric symptoms and the tendency to amplify bodily sensation, measured at inception, were significant but modest predictors of subsequent palpitations. The authors concluded that patients with palpitations remained symptomatic and functionally impaired and had increased rates of physician visits in the 6 months following Holter monitoring for palpitations. They also continued to have elevated rates, panic disorder, and to evidence some confusion about the cause of their symptoms.

Ambulatory Electrocardiography

Kessler and associates[78] from Miami, Florida, evaluated the current clinical use and costs of ambulatory electrocardiographic monitoring for arrhythmia detection based on a cost per management decision analysis. Consecutive inpatient and outpatient 24-hour ambulatory electrocardiographic monitoring performed during the calendar year 1991 were retrospectively reviewed for clinical indication, arrhythmia detection, diary information, and whether a management decision that might alter patient outcome was derived from the data. The cost per management decision (based on a representative reimbursement of $550 per ambulatory electrocardiographic monitoring) and the cost index (all tests divided by useful tests) were calculated. Although arrhythmias were identified in 91% of the patients, management decisions were indicated in only 18% (cost per decision, $2974). Management decisions were most often derived from the data in patients being evaluated for arrhythmia therapy (37 of 37 patients; cost per decision, $550). Symptoms and arrhythmias were correlated in only 11 patients (2%). More often typical clinical symptoms were present (26 patients) in the absence of an arrhythmia. Of 101 ambulatory electrocardiographic monitorings following a cerebrovascular event, 4 had unsuspected AF (cost per decision, $13 888). Dizziness or lightheadedness associated with other cardiac symptoms were more likely to lead to a management decision than the same symptoms in isolation (29% vs 7%). No patient had central nervous system symptoms correlated with an arrhythmia during the recording period or unsuspected VT. Ambulatory electrocardiography has a highly variable and indication-dependent effectiveness and cost. The results suggest a strategy for improving the use of ambulatory electrocardiography based on knowing what testing indications are more likely to lead to useful clinical information.

Amiodarone

Podrid[79] from Boston, Massachusetts, provided an excellent review of amiodarone. He concluded that amiodarone was unique among the antiarrhythmic drugs in many ways. It is highly effective against a wide range of arrhythmias, and its efficacy appears to be unrelated to the type and severity of the arrhythmia or to the nature and extent of underlying heart disease. Amiodarone has not been reported to aggravate arrhythmia or to increase mortality from sudden death or cardiac mortality in any group of patients studied to date. Unfortunately, it is associated with a wide range of side effects, some of which are potentially serious, such as liver, thyroid gland, pulmonary, and cardiac toxicity. Although many of the minor side effects are dose related, serious toxicity is often unrelated to dose and is unpredictable. Laboratory abnormalities can serve as markers for potential problems and can be observed before symptoms develop. Therefore, close monitoring of chest radiographs, liver and thyroid gland functions, and cardiac status will often show potentially serious toxicity early, permitting discontinuation of amiodarone therapy before any serious symptoms or adverse events develop.

1. Flegel KM: From delirum cordis to atrial fibrillation: Historical development of a disease concept. Ann. Intern Med 1995 (June 1);122:11:867–873.
2. Reimold SC, Lamas GA, Cantillon CA, Antman EM: Risk factors for the development of recurrent atrial fibrillation: Role of pacing and clinical variables. Am Heart J 1995 (June);129:1127–1132.
3. Flaker GC, Fletcher KA, Rothbart RM, Halperin JL, Hart RG: For the stroke prevention in atrial fibrillation investigators: Clinical and electrocardiographic features of intermittent atrial fibrillation that predict recurrent atrial fibrillation. Amer J Cardiol 1995 (August 15);76:355–358.
4. Feinberg WM, Blackshear JL, Laupacis A, Kromnal R, Hart RG: Prevalence, age distribution and gender of patients with atrial fibrillation. Arch Intern Med 1995 (March 13);155:469–473.
5. Krahn AD, Manfreda J, Tate RB, Mathewson FAL, Cuddy TE: The natural history of atrial fibrillation: incidence, risk factors, and prognosis in the Manitoba follow-up study. Am J Med 1995 (May);98:476–484.
6. Ezekowitz MD, James KE, Nazarian SM, Davenport J, Broderick JP, Gupta SR, Thadani V, Meyer ML, Bridgers SL, for the Veterans Affairs Stroke Prevention in Nonrheumatic Atrial Fibrillation Investigators: Silent cerebral infarction in patients with nonrheumatic atrial fibrillation. Circulation 1995 (October);92:2178–2182.
7. Collins LJ, Silverman DI, Douglas PS, Manning WJ: Cardioversion of nonrheumatic atrial fibrillation: Reduced thromboembolic complications with 4 weeks of precardioversion anticoagulation are related to atrial thrombus resolution. Circulation 1995 (July);92:160–163.
8. The European Atrial Fibrillation Trial Study Group. Optimal oral anticoagulant therapy in patients with nonrheumatic atrial fibrillation and recent cerebral ischemia. N Eng J Med 1995 (July 6);333:1:5–10.
9. Gage BF, Cardinalli AB, Albers GW, Owens DK: Cost-effectiveness of warfarin and aspirin for prophylaxis of stroke in patients with nonvalvular atrial fibrillation. JAMA 1995 (December 20);274:1839–1845.
10. Middlekauff HR, Stevenson WG, Cornbein JA: Antiarrhythmic prophylaxis vs warfarin anticoagulation to prevent thromboembolic events among patients with atrial fibrillation. Arch Intern Med 1995 (May);155:913–920.
11. Ellenbogen KA, Dias VC, Cardello FP, Strauss WE, Simonton CA, Pollak SJ, Wood MA, Stambler BS: Safety and efficacy of intravenous diltiazem in atrial fibrillation or atrial flutter. Am J Cardiol 1995 (January 1);75:45–49.
12. Murgatroyd FD, Slade AKB, Sopher SM, Rowland E, Ward DE, Camm AJ: Efficacy and tolerability of transvenous low energy cardioversion of paroxysmal atrial fibrillation in humans. J Am Coll Cardiol 1995 (May);25:1347–1353.
13. Manning WJ, Silverman DI, Keighley CS, Oettgen P, Douglas PS: Transesophageal echocardiographically facilitated early cardioversion from atrial fibrillation using short-term anticoagulation: Final results of a prospective 4.5-year study. J Am Coll Cardiol 1995 (May);25:1354–1361.
14. Stoddard MF, Dawkins PR, Prince CR, Longaker RA: Transesophageal echocardiographic guidance of cardioversion in patients with atrial fibrillation. Am Heart J 1995 (June);129:1204–1215.

15. Della Bella P, Carbucicchio C, Tondo C, Riva S: Modulation of atrioventricular conduction by ablation of the "slow" atrioventricular node pathway in patients with drug-refractory atrial fibrillation or flutter. J Am Coll Cardiol 1995 (January);25:39–46.

16. Fischer B, Haissaguerre M, Garrigues S, Poquet F, Gencel L. Clementy J, Marcus FI: Radiofrequency catheter ablation of common atrial flutter in 80 patients. J Am Coll Cardiol 1995 (May);25:1365–1372.

17. Steinberg JS, Prasher S, Zelenkofske S, Ehlert FA: Radiofrequency catheter ablation of atrial flutter: Procedural success and long-term outcome. Am Heart J 1995 (July);130:85–92.

18. Poty H, Saoudi N, Aziz AA, Nair M, Letac B: Radiofrequency catheter ablation of type 1 atrial flutter: Prediction of late success by electrophysiological criteria. Circulation 1995 (September);92:1389–1392.

19. Zarembski DG, Nolan PE Jr, Slack MK, Caruso AC: Treatment of resistant atrial fibrillation. Arch Intern Med 1995 (September 25);155:1885–1891.

20. Manning, WJ, Silverman DI, Waksmonski CA, Oettgen P, Douglas PS: Prevalence of residual left atrial thrombi among patients with acute thromboembolism and newly recognized atrial fibrillation. Arch Intern Med 1995 (November 13);155:2193–2197.

21. Ganz LI, Friedman PL: Supraventricular tachycardia. N Eng J Med 1995 (January 19);332:162–173.

22. Hamer ME, Wilkinson WE, Clair WK, Page RL, McCarthy EA, Pritchett ELC: Incidence of symptomatic atrial fibrillation in patients with paroxysmal supraventricular tachycardia. J Am Coll Cardiol 1995 (April);25:984–988.

23. UK Propafenone PSVT Study Group: A randomized, placebo-controlled trial of propafenone in the prophylaxis of paroxysmal supraventricular tachycardia and paroxysmal atrial fibrillation. Circulation 1995 (November);92:2550–2557.

24. Sung RJ, Tan HL, Karagounis L, Hanyok JJ, Falk R, Platia E, Das G, Hardy SA, and the Sotalol Multicenter Study Group: Intravenous sotalol for the termination of supraventricular tachycardia and atrial fibrillation and flutter: A multicenter, randomized, double-blind, placebo-controlled study. Am Heart J 1995 (April);129:739–748.

25. Goldstein S, Brooks MM, Ledingham R, Kennedy HL, Epstein AE, Pawitan Y, Bigger JT: Association between ease of suppression of ventricular arrhythmia and survival. Circulation 1995 (January);91:79–83.

26. Berntsen RF, Gjestvang FT, Rasmussen K: QRS prolongation as an indicator of risk of ischemia-related ventricular tachycardia and fibrillation induced by exercise. Am Heart J 1995 (March);129:542–548.

27. Hernández M, Taylor J, Marinchak R, Rials S, Rubin A, Kowey P: Outcome of patients with nonsustained ventricular tachycardia and severely impaired ventricular function who have negative electrophysiologic studies. Am Heart J 1995 (March);129:492–496.

28. Eisenberg SJ, Scheinman MM, Dullet NK, Finkbeiner WE, Griffin JC, Eldar M, Franz MR, Gonzalez R, Kadish AH, Lesh MD: Sudden cardiac death and polymorphous ventricular tachycardia in patients with normal QT intervals and normal systolic cardiac function. Am J Cardiol 1995 (April 1);75:687–692.

29. Szabó BM, Crijns HJGM, Wiesfeld ACP, van Veldhuisen DJ, Hillege HL, Lie KI: Predictors of mortality in patients with sustained ventricular tachycardias or ventricular fibrillation and depressed left ventricular function: Importance of β-blockade. Am Heart J 1995 (August);130:281–286.

30. Reese DB, Silverman ME, Gold MR, Gottlieb SS: Prognostic importance of the length of ventricular tachycardia in patients with nonischemic congestive heart failure. Am Heart J 1995 (September);130:489–493.

31. Jadonath RL, Schwartzman DS, Preminger MW, Gottlieb CD, Marchlinski FE: Utility of the 12-lead electrocardiogram in localizing the origin of right ventricular outflow tract tachycardia. Am Heart J 1995 (November);130:1107–1113.

32. Berntsen RF, Gunnes P, Rasmussen K: Pattern of coronary artery disease in patients with ventricular tachycardia and fibrillation exposed by exercise-induced ischemia. Am Heart J 1995 (April);129:733–738.

33. Ammar A, Wong M, Singh BN: Divergent effects of chronic amiodarone administration on systolic and diastolic function in patients with heart disease. Am J Cardiol 1995 (March 1);75:465–469.

34. Ferrick KJ, Singh S, Roth JA, Kim SG, Fisher JD: Prediction of electrophysiologic study results in patients treated with amiodarone. Am Heart J 1995 (March);129:496–501.

35. Garguichevich JJ, Ramos JL, Gambarte A, Gentile A, Hauad S, Scapin O. Sirena J, Tibaldi M, Toplikar J: Effect of amiodarone therapy on mortality in patients with left ventricular dysfunction and asymptomatic complex ventricular arrhythmias: Argentine pilot study of sudden death and amiodarone (EPAMSA*). Am Heart J 1995 (September);130:494–500.

36. Kowey PR, Levine JH, Herre JM, Pacifico A, Lindsay BD, Plumb VJ, Janosik DL, Kopelman HA, Scheinman MM, for the Intravenous Amiodarone Multicenter Investigators Group: Randomized, double-blind comparison of intravenous amiodarone and bretylium in the treatment of patients with recurrent, hemodynamically destabilizing ventricular tachycardia or fibrillation. Circulation 1995 (December);92:3255–3263.

37. Singh BN, Kehoe R, Woosley RL, Scheinman M, Quart B, and the Sotalol Multicenter Study Group: Multicenter trial of sotalol compared with procainamide in the suppression of inducible ventricular tachycardia: A double-blind, randomized parallel evaluation. Am Heart J 1995 (January);129:87–97.

38. Zhu DWX, Maloney JD, Simmons TW, Nitta J, Fitzgerald DM, Trohman RG, Khoury DS, Saliba W, Belco KM, Rizo-Patron C, Pinski SL: Radiofrequency catheter ablation for management of symptomatic ventricular ectopic activity. J Am Coll Cardiol 1995 (October);26:843–849.

39. Karetzky M, Zubair M, Parikh J: Cardiopulmonary resuscitation in intensive care unit and non-intensive care unit patients. Arch Intern Med 1995 (June 26);155:1277–1280.

40. Grubb NR, Elton RA, Fox KAA: In-hospital mortality after out-of-hospital cardiac arrest. Lancet 1995 (August 12);346:417–421.

41. Heller RF, Steele PL, Fisher JD, Alexander HM, Dobson AJ: Success of cardiopulmonary resuscitation after heart attack in hospital and outside hospital. Br Med J 1995 (November 18);311:1332–1336.

42. Duflou J, Virmani R, Rabin I, Burke A, Farb A, Smialek J: Sudden death as a result of heart disease in morbid obesity. Am Heart J 1995 (August);130:306–313.

43. Peters RW, Brooks MM, Todd L, Liebson PR, Wilhelmsen L: Smoking cessation and arrhythmic death: The CAST experience. J Am Coll Cardiol 1995 (November 1);26:1287–1292.

44. Shen W-K, Edwards WD, Hammill SC, Bailey KR, Ballard DJ, Gersh BJ: Sudden unexpected nontraumatic death in 54 young adults: A 30-year population-based study. Am J Cardiol 1995 (July 15);76:148–152.

45. Kendall MJ, Lynch KP, Hjalmarson A, Kjekshus J: β-Blockers and sudden cardiac death. Ann Intern Med 1995 (September 1);123:358–367.

46. Siscovick DS, Raghunathan TE, King I, Weinmann S, Wicklund KG, Albright J, Bovbjerg V, Arbogast P, Smith H, Kushi LH, Cobb LA, Copass MK, Psaty BM, Lemaitre R, Retzlaff B, Childs M, Knopp RH: Dietary intake and cell membrane levels of long-chain n-3 polyunsaturated fatty acids and the risk of primary cardiac arrest. JAMA 1995 (November 1);274:1363–1367.

47. Kawachi I, Sparrow D, Vokonas PS, Weiss ST: Decreased heart rate variability in men with phobic anxiety (data from the Normative Aging Study). Am J Cardiol 1995 (May 1);75:882–885.

48. Farb A, Tang AL, Burke AP, Sessums L, Liang Y, Virmani R: Sudden coronary death: Frequency of active coronary lesions, inactive coronary lesions, and myocardial infarction. Circulation 1995 (October);92:1701–1709.

49. Calkins H, Shyr U, Frumin H, Schork AN, Morady F: The value of the clinical history in the differentiation of syncope due to ventricular tachycardia, atrioventricular block, and neurocardiogenic syncope. Am J Med 1995 (April);98:365–373.

50. Dhala A, Natale A, Sra J, Deshpande S, Blanck Z, Jazayeri MR, Akhtar M: Relevance of asystole during head-up tilt testing. Am J Cardiol 1995 (February 1);75:251–254.

51. Morillo CA, Klein GJ, Zandri S, Yee R: Diagnostic accuracy of a low-dose isoproterenol head-up tilt protocol. Am Heart J 1995 (May);129:901–906.
52. Natale A, Akhtar M, Jazayeri M, Dhala A, Blanck Z, Deshpande S, Krebs A, Sra JS: Provocation of hypotension during head-up tilt testing in subjects with no history of syncope or presyncope. Circulation 1995 (July);92:54–58.
53. Hou Z-Y, Yang C-Y, Ko C-C, Lee S S-J, Chiang H-T, Chen C-Y: Upright postures and isoproterenol infusion for provocation of neurocardiogenic syncope: A comparison of standing and head-up tilting. Am Heart J 1995 (December);130:1210–1215.
54. Calkins H, Seifert M, Morady F: Clinical presentation and long-term follow-up of athletes with exercise-induced vasodepressor syncope. Am Heart J 1995 (June);129:1159–1164.
55. Cohen MB, Snow JS, Grasso V, Lehnert L, Goldner BG, Jadonath RL, Cohen TJ: Efficacy of pindolol for treatment of vasovagal syncope. Am Heart J 1995 (October);130:786–790.
56. Benditt DG, Petersen M, Lurie KG, Grubb GP, Sutton R: Cardiac pacing for prevention of recurrent vasovagal syncope. Ann Intern Med 1995 (February 1);122:204–209.
57. Tan HL, Hou CJY, Lauer MR, Sung RJ: Electrophysiologic mechanisms of the long QT interval syndromes and torsade de pointes. Ann Intern Med 1995 (May 1);122:701–714.
58. Schwartz PJ, Priori SG, Locati EH, Napolitano C, Cantù F, Towbin JA, Keating MT, Hammoude H, Brown AM, Chen L-S K, Colatsky TJ: Long QT syndrome patients with mutations of the *SCN5A* and *HERG* genes have differential responses to Na$^+$ channel blockade and to increases in heart rate: Implications for gene-specific therapy. Circulation 1995 (December);92:3381–3386.
59. Moss AJ, Zareba W, Benhorin J, Locati EH, Hall WJ, Robinson JL, Schwartz PJ, Towbin JA, Vincent GM, Lehmann MH, Keating MT, MacCluer JW, Timothy KW: ECG T-wave patterns in genetically distinct forms of the hereditary long QT syndrome. Circulation 1995 (November);92:2929–2934.
60. Mairesse GH, Marwick TH, Arnese M, Van Overschelde JJ, Cornel JH, Detry JR, Melin JA, Fioretti PM: Improved identification of coronary artery disease in patients with left bundle branch block by use of Dobutamine stress echocardiography and comparison with myocardial profusion tomography. Am J Cardiol 1995 (August 15);76:321–325.
61. Brink PA, Ferreira A, Moolman JC, Weymar HW, van der Merwe P-L, Corfield VA: Gene for progressive familial heart block type I maps to chromosome 19q13. Circulation 1995 (March);91:1633–1640.
62. Leclercq C, Gras D, Le Helloco A, Nicol L, Mabo P, Daubert C: Hemodynamic importance of preserving the normal sequence of ventricular activation in permanent cardiac pacing. Am Heart J 1995 (June);129:1133–1141.
63. Pinski SL, Trohman RG: Implantable cardioverter-defibrillators. Ann Intern Med 1995 (May 15);122:770–788.
64. Brooks R, Garan H, McGovern BA, Ruskin JN: Implantation of transvenous nonthoracotomy cardioverter-defibrillator systems in patients with permanent endocardial pacemakers. Am Heart J 1995 (January);129:45–53.
65. Trappe H-J, Pfitzner P, Heintze J, Kielblock B. Wenzlaff P, Fieguth H-G, Demertzis S, Lichtlen PR, Panning B, Piepenbrock S: Cardioverter-defibrillator implantation in the catheterization laboratory: Initial experiences in 48 patients. Am Heart J 1995 (February);129:259–264.
66. Jordaens L, Vertongen P, Provenier F, Trouerbach JW, Poelaert J, Herregods L: A new transvenous internal cardioverter-defibrillator: Implantation technique, complications, and short-term follow-up. Am Heart J 1995 (February);129:251–258.
67. Osswald S, Roelke M, O'Nunain SS, Trouton TG, Sosa Suarez GE, Perez IE, Torchiana D, McGovern BA, Garan H, Ruskin JN, Brooks R: Electrocardiographic pseudoinfarct patterns after implantation of cardioverter-defibrillators. Am Heart J 1995 (February);129:265–272.
68. Wood MA, Simpson PM, London WB, Stambler BS, Herre JM, Bernstein RC, Ellenbogen KA: Circadian pattern of ventricular tachyarrhythmias in patients with implantable cardioverter-defibrillators. J Am Coll Cardiol 1995 (March 15);25:901–907.
69. Raitt MH, Dolack GL, Kudenchuk PJ, Poole JE, Bardy GH: Ventricular arrhythmias detected after transvenous defibrillator implantation in patients with a clinical

history of only ventricular fibrillation: Implications for use of implantable defibrillator. Circulation 1995 (April);91:1996–2001.

70. Wever EFD, Hauer RNW, van Capelle FJL, Tijssen JGP, Crijns HJGM, Algra A, Wiesfeld ACP, Bakker PFA, Robles de Medina EO: Randomized study of implantable defibrillator as first-choice therapy versus conventional strategy in postinfarct sudden death survivors. Circulation 1995 (April);91:2195–2203.

71. Nunain SO, Roelke M, Trouton T, Osswald S, Kim YH, Sosa-Suarez G, Brooks DR, McGovern B, Guy M, Torchiana DF, Vlahakes GJ, Garan H, Ruskin JN: Limitations and late complications of third-generation automatic cardioverter-defibrillators. Circulation 1995 (April);91:2204–2213.

72. Kim SG, Roth JA, Fisher JD, Chung J, Nagabhairu R, Ferrick KJ, Ben-Zur U, Gross J, Furman S: Long-term outcomes and modes of death of patients treated with nonthoracotomy implantable defibrillators. Am J Cardiol 1995 (June 15);75:1229–1232.

73. Curtis AB, Conti JB, Tucker KJ, Kubilis PS, Reilly RE, Woodard DA: Motor vehicle accidents in patients with an implantable cardioverter-defibrillator. J Am Coll Cardiol 1995 (July);26:180–184.

74. Zipes DP, Roberts D, for the Pacemaker-Cardioverter-Defibrillator Investigators: Results of the international study of the implantable pacemaker cardioverter-defibrillator: A comparison of epicardial and endocardial lead systems. Circulation 1995 (July);92:59–65.

75. Daoud EG, Niebauer M, Kou WH, Man C, Horwood L, Morady F, Strickberger SA: Incidence of implantable defibrillator discharges after coronary revascularization in survivors of ischemic sudden cardiac death. Am Heart J 1995 (August);130:277–280.

76. Sweeney MO, Ruskin JN, Garan H, McGovern BA, Guy ML, Torchiana DF, Vlahakes GJ, Newell JB, Semigran MJ, Dec GW: Influence of the implantable cardioverter/defibrillator on sudden death and total mortality in patients evaluated for cardiac transplantation. Circulation 1995 (December);92:3273–3281.

77. Barsky AJ, Cleary PD, Coeytaux RR, Ruskin JN: The clinical course of palpitations in medical outpatients. Arch Intern Med 1995 (September 11);155:1782–1788.

78. Kessler DK, Kessler KM, Myerburg RJ. Ambulatory electrocardiography. Arch Intern Med 1995 (January 23);155:165–169.

79. Podrid PJ: Amiodarone: reevaluation of an old drug. Ann Intern Med 1995 (May 1);122:9:689–700.

5
Systemic Hypertension

General Topics

Drugs, Poisons, and Foods Increasing Blood Pressure

Grossman and Messerli[1] from New Orleans, Louisiana, reviewed the variety of therapeutic agents or chemical substances that could induce either a transient or sustained increase in BP. These agents increase BP either by causing sodium retention and extracellular body expansion, or directly or indirectly activating the sympathetic nervous system. Some agents act directly on arteriolar smooth muscle. For certain agents, the mechanism of BP elevation is mixed or unknown. Paradoxically, some agents that are used to lower BP may acutely increase arterial BP. Also, a rebound increase in BP may be encountered after discontinuation of certain antihypertensive agents. In general, these chemically-induced increases in arterial BP are small and transient; however, severe hypertension involving encephalopathy, stroke, and irreversible renal failure has been reported. Careful evaluation of a patient's drug regimen may identify chemically-induced hypertension and prevent the need for evaluation and therapy. This study reviews the therapeutic agents or chemical substances that elevate BP and their mechanisms of action.

Effects of Nonsteroidal Anti-inflammatory Drugs on Blood Pressure

Nonsteroidal anti-inflammatory drugs may attenuate the antihypertensive effects of diuretics, β-blockers, ACE inhibitors, central α-agonists, and other vasodilators. Their effects on the antihypertensive efficacy of calcium antagonists are inadequately studied. Houston and associates[2] from several medical centers in the USA performed a three-phase randomized, double-blind, placebo-controlled, multicenter study that included 162 patients (age, 18–75 years) with essential systemic hypertension. After diastolic BP was controlled to ≤90 mm Hg with once-daily verapamil hydrochloride, patients received ibuprofen, naproxen, or placebo matching capsules for 3 weeks, and BP, heart rate, weight, and adverse effects were evaluated. A general linear model with 95% CIs was used to compare each nonsteroidal anti-inflammatory drug treatment group with the placebo group. No significant differences in sitting, standing, or supine BP were noted with naproxen or ibuprofen compared with placebo. The percentages of patients in each treatment group with increases of 10 mm Hg or more in either systolic or diastolic BP were similar. Statistically significant increases in weight were seen with both nonsteroidal anti-inflammatory drug therapies. Changes in pulse rate were not significant. The incidence of adverse effects was similar across all 3 treatment groups. The addition of naproxen or ibuprofen to the treatment of hypertensive patients in whom BP is controlled by once-daily verapamil does not cause an increase in BP. Verapamil may therefore offer considerable advantages in maintaining control of BP in patients who regularly receive nonsteroidal anti-inflammatory drug therapy.

Implications of Small Reductions

To estimate the impact of small reduction in the population distribution of diastolic BP, such as those potentially achievable by population-wide lifestyle modification, on the incidence of CAD and stroke, Cook and associates[3] from Boston, Massachusetts, and St. Louis, Missouri, used published data from the Framingham Heart Study and from the National Health and Nutrition Examination Survey II to examine the impact of a population-wide strategy aimed at reducing diastolic BP by an average of 2 mm Hg in a population including normotensive individuals. The subjects included white men and white women aged 35–64 years living in the USA. Data from overviews of observational studies and randomized trials suggest that a 2–mm Hg reduction in diastolic BP would result in a 17% decrease in the prevalence of hypertension as well as a 6% reduction in the risk of CAD and a 15% reduction in risk of stroke and transient ischemic attacks. From an application of these results to US white men and women aged 35–64 years, it is estimated that a successful population intervention alone could reduce CAD incidence more than could medical treatment for all those with a diastolic BP of 95 mm Hg or higher. It could prevent 84% of the number prevented by medical treatment for all those with a diastolic BP ≥90 mm Hg. For stroke (including transient ischemic attacks) a population-wide 2–mm Hg reduction could prevent 93% of events prevented by medical treatment for those with a diastolic BP of 95 mm Hg or higher and 69% of events for treatment for those with a diastolic BP of 90 mm Hg or higher. A combination strategy of both a population reduction in diastolic BP and targeted medical intervention is most effective and could double or triple the impact of medical treatment alone. Adding a population-based intervention to existing levels of hypertension treatment could prevent an estimated additional 67 000 CAD events (6%) and 34 000 stroke and TIA events (13%) annually among all those aged 35–64 years in the USA. A small reduction of 2 mm Hg in diastolic BP in the mean of the population distribution, in addition to medical treatment, could have a great public health impact on the number of CAD and stroke events prevented. Whether such diastolic BP reductions can be achieved in the population through lifestyle interventions, in particular through sodium reduction, depends on the results of ongoing primary prevention trials as well as the cooperation of the food industry, government agencies, and health education professionals.

Relation of Blood Pressure and Mortality

Many studies of BP in the elderly have found higher death rates in groups with the lowest BP than in those with intermediate values. In a large community study, Glynn and associates[4] from Boston, Massachusetts, assessed drug use, medical history, disability, physical function, and BP in 3657 residents of East Boston, Massachusetts, aged 65 and older. The authors identified all deaths (1709) up to 1992 and followed up survivors for an average of 10.5 (range, 9.5–11.0) years. After adjustment for confounding variables (including frailty and

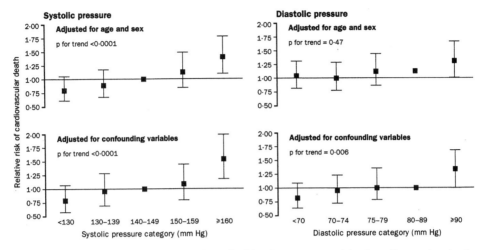

Figure 5-1. Relation of systolic and diastolic blood pressure to risk of cardiovascular death. Only deaths that occurred more than 3 years after baseline assessment are included. Reprinted by permission from Glynn et al.[4]

disorders such as CHF and AMI) and exclusion of deaths within the first 3 years of follow-up, higher systolic BP predicted linear increases in cardiovascular but not total mortality (Figure 5-1). These results differed from those for the first 3 years, during which groups with the lowest systolic and diastolic BP had the highest death rates. In the long term, lower BP in old age, as in middle age, is associated with better survival. Short-term findings may differ because of associations of comorbidity and frailty with BP near death. Overall, the findings support recommendations to treat high BP in elderly people.

Association of Midlife Pressure and Late-Life Cognition

To assess the long-term relation of midlife BP levels to late-life cognitive function, Launer and associates[5] from Bilthoven, the Netherlands; Honolulu, Hawaii; and Bethesda, Maryland, examined the 4678 surviving cohort members of the prospective Honolulu Heart Program (baseline, 1965–1968) a fourth time from 1991–1993 and gave the survivors a cognitive test. Their average age was 78 years at the fourth examination and 3735 were Japanese-American men living in Hawaii in the community or in institutions. Cognitive function, measured by the 100 point Cognitive Abilities Screening Instrument, was categorized into good (score, 92–100), intermediate (<92–82), and poor (<82). Midlife systolic BP and diastolic BP values were measured in 1965, 1968, and 1971. When controlled for age and education, the risk for intermediate and poor cognitive function increased progressively with increasing levels of midline systolic BP. For every 10–mm Hg increase in systolic BP there was an increase in risk for intermediate cognitive function of 7% and for poor cognitive function of 9%. Adjustment for prevalent stroke, CAD, and subclinical atherosclerosis reduced the risks of the relation between midlife systolic BP and poor cognitive function to 5%. The level of cognitive function was not associated with midlife diastolic BP. Thus, midlife systolic BP is a significant predictor of reduced cognitive function in later life. Early control of systolic BP levels may reduce the risks of cognitive impairment in old age.

Atrial Natriuretic Peptide

Flickenger and associates[6] from Rochester, Minnesota, performed a cross-sectional study of the relation between atrial natriuretic peptide levels and BP levels, a diagnosis of systemic hypertension, and family history of hypertension in white persons from Rochester, Minnesota Plasma atrial natriuretic peptide and BP levels were measured in 1338 white people who were members of 301 three-generation families from the population. Hypertension was defined as systolic BP of 140 mm Hg or more or diastolic BP of 90 mm Hg or more. Each subject in the parental generation was categorized as having 0, 1, or 2 parents with hypertension. Analyses were done separately for each generation and gender stratum. Within gender and generation strata, the authors noted no consistent pattern of positive or negative correlation of plasma atrial natriuretic peptide levels with systolic BP, diastolic BP, or heart rate. Within the grandparental generation, mean plasma atrial natriuretic peptide levels did not differ between those with normal BP and those with hypertension. In the parental generation, mean plasma atrial natriuretic peptide levels did not differ between subjects with 0, 1, or 2 parents with hypertension. In white people, interindividual differences in plasma atrial natriuretic peptide levels are not associated with interindividual differences in BP levels, the diagnosis of hypertension, or family history of hypertension.

Endothelial Function

Panza and colleagues[7] in Bethesda, Maryland, determined whether patients with essential hypertension have abnormal endothelium-dependent vascular relaxation largely related to reduced availability of nitric oxide. The responses of the forearm vasculature to acetylcholine and bradykinin (endothelium-dependent agents) and to sodium nitroprusside (a direct dilator of vascular smooth muscle) were studied in 10 hypertensive patients and 12 control individuals. To determine the contribution of nitric oxide to bradykinin-induced vasodilation, the vascular responses to bradykinin were measured after administration of N^G-monomethyl-L-arginine, an arginine analogue that inhibits the synthesis of nitric oxide. Drugs were infused into the brachial artery and the forearm blood flow was measured by strain-gauge plethysmography. The response to acetylcholine was blunted in hypertensive patients. The vasodilator effect of bradykinin was significantly reduced in these same individuals compared with normal controls. A significant correlation was found between maximal blood flow with acetylcholine and that with bradykinin. No significant differences were found between the two groups for vascular responses to sodium nitroprusside. The N^G-monomethyl-L-arginine significantly blunted the response to bradykinin in control subjects. Thus, inhibition of nitric oxide synthesis did not modify the response to bradykinin in hypertensive patients. The response to bradykinin after inhibition of nitric oxide synthesis was not significantly different between the two groups. These data indicate that patients with essential hypertension have impaired endothelium-dependent vasodilator responses to both acetylcholine and bradykinin. However, these findings also indicate that the endothelial dysfunction is not related to a specific defect of a single intracellular signal-transduction pathway, but instead suggests a more generalized abnormality of endothelial vasodilator function.

Taddei and colleagues[8] in Rome, Italy, evaluated the effect of age on endothelial responsiveness in the forearm vessels of either normotensive control subjects or those with essential hypertension. Within the normotensive or hypertensive group, including 53 and 57 patients, respectively, the patients were selected with similar blood pressure, plasma cholesterol, and glucose values, and hypercholesterolemic subjects, diabetics, and smokers were excluded. Forearm blood flows were evaluated by strain-gauge plethysmography and modifications induced by intrabrachial acetylcholine infusion at rates of 0.15, 0.45, 1.5, 4.5, and 15 μg/100 mL per minute. Acetylcholine is an endothelium-dependent vasodilator, and sodium nitroprusside, given as 1, 2, and 4 μg/100 mL per minute, an endothelium-independent vasodilator. Acetylcholine caused a dose-dependent vasodilation that was lower in patients with essential hypertension than in normotensive control subjects. A significant negative correlation was observed between acetylcholine-induced vasodilation and patient age in both normotensive and hypertensive patients. Vasodilation to sodium nitroprusside was similar in normotensive control subjects and those with hypertension. Thus, these data indicate that there is a blunted response to acetylcholine with advancing age in both normotensive control subjects and essential hypertensive patients suggesting that aging is associated with a reduced endothelium-dependent vasodilation in humans.

Treatment

Regular Exercise

The prevalence of systemic hypertension and its cardiovascular complications is higher in African-Americans than in whites. Interventions to control BP in this population are particularly important. Regular exercise lowers BP in patients with mild to moderate hypertension, but its effects in patients with severe hypertension have not been studied. Kokkinos and associates[9] from Washington, DC, examined the effects of moderately intense exercise on BP and LV hypertrophy in African-American men and with severe systemic hypertension. The authors randomly assigned 46 men 35–76 years of age to exercise plus antihypertensive medication (23 men) or antihypertensive medication alone (23 men). A total of 18 men in the exercise group completed 16 weeks of exercise, and 14 completed 32 weeks of exercise, which was performed three times a week at 60–80% of the maximal heart rate. After 16 weeks, mean ($\pm$SD) diastolic BP had decreased from 88$\pm$7 to 83$\pm$8 mm Hg in the patients who exercised, whereas it had increased slightly, from 88$\pm$6 to 90$\pm$7 mm Hg, in those who did not exercise. Diastolic BP remained significantly lower after 32 weeks of exercise, even with substantial reductions in the dose of antihypertensive medication. In addition, the thickness of the ventricular septum, the LV mass, and the LV mass index had decreased significantly after 16 weeks in the patients who exercised, whereas there was no significant change in the nonexercisers. Regular exercise reduced BP and LV hypertrophy in African-American men with severe hypertension.

Trends in Management

Two new classes of antihypertensive agents were introduced in the 1980s, but their effectiveness in preventing heart disease and stroke has not been

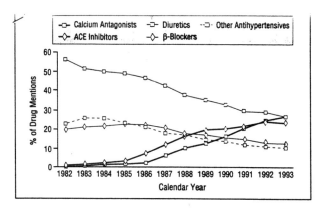

Figure 5-2. Percentage of drug mentions by class of antihypertensive agent, 1982 through 1993. ACE indicates angiotensin-converting enzyme. Data from IMS America. Reproduced with permission from Manolio et al.[10]

demonstrated. Lack of evidence of their efficacy might reasonably be expected to discourage their widespread use in management of hypertension. Manolio and associates[10] from 5 medical centers in the USA estimated use of various classes of antihypertensive agents from published drug use information in an effort to estimate trends in antihypertensive drug use and evaluate the impact of these trends on antihypertensive therapy in the United States (Figure 5-2). Proportionate use of the 5 major antihypertensive drug classes shifted markedly between 1982 and 1993. Diuretics accounted for 56% of all hypertensive drug mentions in 1982 but only 27% in 1993, a relative decline of 52%. Use of β-blockers and central agents also declined during this period. Proportionate use of calcium antagonists showed the greatest gains, increasing from 0.3% to 27%, while the use of ACE inhibitors increased from 0.8% to 24%. Given the higher costs of the newer agents, and assuming an estimated total cost of antihypertensive medications in 1992 of $7 billion, approximately $3.1 billion would have been saved had 1982 prescribing practices remained in effect in 1992 (Table 5-1). Use of calcium antagonists and ACE inhibitors in hypertension has increased dramatically in the past 10 years. Without convincing evidence of the advantages of these agents, it is difficult to explain the continued decline in the use of less expensive agents, such as diuretics and β-blockers, which are the only antihypertensive agents proved to reduce stroke and CAD in hypertensive patients.

Risk of Myocardial Infarction from Antihypertensive Agents

To assess the association between first AMI and the use of antihypertensive agents, Psaty and associates[11] from multiple medical centers in the United States conducted a population-based case-control study among enrollees of the Group Health Cooperative of Puget Sound (GHC). The cases were hypertensive patients who sustained a first fatal or nonfatal AMI from 1986–1993 among women and from 1989–1993 among men. The control patients were a stratified random sample of hypertensive GHC enrollees, frequency matched to the cases on age, sex, and calendar year. All 623 cases and 2032 control patients had pharmacologically treated hypertension. Antihypertensive therapy was assessed using the GHC's computerized pharmacy database. The first analysis included only the 35 cases and 1395 control patients initially free of cardiovascular disease. Compared with users of diuretics alone, the adjusted RR of myocardial infarction was increased by about 60% among users of calcium channel blockers with or without diuretics. The second analysis was restricted to 384 cases and 1108 control subjects who were taking either a calcium channel blocker or a β-blocker. Among these subjects, the use of calcium channel blockers compared with β-blockers was associated with about a 60% increase in the adjusted risk of AMI (RR, 1.57). While high doses of β-blockers were associated with a decreased risk of AMI, high doses of calcium channel blockers were associated with an increased risk. In this study of hypertensive patients, the use of short-acting calcium channel blockers, especially in high doses, was associated with an increased risk of AMI. Ongoing large-scale clinical trials will assess the effect of various antihypertensive therapies, including calcium channel blockers, on several important cardiovascular end points. Until these results are available, the findings of this study support the current guidelines from the Joint National Committee on the Detection, Evaluation and Treatment of High Blood Pressure that recommend diuretics and β-blockers as first-line agents unless contraindicated, unacceptable, or not tolerated.

Change of Treatment

To evaluate the incidence of discontinuation of and changes in treatment after newly prescribed courses of antihypertensive drugs of the 3 primary therapeutic classes (β-blockers, calcium antagonists, and ACE inhibitor), Jones and associates[12] from Arlington, Virginia, conducted a retrospective analysis of patients on an automated database of 1.2 million patients seen between October 1, 1992, and September 30, 1993, by a number of general practitioners in the United Kingdom. A total of 37 643 patients with systemic hypertension were receiving a relevant drug in the time period. A new course of treatment in at least 1 of the 4 therapeutic classes, defined as a drug not prescribed in the previous 4 months, was observed in 10 222 patients age ≥40 years. Patients changing to other treatment or discontinuing after initiating a new course of treatment, defined as the absence of a refill prescription for the new drug or another in its category within a 6-month observation period. Changes in or discontinuation of treatment were frequently observed, and by month 6 continuation rates ranged between 40% and 50% for all 4 classes of drugs. Low rates of continuation with a newly prescribed antihypertensive drug exist regardless of which drug is prescribed.

To analyze the antihypertensive response of patients who had failed to achieve their diastolic BP goal (<90 mm Hg at the end of 8–12 weeks of titration) with 1 of 6 randomly allocated drugs or placebo to the random allocation of an alternate drug, Materson and associates[13] for the Department of Veterans Affairs Cooperative Study Group on Antihypertensive Agents initially randomly assigned 1292 men with diastolic BP 95–105 mm Hg to treatment with hydrochlorazide, atenolol, captopril, clonidine hydrochloride, diltiazem hydrochloride (sustained release), prazosin hydrochloride, or placebo. Of 410 men in whom initial treatment failed, 352 qualified for randomization to the alternate drug. Of the 352 patients, 173 (49%) achieved their goal diastolic BP, in 133

Table 5-1. Estimated Cost per Month of Therapy for Antihypertensive Agents, Weighted by Reported Uses, 1992*

Class/Agent	Proprietary Name†	Usual Daily Dose, mg	Usual Frequency	Uses (×1000)	Cost, $/mo
Calcium antagonists				23 623‡	47.63§
Nifedipine SR	Procardia XL, Pfizer Inc, New York, New York	60	QD	7213	56.13
Nifedipine	Procardia, Pfizer	20	TID	952	82.83
Nicardipine	Cardene, Syntex Laboratories Inc. Palo Alto, California	30	TID	420	52.21
Felodipine	Plendil, Merck & Co Inc, West Point, Pennsylvania	10	QD	698	43.73
Isradipine	DyneCirc, Sandoz Pharmaceuticals Corp, Hanover, New Jersey	5	BID	1117	38.03
Diltiazem CD	Cardizem CD, Marion Merrell Dow Pharmaceuticals Inc, Cincinnati, Ohio	240	QD	1795	49.48
Diltiazem SR	Cardizem SR, Marion Merrell Dow	120	BID	1134	63.65
Diltiazem	Cardizem, Marion Merrell Dow	60	TID	910	55.07
Verapamil SR	Calan SR, GD Searle & Co, Skokie, Illinois	240	QD	4943	32.86
Verapamil SR	Isoptin SR, Knoll Pharmaceuticals, Whippany, New Jersey	240	QD	1115	33.69
Verapamil	Calan, Searle	120	BID	300	32.54
Verapamil	Verelan, Lederle Laboratories, Pearl River, New York	120	BID	1502	50.04
Verapamil HCl	· · ·	120	BID	747	18.12
ACE inhibitors				22 713	36.14
Enalapril	Vasotec, Merck	5	BID	7037	46.34
Enalapril/HCTZ	Vaseretic, Merck	5	BID	593	46.90
Captopril	Capoten, Bristol-Myers Squibb, New Brunswick, New Jersey	50	BID	3131	53.17
Captopril	· · ·	50	BID	245	53.17
Captopril/HCTZ	Capozide, Bristol-Myers Squibb	50	BID	616	56.18
Lisinopril	Prinivil, Merck	10	QD	2008	21.92
Lisinopril	Zestril, Zeneca Pharmaceuticals, Wilmington, Delaware	10	QD	3596	22.98
Lisinopril	· · ·	10	QD	482	22.45
Lisinopril/HCTZ	Prinzide, Merck	10	QD	340	22.94
Lisinopril/HCTZ	Zestoretic, Zeneca	10	QD	519	22.98
Benazepril	Lotensin, Ciba-Geigy Corp, Summit, New Jersey	20	QD	1022	19.36
Fosinopril	Monopril, Bristol-Myers Squibb	20	QD	979	23.07
Quinapril	Accupril, Parke-Davis Pharmaceuticals, Morris Plains, New Jersey	20	QD	1182	23.89
Ramipril	Altace, Hoechst-Roussel Pharmaceuticals Inc, Somerville, New Jersey	5	QD	720	22.57
β-Blockers				12 680	23.77
Propranolol SR	Inderal LA, Wyeth-Ayerst Laboratories, Philadelphia, Pennsylvania	120	QD	616	19.69
Propranolol	Inderal, Wyeth-Ayerst	40	BID	958	25.63
Propranolol		40	BID	272	5.41
Atenolol	Tenormin, ICI Americas Inc, Wilmington, Delaware	50	QD	4232	23.64
Atenolol		50	QD	443	18.61
Metoprolol	Lopressor, Ciba-Geigy	200	QD	2927	21.57
Nadolol	Corgand, Bristol-Myers Squibb	80	QD	821	24.17

		Dose (mg)	Frequency	No.	Cost
Pindolol	Visken, Sandoz	10	BID	299	51.25
Betaxolol	Kerlone, Searle	10	QD	246	55.83
Diuretics				24 811	8.25
Thiazide and related					
HCTZ	HCTZ, generic	25	QD	4902	0.95
HCTZ	HydroDIURIL, Merck	25	QD	590	3.35
Enalapril/HCTZ	Vaseretic, Merck	5	BID	593	0.96
Captopril/HCTZ	Capozide, Bristol-Myers Squibb	50	BID	616	1.00
Lisinopril/HCTZ	Prinzide, Merck	10	QD	340	1.02
Lisinopril/HCTZ	Zestoretic, Merck	10	QD	519	0.97
Chlorthalidone	Hygroton, Rhone-Poulenc Rorer Pharmaceuticals Inc, Fort Washington, Pennsylvania	25	QD	540	13.68
Other noninjectable					
Furosemide	Lasix, Hoechst-Roussel	80	QD	3532	1.80
Indapamide	Lozol, Rhone-Poulenc Rorer	2.5	QD	2393	20.04
Bumetanide	Bumex, Hoffmann-LaRoche Inc, Nutley, New Jersey	2.5	QD	541	17.17
Potassium-sparing					
Triamterene/HCTZ	Dyazide, SmithKline Beecham Pharmaceuticals, Philadelphia, Pennsylvania	25/50	QD	5709	11.00
Triamterene/HCTZ	Maxzide, Lederle	50/75	QD	1969	18.64
Triamterene/HCTZ	Maxzide-25, Lederle	25/37	QD	1542	9.32
Amiloride	Moduretic, Merck	5	QD	714	12.79
Spironolactone/HCTZ	Aldactazide, Searle	25/25	QD	345	10.49
Other antihypertensives				10 897	26.84
Prazosin	Minipress, Pfizer	5	BID	787	53.87
Terazosin	Hytrin, Abbott Laboratories, North Chicago, Illinois	5	QD	2203	27.46
Doxazosin	Cardura, Pfizer	4	QD	983	24.35
Guanfacine	Tenex, AH Robins Co Inc, Richmond, Virginia	1	QD	1168	25.93
Guanabenz	Wytensin, Wyeth-Ayerst	8	BID	235	48.45
Methyldopa	Aldomet, Merck	500	BID	1055	17.81
Clonidine	Catapres, Boehringer Ingelheim Pharmaceuticals Inc, Ridgefield, Connecticut	0.2	BID	678	44.26
Clonidine	···	0.2	BID	562	6.43
Clonidine	Catapres-TTS,‖ Boehringer Ingelheim	0.3	Weekly	432	9.73
Hydralazine	···	25	QID	347	4.95

*SR indicates sustained release; CD, extended release; HCl, hydrochloride; HCTZ, hydrochlorothiazide; ACE, angiotensin-converting enzyme; QD, daily; TID, three times daily; BID, twice daily; and QID, four times daily.

†Proprietary names are included only if the National Disease and Therapeutic Index (NDTI) listed drug by proprietary and not generic name. Multiple listings for a single generic agent reflect separate NDTI listings for specific brand names.

‡Total mentions for each class slightly exceed the sum of individual mentions within class because of deletion of infrequent listings in published NDTI data.

§Average cost per month estimated as weighted average of cost per month multiplied by uses.

‖Clonidine transdermal preparation.

Reproduced with permission from Manolio et al.[10]

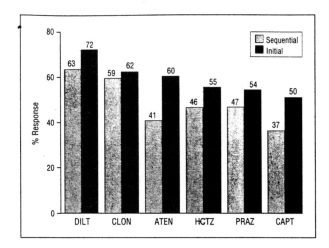

Figure 5-3. Percentage response (diastolic blood pressure <90 mm Hg at the end of the titration period) achieved by each of the initial drugs compared with that achieved by each of the sequential single drugs. All of the patients who received the sequential drug had failed to achieve a response to an initial drug. DILT indicates diltiazem hydrochloride (sustained release); CLON, clonidine hydrochloride; ATEN, atenolol; HCTZ, hydrochlorothiazide; PRAZ, prazosin hydrochloride; CAPT, captopril. Reproduced with permission from Materson et al.[13]

(38%) the alternate drug failed, and 46 (13%) left the study for various reasons. Overall response rates were as follows: diltiazem, 63%; clonidine, 59%; prazosin, 47%; hydrochlorothiazide, 46%; atenolol, 41%; and captopril, 37% (Figure 5-3). The best response rate for patients in whom hydrochlorothiazide failed was achieved with diltiazem (70%); after atenolol failure, clonidine (86%); after captopril failure, prazosin (54%); after clonidine failure, diltiazem (100%); after diltiazem failure, captopril (67%); and after prazosin failure, clonidine (53%). The combined response rate for patients initially randomized to an active treatment was 76%, which is similar to that achieved by the combination of 2 drugs in previous studies. The authors concluded that sequential single-drug therapy is rational approach for treatment of hypertension in patients in whom initial drug therapy has failed.

Effects of Drugs on Serum Lipids

Kasiske and associates[14] from Minneapolis, Minnesota, investigated 474 controlled and uncontrolled clinical trials on the effects of 85 antihypertensive agents on lipids and BP in more than 65 000 patients. **Diuretics** caused relative increases in cholesterol levels that were greater with higher doses and were worse in blacks than in nonblacks (Figure 5-4). **β-Blockers** caused increases in triglyceride levels that were substantially smaller with agents with intrinsic sympathomimetic activity. When combined with cardioselectivity, β-blockers with intrinsic sympathomimetic activity favorably affected lipids and reduced both total and LDL cholesterol levels. β-Blockers beneficially affected total cholesterol, LDL cholesterol, triglycerides, and in younger persons HDL cholesterol. **Converting enzyme inhibitors** reduced triglycerides and in patients with diabetes total cholesterol. **Vasodilators** reduced total and LDL cholesterol and

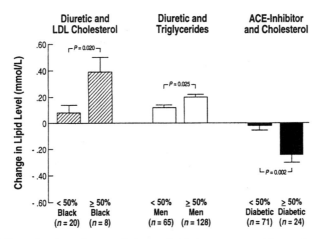

Figure 5-4. Effect of patient characteristics on lipid changes caused by antihypertensive therapy. The effect of race on diuretic-associated changes in low density lipoprotein (LDL) cholesterol levels (mean ± SEM) is shown in the left panel. Only groups for which race was reported in the study are included. Numbers in parentheses refer to the number of experimental groups with fewer than 50% blacks (15±16%) or 50% or more blacks (86±20%). The effect of sex on diuretic-associated changes in triglycerides is shown in the middle panel. Numbers in parentheses refer to the number of experimental groups with fewer than 50% men (27±18%) or 50% or more men (82±19%). The effect of diabetes on changes in cholesterol levels after treatment with an angiotensin-converting enzyme (ACE) inhibitor is shown in the right panel. Numbers in parentheses refer to the number of experimental groups with fewer than 50% patients with diabetes (1±5%) or 50% or more patients with diabetes (100%). Significance was tested using an unweighted *t*-test. Reproduced with permission from Kasiske et al.[14]

increased HDL cholesterol. Thus, with the exception of **calcium antagonists,** nearly all antihypertensive agents affect serum lipids.

Effect on Proteinuria and Renal Function

Although many studies have examined the effects of antihypertensive agents on proteinuria and glomerular filtration rate in patients with kidney disease, many questions remain unresolved. These questions include whether the effects of agents differ, whether their effects are similar in diabetic and nondiabetic patients with renal disease, and whether the effects of any agents are independent of BP reductions. Maki and associates[15] from Minneapolis, Minnesota, conducted a meta-analysis of studies obtained with MEDLINE and bibliographies from comprehensive reviews but included only investigations with follow-up times of at least 6 months. The authors combined data 1) in an analysis of randomized controlled trials, 2) in a separate univariate analysis of controlled and uncontrolled trials, and 3) using weighted multiple linear regression. In 14 randomized controlled trials, ACE inhibitors caused a greater decrease in proteinuria (pooled mean, 0.51, in improvement in glomerular filtration rate   (0.13 mL/min per month vs. 0.10–0.16 mL/min per month), and decline in mean arterial pressure (–4.0 mm Hg) compared with controls. In a multivariate analysis of controlled and uncontrolled trials, each 10–mm Hg reduction in blood pressure decreased proteinuria (regression coefficient (–0.14), but ACE inhibitors (–0.45) and nondihydropyridine calcium antagonists (–0.38) were associated with additional decklines in proteinuria that were independent of BP changes and diabetes. Each 10–mm Hg reduction in BP caused a relative improvement in glomerular filtration rate (0.18 mL/min per month), but among diabetic patients there was a tendency for dihydropyridine calcium antagonists to cause a relative reduction in glomerular filtration rate (–0.68 mL/min per month). Long-term beneficial effects of antihypertensive agents on proteinuria and glomerular filtration rate are proportional to BP reductions and are similar in diabetic and nondiabetic patients with renal disease. In addition, ACE inhibitors, and possibly nondihydropyridine calcium antagonists, have additional beneficial effects on proteinuria that are independent of BP reductions.

Thiazides

Edward D. Freis[16] Washington, DC, reviewed the efficacy of thiazides and related diuretics in preventing most of the complications of systemic hypertension. Freis was the first to recognize the antihypertensive effects of diuretics which had been introduced for treatment of CHF. Freis recommended beginning patients with systemic hypertension with a low-dose diuretic. He recommended a potassium-sparing diuretic for patients requiring increased doses or patients who had signs of myocardial ischemia.

Elliott[17] from Chicago, Illinois, determined fasting serum glucose, potassium, and cholesterol levels before therapy and yearly thereafter in 634 consecutive patients treated for more than 1 year, treated with thiazide (hydrochlorothiazide in 98% of patient years) to maintain target diastolic BP <90 mm Hg. Of the 634 patients, 310 were treated with a thiazide diuretic. The changes during the 5-year period are summarized in Tables 5-2 and 5-3. Thus, when the data were analyzed by actual on-therapy experience compared with reported randomized trials by which the data are analyzed by intention to treat methods, the thiazide therapy had a significant effect on both cholesterol and glucose levels for all 5 years studied.

Enalapril

The appropriate dose of intravenous enalaprilat to be used in the treatment of hypertensive crisis is controversial. There has been no comparative study of the efficacy and safety of different dosages of enalaprilat in hypertensive patients. Hirschl and associates[18] from Vienna, Austria, studied 65 consecutive patients with hypertensive urgencies (systolic BP > 210 mm Hg and/or diastolic BP > 100 mm Hg and evidence of end-organ damage, i.e., angina pectoris, hypertensive encephalopathy, or CHF) who were admitted to an emergency department from January 1, 1994, to September 30, 1994. The patients were randomized to receive different doses of enalaprilat (0.625, 1.25, 2.5, and 5 mg). Response to treatment was defined as a stable reduction of systolic BP to below 180 mm Hg and diastolic BP to below 95 mm Hg within 45 minutes after the start of treatment and relief of symptoms in patients with hypertensive emergencies. In 41 (63%) of 65 patients, the treatment goal was reached. Twenty-four patients (37%) failed to achieve the goal of treatment within 45 minutes after administration of enalaprilat. The response rates in the 0.625-mg, 1.25-mg, 2.5-mg, and 5-mg groups were 67%, 65%, 59%, and 62%, respectively. The proportion of patients initially randomized who responded to treatment

Table 5-2. Changes (Compared with Baseline) in Blood Levels in Treated Hypertensive Patients Analyzed by the Intention-To-Treat Method

	Year 1		Year 2		Year 3		Year 4		Year 5	
	Thiazide	Other	Thiazide	Other	Thiazide	Other	Thiazide	Other	Thiazide	Other
[Potassium] (mEq/L)	−0.08±0.04**	+0.06±0.04†	−0.09±0.06*	+0.09±0.06†	−0.02±0.06	+0.09±0.05	−0.01±0.05	+0.12±0.08*†	−0.09±0.07	+0.12±0.09†
[Glucose] (mg/dL)	+10.3±4.7**	+1.0±1.5†	+7.9±5.7	−0.1±2.1	+2.4±3.8	+1.5±2.1	+2.1±2.2	−0.9±2.6	1.8±2.7	−2.1±2.9
[Cholesterol] (mg/dL)	+14.3±2.9**	−4.8±2.0†	+7.4±3.5*	−4.7±2.5	+4.6±3.1	−5.8±4.7	+3.8±3.1	−6.5±4.1	+3.2±4.1	−9.0±5.6
Number	310	324	274	263	225	194	190	142	156	107

*P < 0.05 versus baseline.
**P < 0.005 versus baseline.
†P < 0.05 versus thiazide (same year).
‡P < 0.005 versus thiazide (same year).
Thiazide = thiazide monotherapy; other = other antihypertensive monotherapy (no diuretic).
Reproduced with permission from Elliott.[17]

Table 5-3. Changes (Compared with Baseline) in Blood Levels in Treated Hypertensive Patients Analyzed by the Actual On-Therapy Experience Method

	Year 1		Year 2		Year 3		Year 4		Year 5	
	Thiazide	Other	Thiazide	Other	Thiazide	Other	Thiazide	Other	Thiazide	Other
[Potassium] (mEq/L)	−0.08±0.04**	+0.06±0.04†	−0.13±0.05*	+0.10±0.04*‡	−0.04±0.05	+0.10±0.05	−0.02±0.06	+0.17±0.08*†	−0.12±0.07	+0.15±0.08*‡
[Glucose] (mg/dL)	+10.3±4.7**	+1.0±1.5†	+16.8±4.7**	−0.4±1.7†	+8.6±3.2*	+1.9±2.0†	+6.5±3.3*	−0.8±2.5†	+3.4±2.5	−4.9±2.6†
[Cholesterol] (mg/dL)	+14.3±2.9**	−4.8±2.0†	+13.8±2.5**	−6.8±2.5*‡	+12.6±2.7**	−8.8±3.3**‡	+12.4±2.9**	−9.6±3.8*‡	+7.9±3.8*	−11.3±4.7†
Number	310	324	243	246	184	179	150	129	118	95

*P < 0.05 vs. baseline.
**P < 0.005 vs. baseline.
†P < 0.05 vs. thiazide (same year).
‡P < 0.005 vs. thiazide (same year).
Thiazide indicates thiazide monotherapy; other, other antihypertensive monotherapy (no diuretic).
Reproduced with permission from Elliott.[17]

was not different between any of the 4 groups of enalaprilat doses. There were no significant differences according to enalaprilat dose with respect to changes in systolic, diastolic, and mean arterial BP. No severe side effects were observed. Enalaprilat is a safe antihypertensive drug with moderate efficacy in the treatment of hypertensive crisis. As doses above 0.625 mg alter neither response rates nor the magnitude of BP reduction, the authors recommend 0.625 mg as the initial dose in the treatment of hypertensive crisis.

Losartan

A good review on the new angiotensin-receptor antagonist, namely losartan, was provided by Colin I. Johnston in the November 25, 1995, issue of *The Lancet*.[19] This class of drugs is an important advance and losartan is the prototype of this new class of cardiovascular drug.

Losartan potassium, the first nonpeptide selected blocker of angiotensin II at the AT1 receptor, has been shown to exhibit clinical antihypertensive effects. Weber and associates[20] from several US medical centers characterized the efficacy and duration of action of losartan by ambulatory BP monitoring. The study was performed in nonblack hypertensive patients whose baseline untreated clinical diastolic BP were 95 mm Hg or higher and whose average 24-hour ambulatory diastolic BP were 85 mm Hg or higher. Patients were randomized, double-blind, into 4 treatment groups: placebo (n = 32) or losartan, 50 mg once day (n = 29), 100 mg once day (n = 30), or 50 mg twice daily (n = 31) (Table 5-4). Clinical and 24-hour ambulatory BP were measured at baseline (off treatment for at least 4 weeks) and after 4 weeks of treatment. By clinical sphygmomanometer measurements at the end of the 24-hour of 12-hour dosing intervals (trough), all 3 losartan dosages were significantly more effective than placebo at decreasing systolic and diastolic BP. By average 24-hour ambulatory systolic/diastolic BP measurements, the decreases produced were 0.0/0.2 mm Hg for placebo and 9.2/6.9, 9.9/6.4, and 13.2/8.5 mm Hg, respectively, for losartan, 50 mg once daily, 100 mg once daily, and 50 mg twice daily. All drug effects were different from placebo. The effects of losartan, 50 mg twice daily, were not significantly different from those of 100 mg once daily, but as expected, the effects were greater than those of 50 mg once daily. Addition of hydrochlorothiazide, 12.5 mg/d, during an additional 2-week treatment period in patients whose clinical diastolic BP remained at 85 mm Hg or higher while receiving monotherapy, produced additional and clinically meaningful BP decrements that were similar in all 4 treatment groups. There were no clinical adverse events in any group. Ambulatory BP monitoring, which virtually eliminated antihypertensive placebo responses, demonstrated clear 24-hour efficacy for losartan, 50 mg once daily, as well as for higher doses of 100 mg once daily and 50 mg twice daily. This angiotensin I–receptor blocker had antihypertensive effects that appeared additive when combined with low-dose diuretic therapy. Losartan was generally well tolerated.

Bauer and Reams[21] from Columbia, Missouri, provided a review of the angiotensin II type I receptor antagonists (Table 5-5). Initial clinical trials suggested that these drugs are effective in the treatment of essential systemic hypertension and hypertensive patients with transient renal disease. They are

Table 5-4. Effects on Systolic and Diastolic Blood Pressures of Monotherapy with Placebo or Various Dosages of Losartan Followed by Combination Therapy With Hydrochlorothiazide

| Treatment | No. of Patients | Mean (SD) Systolic/Diastolic Blood Pressure | | Additional Decrease After 2 wk of Combination Therapy With Hydrochlorothiazide, 12.5 mg/d |
		Baseline	After 4 wk of Monotherapy	
Placebo	26	148.5 (14.7)/100.5 (3.8)	150.8 (12.9)/99.9 (5.9)	8.7 (11.4)/4.0 (6.4)
Losartan, 50 mg once per day	21	159.3 (16.6)/101.0 (4.9)	148.9 (16.5)/96.2 (7.9)	5.5 (14.0)/5.1 (7.8)
Losartan, 100 mg once per day	16	150.9 (14.0)/102.3 (4.7)	140.9 (15.7)/95.6 (7.6)	6.0 (7.5)/4.0 (6.1)
Losartan, 50 mg twice per day	20	155.2 (13.8)/101.7 (4.1)	146.2 (12.6)/95.6 (6.4)	7.3 (10.4)/4.0 (6.9)

Reproduced with permission from Weber et al.[20]

Table 5-5. Evolving Class of Angiotensin II Receptor Antagonists

Pharmaceutical Company	Drug Name/Code Designation	Chemical Formula
Biphenyl Tetrazoles Angiotensin II Antagonists		
DuPont Merck, Wilmington, Delaware	Losartan potassium/DuP 753, MK-954*	2-n-butyl-4-chloro-5-hydroxymethyl-1-[(2′-(1 H-tetrazol-5-yl)biphenyl-4-yl) methyl] imidazole
	EXP-3174, L-158,641†	2-n-butyl-4-chloro-1-[(2′-(1 H-tetrazol-5-yl) biphenyl-4-yl) methyl] imidazole
	DuP 532†	2-propyl-4-pentafluoroethel-1-[(2′-(1 H-tetrazol-5-yl) biphenyl-4-yl) methyl] imidazole-5-carboxylic acid
	L-158,809†	5,7-dimethyl-2-ethyl-3-[(2′-(1 H-tetrazol-5-yl)[1,1′]-biphenyl-4-yl)methyl]-3H-imidazol[4,5-b] pyridine
Takeda Chemical Industries Ltd, Osaka, Japan	Candesartan, TCV-116 (inactive ester prodrug of CV-11974†)	(±)-1-(cyclohexyloxycarbonyloxy)ethyl-2-ethoxy-1-[(2′-(1 H-tetrazol-5-yl)biphenyl-4-yl)-methyl]-1 H-benzimidazole-7-carboxylate]
ICI Pharmaceuticals, Inc, Wilmington, Delaware	ICI D8731*	2-ethyl-4-[(2′-(1 H-tetrazol-5-yl)biphenyl-4-yl)methoxy]quinolone
G. D. Searle & Co, Skokie, Illinois	SC-52458*	5-[(3,5-dibutyl-1 H-1,2,4-triazol-1-yl)methyl]-2-[2-(1 H-tetrazol-5-ylphenyl)] pyridine
Sanofi Recherche, Montpellier Cedex, France	Irbesartan, SR47436, BMS 186295*	2-n-butyl-3-[(2′-(1 H-tetrazol-5-yl)biphenyl-4-yl) methyl]-1,3-diazaspiro-[4,4]-non-1-en-4-one
Fujisawa Pharmaceutical Co, Deerfield, Illinois	FK 739*	2-butyl-3-[(2′-(1 H-tetrazol-5-yl)biphenyl-4-yl) methyl]-3H-imidazo-[4,5-b]pyridine
Non-Biphenyl Tetrazoles Angiotensin II Antagonists		
SmithKline Beecham Pharmaceuticals, Philadelphia, Pennsylvania	Eprosartan, SK&F 108566*	(E)-3-[2-butyl-1-(4-carboxybenzyl)-1 H-imidazol-5-yl]-2-[(2-thienyl)methyl] propenoic acid
Pharma Research, Biberach, Germany	BIBR-277†	4′-[(1,4′-dimethyl-2′-propyl[2,6′-bi-1 H-benzimidazol]-1′-y)methyl]-[1-1′-biphenyl]-2-carboxylic acid
Non-Heterocyclic Angiotensin II Antagonists		
CIBA-Geigy Corp, Summit, New Jersey	Valsartan, CGP 48933†	(S)-N-valeryl-N-[(2′-(1 H-tetrazol-5-yl)biphenyl-4-yl)-methyl]-valine

*Competitive antagonism.
†Noncompetitive antagonism.
Reproduced with permission from Bauer and Reams.[21]

the newest addition to the therapeutic armamentarium for the treatment of hypertensive diseases.

Losartan ± Captopril

Azizi and colleagues[22] in Paris, France, tested the hypothesis that a combination of angiotensin-converting enzyme inhibition and angiotensin II receptor blockade may have additive biological and hemodynamic effects in a single-dose, double-blind, randomized, four-way, crossover study using the angiotensin II antagonist losartan (50 mg) and the ACE inhibitor captopril (50 mg) and their combination. Matched placebos were orally administered to 12 normotensive male volunteers maintained in sodium depletion. When 50 mg captopril and 50 mg losartan were given alone, the magnitude of their effects on BP, plasma renin, angiotensin I, and aldosterone was similar, whereas the kinetics of their effects were different, reflecting different pharmacokinetics. The losartan-captopril combination suppressed the rise in plasma angiotensin II induced by losartan 2 hours after drug intake. Six hours after drug intake, the losartan-captopril combination caused a significantly greater decrease in mean BP than has been produced by either losartan or captopril alone. After combined losartan-captopril therapy, the plasma active renin vs. time curve was significantly increased when compared with the use of either agent alone. The combination had no adverse effects on plasma aldosterone when compared with either agent alone.

Dexamethasone (for Alcohol-Induced Hypertension)

Alcohol consumption is associated with an increased incidence of systemic hypertension and stroke, but the triggering mechanisms are unclear. In non-human animals, alcohol causes activation of the sympathetic nervous system and also stimulates the release of corticotropin-releasing hormone, which has sympatho-excitatory effects when administered centrally. To determine whether alcohol evokes sympathetic activation and whether such activation is attenuated by the inhibition of corticotropin-releasing hormone release, Randin and associates[23] from Lausanne, Switzerland, measured BP, heart rate, and sympathetic nerve action potentials (using intraneural microelectrodes), in 9 normal subjects before and during intravenous infusion of alcohol (0.5 g per kg of body weight over a period of 45 minutes) and for 75 minutes after the infusion. Each subject received 2 infusions, 1 after the administration of dexamethasone (2 mg/d) and 1 after the administration of a placebo for 48 hours. The infusion of alcohol alone evoked a marked and progressive increase in the mean ($\pm$SD) rate of sympathetic discharge, from 16 ± 3 bursts per minute at baseline to 30 ± 8 bursts per minute at the end of the 2-hour period. This sympathetic activation was accompanied during the second hour by an increase in mean arterial pressure of 10 ± 5 mm Hg. After the administration of dexamethasone, the alcohol infusion had no detectable sympathetic effect. The dexamethasone-induced suppression of sympathetic activation was associated with a decrease in mean arterial pressure of 7 ± 8 mm Hg during the alcohol infusion and with suppression of the pressor effect during the second hour. Alcohol induces pressor effects by sympathetic activation that appear to be centrally mediated. It is possible that these alcohol-induced hemodynamic and sympathetic actions could participate in triggering cardiovascular events.

1. Grossman E, Messerli FH: High blood pressure. Arch Intern Med 1995 (March 13);155:450–460.
2. Houston MC, Weir M, Gray J, Ginsberg D, Szeto C, Kaihlenen PM, Sugimoto D, Runde M, Lejkowitz M: The effects of nonsteroidal anti-inflammatory drugs on blood pressures of patients with hypertension controlled by verapamil. Arch Intern Med 1995 (May 22);155:1049–1054.
3. Cook NR, Cohen J, Hebert PR, Taylor JO, Hennekens CH: Implications of small reductions in diastolic blood pressure for primary prevention. Arch Intern Med 1995 (April 10);155:701–709.
4. Glynn RJ, Field TS, Rosner B, Hebert PR, Taylor JO, Hennekens CH: Evidence for a positive linear relation between blood pressure and mortality in elderly people. Lancet 1995 (April 1);345:825–829.
5. Launer LJ, Masaki K, Petrovitch H, Foley D, Havlik RJ: The association between midlife blood pressure levels and late-life cognitive function. JAMA 1995 (December 20);274:1846–1851.
6. Flickinger AL, Burnett JC, Turner ST: Atrial natriuretic peptide and blood pressure in a population-based sample. Mayo Clin Proc 1995 (October);70:932–938.
7. Panza JA, García CE, Kilcoyne CM, Quyyumi AA, Cannon RO III: Impaired endothelium-dependent vasodilation in patients with essential hypertension: Evidence that nitric oxide abnormality is not localized to a single signal transduction pathway. Circulation 1995 (March);91:1732–1738.
8. Taddei S, Virdis A, Mattei P, Ghiadoni L, Gennari A, Fasolo CB, Sudano I, Salvetti A: Aging and endothelial function in normotensive subjects and patients with essential hypertension. Circulation 1995 (April);91:1981–1987.
9. Kokkinos PF, Narayan P, Colleran JA, Pittaras A, Notargiacomo A, Reda D, Papademetriou V: Effects of regular exercise on blood pressure and left ventricular hypertrophy in African-American men with severe hypertension. N Eng J Med 1995 (November 30);333:1462–1467.
10. Manolio TA, Cutler JA, Furberg CD, Psaty BM, Whelton PK, Applegate WB: Trends in pharmacologic management of hypertension in the United States. Arch Intern Med 1995 (April 24);155:829–837.
11. Psaty BM, Heckbert SR, Koepsell TD, Siscovick DS, Raghunathan TE, Weiss NS, Rosendaal FR, Lemaitre RN, Smith NL, Wahl PW, Wagner EH, Furgerb CD: The risk of myocardial infarction associated with antihypertensive drug therapies. JAMA 1995 (August 23/30);274:620–625.
12. Jones JK, Gorkin L, Lian JF, Staff JA, Fletcher AP: Discontinuation of and changes in treatment after start of new courses of antihypertensive drugs: A study of a United Kingdom population. Br Med J 1995 (July 29);311:293–295.
13. Materson BJ, Reda DJ, Preston RA, Cushman WC, Massie BM, Freis ED, Kochar MS, Hamburger RJ, Fye C, Lakshman R, Gottdiener J, Ramirez EA, Henderson WG, for the Department of Veterans Affairs Cooperative Study Group on Antihypertensive Agents: Response to a second single antihypertensive agent used as monotherapy for hypertension after failure of the initial drug. Arch Intern Med 1995 (September 11);155:1757–1762.
14. Kasiske BL, Ma JZ, Kalil RSN, Louis TA: Effects of antihypertensive therapy on serum lipids. Ann Intern Med 1995 (January 15);122:133–141.
15. Maki DD, Ma JZ, Louis TA, Kasiske BL: Long-term effects of antihypertensive agents on proteinuria and renal function. Arch Intern Med 1995 (May 22);155:1073–1080.
16. Freis ED: The efficacy and safety of diuretics in treating hypertension. Ann Intern Med 1995 (February 1);122:223–226.
17. Elliott WJ: Glucose and cholesterol elevations during thiazide therapy: Intention-to-treat versus actual on-therapy experience. Am J Med 1995 (September);99:261–269.
18. Hirschl MM, Binder M, Bur A, Herkner H, Brunner M, Müllner M, Sterz F, Laggner AN: Clinical evaluation of different doses of intravenous enalaprilat in patients with hypertensive crises. Arch Intern Med 1995 (November 13);155:2217–2223.
19. Johnston CI: Angiotensin receptor antagonists: Focus on losartan. Lancet 1995 (November 25);346:1403–1407.
20. Weber MA, Byyny RL, Pratt JH, Faison EP, Snavely DB, Goldberg AI, Nelson EB: Blood pressure effects of the angiotensin II receptor blocker, losartan. Arch Intern Med 1995 (February 27);155:405–411.

21. Bauer JH, Reams GP: The angiotensin II type I receptor antagonists. Arch Intern Med 1995 (July 10);155:1361–1369.
22. Azizi M, Chatellier G, Guyene T-T, Murieta-Geoffroy D, Ménard J: Additive effects of combined angiotensin-converting enzyme inhibition and angiotensin II antagonism on blood pressure and renin release in sodium-depleted normotensives. Circulation 1995 (August);92:825–834.
23. Randin D, Vollenweider P, Tappy L, Jequier E, Nicod P, Shcerrer U: Suppression of alcohol-induced hypertension by dexamethasone. N Engl J Med 1995 (June 29);332:26:1733–1737.

6
Valvular Heart Disease

Mitral Stenosis

Massive Calcium in Left Atrial Wall

Between January 1988 and June 1993, Vallejo and associates[1] from Madrid, Spain, investigated 971 patients who underwent valvular operations at their institution; 21 patients showed extensive LA calcium. In 8 patients the calcification was massive, involving almost all the atrial surface. The diagnoses were established by radiology and were confirmed at surgery. The mean age of these patients (4 men, and 4 women) was 55 ± 9.6 years. All had rheumatic valve disease, experienced AF, and had undergone at least 1 operation previously. PA pressure was severely increased, even up to systemic levels, in all patients except 1. Total endoatriectomy of the left atrium and mitral valve replacement were performed. No patient was lost during the follow-up. Hospital mortality rate was 12.5% (1 patient) and 2 patients died in the late postoperative period. No deaths were attributable to the surgical procedure. In toto endoatriectomy of a massively calcified atrium is an easy to perform technique that helps to replace the mitral valve and close the atrial wall.

Percutaneous Balloon Valvuloplasty

Palacios and colleagues[2] in Boston, Massachusetts, followed 327 patients who had percutaneous mitral balloon valvotomy during a period of 6 to 49 months. There were 7 in-hospital deaths. The patients were divided into 2 groups according to their echocardiographic scores; 211 patients had echocardiographic scores ≤8, and 116 had echocardiographic scores >8. Compared with patients with echocardiographic scores ≤8, patients with echocardiographic scores >8 were older (64 vs. 48 years) had more AF (65% vs. 40%), calcium detected by fluoroscopy (81% vs. 29%), and previous surgical commissurotomy (30% vs. 16%). With the mitral valvulotomy, mitral valve area increased from 1 to 2 cm^2 in patients with echocardiographic scores ≤8 and from 1 to 1.7 cm^2 in those with echocardiographic scores >8. Rates of survival, survival with freedom from mitral valve replacement, and survival with freedom from combined events at follow-up were greater in patients with echocardiographic scores ≤8 (Figure 6-1). Cox regression analysis identified the echocardiographic score as the most important unfavorable intermediate long-term follow-up predictive factor after percutaneous mitral valvulotomy.

Zhang and associates[3] from Loma Linda, California, assessed immediate and late outcome in 55 patients with significantly calcified valves (group 1) after balloon mitral valvotomy and compared the results with those from 60 patients with noncalcified or minimally calcified valves (group 2). After valvotomy, mitral valve area increased from 1.03 ± 0.30 cm^2 to 1.64 ± 0.35 cm^2 by echo planimetry in group 1 but was significantly smaller than the mitral valve area in group 2 after valvotomy (1.94 ± 0.38 cm^2). At a mean follow-up period of 30

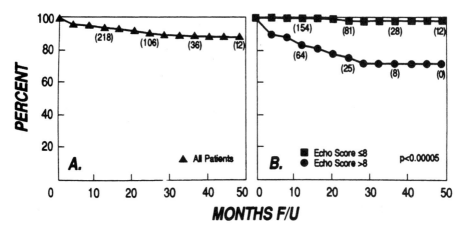

Figure 6-1. Line graphs of actuarial survival estimated from life-table analysis. Numbers in parentheses represent patients alive and uncensored at the end of each of the 4 years. Panel A: All patients, with 95% confidence intervals (CIs) for 1-, 2-, 3-, and 4-year survival at (92%, 96%), (87%, 95%), (86%, 94%), and (86%, 94%), respectively. Panel B; Comparative survival for the two echocardiographic (echo) score groups. For the group with echocardiographic scores ≤8 (211 patients at the outset of the study), the 95% CIs for percent survival at the end of years 1 through 4 were (98%, 100%), (97%, 100%), (96%, 100%), and (96%, 100%), respectively. For the group with echocardiographic score >8, the corresponding 95% CIs were (76%, 90%), (66%, 86%), (61%, 83%), and (61%, 83%). One hundred sixteen patients in this group were entered at the outset. F/U indicates follow-up. Reproduced with permission from Palacios et al.[2]

months (range, 2 to 81 months), 51% of patients in group 1 and 83% in group 2 were symptom free. Fifteen (27%) patients in group 1 and 4 (7%) patients in group 2 had cardiac events. The RR for cardiac events was 4.3 times greater in group 1 than in group 2. In group 1, the RR for cardiac events was 3.2 times higher in patients aged ≥65 years and in patients with AF. The 6-year cumulative cardiac event-free survival rate was 64% in group 1 and 90% in group 2. In 75 (65%) patients who had follow-up echocardiography study (35 in group 1 and 40 in group 2), mitral valve area decreased to 1.48±0.42 cm^2 at follow-up in group 1 and to 1.77±0.50 cm^2 group 2. It was concluded that significant valve calcification affects the immediate results of balloon mitral valvotomy and greatly increases the risk of later cardiac events. However, more than half of such patients may still derive long-term benefits from balloon mitral valvotomy, especially if they are young and have normal sinus rhythm.

Percutaneous balloon mitral valvotomy has become the procedure of choice for many patients with acquired mitral stenosis. Post et al.[4] from Philadelphia, Chicago, Illinois, and Boston, Massachusetts, evaluated the immediate and long-term results of percutaneous Inoue balloon mitral valvotomy in 72 patients with severe valvular and subvalvular deformity. An immediate optimal result, defined as a >50% increase in mitral valve area or final area >1.5 cm^2 with no major complications was achieved in 64% of patients. At a mean follow-up of 23 months, 31% required mitral valve replacement or a second valvotomy, 13% died, and 45% were in New York Heart Association functional class I or II. Only sinus rhythm predicted an optimal result by multivariate analysis. Actuarial 3-year event-free survival was 42%. These authors concluded that Inoue mitral valvotomy in patients with severe valvular and subvalvular deformity has a high technical success rate and good immediate hemodynamic result but a high cardiovascular event rate in follow-up. Balloon valvotomy remains a reasonable palliative therapeutic option for some patients with severe valvular deformity and high surgical risk.

Chen and Cheng[5] from Guangzhou, China, and Washington, DC, between November 1985 and January 1994, performed percutaneous balloon mitral valvuloplasty by the Inoue technique in 4832 patients with rheumatic MS from 120 medical centers in China. There were 1440 men and 3392 women with a mean age of 37 ± 12 years. The procedure success rate was 99%. Major complications included death in 0.12%, $\geq 3+/4+$ MR in 1.4%, cardiac tamponade in 0.81%, and thromboembolism in 0.48%. After percutaneous balloon mitral valvuloplasty, the mean LA pressure decreased from 26 ± 7.6 to 11 ± 6 mm Hg; mean mitral diastolic gradient decreased from 18 ± 5 to 5.4 ± 3.1 mm Hg; PA systolic pressure decreased from 51 ± 15 to 34 ± 9 mm Hg; cardiac output increased from 3.8 ± 1.3 to 4.8 ± 1.2 L/min; and mitral valve area expanded from 1.1 ± 0.3 to 2.1 ± 0.2 cm^2. Functional status was New York Heart Association class IV in 5.6%, class III in 39%, class II in 56%, and class I in 0.1% of patients before percutaneous balloon mitral valvuloplasty and improved to class I in 76%, class II in 23%, and class III in 1.2% after percutaneous balloon mitral valvuloplasty. The rate of restenosis was 5.2% over a follow-up period of 32 ± 14 months in the entire group and 4.6% over a follow-up period of 5.1 ± 1.0 years in the Guangdong Cardiovascular Institute, where percutaneous balloon mitral valvuloplasty was begun in China. Thus, percutaneous balloon mitral valvuloplasty by the Inoue technique is a safe and effective nonsurgical method of treatment for symptomatic MS and has long-lasting results.

Mitral Regurgitation

Quantification by Echocardiography

Pu and colleagues[6] from Cleveland, Ohio, evaluated 85 patients intraoperatively with transesophageal echocardiography and divided them into two groups: central convergence (no constraining wall) and eccentric convergence (at least one constraining wall) to determine whether proximal flow convergence allows the quantification of MR. Regurgitant stroke volume (RSV) and orifice area (ROA) were calculated by $ROA = 2\pi \, r^2 \, V_a/V_p$ and $RSV = ROA \times VTI_{cw}$, where r and v_a are the radius and velocity of the aliasing contour and v_p and VTI_{cw} are the peak and integral of regurgitant velocity. In eccentric convergence patients, convergence angle was measured from two-dimensional Doppler color flow maps and ROA and RSV were corrected by mutiplying by $\alpha/180$. RSV was the difference between thermodilution and pulsed Doppler stroke volumes. In central convergence patients (n = 45), RSV and ROA were accurately calculated, but significant overestimation was noted in the eccentric convergence patients, a significant number of whom had leaflet prolapse or flail leaflet. After correction by $\alpha/180$, overestimation was largely eliminated and excellent correlation for the whole group was found. Thus, a simple geometric correction factor largely eliminates overestimation caused by flow constraint with the proximal convergence method and should extend the clinical utility of this technique in allowing noninvasive estimation of the severity of MR using transesophageal echocardiography.

Quantification by Magnetic Resonance Imaging

Hundley and colleagues[7] in Dallas, Texas, determined whether MRI provides a rapid, noninvasive method of identifying and quantifying MR in 23 subjects (14 women and 9 men ranging in age from 18 to 72 years) with (n = 17) or without (n = 6) MR underwent MRI scanning followed immediately by cardiac catheterization. The presence (or absence) of valvular regurgitation was determined and LV volume and regurgitant fraction quantified during each procedure. There was an excellent correlation between invasive and MRI assessments of LV end-diastolic and end-systolic volumes and regurgitant fraction. All magnetic resonance imaging studies were completed in <28 minutes. In the patient with MR, magnetic resonance imaging compares favorably with cardiac catheterization for assessment of the magnitude of MR and its influence on LV volumes and systolic function.

Operative Valve Repair

Enriquez-Sarano and colleagues[8] in Rochester, Minnesota, evaluated the outcomes in 195 patients with mitral valve repair and 214 with replacement for organic MR. All patients had preoperative echocardiographic assessment of LV function. Before surgery, patients with valve repair were less symptomatic than those with replacement, had less AF, and had a better LVEF. After valve repair, compared with valve replacement, overall survival at 10 years was 68% vs. 52%, overall operative mortality was 3% vs. 10%, operative mortality in patients under age 75 was 1% vs. 6%, and late survival at 10 years was 69% vs. 58%. Late survival after valve repair was not different from expected survival. After surgery, LVEF decreased in both groups, but was higher after valve repair. Multivariate analysis indicated an independent beneficial effect of valve repair on overall survival, operative mortality, late survival, and postoperative LVEF. Thus, valve repair significantly improves postoperative outcome in patients with MR and should be the preferred type of surgical correction.

Mitral Valve Prolapse

Mitral regurgitation in patients with MVP identifies a subset of patients at higher risk for morbid events. However, MR may be intermittent and go unrecognized. Stoddard and associates[9] from Louisville, Kentucky, evaluated the development of MR in patients with MVP during supine bicycle ergometry. Thirty of 94 patients had exercise-induced MR. Prospective follow-up over a mean of 38 months showed more morbid events in the group with MR than those without. This included syncope (43% vs. 5%), CHF (17% vs. 0%), and progressive MR requiring MVR (10% vs. 0%). These authors concluded that in patients with MVP and no MR at rest, exercise-provoked MR occurs in a moderate percent of patients and predicts a higher risk of morbid events.

To assess the rate and predictors of complications in patients with MVP, 316 subjects with echocardiographic MVP were followed prospectively by Zuppiroli and coworkers[10] in New York, New York, for a mean of 102 months: 220 (70%) were women, 225 (71%) had clinically recognized MVP, and 91 (29%) were detected in family studies. During follow-up, 11 patients required mitral valve surgery, 6 died of cardiac causes, 7 developed cerebral ischemia, and 2 developed active infective endocarditis. The overall rate of fatal and nonfatal complications (1 per 100 patient-years) was higher in men than in women, in subjects aged >45 than ≤45 years, in clinically recognized patients than in affected family members, and in those with a holosystolic murmur; the overall rate was lower in those with a midsystolic click. Echocardiographic LV or atrial diameter ≥6.0 or ≥4.0 cm, respectively, was associated with a 17- and 15-fold higher likelihood, respectively, of subsequent complications. In conclusion, the risk of morbid and mortal complications of MVP 1) is low (1%/year vs. 2% to 4%/year in previous echocardiographic series); 2) is higher in men, older patients, and patients with evidence of significant MR (holosystolic murmurs and left-sided chamber enlargement); and 3) may only be about one fourth as high in unselected patients with MVP as in MVP patients referred to university hospitals.

Aortic Valve Stenosis

Villari and colleagues[11] in Zurich, Switzerland, and Naples, Italy, studied 22 patients with severe aortic stenosis prior to surgery, within 22 months after surgery, and in a late study 81 months following AVR using LV biplane angiograms, high-fidelity pressure measurements, and endomyocardial biopsies. Ten healthy subjects were used as controls. LV systolic function was assessed by biplane EFs and diastolic function from the time constant of relaxation, the peak filling rate, and the myocardial stiffness constant. LV structure was evaluated from interstitial fibrosis, fibrous content, and muscle fiber diameter. LV muscle mass was significantly increased before surgery in patients with AS and remained increased early after surgery, although there was a 35% decrease. Late after AVR, muscle mass decreased significantly but remained slightly elevated. LVEF increased slightly after AVR. LV relaxation was significantly prolonged before surgery and returned toward normal early and later after AVR. Peak filling rates remained unchanged before and after surgery. Myocardial stiffness constant was increased before surgery in patients with AS compared with controls and increased even further early after AVR, but was normalized late after surgery. Muscle fiber diameter was elevated in patients with AS before and after surgery compared with controls. However, it decreased significantly early and late after AVR with respect to preoperative data, but remained hypertrophied even late after surgery. Interstitial fibrosis and fibrous contents were larger before surgery than in controls and increased more early but decreased significantly late after AVR. Thus, diastolic stiffness increases in AS early after AVR parallel with the increase in interstitial fibrosis, whereas relaxation rate decreases with a reduction in LV muscle mass. Late after AVR, both diastolic stiffness and relaxation are normalized due to a regression of both muscular and nonmuscular tissue. Therefore, reversal of diastolic dysfunction in the patient with AS takes years and is accompanied by a slow regression of interstitial fibrosis.

Lieberman and colleagues[12] from Durham, North Carolina, evaluated the long-term outcome of 165 patients undergoing balloon aortic valvuloplasty. The median duration of follow-up was 3.9 years. During this 6-year period, 93% of patients died or underwent AVR and 60% died of cardiac related causes. The probability of event-free survival (freedom from death, AVR, or repeat balloon aortic valvuloplasty) 1, 2, and 3 years after valvuloplasty was 40%,

19%, and 6%, respectively. By contrast, the probability of survival 3 years after balloon aortic valvuloplasty in the subset of 42 patients who underwent subsequent AVR was 84%. These authors concluded that AVR may be performed in selected subjects who have undergone balloon aortic valvuloplasty with good results. However, the prognosis for the remainder of the patients who undergo balloon aortic valvuloplasty and who were not candidates for AVR is particularly poor.

Aortic Regurgitation

Tornos and associates[13] from Barcelona, Spain, monitored 101 patients with asymptomatic chronic severe AR and normal EF for up to 10 years (mean, 55 ± 34 months). Predefined surgical indications were the development of cardiac symptoms or the documentation of impaired basal LV function. During the follow-up period there were no cardiac deaths; 14 patients needed surgery, 8 because of development of symptoms and 6 because of LV impairment. The risk of surgery was 12% at 5 years and 24% at 10 years. Baseline end-systolic diameter >50 mm and radionuclide EF <60% were independent predictors of either cardiac symptoms or LV dysfunction. In patients needing surgery, a pattern of progressive LV dilatation was demonstrated. There were no deaths during surgery, and echocardiographic and radionuclide parameters normalized in the first year of follow-up. These data confirm that the prognosis of severe AR in patients with no symptoms is good and that the occurrence of asymptomatic LV dysfunction is an uncommon event. Surgery can be safely postponed until the appearance of cardiac symptoms or the documentation of LV dysfunction at rest.

David and associates[14] from Toronto, Canada, reported on 45 patients who had either reimplantation of the aortic valve (19 patients) or remodeling of the aortic root (26 patients) because of AR and aortic root aneurysm. Fourteen of the 45 patients had the Marfan syndrome, 11 had acute and 5 had chronic type A dissection, and 9 also had transverse heart aneurysm. There were 2 operative deaths, both in the remodeling group. One patient who had reimplantation needed composite replacement of the aortic valve and ascending aorta because of persistent AR after the repair. A young patient with the Marfan syndrome and progressive aortic valve dysfunction during a growth spurt and had AVR 2 years after the initial surgery. No other valve-related complication has occurred. The remaining 41 patients have only mild or no AR, and the repair remains stable from 1–58 months (mean, 18 months). These 2 types of aortic valve reconstruction have provided excellent clinical results in carefully selected adult patients.

Infective Endocarditis

To describe a 30-year experience with surgically treated culture-positive active endocarditis, Mullany and associates[15] from Rochester, Minnesota, retrospectively reviewed the microbiologic, clinical, and operative findings and survival data in 151 patients with culture-positive active endocarditis encountered in the Mayo Clinic between 1961 and 1991. The mean age of the 110 male and 41 female patients was 49.8 years. Native valve endocarditis was present in 86 patients, and prosthetic valve endocarditis was diagnosed in 65. The aortic valve was involved in 62% of patients, the mitral valve in 25%, and both valves in 10%. The operative mortality was 26%. The most important univariate determinants of mortality were an abscess at operation and renal failure. A trend toward a higher mortality with prosthetic valve endocarditis and staphylococcal infection was noted. For hospital survivors, the 5- and 10-year survival was 71% and 60%, respectively. Univariate determinants of an adverse long-term survival were annular abscess, renal impairment, heart failure, and aortic valve involvement. On multivariate analysis, the most important adverse determinants of long-term survival were heart failure, renal impairment, and prosthetic valve endocarditis. Thirty patients required a subsequent reoperation of these, 7 required a second and 2 a third operation. The most common reason for reoperation was periprosthetic regurgitation without infection (n = 19). Four operations were performed for recurrent endocarditis. At 5 and 10 years, the risk of reoperation was 23% and 36%, respectively. Although surgical treatment of culture-positive active endocarditis is still associated with substantial mortality, the long-term outcome of hospital survivors is excellent. Subsequent reoperations for periprosthetic leak are common, but recurrent infection is uncommon.

Tingleff and associates[16] from Aarhus and Copenhagen, Denmark, studied the appearance of perivalvular cavities in patients with infectious endocarditis by transesophageal echocardiography color Doppler examinations to determine whether the color Doppler transesophageal echocardiography presentation was in keeping with the current concept of perivalvular cavities representing abscesses. Two heart centers participated in the study. Videotape recordings of transesophageal echocardiography examinations in patients with infectious endocarditis were analyzed retrospectively for 18 months in both centers, and 1 center included patients prospectively for an additional 18 months. A total of 118 patients with a diagnosis of infectious endocarditis based on transesophageal echocardiography, and clinical and laboratory findings were seen during the study period. Transesophageal echocardiography showed perivalvular cavities in 34 patients. In 3 patients who died, no autopsy was performed; the perivalvular cavities were proved at autopsy or surgery in the remaining 31 patients, who constituted the study population. All perivalvular cavities were echo free at transesophageal echocardiography. Apart from 1 technically inadequate examination, all perivalvular cavities contained color Doppler signals indicating intracavitary blood flow; the perivalvular cavities communicated through a narrow channel with high-pressure regions (the left ventricle or the ascending aorta). At surgery or autopsy, only 2 of the 31 patients had pus accumulations besides the blood-filled perivalvular cavities. At transesophageal echocardiography the pus accumulations presented as echo-rich, shaggy tissue thickening. It is concluded that well-delineated, echo-free perivalvular cavities with intracavitary color Doppler signals at transesophageal echocardiography appear to be pseudoaneurysms, and therefore the term abscess should not be used in these cases. Although further studies are needed, our findings suggest that perivalvular cavities more likely occur by infectious tissue weakening and subsequent dissection rather than as a result of primary abscess formation with secondary rupture. Perivalvular cavities are nevertheless a result of severe infectious endocarditis, and an aggressive surgical approach is still recommended.

Mathew and associates[17] from Chicago, Illinois, studied 125 cases of infective endocarditis in 114 patients (84 men and 41 women) aged 37 ± 7 years. The tricuspid valve was involved in 58 cases (46%), the mitral valve in 40 cases (32%), and the aortic valve in 24 cases (19%). The microorganisms identified included *Staphylococcus* in 82 cases (66%) and *Streptococcus* in 32 cases (26%). Twenty-three patients (18%) underwent surgery, and 2 (9%) of them died. One hundred two patients (82%) were treated medically, and 9 (9%) of them died. Fifteen patients (63%) with aortic valve involvement vs. 17 patients (17%) without aortic valve involvement underwent surgery or died without surgery (OR, 89.24). Among the survivors, at least 1 major cardiovascular complication occurred in 79 cases (69%). Infective endocarditis in intravenous drug users affects the right and left sides of the heart with approximately equal frequency. At present, more than 90% of cases of infective endocarditis in intravenous drug users in Chicago are caused by staphylococci or streptococci. Involvement of the aortic valve is predictive of increased morbidity and mortality in intravenous drug users with infective endocarditis. With medical treatment, and surgery when medical treatment fails, intravenous drug users with infective endocarditis have an in-hospital survival rate of 91%.

Valve Replacement

St. Jude Medical Prosthesis

To assess long-term results of valve replacement with the St. Jude Medical Prosthesis, Baudet and associates[18] from Bordeaux, France, reviewed the case histories of the first 1112 patients undergoing 1244 valve replacements with this valve between June 12, 1978 and June 12, 1987: 690 male (62%) and 422 female patients (mean age, 56 years) (Figure 6-2). A total of 773 patients (69%) had the aortic valve replaced, 2307 (19%) the mitral valve, and 132 (12%) the aortic and mitral valves. There were 42 hospital deaths (3.8%). Follow-up was 97.5% complete (8988 patient-years). There were 213 late deaths. Ninety-one (43%) were considered valve-related: sudden death, n = 27; anticoagulant-related hemorrhage, n = 22; thromboembolism, n = 19; prosthetic valve endocarditis, n = 13; valve thrombosis, n = 9; and noninfectious perivalvular leak, n = 1. Overall actuarial survival, including hospital mortality, was $68\pm6\%$ 14 years after the operation. Linearized rates of late valve-related events were as follows: thromboembolism, 1.09%/patient-year; anticoagulant-related hemorrhage, 0.94%/patient-year; prosthetic valve endocarditis, 0.32/patient-year; valve thrombosis, 0.33%/patient-year; and perivalvular leak, 0.19%/patient year. Actuarial freedom from all valve-related deaths and valve-related morbidity and mortality, at 14 years, was $84\pm6\%$ and $61\pm8\%$, respectively. The authors conclude that, because of its low thrombogenicity, low incidence of valve-related events, and low valve-related mortality, the St. Jude Medical valve is one of the best performing mechanical prosthesis currently available. Nevertheless, the late valve-related complications and deaths illustrate that the quest for a "perfect" prosthesis remains unfulfilled.

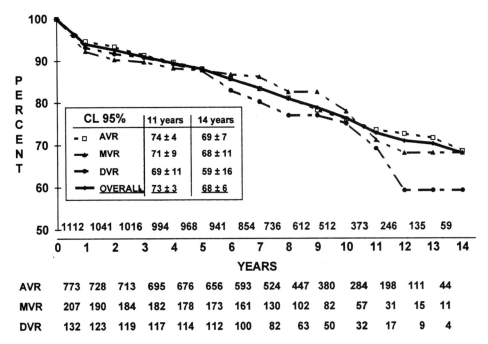

Figure 6-2. Actuarial patient survival at 14 years including hospital mortality (overall and stratified according to valve position). Numbers below figure indicate AVR, MVR, and DVR patients at risk during follow-up. CL indicates confidence limits. Reproduced with permission from Baudet et al.[18]

Porcine Bioprostheses

Long-term results after replacement of the aortic valve with a Carpentier-Edwards bioprosthesis have shown identical survival event-free status to that of mechanical prostheses in the aortic valve position. Some discrepancy exists as to the need for and duration of systemic anticoagulation in the bioprostheses, and some evidence exists to contraindicate anticoagulation because of a high late mortality in patients with an aortic valve prosthesis. Orszulak and associates[19] from Rochester, Minnesota, reviewed the records of 561 patients having the Carpentier-Edwards bioprosthesis in the aortic valve position as an isolated valve procedure. The overall rate of bioprosthetic failure events was low (0.23%/patient-year) and the survival (5-year, 74.8±2.4%; 10-year, 52.9±4.9%) and event-free statistics (5-year, 67.9±2.6%; 10-year, 42.4±5.1%) were excellent (Figure 6-3). No gender difference was present. A vulnerable period for neurological events was identified by hazard function whereby the incidence of stroke was high; these were increased in the patient variables of compromised ejection fraction (0.54), order age (≤73 years), and preoperative AF or paced rhythm. This pattern was similar for both transient ischemic events and strokes and rapidly decreased over the first few months of the first year and the first few years of the 12-year follow-up. These patients were not routinely anticoagulated. Although, in general, patients receiving a bioprosthesis in the aortic position do not require anticoagulants, a subset of patients have been identified who should receive short-term anticoagulation in an attempt to reduce the high early incidence of neurological events.

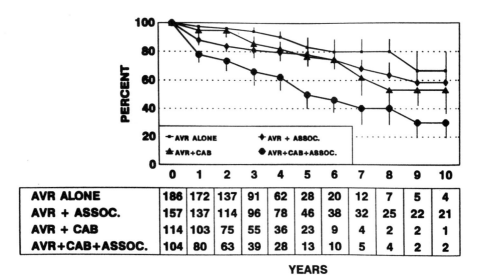

	0	1	2	3	4	5	6	7	8	9	10
AVR ALONE	186	172	137	91	62	28	20	12	7	5	4
AVR + ASSOC.	157	137	114	96	78	46	38	32	25	22	21
AVR + CAB	114	103	75	55	36	23	9	4	2	2	1
AVR+CAB+ASSOC.	104	80	63	39	28	13	10	5	4	2	2

YEARS

Figure 6-3. Comparative actuarial survival of various procedural cohorts. Assoc indicates associated procedures; AVR, aortic valve replacement; CAB, coronary artery bypass. Reproduced with permission from Orszulak et al.[19]

Jamieson and associates[20] from Vancouver, Canada, describe results of using Carpentier-Edwards porcine bioprostheses in 1195 patients (1214 operations, 1315 valves) commencing in 1975. The early mortality was 7.6% (92 patients). The early mortality without concomitant procedures was 6.1% and 11.7% with concomitant procedures. The late mortality was 5.3%/patient-year; 4.6%/patient-year without and 7.5%/patient-year with concomitant procedures. The valve-related causes of late mortality (131) were thromboembolism (41), antithromboembolic hemorrhage (14), prosthetic valve endocarditis (20), nonstructural dysfunction (12), and structural valve deterioration (44). The valve-related deaths (early, 7, and late, 124) were 21.2% of the total 617 total deaths. Reoperation for valve-related complications was performed in 406 patients (4.1%/patient-year), of which 327 were for structural valve deterioration (3.3%/patient-year). Mortality for reoperation was 0.5%/patient-year (49 patients) or 12.1%. Of the 49 deaths, 33 were caused by structural valve deterioration. The linearized occurrence rate for thromboembolism was 1.6%/patient-year (major, 0.9%/patient-year, and minor, 0.7%/patient-year). The fatal thromboembolic rate was 0.4%/patient-year (41), undifferentiated by valve position. The freedom from thromboembolism was 76% at 17 years (major, 87%; fatal, 93%). The freedom from prosthetic valve endocarditis was 92% at 17 years. The freedom from reoperation, at 15 years, was 38%; aortic (AVR), 55%; mitral (MVR), 20%; and multiple valve replacement, 24%. The freedom from structural valve deterioration, at 15 years, was 41%; AVR, 58%; MVR, 21%; multiple valve replacement 36%. The freedom from structural valve deterioration was greater for advancing age groups (AVR ≥ 70 years 96% at 12 years, and 65–69 years 94% at 12 years and 82% at 15 years; MVR ≥ 70 years 85% at 12 years, and 65–69 years 54% at 12 years. The freedom from valve-related mortality was 73% at 17 years: AVR, 80%; MVR, 61%; and multiple valve replacement, 67% (AVR > MVR, multiple valve replacement). The freedom from valve-related residual morbidity was 94%. The Carpentier-

Edwards standard porcine bioprosthesis continues to provide satisfactory clinical performance to 17 years. Thromboembolism is a more serious problem than structural failure: 92 major thromboembolic events with 41 fatalities compared with 44 fatalities, of which 33 occurred with reoperation. The prosthesis is especially recommended for patients more than 65 years of age for AVR and more than 70 years of age for MVR.

Thromboembolism appears to occur early after bioprosthetic replacement of aortic or mitral valves. Heras et al.[21] from Rochester, Minnesota; New York, New York, and Cardiff, Wales, evaluated the rate of thromboembolism at 3 time intervals in 816 patients who underwent bioprosthetic replacement of the aortic or mitral valve. The median follow-up of surviving patients was 8.6 years. The rate of thromboembolism decreased significantly at each time interval after surgery (1 to 10, 11 to 90, and >90 days). For MVR the numbers were 55%, 10%, and 2.4% per year, respectively. For AVR the numbers were 41%, 3.6%, and 1.9% per year, respectively. Patients with MVR who received anticoagulation had a lower rate of thromboembolism for the entire follow-up period (2.5% per year vs. 3.9% per year without anticoagulation). Patients with bleeding episodes were older and usually underwent anticoagulation. Blood transfusions were required in 1.2% of patients per year. These authors concluded that the thromboembolic risk was especially high for bioprosthetic AVR and MVR for 90 days after operation and was increased with lack of anticoagulation, mitral valve location, previous thromboembolism, and increasing age. Anticoagulation reduced thromboemboli and appears to be indicated in all patients as early as possible for 3 months, and thereafter in those with risk factors.

Tricuspid Valve Replacement

Porcine bioprostheses often are used for tricuspid valve replacement, yet the long-term outcome after this procedure is not well documented. Glower and associates[22] from Durham, North Carolina, reviewed the records of 129 patients undergoing tricuspid valve replacement with Carpentier-Edwards (n = 88) or Hancock (n = 41) bioprostheses between 1975 and 1993 (Figure 6-4). The operation required a repeat median sternotomy in 66 of 129 (51%) patients,

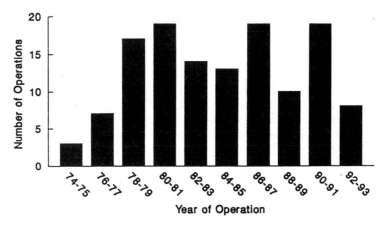

Figure 6-4. Number of porcine tricuspid valve replacements performed at Duke University over the period 1974 to 1993. Reproduced with permission from Glower et al.[22]

whereas 67 of 129 (52%) underwent double or triple valve replacement. Operative mortality was 14% (2 of 14) in patients undergoing first-time isolated tricuspid valve replacement and 27% (35 of 129) overall. Survival at 5, 10, and 14 years was 56±5%, 48±5%, and 31±9%, and freedom from tricuspid reoperation at 5, 10, and 14 years was 96±3%, 93±4%, and 49±17%. No valve thrombosis was observed. In this largest reported series of porcine bioprostheses in the tricuspid position, long-term freedom from valve-related events was excellent because of a low incidence of valve thrombosis and a valve durability of 13–15 years in a population with limited life expectancy.

Tricuspid valve replacement is not a common operation. Scully and Armstrong[23] from Toronto, California, examined the early and late results in 60 patients who underwent 28 (47%) bioprosthetic and 42 (53%) mechanical tricuspid valve replacements. All operations took place between January 1978 and June 1993 during a period in which a total of 4741 patients underwent replacement of 1 or more cardiac valves. Mean patient ages was 50±15 (18 to 75) years. Forty-one patients (68%) were female and 19 patients (32%) were male. Forty-nine patients (82%) were in New York Heart Association class III or IV before surgery. Forty-five patients (75%) were undergoing repeat cardiac valve operation. Seventeen patients (28%) had complex congenital cardiac problems. Operation was urgent in 15 patients (15%). The hospital mortality rate was 27% (16 patients). All patients with hospital death were in New York Heart Association class III or IV, were having repeat operations, or had complex congenital disease. Low output syndrome was observed in 21 patients (5%). Reoperation because of bleeding was required in 7 patients (12%). Thirteen patients (22%) required permanent (epicardial lead) pacemaker implantation. Mean follow-up is 75±45 months (maximum, 173 months) and 100% complete for the 44 patients who left the hospital. There have been 14 deaths (32%). Nine of these patients (64%) had mechanical valves, and 5 (36%) had bioprostheses. Of the 11 cardiac deaths, 3 were valve related (bioprostheses). Three patients (10%) required reoperation because of tricuspid valve prosthetic failure (1 thrombosed mechanical valve and 2 failed porcine valves). Of the remaining 30 patients, 20 (67%) are in New York Heart Association class I or II. Seventeen patients have mechanical valves and 13 have bioprostheses. Twenty-six patients (90%) are receiving warfarin. Thromboembolism has occurred in 1 patient with a mechanical valve who also had a previous cerebrovascular accident. In this group there has been no hemorrhage, endocarditis, or new pacemaker requirement. Actuarial survival for the whole series is 37±9%, and for the hospital survivors is 50±12% at 15 years. Linearized rates of valve-related complications are not different between groups. Tricuspid valve replacement is a beneficial procedure for patients with structural tricuspid valve disease, many of whom have other valvular or congenital diseases. Contemporary mechanical prostheses and bioprostheses are equally effective in the tricuspid position. Mechanical valves should be considered for tricuspid replacement in young patients and in patients with mechanical valves implanted in the left side of the heart.

Aortic Valve Replacement With Small Aortic "Root"

AVR in the small aortic root has been reported to be associated with obstruction of LV output. He and associates[24] from Portland, Oregon, designed a study to investigate the determinants of long-term survival after the implantation of small-sized prostheses. From September 1961 to December 1993, 2977 patients underwent isolated AVR at our institution. Of these patients, 447 who were older than 18 years received small-size (21 mm or less) prostheses. Long-term survival was investigated in the 404 patients who survived operation (more than 30 days) with 92% follow-up completeness (mean±SD, 7.1±6.4; maximum, 31 years). The age was younger than 50 years in 62 patients, 50–59 years in 60, 60–69 years in 99, 70–79 years in 138, and 80–94 years in 45; 67% were men. Thirty patients (7%) had previous AVR. Prosthesis usage included early Starr-Edwards models in 130 (32%), current Starr-Edwards (model 1260 since 1969) in 50 (12%), Carpentier-Edwards (porcine) in 113 (28%), and other prostheses in 111 patients (27%). One hundred sixteen patients (26%) had concomitant CABG. Eleven variables (age divided as above, sex, preoperative functional class, body surface area, small body surface area ([<1.6, 1.7, 1.8, or $1.9 m^2$] period of operation, previous AVR, type of prosthesis, size of prosthesis, concomitant CABG, and re-replacement) were investigated with regard to the long-term survival by the Kaplan-Meier method, and age, concomitant CABG, and type of prosthesis were significant. Multivariable analyses (Cox proportional hazard regression) were performed for the whole group as well as subsets of patients. The multivariable analyses reveal that concomitant CABG and age are independent variables to determine the long-term survival. In the subgroup of patients without concomitant CABG, age was the only independent variable found to determine long-term survival, and in the subgroup of the patients with concomitant CABG, body surface area < $1.7 m^2$ is the only independent variable. The authors conclude that patients with small aortic root and small body surface area may have satisfactory long-term results after isolated AVR and that old age and concomitant CABG are the risk factors for long-term survival in those patients. However, mismatch determinant for long-term survival in the subgroup of patients who receive small size of prostheses with concomitant CABG.

Pericardial Aortic Valve

To evaluate the function of the Carpentier-Edwards pericardial valve in the aortic position, Cosgrove and associates[25] from Cleveland, Ohio, analyzed the results of 310 AVRs performed between 1982–1985. Mean age was 64±11 years (range, 22–95 years); 190 patients (61%) were males. There were 18 hospital deaths (6%), none valve related. Follow-up of the 292 survivors was 100% complete at a mean of 8±3 years; 2290 patient-years of follow-up were available for analysis. There were 133 late deaths (46%). Actuarial survivals at 5 and 10 years were 83% and 46%, respectively. The 10-year actuarial freedom from events was 89±2% for thromboembolism, 91±2% for hemorrhage, 94±2% for endocarditis, and 91±3% for structural deterioration. The 153 hospital survivors 65 years of age or older had an extremely low incidence of structural valve deterioration, with only 4 explants and 96% actuarial freedom from explanation at 10 years, and a linearized rate of 0.3±0.2/patient-year compared with 87% and 0.7±0.2 for patients younger than 65 years of age. Twelve valves were explanted for structural deterioration. Of these, 11 (93%) had leaflet calcification causing stenosis, and 1 had a wear-related leaflet tear. The Carpentier-Edwards pericardial valve has a low incidence of valve-related complications.

The freedom from structural valve deterioration is low at 10 years, particularly in patients 65 years of age and older.

Homovital Homografts for Aortic Valve Replacement

Yacoub and associates[26] from London, UK, reported results of using viable homograft ("homovital") aortic valves for AVR in 275 patients aged 1.5–79 years (mean, 46±19) with maximum follow-up of a 14-year period (mean, 4.8 years). Ninety-two percent (252 patients) had New York Heart Association class II or IV functional status before surgery and 25 underwent emergency surgery. Valves were harvested under sterile conditions and kept in nutrient medium-199. Freehand (subcoronary) technique was used in 147 patients, and freestanding root replacement was used in 128. Cumulative survival rates for the whole group were 92±2% at 5 years and 85±3% at 10 years, compared with 96±2% and 94±4%, respectively, for the 98 patients who underwent isolated root replacement. Multivariate analysis determined that root replacement with associated procedures and surgery for prosthetic endocarditis were risk factors for death, whereas previous xenograft valve and surgery for endocarditis or for AR were risk factors for reoperation. Actuarial rates for freedom from degenerative valve failure diagnosed at surgery, by postmortem examination, or by routine echocardiography were 94±2% at 5 years and 89±3% at 10 years. Recipient age younger than 30 years and previous xenograft valve were risk factors for late degeneration. The authors concluded that homovital valves demonstrate good durability, particularly in patients older than 30 years, who had a 10-year freedom from degeneration rate of 97%.

Warfarin ± Dipyridamole

The addition of dipyridamole, an antiplatelet agent, to conventional anticoagulant regimens has been shown to reduce the frequency of embolization after valve replacement with a mechanical prosthesis. Pouleur and Buyse[27] from Brussels, Belgium, did a meta-analysis to reevaluate the benefit of dipyridamole by analyzing the evidence from all randomized clinical trials. Summary data were extracted from the application to the Food and Drug Administration. Six randomized clinical trials had accrued 1141 patients, of whom 582 received anticoagulant therapy alone and 559 received additional dipyridamole at dosages ranging from 225–400 mg/d. The events analyzed were all thromboembolic events, both fatal and nonfatal; hemorrhagic events, both fatal and nonfatal; and the overall mortality. The combination of dipyridamole with anticoagulants reduced the risk of thromboembolic events (fatal or nonfatal) by 56% compared with the use of anticoagulants alone. The risk reduction was seen in fatal and in nonfatal thromboembolic events (risk reduction for fatal events, 64%; for nonfatal events, 50%). The overall mortality rate was also significantly reduced by 40% in the group receiving dipyridamole. There was no difference between treatment groups with respect to hemorrhagic events (risk reduction, –1%). This meta-analysis supports the use of dipyridamole in this setting and warrants further trials with new antiplatelet agents.

The optimal intensity of oral anticoagulant therapy for patients with mechanical heart valves (i.e., the level at which thromboembolic complications are affectively prevented without excessive bleeding) is not known.

Cannegieter and associates[28] from Leiden, the Netherlands, attempted to determine the optimal intensity by calculating the incidence of both complications at different levels of anticoagulation. Data were collected on all patients with mechanical heart valves who have been seen at 4 regional Dutch anticoagulation clinics since 1985. The primary outcome events were episodes of thromboembolism or major bleeding. The intensity-specific incidence of each type of event was calculated as the number of events that occurred at a certain intensity of anticoagulation (expressed in terms of the INR) divided by the number of patient-years during which the INR was at this level in the total patient population. A total of 1608 patients were followed during 6475 patient-years. Cerebral embolism occurred in 43 patients (0.68/100 patient-years) and peripheral embolism in 2 (0.03/100 patient-years). Intracranial and spinal bleeding occurred in 36 patients (0.57/100 patient-years) and major extracranial bleeding in 128 (2.1/100 patient-years). The optimal intensity of anticoagulation, at which the incidence of both complications was lowest, was achieved when the INR was between 2.5 and 4.9 (Figure 6-5). The intensity of anticoagulant therapy for patients with prosthetic heart valves is optimal when the INR is between 2.5 and 4.9. To achieve this level of anticoagulation, a target INR of 3.0 to 4.0 is recommended.

Mechanical Valve Thrombosis

Gueret and colleagues[29] in Limoges, France, defined the role of transesophageal echocardiography in identifying nonobstructive thrombi in patients with mitral mechanical valve prostheses. Examinations were performed for recent systemic emboli in 15 patients, fever of unknown origin in 11 patients, routine postoperative evaluation in 56 patients, and for other reasons in 32 patients. All prostheses were considered normal based on transthoracic echocardiographic evaluations. However, in 20 patients, transesophageal echocardiography revealed the presence of a 2- to 15-mm long mobile thrombus localized on the atrial surface of the prosthesis. When compared with the remaining 94 patients with no visible thrombus, there was no significant difference between the 2 groups in terms of incidence of AF, LA size, LV end-diastolic diameter and fractional shortening, presence of spontaneous contrast in the LA, transprosthetic mean pressure gradient, or the type of prosthesis used. If a nonobstructive thrombus was discovered, patients were treated with heparin (n = 9) or oral anticoagulation (n = 11). The presence of a localized thrombus was confirmed in 3 patients who had subsequent operations. Clinical course appeared to depend on thrombus size: in 14 patients with a small (<5 mm) thrombus, 10 had an uneventful course, whereas 5 of 6 patients with a large (≥5 mm) thrombus developed complications or died. Thus, transesophageal echocardiography is useful in the diagnosis of thrombi on a mechanical mitral valve prosthesis, even when transthoracic Doppler echocardiographic variables appear to be normal. The transesophageal echo assessment of thrombus size may be helpful in deciding whether a patient with a mitral prosthesis should be treated by anticoagulation, thrombolysis, or valve replacement.

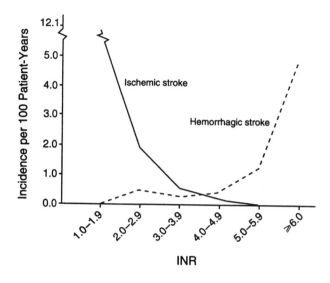

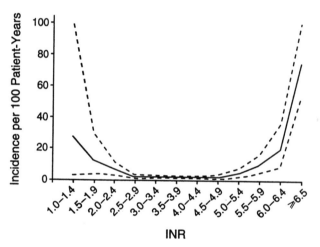

Figure 6-5. INR-Specific Incidence of All Adverse Events (All Episodes of Thromboembolism, All Major Bleeding Episodes, and Unclassified Stroke). The dotted lines indicate the 95 percent confidence interval. Reproduced with permission from Cannegieter et al.[28]

Mechanical Valve Strut Fracture

The outlet struts of Bjork-Shiley convexoconcave heart valves can occasionally fracture. By December 31, 1994, 564 complete strut fractures had been reported to the manufacturer, approximately two-thirds of which were fatal. There are no reliable diagnostic methods to detect valves that may be at risk for a strut fracture. The outlet strut has 2 legs, and 1 leg often appears to break before the other, offering potential detection of the single leg separation while the valve is still functionally intact. O'Neill and associates[30] from Royal Oak, Michigan, used high-resolution cineradiography and defined valve profiles to evaluate 315 patients who had mitral convexoconcave valves with an estimated fracture rate of 0.46% or higher per year. Two examinations were scheduled 6 months apart, with early reimaging performed when initial ratings were inconclusive. Three patients had unsatisfactory studies; the most recent examinations in 277 patients were rated as apparently normal, 23 had findings considered minimally suspicious, and 1 had findings termed suspicious. The number of false-negative results in this study group is unknown. Eleven cineradiograms were rated as showing probable or definite single-leg separations. All 5 "definite" ratings and 5 of the 6 "probable" ratings were confirmed by removal of the valves. One valve with a "probable" rating was intact. Two complete outlet-strut fractures occurred 3 and 7 months after apparently normal radiographic examinations. Unsuspected new positive findings were not found at 6 months among 288 patients who completed the examination cycle. Cineradiographic imaging can detect some single-leg separations in mitral convexoconcave valves and may help the estimated 47 000 patients with these valves worldwide and their physicians decide about elective valve removal.

Reoperations

Reoperation on prosthetic heart valves is increasingly more common. To determine the correlates of hospital events, including in-hospital mortality, new persisting neurological deficit, and length of hospital stay, a 3-institution study of 2246 consecutive prosthetic valve reoperations performed on 1984 patients between 1963 and 1992 was reported by Piehler and associates.[31] The combined experience ranged from high-risk patients coming moribund to the operating room to an important number of well individuals undergoing prophylactic reoperations on potentially failing valves. The risk-unadjusted hospital mortality was 10.8%; neurological deficit at hospital discharge, 1.1%; and median length of stay, 10 days. Multivariably determined correlates of outcome included age at reoperation; degree, severity, and acuity of impairment of cardiac function; extensiveness of valvular heart disease; coexisting morbid conditions; number of previous heart operations; and concomitant procedures. The risk-adjusted hospital mortality for the first elective reoperation in a good-risk patient was 1.3%; neurological deficit, 0.3%; and length of postoperative stay, 7 days, emphasizing the wide variance in outcome events. Equations were developed to permit wide application of the results of the study for quantitatively estimating the risk of outcome events based on individual preoperative patient characteristics. These estimates should be useful for informed patient consent, considerations of prophylactic valve replacement, and cost and resource use.

1. Vallejo JL, Merino C, González-Santos JM, Bastida E, Albertos J, Riesgo MJ, de Diego FG: Massive calcification of the left atrium: surgical implications. Ann Thorac Surg 1995 (November);60:1226–1229.
2. Palacios IF, Tuzcu ME, Weyman AE, Newell JB, Block PC: Clinical follow-up of patients undergoing percutaneous mitral balloon valvotomy. Circulation 1995 (February);91:671–676.
3. Zhang HP, Allen JW, Lau FYK, Ruiz CE: Immediate and late outcome of percutaneous balloon mitral valvotomy in patients with significantly calcified valves. Am Heart J 1995 (March);129:501–506.

4. Post JR, Feldman T, Isner J, Herrmann HC: Inoue balloon mitral valvotomy in patients with severe valvular and subvalvular deformity. J Am Coll Cardiol 1995 (April);25:1129–1136.

5. Chen C-R and Cheng TO: Percutaneous balloon mitral valvuloplasty by the Inoue technique: A multicenter study of 4832 patients in China. Am Heart J 1995 (June);129:1197–1203.

6. Pu M, Vandervoort PM, Griffin BP, Leung DY, Stewart WJ, Cosgrove DM III, Thomas JD: Quantification of mitral regurgitation by the proximal convergence method using transesophageal echocardiography: Clinical validation of a geometric correction for proximal flow constraint. Circulation 1995 (October);92:2169–2177.

7. Hundley WG, Li HF, Willard JE, Landau C, Lange RA, Meshack BM, Hillis LD, Peshock RM: Magnetic resonance imaging assessment of the severity of mitral regurgitation. Comparison with invasive techniques. Circulation 1995 (September);92:1151–1158.

8. Enriquez-Sarano M, Schaff HV, Orszulak TA, Tajik AJ, Bailey KR, Frye RL: Valve repair improves the outcome of surgery for mitral regurgitation. A multivariate analysis. Circulation 1995 (February);91:1022–1028.

9. Stoddard MF, Prince CR, Dillon S, Longaker RA, Morris GT, Liddell NE: Exercise-induced mitral regurgitation is a predictor of morbid events in subjects with mitral valve prolapse. J Am Coll Cardiol 1995 (March 1);25:693–699.

10. Zuppiroli A, Rinaldi M, Kramer-Fox R, Favilli S, Roman MJ, Devereux RB: Natural history of mitral valve prolapse. Am J Cardiol (May 15);75:1028–1032.

11. Villari B, Vassalli G, Monrad ES, Chiariello M, Turina M, Hess OM: Normalization of diastolic dysfunction in aortic stenosis late after valve replacement. Circulation 1995 (May);91:2353–2358.

12. Lieberman EB, Bashore TM, Hermiller JB, Wilson JS, Pieper KS, Keller GP, Pierce CH, Kisslo KB, Harrison JK, Davidson CJ: Balloon aortic valvuloplasty in adults: Failure of procedure to improve long-term survival. JACC 1995 (Nov 15); 26:1522–1528.

13. Tornos MP, Olona M, Permanyer-Miralda G, Herrejon MP, Camprecios M, Evangelista A, Garcia del Castillo H, Candell J, Soler-Soler J: Clinical outcome of severe asymptomatic chronic aortic regurgitation: A long-term prospective follow-up study. Am Heart J 1995 (August);130:333–339.

14. David TE, Feindel CM, Bos J: Repair of the aortic valve in patients with aortic insufficiency and aortic root aneurysm. J Thorac Cardiovasc Surg 1995 (February);109:2:345–352.

15. Mullany CJ, Chua YL, Schaff HV, Steckelberg JM, Ilstrup DM, Orszulak TA, Danielson GK, Puga FJ: Early and late survival after surgical treatment of culture-positive active endocarditis. Mayo Clin Proc 1995; (June);70:517–525.

16. Tingleff J, Egeblad, Gotzsche C-O, Baandrup U, Kristensen BO, Pilegaard H, Pettersson G: Perivalvular cavities in endocarditis: Abscesses versus pseudoaneurysms? A transesophageal Doppler echocardiographic study in 118 patients with endocarditis. Am Heart J 1995 (July);130:934–100.

17. Mathew J, Addai T, Anand A, Morrobel A, Maheshwari P, Freels S: Clinical features, site of involvement, bacteriologic findings, and outcome of infective endocarditis in intravenous drug users. Arch Intern Med 1995 (August 7/21);155:1641–1648.

18. Baudet EM, Puel V, McBride JT, Grimaud JP, Roquex, F, Clerc F, Roques X, Laborde N: Long-term results of valve replacement with the St. Jude Medical Prosthesis. J Thorac Cardiovasc Surg 1995 (May);109:5:858–870.

19. Orszulak TA, Schaff HV, Mullany CJ, Anderson BJ, Ilstrup DM, Puga FJ, Danielson GK: Risk of thromboembolism with the aortic Carpentier-Edwards bioprosthesis. Ann Thor Surg 1995 (February);59:2:462–468.

20. Jamieson WRE, Munro AI, Miyagishima RT, Allen P, Burr LH, Tyers GFO: Carpentier-Edwards standard porcine bioprosthesis: Clinical performance to seventeen years. Ann Thorac Surg 1995 (October);60:999–1007.

21. Heras M, Chesebro JH, Fuster V, Penny WJ, Grill DE, Bailey KR, Danielson GK, Orszulak TA, Pluth JR, Puga FJ, Schaff HV, Larsonkeller JJ: High risk of thromboemboli early after bioprosthetic cardiac valve replacement. J Am Coll Cardiol 1995 (April);25:1111–1119.

22. Glower DD, White WD, Smith R, Young WG, Oldham HN, Wolfe WG, Lowe JE: In-hospital and long-term outcome after porcine tricuspid valve replacement. J Thorac Cardiovasc Surg 1995 (May);109:877–884.
23. Scully HE, Armstrong CS: Tricuspid valve replacement. J Thorac Cardiovasc Surg 1995 (June);109:1035–1041.
24. He GW, Grunkemeier GL, Tagely HL, Furnary AP, Starr A: Up to thirty-year survival after aortic valve replacement in the small aortic root. Ann Thor Surg 1995 (May);59:5:1056–1062.
25. Cosgrove DM, Lytle BW, Taylor PC, Camacho MT, Stewart RW, McCarthy PM, Miller DP, Piedmonte MR, Loop FD: The Carpentier-Edwards pericardial aortic valve. J Thorac Cardiovasc Surg 1995 (September);110:651–662.
26. Yacoub M, Rasmi NRH, Sundt TM, Lund O, Boyland E, Radley-Smith R, Khaghani A, Mithcell A: Fourteen-year experience with homovital homografts for aortic valve replacement. J Thorac Cardiovasc Surg 1995 (July);110:186–194.
27. Pouleur H, Buyse M: Effects of dipyridamole in combination with anticoagulant therapy on survival and thromboembolic events in patients with prosthetic heart valves. J Thorac Cardiovasc Surg 1995 (August);110:463–472.
28. Cannegieter SC, Rosendaal FR, Wintzen AR, VanDerMeer FJM, Vandenbroucke JP, Briet E: Optimal oral anticoagulant therapy in patients with mechanical heart valves. N Eng J Med 1995;333:1:11–17.
29. Gueret P, Vignon P, Fournier P, Chabernaud J-M, Gomez M, LaCroix P, Bensaid J. Transesophageal echocardiography for the diagnosis and management of nonobstructive thrombosis of mechanical mitral valve prosthesis. Circulation 1995 (January);91:103–110.
30. O'Neill WW, Chandler JG, Gordon RE, Bakalyar DM, Abolfathi AH, Castellani MD, Hirsch JL, Wieting DW, Bassett JS, Beatty KC, Soltis MA, Timmis GC, Grines CL: Radiographic detection of strut separations in Bjork-Shiley convexo-concave mitral valves. N Engl J Med 1995 (August 17);333:414–419.
31. Piehler JM, Blackstone EH, Bailey KR, Sullivan ME, Pluth JR, Weiss NS, Brookmeyer RS, Chandler JG: Reoperation on prosthetic heart valves. J Thorac Cardiovasc Surg 1995 (January);109:1:30–48.

7

Myocardial Heart Disease

Idiopathic Dilated Cardiomyopathy

Risk of Alcoholic Type by Gender

To compare the cardiac and muscular status of male and female alcoholics to determine if the response of women to alcohol is different from that of men, Urbano-Márquez and associates[1] studied 50 asymptomatic alcoholic women, 100 asymptomatic alcoholic men, and 50 female nonalcoholic control subjects. The mean strength of the deltoid muscle in alcoholic women was significantly lower than that of the control subjects, and half suffered clinical weakness. Muscle biopsy specimens from half of all asymptomatic women showed histological evidence of myopathy. LVEF tended to be depressed, and a third of the alcoholic women had evidence of cardiomyopathy. Muscular strength and EF in women were inversely correlated with the total lifetime dose of ethanol. However, the threshold dose for the development of cardiomyopathy was considerably less in women than in men, and the decline of the EF with increasing alcohol dose was significantly steeper. Despite the fact that the mean lifetime dose of alcohol in female alcoholics was only 60% that in male alcoholics, cardiomyopathy and myopathy were as common in female alcoholics as in male alcoholics. This finding, together with a more pronounced response of the EF to the dose of ethanol, indicates that women are more sensitive than men to the toxic effects of alcohol on striated muscle.

With Ventricular Tachycardia

Kottkamp and colleagues[2] in Münster, Germany, investigated the feasibility of radiofrequency catheter ablation in patients with idiopathic dilated cardiomyopathy in the treatment of sustained VT in patients who could not be adequately treated by conventional treatment modalities. Radiofrequency current ablation for ablation of 9 VTs was attempted in 8 patients with idiopathic dilated cardiomyopathy (mean age, 54 years; mean LVEF, 30%). Inclusion criteria for ablation were incessant VT or frequent, recurrent VT reproducibly inducible with programmed electrical stimulation. Three patients had suffered aborted sudden cardiac death, and 2 had experienced syncope. Two patients were artificially ventilated and catecholamine dependent for hemodynamic reasons at the time of attempted ablation. Potential target sites for radiofrequency catheter ablation are identified by detailed endocardial mapping during sinus rhythm, activation, and entrainment mapping during VT and pace mapping. After 7 radiofrequency pulses applied with 32 W for 39 seconds, 6 of the 9 target VTs were made noninducible. In 6 patients, VTs with electrocardiographic morphologies other than the target VTs were inducible after radiofrequency catheter ablation. Seven patients were on antiarrhythmic drugs during the ablation procedure and during the follow-up period of 8 months. One patient received an implantable cardioverter defibrillator before radiofrequency ablation, 4 patients after radiofrequency ablation, and 1 patient after ablation of an incessant VT and before attempted ablation of frequent, recurrent VTs. One patient underwent heart transplantation 5 months after ablation in end-stage CHF. There were no acute complications during the mapping and ablation procedure. During the follow-up period, 1 patient had been resuscitated from VF 6 weeks after ablation and finally died of CHF 2 weeks later. No further episodes of incessant VT occurred in the patients who had undergone radiofrequency current application for ablation of incessant VT. A complete prevention of VT could be achieved in 2 of 8 patients, whereas in 5 patients, VT episodes were stored in the implantable cardioverter defibrillator during follow-up. The results of this study indicate that radiofrequency current ablation may be used for ablation of VT in a select group of patients with idiopathic dilated cardiomyopathy.

Effect of Exercise Training

Belardinelli and colleagues[3] determined whether exercise training may induce changes in LV diastolic filling that allow an increase in exercise capacity and whether these changes influence prognosis in patients with dilated cardiomyopathy. Fifty-five consecutive patients with a mean age of 55 years with dilated cardiomyopathy were evaluated. They were randomly assigned into a training group (36 patients) or a control untrained group (19 patients) and matched for clinical and functional characteristics. All patients underwent a pulsed Doppler echocardiographic study, a radionuclide angiographic study, and a cardiopulmonary exercise test before and after a 2-month exercise program. On the basis of the Doppler LV diastolic filling pattern at the beginning of the study, patients were prospectively divided into three subgroups: A (restrictive pattern), B ("normal" pattern), and C (abnormal relaxation pattern). In the trained group, peak myocardial oxygen consumption, peak workload, and lactic acidosis threshold were significantly increased after training without changes in LVEF. However, only subgroup C demonstrated significant improvement in peak myocardial oxygen consumption. No changes were observed in the untrained group. In the trained subgroups, significant increase in rapid filling fraction, peak filling rate, peak early filling velocity, and E/A ratio of diastolic filling were noted. A significant decrease in atrial filling fraction, peak atrial filling velocity, deceleration time of early filling velocity, and isovolumic relaxation time were observed only in subgroup C. No changes were found in the untrained subgroups. A good correlation was found between Doppler and radionuclide LV diastolic filling variables before and after training. Multiple stepwise regression analysis demonstrated that pretraining diastolic relaxation ratio and peak heart rate were positive predictors of pretraining peak myocardial oxygen consumption. Post-training increase in exercise tolerance and increase in diastolic relaxation were the strongest predictors of an increase in peak myocardial oxygen consumption. The independent predictors of cardiac events were greater rapid filling fraction and a shorter isovolumic relaxation time and deceleration time of early filling velocity. Stepwise logistic regression showed that the Doppler LV diastolic filling patterns are independent predictors of overall cardiac events. The restrictive pattern had a worse prognosis compared with the "normal" and abnormal relaxation pattern (groups B and C, respectively). However, exercise training did not reach statistical significance as a predictor of cardiac events. Thus, these data demonstrate that exercise training induces significant improvement in exercise capacity in patients with dilated cardiomyopathy with abnormal LV relaxation. An improvement in myocardial oxygen consumption is correlated with an increase in peak early filling rate and a decrease in atrial filling rate. Doppler echocardiography is a valuable tool in the prognostic assessment of patients with dilated cardiomyopathy who will benefit from exercise training.

Location of Gene in the Familial Variety

Durand and colleagues[4] studied a family of 46 members with hereditary dilated cardiomyopathy. Among these family members, there were 4 generations of patients who had medical histories and physical examinations, echocardiographic analyses, and blood sampling for genotyping. Diagnostic criteria from echocardiography, consisted of ventricular dimensions ≥2.7 cm/m^2 with LVEFs ≤50% in the absence of other causes for cardiomyopathy. DNA from all family members was analyzed by polymerase chain reaction for amplification of short tandem-repeat polymorphic markers located every 10 cM throughout the human genome. Assuming a penetrance of 90%, linkage analysis was performed to map the responsible chromosomal locus. Linkage analysis, after 412 markers were analyzed, indicated the locus to be on chromosome 1q32 with a peak multipoint logarithm of the odds score at D1S414 of 6.37. These data suggest a locus, 1q32, is rich in candidate genes for familial dilated cardiomyopathy.

Interleukin-2 Receptor Levels

Limas and colleagues[5] in Minneapolis, Minnesota, explored the possibility that activation of cellular immunity is frequent in patients with idiopathic dilated cardiomyopathy. Serum soluble interleukin-2 receptors were determined with an enzyme-linked immunosorbent assay in 50 patients with dilated cardiomyopathy, 30 patients with CAD, and 22 normal control subjects. The presence of an anti–β-receptor and antimyosin antibodies were also sought in the serum of the cardiomyopathic patients. Elevated soluble interleukin-2 receptor levels were found in 38% of the patients with dilated cardiomyopathy but in only 6% of the CAD patients. The patients with soluble interleukin-2 receptors were characterized by being older, having more women, and more severe heart muscle disease. Although the prevalence of cardiac autoantibodies did not correlate with the presence of high soluble interleukin-2 receptor levels, higher titers of autoantibodies were found predominantly in the soluble interleukin-2–receptor positive patients. These results suggest that T-lymphocyte activation as reflected in elevated soluble interleukin-2 receptor levels is frequent in patients with dilated cardiomyopathy and is associated with more severe disease.

Hypertrophic Cardiomyopathy

Prevalence

Maron and colleagues[6] as part of the Coronary Artery Risk Development in Young Adults (CARDIA) study estimated the prevalence of HC in young people, including competitive athletes. In this epidemiological study of coronary risk factors, 4111 men and women (age, 23 to 35 years) selected from the general population of four urban centers had technically satisfactory echocardiographic studies during 1987 through 1988 to make these determinations. Probable or definite echocardiographic evidence of HC was present in 7 subjects (0.17%) on the basis of identification of a hypertrophied, nondilated LV and maximal wall thickness ≥15 mm that were not associated with systemic hypertension. Prevalence in men and women was 0.26:0.09%; in blacks and whites, 0.24:0.10%. Ventricular septal thickness was 15 to 21 mm (mean, 17 mm) in the 7 subjects. Only 1 of the 7 individuals had ever experienced important cardiac symptoms or had been previously suspected of having cardiovascular disease or obstruction to LV outflow. Four other individuals had relatively mild systolic anterior motion of the mitral valve that was insufficient to produce dynamic basal outflow obstruction. Electrocardiograms were abnormal in 5 of the 7 subjects. Thus, HC was present in approximately 2 of 1000 young adults.

Natural History

Cannan and colleagues[7] in Washington, DC, and Rochester, Minnesota, undertook a population-based study to examine the natural history of HC among unselected residents of Olmsted County, Minnesota. Patients with HC confirmed by echocardiography were identified by use of the resources of the Rochester Epidemiology Project. Patients with echocardiographic features of HC but with long-standing increases in BP requiring drug therapy were categorized as having hypertensive HC. Baseline clinical details and follow-up events were obtained by retrospective chart review. Thirty-seven patients were diagnosed with HC and 24 with hypertensive HC. Eight additional patients were first recognized at autopsy. The mean age of the 37 patients with HC was 59 years. Follow-up was obtained for a median of 8 years. The 1- and 5-year survival rates were 95% and 92%, respectively; these results did not differ from those of an age- and sex-matched population. The annual risk of cardiac death was 0.7%. The mean age of patients with HC was 79 years, and the mean ventricular septal thickness was 19 mm. Follow-up was obtained for a median of 3 years. The 1- and 5-year survival rates were 75% and 43%, respectively, differing from the expected rates of 94% and 70%. The annual rate of cardiac death was 5%. AF and evidence for AMI on the electrocardiogram, use of digoxin and diuretics, and a high New York Heart Association functional class at presentation were associated with decreased survival by multivariate analysis for both groups combined. A history of AMI, AF, and mitral annular calcium at presentation were associated with cardiac death. These data suggest that HC is a more benign disease than previously reported from tertiary referral centers. Patients found to have hypertensive HC are at higher risk of cardiac and noncardiac death and have overall decreased survival rate.

Response to Isoproterenol

In most patients with HC, LV systolic function is normal or supernormal. In a few patients, however, HC progresses to a state that is characterized by systolic dysfunction and LV dilation, and resembles dilated cardiomyopathy. Kawano and associates[8] from Ibaraki, Japan, did echocardiograms before and immediately after the intravenous infusion of isoproterenol (0.02 μg/kg body weight per minute) for 5 minutes in 18 patients with typical HC. In the good-response group neither end-diastolic diameter nor fractional shortening changed significantly. In the poor-response group end-diastolic diameter significantly increased from a mean of 41–53 mm, and fractional shortening decreased from 40% to 29% during an average follow-up period of 5.4 years. One of these patients developed CHF due to systolic dysfunction. These authors concluded that the response of patients with HC to isoproterenol is predictive of those who will go on to develop future deterioration of LV systolic function.

Paced Electrogram Fractionation

Saumarez and colleagues[9] in London, United Kingdom, have evaluated the ultimate significance of an increased duration of paced RV electrograms in 64 patients with HC to correlate the risk of VF with changes in electrogram duration. Preliminary studies had suggested that the change in electrogram duration with pacing stimulus prematurity discriminated patients into three groups: VF survivors; an intermediate group with either nonsustained VT on ambulatory monitoring or a family history of sudden death; and those with none of these risk factors for sudden death. Among the 64 patients with HC, 3 had documented VT, 1 had witnessed sudden death and was assumed to have had VF, 25 had nonsustained VT, 21 had a familial history of sudden death, and 14 had no risk factors. Nineteen patients had syncope. They were studied by pacing one RV site with a decremental sequence and recording high-pass filtered electrograms from three other RV sites. The delay of each fractionated potential in the electrogram was determined relative to a pacing stimulus of increasing prematurity. These measurements were repeated by pacing each ventricular site in turn. The electrograms were characterized by two variables: the extrastimulus coupling interval (S_1S_2) at which the delay increased by more than 0.75 msec/ 20 msec decrease in S_1S_2 interval and the change in electrogram duration between an S_1S_2 of 350 msec and ventricular effective refractory period. Four VF patients had a mean increase in electrogram duration of 16 ms and an increase in delay at a mean S_1S_2 of 368 msec. Three VF patients were within the original VF group, whereas only 6 of 60 non-VF patients were within this group, discriminating between VF patients and the remainder of the individuals evaluated. The 14 without risk factors had a mean change in electrogram duration of 4.5 msec and an increase in delay at a mean S_1S_2 of 301 msec. Eleven patients were within the original no risk factor group, and only 8 of the remaining 50 patients were also within that group, discriminating between the group with no risk factors and the remainder of the patients. Most of the nonsustained VT and familial history sudden death patients were between the original VF and no risk factor groups with 5 of the 25 nonsustained VT and 1 of 31 with familial history of sudden death patients in the original VF group. There was no relation between syncope and electrophysiological characteristics. Programmed electrical stimulation was performed in the first 15 patients in this study. Of the total 52 patients from the original and current studies, programmed electrical stimulation identified 2 of 6 VF patients, and there was no correlation between VF inducibility and intraventricular conduction delay. Thus, these data are consistent with the data described in the original VF and no risk factor groups.

Most patients with familial history of sudden death or nonsustained VT were between these two groups. Pooled data from the original and current groups allow definition of the new VF group, which includes all patients with VF, 8 of 30 patients with VT, and 3 of 31 patients with a familial history of sudden death. These insights may be helpful in identifying patients who may benefit from an implantable cardioverter-defibrillator.

Genetic Studies

Familial HC can be caused by mutations in the genes for β-cardiac myosin heavy chain, α-tropomyosin, or cardiac troponin T. It is not known how often HC is caused by mutations in the tropomyosin or troponin genes and the associated phenotypes have not been studied. Watkins and associates[10] from multiple medical centers assessed linkage between polymorphism of the α tropomyosin gene or the cardiac troponin T gene and HC in 27 families. In addition, 100 probands were screened for mutations in the α-tropomyosin gene, and 26 were screened for mutations in the cardiac troponin T gene. Life expectancy, the incidence of sudden death, and the extent of LV hypertrophy were compared in patients with different mutations. Genetic analyses identified only one α-tropomyosin mutation, identical to one previously described. Five novel mutations in cardiac troponin were identified, as well as a further example of a previously described mutation. The clinical phenotype of 4 troponin T mutations in 7 unrelated families was similar and was characterized by a poor prognosis (life expectancy, approximately 35 years) and a high incidence of sudden death. The mean (±SD) maximal thickness of the LV wall in subjects with cardiac troponin T mutations (16.7±5.5 mm) was significantly less than that in subjects with β-cardiac myosin heavy-chain mutations (23.7±7.7 mm).

Watkins and colleagues[11] in Boston, Massachusetts, investigated 2 missense mutations in the gene for α-tropomyosin by evaluating the origins of one of these mutations, Asp175Asn, in a third and unrelated family. The presence or absence of an α-tropomyosin mutation and the haplotypes of the flanking chromosomal regions were determined for members of the family with HC. Haplotypes were constructed by use of an intragenic polymorphism and 10 flanking polymorphisms spanning a region of 35 cM. The Asp175Asn missense mutation was present in the proband and his 2 affected offspring but not in any of the proband's 3 siblings. Although both parents were deceased, the haplotypes of the 4 parental chromosomes could be reconstructed. One parental chromosome was transmitted to 2 offspring, 1 bearing the Asp175Asn mutation (affected proband) and 1 clinically unaffected sibling who lacked the α-tropomyosin mutation. Thus, the Asp175Asn mutation must have arisen de novo. Therefore, de novo mutations in the α-tropomyosin gene may result in HC, and it may appear to be sporadic but in subsequent generations give rise to familial disease. Individuals with sporadic HC should be advised of the risk of transmission to offspring. These data provide strong genetic evidence that mutations in the α-tropomyosin gene are directly responsible for HC.

Nishi and colleagues[12] from Tokyo, Japan, analyzed the nature of the cardiac beta myosin heavy chain gene from patients with HC using polymerase chain reaction–DNA conformation polymorphism analysis and found two sequence variations in exons 3 and 22 in 1 patient. These sequence variations at codons

54 and 870 were identified by direct sequencing and dot-blot hybridization with allele-specific oligonucleotide probes. Relatives of this patient were examined for the mutations. Examination of the patient's revealed that the missense mutation was inherited from the affected father and the nonsense mutation from the unaffected grandmother through the unaffected mother. The missense mutation was also found in 7 other patients from 2 other unrelated multiplex HC families. These data suggest that the Arg[870]His mutation was causally related to HC in this patient. The gene with a nonsense mutation encoded for a cardiac beta myosin heavy chain protein of only 53 amino acid residues which may be too short to be incorporated into the thick filament assembly of cardiac myosin chains and showed no dominant phenotype of heart disease. This may be the first report of a nonsense mutation in the human cardiac β-myosin heavy chain gene leading to HC.

Nonsurgical Reduction of Septum

Surgery has been the only therapeutic option for patients with obstructive HC who are resistant to drug therapy and sequential pacemaker therapy. Sigwart[13] from London, UK, described a novel catheter-based technique that may replace surgical myocardial reduction in some patients. The technique aims at selective destruction of the hypertrophied part of the left side of the ventricular septum. If temporary occlusion of the first major septal artery is shown to reduce the intraventricular pressure gradient significantly, absolute alcohol is injected through the inflated balloon catheter to produce a localized infarct. In the first 3 patients treated with this method, the size of the septal infarct was sufficient to eliminate any subaortic stenosis immediately. Clinical improvement was maintained up to 12 months. The author concluded that non-surgical reduction of the ventricular septum in obstructive HC warrants further clinical evaluation.

Operative Treatment

Heric and associates[14] from Tacoma, Washington; Cleveland, Ohio; and Buffalo, New York, reported results of surgical operations for obstructive HC in 178 patients operated on from 1975–1993. Operations included isolated septal myectomy (n=95); septal myectomy and CABG (n=41); septal myectomy plus a valve procedure (n=25); septal myectomy, valve procedure, and CABG (n=14); and mitral valve replacement without septal myectomy (n=3). Recent myectomy results were monitored with transesophageal echocardiography. After initial myectomy, 32 patients (20%) underwent a second pump run for more extensive myectomy only (n=22), MVR only (n=5), or both (n=2). In-hospital mortality was 6% (n=11) and 4% (n=6) for patients undergoing septal myectomy or septal myectomy plus CABG, respectively. Heart block occurred in 17 patients (10%). LV outflow tract systolic gradients decreased from a mean of 93 to 21 mm Hg after myectomy. Late survival was 86% and 70% at 5 and 10 postoperative years, respectively, and 93% and 79% for patients undergoing septal myectomy alone or septal myectomy plus CABG. Only 3 of 131 in-hospital survivors of septal myectomy or septal myectomy plus CABG died late of cardiac causes, for a yearly mortality of 0.6%. However, the 5-year late survival of patients undergoing valve operation plus septal myectomy was 51%, and multivariate testing confirmed the adverse influence on late survival, as well as adverse influences of increasing age and return to cardiopulmonary bypass for MVR. At follow-up 136 patients (94%) had New York Heart Association class I or II symptoms. For patients with HC, septal myectomy alone or in combination with CABG produces effective symptom relief, excellent long-term survival and a low risk of late cardiac death.

Pseudoform After Tacrolimus Therapy

Reported side-effects of tacrolimus, a potent immunosuppressive agent, have not included cardiotoxicity. Atkison and associates[15] from Dallas, Texas, describe 5 consecutive pediatric transplant recipients (3 small bowel with or without liver and 2 liver) who received tacrolimus. Two developed CHF and obstructive HC, which resolved after changing to cyclosporin. In the other 3 patients the cardiomyopathy regressed or improved with a lower dose of tacrolimus or after stopping the drug.

Association with a Condition Affecting Primarily a Noncardiac Structure(s)

HIV Involvement

Lipshultz and associates[16] from Boston, Massachusetts, studied the effect of intravenous immunoglobulin therapy on cardiac function in children with HIV infection. Progressive LV dilation is common in children infected with HIV-1 and may be a harbinger of CHF. In many such children, dilation is associated with inadequate LV hypertrophy, elevated afterload, and reduced LV function. Intravenous immunoglobulin has been observed empirically to improve CHF in other conditions, and therefore the effect of infusion was examined retrospectively in HIV children with and without CHF. A total of 106 echocardiograms were performed in 49 children within 30 days of serum immunoglobulin measurements, including 12 children treated with IVIG therapy. All parameters were adjusted for age and body surface area and subjected to repeated measures regression. High endogenous serum IgG levels and IVIG treatment were associated with significantly greater wall thickness and lower peak stress. High endogenous serum IgA levels were associated with more normal LV wall thickness and LV thickness-to-dimension ratios. LV contractility, fractional shortening, end-systolic wall stress, and thickness-to-dimension ratio all showed a trend toward more normal values with higher endogenous immunoglobulin values or during IVIG treatment. These results suggest that both the impaired myocardial growth and the LV dysfunction observed may be immunologically mediated and responsive to immunomodulatory therapy.

To determine the natural course of muscle disease in patients infected with HIV, Currie and associates[17] from Edinburgh, U.K., studied 296 adults infected with HIV. Their ages ranged from 21 to 68 years (mean, 33 years). Cardiac dysfunction was identified in 44 subjects (dilated cardiomyopathy, 13; isolated RV dysfunction, 12; borderline LV dysfunction, 19). Dilated cardiomyopathy was strongly associated with a CD4 cell count of $<100\times10^6$/L, in contrast with the other forms of cardiac dysfunction. During the study 12 of 13 (92%) subjects with dilated cardiomyopathy, 5 of 12 (42%) with RV dysfunction, and 8 of 19

(42%) with borderline LV function died of conditions related to AIDS. Survival was significantly reduced in the subjects with dilated cardiomyopathy compared with those with normal hearts. The median survival form the index echocardiogram was 101 days for the subjects with cardiomyopathy compared with 472 days (383 to 560) for those with normal hearts and a CD4 cell count of <20×10⁶. No significant difference existed in survival for subjects with borderline LV or isolated RV dysfunction. Even after adjustment for the significantly reduced CD4 cell count with which dilated cardiomyopathy is associated, the outlook for patients with HIV infection and dilated cardiomyopathy is poor. Isolated RV and borderline LV dysfunction are not associated with reduced CD4 cell counts and do not carry adverse prognostic implications.

Myotonic Dystrophy

Child and Perloff[18] from Los Angeles, California, determined whether and to what degree myocardial myotonia might occur in myotonic muscular dystrophy. Cardiac involvement in this disease manifests itself chiefly as abnormalities of specialized tissues. Current echocardiographic techniques permit assessment of LV diastolic filling properties and thereby detection of subtle myocardial myotonia. Twenty patients (mean age, 37±13 years) with myotonic muscular dystrophy were studied. Twenty normal individuals (mean age, 34±12 years) served as control subjects. Each individual had 2-dimensional targeted M-mode echocardiograms of the posterior LV wall to measure the rate of early diastolic relaxation, which was defined as diastolic endocardial velocity maximum. Global LV function was quantified. Doppler recordings of mitral inflow measured peak E and A velocities, ratio of E to A, mitral deceleration time and isovolumic relaxation time. Normal control subjects had diastolic endocardial velocity maximum, 19±3 cm/sec; isovolumic relaxation, 72±7 msec; ratio of E to A, 1.6±0.5; and mitral deceleration time, 193±18 msec. Two standard deviations below the mean normal diastolic endocardial velocity maximum was 13 cm/sec. Two patient groups emerged: group A (10 patients) had abnormally slow diastolic endocardial velocity maximum (≤13 cm/sec) and group B (10 patients) had normal diastolic endocardial velocity maximum >13 cm/sec) with diastolic endocardial velocity maximum 11±2 cm/sec and 20±4 cm/sec, respectively. Mitral inflow parameters showed a longer mitral deceleration time and isovolumic relaxation, with lower E to A ratios for group A vs. group B, with mitral deceleration time, 203±48 msec and 175±21 msec; isovolumic relaxation, 87±15 msec and 74±7 msec; and ratio of E to A 1.7±0.7 and 2.3±0.9, respectively. This is the first study in which measurements of posterior LV wall early relaxation rates and Doppler evaluation of mitral inflow profiles provide evidence of occult myocardial myotonia in myotonic dystrophy.

To evaluate and quantitate cardiac involvement in myotonic dystrophy, Tokgozoglu and associates[19] from Ankara, Turkey, compared 25 patients with myotonic dystrophy with age-matched normal control subjects, and found that the latter patients were more likely to have conduction abnormalities (52% vs. 9%), MVP (32% vs. 9%), and wall motion abnormalities (28% vs. 0%). LVEF and stroke volume were reduced compared with normals matched for age and heart rate, whereas Doppler indexes of diastolic function were only marginally altered. Patients with more extensive neurological findings (n=12) had a higher incidence of wall motion and/or electrocardiographic conduction abnormalities (83% vs. 43%). The authors concluded that conduction involvement in myotonic dystrophy predominantly affects the conduction system and myocardial function. Alterations in myocardial relaxation and diastolic properties, in contrast to skeletal myotonia, are minor.

β-*Thalassemia Major*

Kremastinos and colleagues[20] in Athens, Greece, conducted a prospective 5-year follow-up study in all patients with β-thalassemia major in whom the diagnosis of acute infectious myocarditis was established between 1977 and 1986. A similar number of age- and sex-matched control subjects with β-thalassemia and normal LVEF and no evidence of myocarditis were followed for 5 years. Among 1048 patients with β-thalassemia major, 47 patients with a mean age of 15 with precordial chest pain were diagnosed as having acute infectious myocarditis. Myocardial biopsy was diagnostic in 26 patients, borderline in 14, and nondiagnostic in 7 patients. Acute CHF with a mean LVEF of 25% developed in 11 patients with myocarditis; 8 died within 1 month to 1 year of diagnosis. Thirteen patients with myocarditis developed chronic CHF with a mean LVEF of 26% within 3 years and 10 of these died within 8 months. LV systolic and diastolic functions in the control subjects did not change significantly during the 5-year period. LV restrictive abnormalities combined with RV dilatation and right-sided CHF developed in 3 patients with high mean serum ferritin levels. In general, however, no significant differences were found in mean levels of serum ferritin between patients with and without myocarditis. These data demonstrate that patients with β-thalassemia may have myocarditis in the pathogenesis of their LV systolic dysfunction and that it is an important cause of death. Iron overload appears to provoke LV restrictive abnormalities combined with RV enlargement and dysfunction.

Miscellaneous Topics

Right Ventricular Dysplasia

To determine the initial clinical manifestations in echocardiographic features of RV dysplasia as encountered in a major cardiovascular referral center, Kullo and associates[21] from Rochester, Minnesota, retrospectively analyzed 20 patients with RV dysplasia diagnosed at the Mayo Clinic between January 1978 and January 1993. The mean duration of follow-up was 7 years. In the 12 females and 8 male patients (mean age, 30 years; range, 3–60), the initial manifestations of RV dysplasia included ventricular arrhythmia (45%), CHF (25%), precordial murmur (10%), asymptomatic heart block (10%), complete heart block (5%), and sudden death (5%). First-order relatives were affected in 30% of the patients. VT with morphologic features of left BBB was inducible in 7 of 9 patients. On Holter monitoring, all but 2 of 15 patients studied had frequent ventricular ectopic activity (Lown grade 2 or more). Characteristic fatty infiltration of the myocardium was present in 7 of 13 RV biopsy specimens. Inordinate RV enlargement was present in 60% of the patients at first echocardiographic assessment and in 2 other patients on follow-up assessment. Variable LV involvement was noted in 50% of the cases. During the follow-up period, 4 patients died: 2 died suddenly, 1 died of CHF, and 1 died of respiratory failure after CABG. Of the 16 living patients, 8 are doing well, 3 have an implanted cardiac defibrillator, 3 are receiving antiarrhythmic agents, and 2 have undergone cardiac transplantation because of progressive biventricular failure. Patients with RV dysplasia have varied initial manifestations and a high frequency of serious cardiovascular symptoms and complications.

Idiopathic Restrictive Cardiomyopathy

To describe the clinical course and outcome of children with idiopathic restrictive cardiomyopathy and to present the Doppler echocardiographic features of this disease in childhood, Cetta and associates[22] from Rochester, Minnesota, reviewed the Mayo Clinic data base for the period of 1975–1993 to identify children who underwent assessment for idiopathic restrictive cardiomyopathy. Clinical records and diagnostic studies, including 2-dimensional, M-mode, and Doppler echocardiograms, were reviewed for each patient. Characteristics were analyzed statistically to determine potential predictors of outcome. Eight children (5 girls and 3 boys) were diagnosed with idiopathic restrictive cardiomyopathy between 1975–1993 at their institution. The median age at diagnosis was 11 years, and the median duration of follow-up was 11.5 years. Of the 8 patients, 5 died (median time from initial examination to death, 1 year). All 5 of these patients had clinical and radiographic evidence of pulmonary venous congestion. In all patients, 2-dimensional and M-mode echocardiography revealed atrial enlargement without ventricular dilatation or hypertrophy. The 4 patients who underwent detailed diastolic Doppler assessment had findings consistent with restrictive filling and increased LV end-diastolic pressure: 1) short mitral deceleration time, 2) increased pulmonary vein atrial reversal velocity and duration, and 3) pulmonary vein atrial reversal duration greater than mitral A-wave duration. The prognosis for children with idiopathic restrictive cardiomyopathy is poor. In this small group of patients, absence of pulmonary venous congestion most consistently predicted extended survival. A combined 2-dimensional and Doppler echocardiographic examination provides a reliable non-invasive means of assessing the physiological and morphological features of idiopathic restrictive cardiomyopathy in children.

Immunosuppression for Myocarditis

Myocarditis is a serious disorder, and treatment options are limited. The Myocarditis Treatment Trial Investigators by Mason and associates[23] from multiple North American medical centers was designed to determine whether immunosuppressive therapy improves LV function in patients with myocarditis. The authors randomly assigned 111 patients with histopathological diagnosis of myocarditis and a LVEF of <45% to receive conventional therapy alone or combined with a 24-week regimen of immunosuppressive therapy consisting of prednisone with either cyclosporine or azathioprine. The primary outcome measure was a change in LVEF at 28 weeks. In the group as a whole the mean LVEF improved from 0.25±0.01 at baseline to 0.34±0.02 at 28 weeks. The mean change in the LVEF at 28 weeks did not differ significantly between the group of patients who received immunosuppressive therapy (a gain of 0.10) and the control group (a gain of 0.97). A higher LVEF at baseline, less intensive conventional drug therapy at baseline, and a shorter duration of disease, but not the treatment assignment, were positive independent predictors of the LVEF at week 28. There was no significant difference in survival between the 2 groups. The mortality rate for the entire group was 20% at 1 year and 56% at 4.3 years. Features suggesting an effective inflammatory response were associated with less severe initial disease. The authors' results do not support routine treatment of myocarditis with immunosuppressive drugs. Ventricular function improved regardless of whether patients received immunosuppressive therapy, but long-term mortality was high.

Hepatitis C Viral Infection

Matsumori and colleagues[24] in Kyoto, Japan, investigated hepatitis C virus infection in patients with dilated cardiomyopathy. The presence, type, and quantity of hepatitis C virus RNA were evaluated in sera, and the presence of positive and negative strands of hepatitis C virus RNA in the heart was investigated with the polymerase chain reaction technique. Anti-hepatitis C virus antibody was present in the sera of 6 of 36 patients (17%) with dilated cardiomyopathy and in 1 of 40 patients (3%) with CAD. Acute myocarditis was suspected in 3 patients with acute onset CHF, and the diagnosis was confirmed by endomyocardial biopsy in 1 patient. Hepatitis C virus RNA was present in the sera of 4 of 6 patients and all 4 had hepatitis C virus type II. The copy number of hepatitis C virus RNA in the serum was 8×10^2 to 2×10^3 genomes per 1 mL serum. Positive strands of hepatitis C virus were found in the hearts of 3 patients, and negative strands of hepatitis C virus were detected in the heart of 1 patient. Thus, these data suggest that hepatitis C virus infection is found in some patients with dilated cardiomyopathy and that hepatitis C virus may be an important causal agent in the pathogenesis of the disease. Antiviral therapy against hepatitis C virus may be indicated in these patients.

1. Urbano-Marquez A, Estruch R, Fernandez-Sola J, Nicholas JM, Pare JC, Rubin E: The greater risk of alcoholic cardiomyopathy and myopathy in women compared with men. JAMA 1995 (July 12);274:149–154.
2. Kottkamp H, Hindricks G, Chen X, Brunn J, Willems S, Haverkapm W, Block M, Breithardt G, Borggrefe M: Radiofrequency catheter ablation of sustained ventricular tachycardia in idiopathic dilated cardiomyopathy. Circulation 1995 (September);92:1159–1168.
3. Belardinelli R, Georgiou D, Cianci G, Berman N, Ginzton L, Purcaro A: Exercise training improves left ventricular diastolic filling in patients with dilated cardiomyopathy. Clinical and prognostic implications. Circulation 1995 (June);91:2775–2784.
4. Durand J-B, Bachinski LL, Bieling LC, Czernuszewicz GZ, Abchee AB, Yu QT, Tapscott T, Hill R, Ifegwu J, Marian AJ, Brugada R, Daiger S, Gregoritch JM, Anderson JL, Quiñones M, Towbin JA, Roberts R: Localization of a gene responsible for familial dilated cardiomyopathy to chromosome 1q32. Circulation 1995 (December);92:3387–3389.
5. Limas CJ, Goldenberg IF, Limas C: Soluble interleukin-2 receptor levels in patients with dilated cardiomyopathy. Correlation with disease severity and cardiac autoantibodies. Circulation 1995 (February);91:631–634.
6. Maron BJ, Gardin JM, Flack JM, Gidding SS, Kurosaki TT, Bild DE: Prevalence of hypertrophic cardiomyopathy in a general population of young adults: Echocardio-

graphic analysis of 4111 subjects in the CARDIA study. Circulation 1995 (August);92:785–789.

7. Cannan CR, Reeder GS, Bailey KR, Melton LJ III, Gersh BJ: Natural history of hypertrophic cardiomyopathy: A population-based study, 1976 through 1990. Circulation 1995 (November);92:2488–2495.

8. Kawano S, Iida K, Fujieda K, Yukisada K, Magdi ES, Iwasaki Y, Tabei F, Yamaguchi I, Sugishita Y: Response to isoproterenol as a prognostic indicator of evolution from hypertrophic cardiomyopathy to a phase resembling dilated cardiomyopathy. J Am Coll Cardiol 1995 (March 1);25:687–692.

9. Saumarez RC, Slade AKB, Grace AA, Sadoul N, Camm AJ, McKenna WJ: The significance of paced electrogram fractionation in hypertrophic cardiomyopathy: A prospective study. Circulation 1995 (June);91:2762–2768.

10. Watkins H, McKenna WJ, Thierfelder L, Suk HJ, Anan R, O'Donoghue A, Spirito P, Matsumori A, Moravec CS, Seidman JG, Seidman CE: Mutations in the genes for cardiac troponin T and α-Tropomyosin in hypertrophic cardiomyopathy. N Engl J Med 1995 (April 20);332:1058–1064.

11. Watkins H, Anan R, Coviello DA, Spirito P, Seidman JG, Seidman CE: A de novo mutation in α-tropomyosin that causes hypertrophic cardiomyopathy. Circulation 1995 (May);91:2302–2305.

12. Nishi H, Kimura A, Harada H, Koga Y, Adachi K, Matsuyama K, Koyanagi T, Yasunaga S, Imaizumi T, Toshima H, Sasazuki T: A myosin missense mutation, not a null allele, causes familial hypertrophic cardiomyopathy. Circulation 1995 (June);91:2911–2915.

13. Sigwart U: Non-surgical myocardial reduction for hypertrophic obstructive cardiomyopathy. Lancet 1995 (July 22);346:211–214.

14. Heric B, Lytle BQW, Miller DP, Rosenkranz ER, Lever HM. Cosgrove DM: Surgical management of hypertrophic obstructive cardiomyopathy. J Thorac Cardiovasc Surg 1995 (July);110:195–208.

15. Atkison P, Joubert G, Barron A, Grant D, Paradis K, Seidman E, Wall W, Rosenberg H, Howard J, Williams S, Stiller C: Hypertrophic cardiomyopathy associated with tacrolimus in paediatric transplant patients. Lancet 1995 (April 8);345:894–896.

16. Lipshultz SE, Orav EJ, Sanders SP, Colan SD: Immunoglobulins and left ventricular structure and function in pediatric HIV infection. Circulation (October 15) 1995;92:2220–2225.

17. Currie PF, Jacob AJ, Foreman AR, Elton RA, Brettle RP, Boon NA: Heart muscle disease related to HIV infection: Prognostic implications. Br Med J 1994 (December 17);309:1605–1607.

18. Child JS and Perloff JK. Myocardial myotonia in myotonic muscular dystrophy. Am Heart J 1995 (May);129:982–990.

19. Tokgozoglu LS, Ashizawa T, Pacifico A, Armstrong RM, Epstein HF, Zoghbi WA: Cardiac involvement in a large kindred with myotonic dystrophy: Quantitative assessment and relation to size of CTG repeat expansion. JAMA 1995 (September 13);274:813–819.

20. Kremastinos DTh, Tiniakos G, Theodorakis GN, Katritsis DG, Toutouzas PK: Myocarditis in β-thalassemia major: A cause of heart failure. Circulation 1995 (January);91:66–71.

21. Kullo IJ, Edwards WD, Seward JB: Right ventricular dysplasia: The Mayo Clinic experience. Mayo Clin Proc 1995;7:541–548.

22. Cetta F, O'Leary PW, Seward JB, Driscoll DJ: Idiopathic restrictive cardiomyopathy in childhood: Diagnostic features and clinical course. Mayo Clin Proc 1995 (July);70:634–640.

23. Mason JW, O'Connell JB, Herskowitz A, Rose NR, McManus BM, Billingham ME, Moon TE, the Myocarditis Treatment Trial Investigators: A clinical trial of immunosuppressive therapy for myocarditis. N Engl J Med 1995 (August 3);333:269–275.

24. Matsumori A, Matoba Y, Sasayama S: Dilated cardiomyopathy associated with hepatitis C virus infection. Circulation 1995 (November);92:2519–2525.

8

Congenital Heart Disease

Atrial Septal Defect

The surgical closure of an ASD is usually recommended for patients over 40 years of age. In a retrospective study, Konstantinides and associates[1] from Freiburg, Bad Krozingen, and Wiesbaden, Germany, examined the clinical courses of 179 consecutive patients with isolated ASD diagnosed after the age of 40 years. The 84 patients (47%) who underwent surgical repair were compared with the 95 patients (53%) who were treated medically. The mean (±SD) follow-up period was 8.90±5.2 years (range, 1–26). Multivariate analysis revealed that surgical closure of the defect significantly reduced mortality from all causes (Figure 8-1). The adjusted 10-year survival rate of surgically treated patients was 95% compared with 84% for the medically treated patients. In addition, surgical treatment prevented functional deterioration, as measured by the New York Heart Association class. However, the incidence of new atrial arrhythmias or of cerebrovascular insults in the 2 groups was not significantly different (Table 8-1). The surgical repair of an atrial septal defect in patients over 40 years of age, as compared with medical therapy, increases long-term survival and limits the deterioration of function due to heart failure. However, surgically treated patients should be followed closely for the onset of atrial arrhythmias so as to reduce the risk of thromboembolic complications.

Marx and associates[2] from Boston, Massachusetts; London, United Kingdom; Ann Arbor, Michigan; and Boulder, Colorado, studied ASDs using 2-dimensional imaging retrieval and reconstruction of 3-dimensional images. There were 16 patients with ASDs with a median age of 18 months and a range of 1 day to 18 years. Images were obtained in 1 patient by transesophageal probe placement, and in the other 15 patients a probe was placed in the transthoracic or subcostal position. A dynamic 3-dimensional echocardiogram of the ASD could be obtained in 13 of 16 patients. How valuable this new imaging data will be in individual lesions remains to be determined.

Holmvang and colleagues[3] in Boston, Massachusetts, used magnetic resonance imaging in the evaluation of 30 patients with ASD. Both spin-echo and phase-contrast cine magnetic resonance imaging were used. Spin-echo images were obtained in 2 orthogonal views perpendicular to the plane of the ASD. Spin-echo major and minor diameters were measured and spin-echo defect area was calculated. Phase-contrast cine magnetic resonance images were obtained in the plane of the ASD and cine major diameter and defect area were measured from the regions of signal enhancement or phase change due to shunt flow across the defect. Magnetic resonance measurements were compared with templates cut during surgery to match the defect or with atrial septal defect diameter determined by balloon sizing at cardiac catheterization. ASD size measured from cine magnetic resonance images agreed closely with cardiac catheteriza-

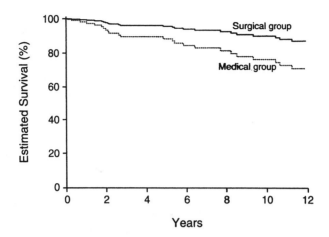

Figure 1. Estimated probability of survival for 179 patients with isolated atrial septal defects. The mean follow-up time was 8.9±5.2 years. Survival data have been adjusted for all important prognostic variables. The adjusted relative risk of death was 0.31 for surgically treated patients as compared with medically treated patients (95% CI, 0.11 to 0.85; *P*=0.02). Reproduced with permission from Konstantinides et al.[1]

Table 8-1. Cardiovascular Events During Follow-up.*

Event	Surgical Group (n=84)		Medical Group (n=95)
	Early	Late	
Death	0	3	21
TIA or stroke	3	9	6
New-onset atrial fibrillation or flutter	6	13	16
Implantation of pacemaker	2	9	2
Total no. of events	11	34	45
Total no. (%) of patients with ≥1 event	9 (11)	25 (30)	37 (39)

*Events occurring within 30 days after surgery were considered early. TIA denotes transient ischemic attack.
Reproduced with permission from Konstantinides et al.[1]

tion and template standards. On average, spin-echo measurements by magnetic resonance imaging overestimated major diameter and area of secundum ASD by 48% and 125%, respectively. Thus, these data indicate that phase-contrast cine magnetic resonance images acquired in the plane of an ASD defined the defect shape by the cross section of the shunt flow stream and allowed noninvasive determination of defect size with sufficient accuracy to permit stratification to closure of the defect by catheter-based techniques or surgery. Spin-echo images do not appear adequate for defining ASD size.

Atrioventricular Septal Defect

Sigfusson and associates[4] from Pittsburgh, Pennsylvania, and London, United Kingdom, studied 8 autopsied specimens with a cleft in the aortic or anterior leaflet of the mitral valve along with echocardiograms from 21 patients with such a cleft. These were compared with specimens and findings typical of the so-called partial AV canal and other forms of atrioventricular septal defect (AVSD). The structure and direction of the cleft, location of the papillary muscles within the left ventricle and AV junctional morphology of the hearts with an otherwise normally structured mitral valve were significantly different from typical findings in hearts with AVSD. It is necessary to distinguish morphologically a cleft in an otherwise normally structured mitral valve in hearts with separate right and left AV junctions from the trifoliate left component of a common AV valve and arch with an AVSD and a common AV junction because the disposition of the conduction tissue varies widely between these lesions. In hearts with an otherwise normal mitral valve, the branching AV bundle and its left bundle branch are intimately related to the points of attachment of the cleft anterior leaflet. In contrast, in hearts with AVSD and common AV junction the conduction axis is displaced posteriorly and is located beneath the inferior bridging leaflet.

van Arsdell and associates[5] from Toronto, Canada, reported 19 children who had operative treatment of subaortic stenosis associated with A-VSD. Specific diagnoses were septum primum defects in 7, Rastelli type A defects in 6, transitional defects in 4, inlet VSD with malattached chordae in 1, and TF with Rastelli type C defect in 1. There were 27 operations for subaortic stenosis and treatment of the outlet lesion was performed at initial repair in 3 children and in the remaining 16 from 1 to 13 years after repair. Fibrous resection and myectomy for relief of obstruction was carried out in 18 of 19 children and 7 had associated left AV valve procedures. Reoperation for subaortic stenosis was required in 7 children. Time to the second procedure was 3 ± 7 years with a mean of 5 years. Follow-up is 0.4 to 14 years with a median of 6 years. Actuarial freedom from reoperation at 6 years is $66\pm15\%$. The outflow tract can be effectively shortened, widened, and the angle between the plane of the outlet septum and the plane of the septal crest increased toward normal by augmenting the left side of the superior bridging leaflet and performing a fibromyectomy. This procedure can decrease the likelihood of reoperation.

Backer and associates[6] from Chicago, Illinois, reported 115 infants and children who underwent repair of complete AV canal defect with a two-patch technique and routine mitral valve cleft closure. Age at repair ranged from 1 month to 108 months, with a mean age of 14 months and a median age of 8 months. Preoperative cardiac catheterization in 113 patients revealed a mean pulmonary to systemic flow ratio of 3.4, mean PA systolic pressure of 71 ± 16 mm Hg, and a mean pulmonary resistance of 5 ± 3 units. Associated anomalies included Down syndrome in 99 patients, PDA in 47, and coarctation in 4. Although there was a trend toward increasing preoperative pulmonary resistance with age from 2 ± 0.9 at 0 to 3 months to 4 ± 3 at 4 to 6 months to 6 ± 3 at 7 to 12 months, this difference was not significant. The operative survival rate was 94% with 7 early deaths and the overall survival rate was 91% with 3 late deaths. Heart block requiring permanent pacemaker was present in 4 patients, and 8 patients required reoperation for MR. These authors present excellent results for AV canal defects using a 2-patch technique with routine mitral valve cleft closure at 4 to 6 months of age with a resulting low operative mortality, low prevalence of permanent heart block, and low reoperation rate for MR.

Bando and associates[7] from Indianapolis, Indiana, reported retrospective analysis of 203 patients who underwent surgical repair of complete AVSD. Overall operative mortality was 8% and operative mortality decreased significantly over the 20 year period of the study. Ten year survival including operative morality was 91% and all survivors are asymptomatic or only mildly symptomatic. Preoperative AV regurgitation was assessed in all patients by angiography or echocardiography and was trivial or mild in 103, moderate in 82, and severe in 18. Left AV valve cleft was closed in 93% and left alone when valve leaflet tissue was inadequate and closure of the cleft might cause significant stenosis. Reoperation for severe postoperative left AV valve regurgitation was necessary in 8 patients, 5 of whom initially did not have closure of the cleft and 3 of whom had cleft closure. Reoperation with annuloplasty was required in 6 patients, and 2 patients required valve replacement. On most recent evaluation by angiography or echocardiography at a mean of 59 months after repair, left AV valve regurgitation was trivial or mild in 94% of those examined and none had moderate or severe left AV valve stenosis. By multiple logistic regression analysis, strong risk factors for early death and need for reoperation included postoperative pulmonary hypertensive crisis, immediate postoperative severe left AV valve regurgitation and double-orifice left AV valve. These results indicate excellent intermediate and long-term results. Routine approximation of the cleft is safe and has a low prevalence of reoperation for left AV valve regurgitation.

Ventricular Septal Defect

Wu and associates[8] form Taipei, Taiwan, reported 63 patients with isolated VSD and anteriorly malaligned outlet septum. Aneurysmal transformation decreased the size of the VSD in 52% of these patients but was also associated with the appearance of a subaortic ridge. Progressive obstruction in the right ventricle was observed in 51%, more often in those without aneurysmal transformation. Aortic valve prolapse was quite common whether or not aneurysmal transformation occurred and this was attributed to the location of the VSD and the anterior malalignment of the outlet septum. Surgery was performed in 28 patients at a median age of 50 months because of significant left to right shunt in 5, the development of RV outflow obstruction in 9, aortic valve prolapse in 3, or combinations in 11. Although VSD with anterior malalignment of the outlet septum toward the RV side is usually seen in TF, it can also be associated with a wide RV outflow tract. It has recently been noted that in such patients, there is a predisposition for the development of a subaortic ridge, aortic valve prolapse, and progressive obstruction in the right ventricle due to a double-chambered RV anatomy. These authors show an excellent summary of a large number of patients with this relatively rare anomaly.

Ramaciotti and associates[9] from Philadelphia, Pennsylvania, retrospectively reviewed all patients with a muscular VSD with and without associated malformations to determine prevalence and rate of spontaneous closure of single defects to relation to location in the muscular septum. Defects were classified into 4 groups: midmuscular, apical, anterior, and posterior. The relative prevalence of singular muscular VSD was: midmuscular 44%, apical 25%, anterior 26%, and posterior 5%. Spontaneous closure occurred in 30 patients, and there was no difference in rate of closure with respect to anatomic location. Patients with multiple muscular VSD were either referred to surgery in the first year of life or had a course similar to patients with a single VSD. Muscular

VSD associated with other malformations was more often encountered in patients with conoventricular VSD and coarctation of the aorta. The distribution of anatomic groups of muscular VSD in association with malformations was similar to the single VSD. The mean age of spontaneous closure in this study was 20 months and 80% of these occurred in the first 18 months of life. The frequency of muscular VSD spontaneous closure in published reports varies from 24% to 76% with differences probably related to population studied, length of follow-up and diagnostic criteria.

Roguin and associates[10] from Nahariya, Israel, used color Doppler echocardiography in 1053 consecutive neonates, 6 to 170 hours old, to identify muscular VSD. Identified patients were followed up to 1 to 10 months or until VSD closure. Muscular VSD was found in 56 of 1053, a prevalence of 53 per 1000 live births. All neonates were asymptomatic, and only 6 had a systolic murmur. Electrocardiographic findings were normal in 44 of 45 neonates followed up and LV hypertrophy occurred in 1. By echocardiography, 50 VSDs (89%) were single and 6 (11%) were multiple. The defects ranged in size from 1 to 5 mm and occurred anywhere along the muscular septum; 43 (77%) were detectable only on color Doppler imaging. Of 45 neonates who were followed for 6 to 10 months or until closure of the defects, 40 (89%) had spontaneous closure. The risk of VSD was not significantly associated with gestational age, birth weight, birth order, maternal age, diabetes, smoking, exposure to drugs or infection, paternal age, familial congenital heart disease, religion or consanguinity. This study indicates a much higher prevalence of muscular VSD than has previously been reported with the majority of these defects not causing a systolic murmur early postnatally. The spontaneous closure rate is quite high, as has been previously reported.

Donofrio and associates[11] from Philadelphia, Pennsylvania, reviewed the pre and postoperative echocardiograms of 18 patients, 15 ± 23 months of age with a diagnosis of single left ventricle who underwent PA banding or cavopulmonary connection. Postoperative studies were performed a mean of 7 ± 7 days after operation and the VSD diameter was measured in 2 orthogonal views and the area calculated using the formula for an ellipse. Mean VSD defect area indexed to body surface area diminished by from 3 ± 3 to 2 ± 2 cm^2/m^2. Mean septal and posterior wall thickness increased significantly and LV diameter and length decreased significantly. A greater diminution in VSD area was noted after cavopulmonary connection ($41 \pm 19\%$) than after PA banding ($25 \pm 28\%$). In the single left ventricle, decrease in VSD size occurs early and is related to acute alteration in ventricular geometry that accompanies the decrease in volume. These authors report interesting data regarding the decrease in VSD size in single left ventricles after cavopulmonary connection. This problem is always one that worries a clinician when volume unloading operations are carried out. The decision about whether or not to combine this operation with one to relieve subaortic stenosis is an important one and these data should help provide data for this management decision.

Zhou and associates[12] from Beijing, China, reported 24 patients with large VSD or large ASD whose ages ranged from 5 to 28 years, with an average age of 16 years, who presented with severe pulmonary hypertension. Cyanosis was present with exercise in 19 patients and clinical evidence of increased pulmonary vascular resistance was evident in the majority of patients. A Dacron patch with a central defect closed with a pericardial patch that allowed right-to-left but not left-to-right shunting was employed. Mean PA pressure decreased from 80±12 to 56±18 following surgery. The unidirectional patch allowed right-to-left shunting in four patients with a systolic PA pressure greater than systolic arterial blood pressure immediately closure of the defect. The patch sealed or was effectively closed by the third postoperative day. There were 2 early deaths and no deaths at intermediate follow-up over a 3-month to 3-year period. This unique unidirectional valve patch may be useful for those rare patients who present with VSD and elevated pulmonary resistance in whom it is felt that a component of their resistance is still reversible.

Pulmonic Valve Stenosis

Fedderly and associates[13] from Ann Arbor, Michigan, reviewed their experience with percutaneous balloon valvotomy in 12 infants with critical PS in 10 or pulmonary atresia with intact septum in 2. There were 2 outcome groups: Group A patients were acyanotic, had residual mild PS, and have not required reintervention; group B patients have required reintervention. Of the 12 infants, 11 had a successful pulmonary valvotomy procedure. Group A patients (n=7) have a residual gradient of 22±19 mm Hg with a follow-up of 3 years. In group B (n=5) operation was required for inability to cross the valve in 1 or persistent severe hypoxemia ≥2 weeks after valvotomy in 4. Significant differences between the 2 groups were identified in pulmonary valve annulus, 8 mm vs. 6 mm (Z – 1 vs. –3); tricuspid valve annulus, 14 mm vs. 9 mm (Z value 0.8 versus –2); RV volume, 65 vs. 29 ml/m^2; and Lewis index, 11 vs. 9. Percutaneous valvotomy is effective and likely to provide definitive therapy in infants who have a tricuspid valve annulus >11 mm, pulmonary valve annulus ≥7 mm and RV volume >30 ml/m^2.

Tetralogy of Fallot

Hornberger and associates[14] from Boston, Massachusetts; Portland, Oregan; and Genolier, Switzerland, studied PA and ascending aortic diameter in prenatal and postnatal echocardiograms of 16 fetuses with TF initially studied at 24±6 weeks gestation. Fetuses were classified retrospectively as having mild and severe TF according to whether the PA circulation was ductal dependent at birth. Initial main PA diameter was small for gestation age in 9, large in 2, and normal in 5 compared with gestationally age-adjusted normal fetal studies. The diameter was significantly smaller in the group with severe TF. The initial main PA/aortic diameter ratio was also smaller for the group with severe TF than the group with mild TF. Initial aortic and branch PAs tended to be normal or near normal for age. In 8 fetuses serially studied, main and branch PA growth was normal or reduced during prenatal follow-up, and PA growth was most reduced in 2 fetuses in the group with severe TF resulting in PA hypoplasia at birth. There were 2 fetuses with valvular pulmonary atresia at birth who had previously shown antegrade pulmonary outflow in midgestation, suggestion progression of TF to pulmonary atresia during fetal life.

Geva and associates[15] from Houston, Texas, studied 21 infants with TF with a median age of 1.6 months and prospectively followed them with serial echocardiograms until the time of first surgical intervention at a median age of 10 months. When compared with age-matched normal control infants, infundibular dimensions in the patients with TF were significantly smaller in length, cross-sectional area, and volume. The angle between infundibular septum and ventricular septum had a greater degree of anterosuperior deviation in TF patients resulting in a larger infundibuloventricular septal angle. During follow-up, infundibular volume in TF patients decreased from 1.24 to 0.81 mL/body surface area correlating with infundibular septal thickness. TF patients who required early surgical intervention at 5 vs. 11 months had a smaller infundibulum at presentation and an accelerated rate of infundibular narrowing. Although these are expected findings in this group, the authors provide a way to quantify the degree of infundibular obstruction in a way that can be useful prognostically.

Sluysmans and associates[16] from Brussels, Belgium, performed balloon dilatation of the pulmonary valve in 19 infants aged 1 to 20 weeks with a median of 10 weeks and a weight from 2.3 to 7 kg with a mean of 4 kg. After dilatation systemic oxygen saturation increased from 79 to 90% but this improvement was short-lasting in 4 patients who required surgery before the age of 6 months. Pulmonary annulus size increased in each case from a mean value 5 to 7 mm, and this gain in size remained stable over time, with a mean Z score of −4.8 before dilatation, −3.1 immediately after the procedure, and −2.7 at preoperative catheterization. PA dimensions remained unchanged immediately after dilatation but increased at follow-up from a mean Z score of −2.5 to −0.06 and −2.2 to 0.04, respectively, for right and left PA at follow-up before surgery. At the time of the reparative surgery the pulmonary annulus was considered large enough to avoid a transannular patch in 69% of the infants. These authors show interesting results for this procedure. The unknown question is whether or not some of these infants would have shown significant growth of the annulus and PAs with nothing being done since most, if not all of them, were without significant symptoms at the time of the catheterization and intervention. If this procedure is used, it should be done only by those physicians who are skilled in interventional cardiology.

Hennein and associates[17] from Ann Arbor, Michigan, reported 30 neonates with symptomatic TF who underwent complete repair. TF and PS was present in 16, TF and nonconfluent PAs in 3, pulmonary atresia in 9, and pulmonary atresia with nonconfluent PAs in 2. The median age at operation was 11 days (mean, 13±3 days) with a mean weight of 3±0.1 kg (range, 2 to 4 kg). Preoperatively, 14 patients were receiving prostaglandin, 13 were mechanically ventilated, and 6 required inotropic support. Outflow tract obstruction was managed by a limited transannular patch in 25 patients, infundibular muscle division with limited resection in 15, and insertion of a right ventricle-PA valved aortic conduit in 5 patients. Follow-up was completed to a median interval of 24 months (range 1 to 62 months). There were no hospital deaths and 2 late deaths, for 1-month, 1-year, and 5-year actuarial survivals of 100%, 93%, and 93%, respectively. Both late deaths occurred in patients with TF and pulmonary atresia who had undergone aortic homograft conduit reconstruction; the only independent risk factor for death was the use of a valved conduit. Reoperation was required in 8 patients resulting in 1-month, 1-year, and 5-year freedom from reoperation rates of 100%, 93%, and 66%, respectively. Indications for reoperation were branch left PA stenosis in 5, residual RV outflow tract obstruction in 2, and severe pulmonary insufficiency in 1. Independent risk factors for reoperation included an intraoperative pressure ratio between right and left ventricles of 0.75 or greater, Doppler residual left PA stenosis of 15 mm Hg or more, or Doppler RV outflow tract obstruction gradient of 40 mm Hg or more at hospital discharge. This series demonstrates the safety of early hemodynamic repair of symptomatic TF in neonates. It also emphasizes the importance of relieving all sources of RV outflow tract obstruction at initial operation, particularly that located at the site of the insertion of the ductus arteriosus, which may be difficult to diagnose in the neonate before ductal closure occurs.

Gatzoulis and associates[18] from London, United Kingdom, studied biventricular function using Doppler echocardiographic examination in 41 patients (age, 15 to 35 years; mean, 29 years) after complete repair of TF. Patients were considered to have evidence of RV restriction if antegrade diastolic flow was detected in the main PA, coincident with atrial systole throughout the respiratory cycle. Exercise function was measured by graded treadmill testing with respiratory mass spectrometry. There were 3 exclusions because of pulmonary outflow obstruction with Doppler gradients >40 mm Hg or residual intracardiac shunts. Of the 38 patients, 37 were in sinus rhythm. Definite evidence of restriction was found in 20, or 53%. In all 20 cases there was superior vena caval flow reversal with atrial systole. Both inspiratory and expiratory transcardiac E-wave deceleration time was significantly shorter in the restrictive group. All patients had Doppler evidence of pulmonary regurgitation, but its duration was shorter in the restrictive group during inspiration. Cardiothoracic ratio was significantly lower in the restrictive group, suggesting less severe pulmonary regurgitation. Both restrictive and nonrestrictive groups had reduced exercise maximum oxygen consumption compared with healthy age- and sex-matched control subjects, but those with restrictive physiology had significantly better maximum oxygen uptake than those in the nonrestrictive group. Isolated RV restriction later after TF repair is common and is associated with less cardiomegaly and improved exercise performance, possibly due to shortening of the duration of pulmonary regurgitation.

Cullen and associates[19] from London, United Kingdom, studied biventricular systolic and diastolic function using Doppler echocardiographic examination during the first postoperative day in 35 patients (age, 6 months to 45 years) who underwent complete repair of TF. Biventricular systolic function was grossly normal in all patients and isolated restrictive RV physiology characterized by pulmonary arterial antegrade flow coincident with atrial systole and associated with prominent retrograde superior vena caval flow was seen in 17 of 35 patients. This flow was augmented during the expiratory phase of positive pressure ventilation and abolished or greatly diminished during the inspiratory phase. An increase in the duration of pulmonary regurgitation occurred during the inspiratory phase of positive pressure ventilation in these patients. All patients with RV restriction had a clinical picture compatible with low cardiac output, requiring prolonged stays in intensive care and the hospital. Clinical improvement was mirrored by resolution of the Doppler markers of RV restriction in most of the patients. These authors suggest that patients with restrictive physiology might benefit from a patent foramen ovale or small ASD to augment systolic output early after TF repair.

Jonsson and associates[20] from Stockholm, Sweden, performed exercise tests and cardiac catheterization in 53 patients, 13 to 26 years after repair of TF. At the time of repair, the median age was 7 years, and 60% of patients with cyanosis had had a previous palliative procedure. The right ventriculotomy was closed without a patch in 40%, a patch restricted to the right ventricle was inserted in 34%, and in 26% the patch extended across the pulmonary annulus. At follow-up, 94% of the patients were free of symptoms and symptom-limited work capacity was 87% of the predicted value. Work capacity was inversely related to age at follow-up, RV systolic pressure at rest, and the presence of moderate or severe pulmonary regurgitation. Cardiac output in relation to oxygen uptake was reduced in 74% of patients during exercise. In 12 patients (23%) systolic pressure at rest in the right ventricle was 50 mm Hg or higher. Systolic pressure during exercise in the right ventricle was lower in patients without a patch than in those with a patch and was abnormally high in all groups compared with healthy subjects. Work capacity was moderately reduced 13 to 26 years after repair of TF and was adversely influenced by RV hypertension and pulmonary regurgitation. Intermittent lifelong surveillance is advocated because patients without symptoms may require invasive intervention, including relief of residual obstruction and/or pulmonary valve insertion.

Okita and associates[21] from Tenri, Nara, Japan, report 511 pediatric patients with TF who underwent repair. There were 78 patients with subpulmonary VSD. Mean age at repair was 6±3 years. The method of RV outflow reconstruction was simple infundibulectomy in 14, RV outflow patch in 36, and transannular patch in 28. There was 9% early deaths as a resulted of low cardiac output and acute renal failure. The pressure ratio of right ventricle to left ventricle was 0.62 during the early postoperative catheterization. Follow-up was achieved for an average of 9±7 years. There were 3 late deaths (2 cardiac and 1 noncardiac). Actuarial survival was 95% at 20 years. Catheterization during late follow-up, an average of 7 years after repair, was done in 53 patients, and the pressure ratio of the right ventricle to left ventricle was 0.48. There were 15 subsequent operations because of residual lesions, including VSD in 4, PS in 9, combined VSD and PS in 1, and pulmonary regurgitation in 1, with no mortality. Actuarial freedom from reoperation was 71% at 10 years and 59% at 20 years. Patients with TF and subpulmonary VSD are more likely to have development of residual obstruction at the level of the pulmonary valve annulus than those with TF repair and perimembranous VSD. Subpulmonary VSD is much more common in oriental rather than occidental countries. These cases account for 10–30% of all TF cases in Japan but only 6–8% in the United States, or western Europe. It appears that more radical management in the relief of RV outflow obstruction in this group frequently is justified.

Meijboom and associates[22] from Rotterdam, the Netherlands, reported long-term results of surgical repair of TF on 77 unselected patients 15±3 years after repair in infancy and childhood. There was a frequent use of a transannular patch in 56% and the prevalence of elevated RV systolic pressure was low at 8%, but the presence of substantial RV dilatation with severe pulmonary regurgitation was high in 58%. The exercise capacity of patients with a substantially dilated right ventricle proved to be significantly decreased at 83±19% of predicted when compared with those of patients with a near normal-sized right ventricle at 96±13%. In 10 patients who required treatment for rhythm disturbance, 8 had supraventricular arrhythmia. Older age at the time of operation and longer duration of follow-up were not associated with an increase in the prevalence or clinical significance of sequelae.

Kondo and associates[23] from Tokyo, Japan, studied 29 patients with TF 16 ± 2 years after intracardiac repair using radionuclide ventriculography and bicycle ergometry. Results were compared with 10 age and sex matched control subjects. Cardiac output of TF patients was normally preserved both at rest and during exercise. The incremental response of the LVEF, however, was depressed in the TF patients. LVEF during exercise was inversely correlated with RV end-diastolic volume and the severity of pulmonary regurgitation. LV diastolic filling was not impaired in the patients compared with control subjects. Late LV dysfunction during exercise is related to an enlarged right ventricle due to pulmonary regurgitation after intracardiac repair of TF.

Pulmonic Valve Atresia

Reddy and associates[24] from San Francisco, California, reported 10 patients (age, 1 month to 37 years, median, 2 years) at the severe end of the morphologic spectrum of pulmonary atresia, VSD, diminutive or absent central PAs, and multiple aorticopulmonary collaterals. These patients underwent a 1-stage complete unifocalization repair from a midline sternotomy approach. The median Nakata index of true PAs was 50 (range, 0 to 103) and they provided vascular supply to up to 9 lung segments (median, 5 segments). The number of collaterals per patient ranged from 2 to 5, with a median of 4. The collaterals provided vascular supply to a median of 15 lung segments per patient (range, 11 to 20). Complete unifocalization was achieved in all patients with emphasis on native tissue to tissue connections via anastomosis of collaterals to other collaterals and to the native PAs. In only 1 patient, age 37 years, was it necessary to use a non-native conduit for peripheral PA reconstruction. The VSD was left open in 1 patient, age 5 years, because of diffuse distal hypoplasia and stenosis of the PAs and collaterals. The postrepair peak systolic RV/LV pressure ratio ranged from 0.31 to 0.58 (median, 0.47). There were no early deaths. Complications were bleeding requiring reoperation in 1 patient, phrenic nerve palsy in 3 patients, and severe bronchospasm in 3 patients. Followup from 2 to 19 months (median, 8 months) was complete in all patients. One patient was reoperated for pseudoaneurysm of the central homograft conduit and then again for stenosis of the left lower lobe collateral. This patient died at 13 months after the initial repair secondary to a pneumothorax. The patient with an open VSD underwent balloon dilatation of the unifocalized PAs with currently pulmonary/systemic flow ratio of 1.4 to 1.8 and is awaiting VSD closure. One other patient underwent balloon dilatation of the reconstructed right PA with a good result. All survivors are clinically well. This approach establishes normal cardiovascular physiology early in life and eliminates the need for multiple systemic PA shunts and the use of prosthetic material and minimizes the number of operations required. Long-term follow-up is essential to determine whether this approach will limit future operations to central homograft conduit changes only. This impressive report details an important new approach to these difficult patients. If these results can be generalized, they represent an important new breakthrough in treating at least a number of these patients with this complex condition.

Pagani and associates[25] from Ann Arbor, Michigan, and Omaha, Nebraska, reported 14 consecutive patients with TF, pulmonary atresia, and diminutive PAs who underwent staged repair. All patients had multiple aortopulmonary collateral arteries and the ductus arteriosus was absent in 11. Mean sizes of the right and left PAs were 2 ± 7 and 2 ± 0.8 mm, respectively. Complete repair has been performed in 8 patients (57%). Age at initial procedure in this group was 5 ± 7 months and the number of operative procedures to achieve complete repair was 3 ± 0.8 per patient. Postrepair peak RV/LV pressure ratio was 0.6 ± 0.2. Additional interventional procedures were required in 6 of 8 patients for angioplasty of peripheral PA stenoses, coil embolization of collateral arteries, or intraoperative insertion of pulmonary arterial stents. Mean follow-up after repair was 9 ± 8 months; there was 1 in-hospital death at 45 days and 1 late cardiac death at 20 months. Initial palliative operations were performed in 6 patients who have not undergone repair. Age at initial procedure in this group was 28 ± 57 months and mean follow-up from initial procedure was 11 ± 11 months. The operative mortality rate was 33%, and there was 1 late death at 5 months. Further interventional or repair is planned in 3 additional patients. This experience suggests that complete repair is feasible even in patients with diminutive PAs and PA growth is facilitated by early (3 to 6 months) establishment of central PA flow by right ventricle/ PA conduit or by direct ascending aorta/PA anastomosis in patients whose PAs are <1.5 mm. Subsequent interventional catheterization procedures allow continued recruitment of central PAs and may obviate or minimize the need for unifocalization procedures.

Gournay and associates[26] from Paris, France, reported 82 newborns with critical PS, and 15 with pulmonary atresia and intact ventricular septum who underwent balloon valvotomy provided that they had a well-developed right ventricle, including an infundibulum close to the PA. In patients with atresia, the outflow tract membrane was perforated with a wire needle or a radiofrequency probe. Balloon valvotomy was performed in 81 patients and was effective in 77. It caused 3 fatal and 16 nonfatal complications; 10 patients had persistent poor RV compliance, despite effective valvotomy, and required a surgical shunt. Among the 81 patients in whom the procedure could be performed, RV surgery was avoided in 5 of 9 (55%) patients with atresia and 55 of 72 (76%) patients with PS. These authors present excellent results for this difficult condition. This is a procedure only for those experienced with infant interventional catheterization, as perforation and serious morbidity and mortality are potential problems even in the most experienced hands.

Dinarevic and associates[27] from London, United Kingdom, evaluated 54 patients with pulmonary atresia and VSD. Ductal supply of confluent PAs was present in 30 patients or 56% (group 1), whereas 24 patients or 44% (group 2) had a pulmonary blood supply that was entirely (31%) or predominantly (13%) dependent on systemic collateral arteries. Over the 20 years there was no significant difference in actuarial survival between the 2 groups. Corrective surgery was performed in 8 of 30 patients in group 1 (27%), significantly more than in group 2 (4 of 24, 17%). Arborization abnormalities of the PAs were almost exclusively present in patients with systemic collateral arteries accounting for the lower probability for corrective surgery. During the first decade of the study, corrective surgery was attempted in 10% of patients, with 42% mortality; during the second decade, surgery was performed in 39% of patients with 26% mortality, a significantly lower figure. This report provides interesting data against which current treatment of patients with pulmonary atresia and VSD can be compared.

Complete Transposition

Wernovsky and associates[28] from Boston, Massachusetts, and Birmingham, Alabama, studied factors influencing early and late outcome of 470 patients who underwent an arterial switch operation. An intact, or virtually intact, ventricular septum was present in 59%, and a VSD was closed in the remaining patients. Survival at 1 month and 1, 5, and 8 years among the 470 patients was 93%, 92%, 91%, and 91%, respectively. The hazard function for death had a rapidly declining single phase that approached 0 by 1 year after surgery. Risk factors for death included coronary artery patterns with a retropulmonary course of the left coronary artery and a pattern in which the right coronary artery and LAD arose form the anterior sinus with a posterior course of the circumflex coronary. Procedural risk factors identified were augmentation of the aortic arch, longer duration of circulatory arrest and earlier date of operation in the case of the senior surgeon. Reinterventions were performed to relieve RV and/or PA stenoses alone in 28 patients. The hazard function for reintervention for PA or valve stenosis revealed an early phase that peaked at 9 months and a constant phase for the duration of follow-up. Incremental risk factors for early phase reintervention included multiple VSDs, the rapid 2-stage arterial switch, and a coronary pattern with a single ostium supplying the right coronary and LAD, with a retropulmonary course of the circumflex. The need for reintervention has decreased with time. The arterial switch operation can currently be performed early in life with a low mortality of <5% and a low incidence of reintervention of <10% for supravalvar PS. The analyses indicate that both the mortality and reintervention risks are lower in patients with favorable coronary anatomy.

Colan and associates[20] from Boston, Massachusetts, studied 330 of 430 hospital survivors by cardiac catheterization at a mean follow-up of 1.6 years after arterial switch operation for TGA. Seventy-eight percent of all survivors, 74% of survivors with VSD, and 82% of patients with a rapid 2-stage repair had catheterization performed. There were only rare abnormalities of LV or RV end diastolic pressure, cardiac index, or pulmonary vascular resistance. Invasive measures of filling pressures, cardiac index, and pulmonary vascular resistance did not differ among the 3 groups. Overall, echocardiographic LV end-diastolic dimension, wall thickness, mass, afterload (as determined by end-systolic wall stress), function (as determined by fractional shortening and rate-corrected velocity of fiber shortening), contractility, and preload were normal, and none of these variables was different between the groups with and without a VSD. Serial evaluation indicated a slight but significant trend toward ventricular dilatation, perhaps related to a relatively high incidence of at least mild AR (30%) In contrast, in the rapid 2-stage group the echocardiographic indices of LV function were found to be mildly but significantly reduced compared with normal subjects and with the other arterial switch operation groups. Over the duration of follow-up encompassed no tendency toward progressive depression of function was seen.

Rhodes and associates[30] from Boston, Massachusetts, obtained electrocardiograms and 24-hour Holter monitor studies in 364 survivors of arterial switch at operation and during follow-up. Limited electrophysiology studies were performed 6 to 12 months after operation. AV node function was preserved in most patients with 2% showing first degree AV block, 0.7% second-degree AV block, and 1.7% having complete AV block (all with coexisting VSD). All 5 patients with complete block received a permanent pacemaker. In those patients not receiving a pacemaker, sinus rhythm was present in 96% on the surface electrocardiogram and 99% during 24-hour Holter monitor studies (1 month to 9 years; mean, 2 years after operation). Intracardiac electrophysiologic studies in 158 patients demonstrated normal corrected sinus node recovery times and AH intervals in 97% of patients. Atrial ectopy was present in 81% of patients with most patients having only occasional premature beats without repetitive forms. Ventricular ectopy was a frequent finding during 24-hour monitoring. At hospital discharge, 70% had ventricular ectopy; these values fell to 57% in patients with intact ventricular septum and 30% in patients with a coexisting VSD at follow-up. In the early postoperative period, there were 25 episodes of SVT, 14 of which required therapy, 6 episodes of junctional ectopic tachycardia, and 9 episodes of VT. The prevalence of SVT had fallen to 5% at follow-up with no atrial flutter or fibrillation noted. VT was noted in 3 patients on follow-up Holter studies. In summary, the results confirm the theoretical advantages of anatomical repair over atrial repair of TGA with respect to preservation of sinus node function and low prevalence of clinically significant tachyarrhythmias.

Turley and associates[31] from San Francisco, California, and Seattle, Washington, presented results of the Congenital Heart Surgeons Society study regarding treatment of TGA. During this study neonatal arterial switch and neonatal or late atrial baffle repair by Senning technique were used in near equal proportion at 1 reporting institution. There were 46 patients enrolled in the study and 44 underwent either neonatal arterial (n=14, or 32%) or neonatal atrial (n=19 or 43%) or late atrial (n=11, or 25%) repair of TGA. Ages ranged form 4 to 80 days and overall survival for the entire series was 91%. The survival of the arterial switch group was 93% and the survival of the Senning group was 90%; late Sennings 91% and neonatal Sennings 92%. Six neonatal Sennings were crossovers from the arterial switch group with an 83% survival (5 of 6). Intermediate follow-up of 5 to 9 years revealed no late deaths. In the arterial switch group there was no ventricular failure, arrhythmias, and 1 reoperation for supravalvular PS. In the Senning group there was no ventricular failure but significant complications developed in 10 patients: cardiac arrhythmias in 7, tachyarrhythmias requiring pharmacologic therapy in 4, and bradyarrhythmias in 3 (2 requiring permanent pacemaker insertion). LV outflow obstruction developed in 3 patients, and 1 required a LV to PA conduit and permanent pacemaker. Systemic AV valve insufficiency has developed in 3 patients. These results during this period of transition from late atrial repair to neonatal arterial repair showed comparable early mortality in all groups. These results at a mean of 7 years revealed fewer arrhythmic and function complications in the arterial switch group.

Wernovsky and associates[32] from Boston, Massachusetts, studied nonneurological postoperative effect of low flow cardiopulmonary bypass and circulatory arrest for infants with TGA and a planned arterial switch operation before the age of 3 months. Of the 171 patients, 129 (66 assigned to circulatory arrest and 63 to low flow bypass) had an intact ventricular septum and 42 (21 assigned to circulatory arrest and 21 to low flow bypass) had an associated VSD. There were 3 hospital deaths. Patients assigned to low-flow bypass had significantly greater weight gain and positive fluid balance compared with patients assigned to circulatory arrest. The duration of mechanical ventilation, stay in the intensive care unit, and hospital stay were similar in both groups. Hemodynamic measurements were made in 122 patients and during the first postoperative night the cardiac index decreased by $32\pm15\%$ while pulmonary and systemic vascular resistance increased. The measured cardiac index was <2 in 24% of the patients, with the lowest measurement typically occurring 9 to 12 hours after surgery. Perfusion strategy assignment was not associated with different postoperative hemodynamics or other nonneurological postoperative events. These comparable postoperative characteristics with different cardiac surgery strategies provide extremely interesting data for study. The known vulnerability of these infants to low output states comes in the middle of the first night after surgery as documented in these patients with the lowest cardiac indices at this time.

Seraff and associates[33] from Le Plessis-Robinson, France, reported 68 of 753 patients who underwent arterial switch operation for TGA and subsequently required 75 reoperations. There were 30 patients requiring early reoperation (<30 days from the original procedure) and 38 requiring late reoperation. Causes for reoperation included pacemaker insertion in 5, left diaphragm plication in 4, revision for hemostasis in 1, mediastinitis in 2, superior vena cava thrombosis in 9, subvalvular PS in 5, supravalvular PS in 16, residual ASD in 2, residual VSD in 8, isolated MR in 2, AR in 2, AS in 1, left coronary artery ostial stenosis in 1, and recurrent aortic or neoaortic obstruction in 10. In all but 27 patients, the residual defects were present immediately after the completion of the arterial switch operation but only patients with critical lesions were reoperated early. Successful relief of superior vena cava thrombosis was achieved by atriojugular bypass grafting in 2 patients, by early open thrombectomy in 6 patients, and by direct patch angioplasty of the superior vena cava in 1 patient. Patch angioplasty for subvalvular or supravalvular PS was carried out in 21 patients, septal defect closure was performed in 9 patients and PA banding was performed in 1 patient with a criss-cross AV relationship and multiple VSDs. One patient with left coronary ostial stenosis underwent a patch enlargement of the ostium. Recoarctation was repaired by end-to-end anastomosis in 8 patients and by a subclavian flap or a patch angioplasty in 1 patient each. A second reoperation was required in 7 patients: supravalvular PS in 3, MVR in 1, VSD in 1, and recurrent coarctation in 2. There were 6 intraoperative and 2 late deaths. Risk factors for intraoperative death at reoperation were early reoperation and multiple VSDs. Mean follow-up of 70 ± 19 months was achieved in all survivors and they are all free of symptoms and need for medication. The authors conclude that most lesions requiring reoperation after arterial switch are detectable early and intraoperative echocardiography may be useful. Most late reoperations can be prevented by primary neonatal repair of almost all forms of TGA.

Lorenz and associates[34] from Nashville, Tennessee, used cine MRI to study ventricular function and mass in 22 patients late after atrial repair of TGA. Results 8 to 23 years after repair were compared with data from 24 age- and sex-matched normal volunteers and revealed markedly elevated RV mass, decreased LV and interventricular septal mass, normal RV size, and only mildly depressed RVEF. Only 1 of 22 patients had clinical RV dysfunction and this patient had increased RV mass. Cine magnetic resonance imaging allows quantitative evaluation of both RV and LV mass and function late after atrial repair of TGA. Longitudinal studies that include these measurements should prove useful in determining the mechanism of late RV failure in these patients. On the basis of these early data, inadequate hypertrophy does not appear to be the cause of late dysfunction in this patient group.

Corrected Transposition

Presbitero and associates[35] from London, United Kingdom, reported 18 patients (age, 16–61 years; follow-up, 1 to 30 years, mean, 10 years) with congenitally corrected TGA. There were no deaths during follow-up, but 6 patients had a worsening ability index. Complications included complete heart block in 3, of whom 2 required pacemaker insertion, and significant left AV valve regurgitation in 50%, appearing only in the third decade with increasing frequency thereafter. Infective endocarditis was responsible for increasing regurgitation in only 1 patient. Supraventricular arrhythmia appeared in the fifth decade and occurred in all patients over 60 years. CHF developed only after 60 years in 66%. There were 7 uneventful pregnancies in 3 of the 9 women in this study. Congenitally corrected TGA is frequently tolerated in the first 4 decades, when there are not associated lesions, as in this report. CHF appears to be extremely common in patients in their 40s, 50s, and 60s, and the exact role of systemic AV regurgitation in precipitating this problem is unclear.

Sano and associates[36] from Melbourne, Australia, reported intermediate-term follow-up of 28 patients after intracardiac repair of congenitally corrected TGA involving closure of VSD with or without additional surgery. VSD closure alone was performed in 7, VSD repair plus PS relief in 5, and VSD repair with conduit insertion between pulmonary ventricle and PA in 16. Hospital mortality was 4% and the 1-, 5-, and 10-year actuarial survival probabilities were 89%, 83%, and 83%, respectively. Twenty-one of 24 survivors were asymptomatic, and 3 were mildly symptomatic. Increasing TR of more than moderate degree occurred within 3 years after surgery in 7 patients. Deterioration of systemic ventricular pump function occurred in 12 of 22 patients (9 of 12 patients within 3 years postoperatively). The pulmonary to systemic flow ratio at the preoperative catheterization was significantly higher in patients who developed systemic ventricular dysfunction than in those with well maintained RV function. Intermediate results of intracardiac repair for congenitally corrected TGA were satisfactory in terms of survival and clinical functional status. There is concern, however, about systemic ventricular dysfunction with development of TR relatively early after operation.

Stumper and associates[37] from Birmingham, United Kingdom, reported use of a combined atrial and arterial switch procedure for 4 symptomatic children ages 9 months to 3 years with congenitally corrected TGA and VSD. Follow-up ranged from 6 to 21 months and averaged 12 months. There were no early or late deaths. Conduction abnormalities worsened in 2 patients. The cardiothoracic ratio decreased from a mean of 0.65 to 0.58 and 3 of 4 patients are without symptoms and 1 child has mild symptoms postoperatively. Although these investigators report small numbers, the use of this procedure has theoretical merit and its application to young patients is encouraging for its more widespread use.

van Son and associates[38] from Rochester, Minnesota, report late results for 40 patients with congenitally corrected transposition and systemic AV valve insufficiency who underwent replacement (n=39) or repair (n=1) of the systemic AV valve. Associated anomalies included Ebstein's malformation of the valve in 22, VSD in 19, and pulmonary stenosis in 14. Preoperatively, 16 patients, or 40%, had complete heart block, and 27 (68%) were moderately or severely symptomatic. Early mortality was 10% (n=4), and 8 patients died subsequently. The principal cause of death in all 12 patients was systemic ventricular failure. Overall survival including early mortality was 78% at 5 years and 61% at 10 years; survival excluding early mortality was 87% at 5 years and 68% at 10 years. Survivorship correlated with preoperative systemic ventricular EF of 44% or more and later interval of operation with 9 deaths in 15 patients before 1981 vs. 3 deaths in 25 patients subsequently. There were no cases of surgically induced complete heart block. Late reoperations related to the systemic AV valve prosthesis were performed in 2 patients. Follow-up extended to 26 years with a median of 5 years. At last follow-up, 18 of 28 survivors were without symptoms; 9 were mildly symptomatic and 1 was moderately symptomatic. These authors suggest early operation to attempt to preserve systemic ventricular function in patients with congenitally corrected transposition. Operation would be performed at the earliest sign of progression of ventricular dysfunction as assessed by serial clinical evaluation and echocardiography.

Truncus Arteriosus

Behrendt and Dick[39] from Ann Arbor, Michigan, reported successful use of 8 and 10 mm nonvalved conduits to connect the right ventricle to the PAs in the repair of truncus arteriosus in 7 neonates ranging in weight from 2 to 3 kg. There were 5 of 7 survivors and conduit replacement was delayed from 3 to 11 years in 4 long-term survivors. These authors conclude that nonvalved conduits can be useful for long-lasting palliation of truncus arteriosus in the neonate. These patients tolerated pulmonary insufficiency exceedingly well.

Valvular Aortic Stenosis

Gaynor and associates[40] from London, United Kingdom, and Durham, North Carolina, examined late outcome after intervention for AS in 73 neonates who underwent intervention during the first 30 days of life at 2 institutions. Procedures performed included closed valvotomy in 12, open valvotomy with inflow occlusion in 14, open valvotomy with cardiopulmonary bypass in 33, balloon valvotomy in 12, and other procedures in 2. The mean age at the first intervention was 8 days, and hospital mortality was 52% with a mean duration of follow-up for survivors of 8±1 year. The actuarial survival for the hospital survivors was 93% at 10 years and 84% at 15 years, whereas event-free survival was 62% at 5 years, 34% at 10 years, and 27% at 15 years. During the follow-up period, 3 patients have died and 11 have required AVR. The age at the initial intervention, the type of initial intervention, and the year of initial intervention were not predictive of early death or the need for reintervention. At late follow-up, 26 of 32 long-term survivors were asymptomatic, and 6 were mildly symptomatic. Critical AS remains a difficult problem with high initial mortality.

Late survival and functional class are excellent for patients surviving initial hospitalization but most require further intervention within 10 years.

Supravalvular Aortic Stenosis

Delius and associates[41] from Iowa City, Iowa, and Salt Lake City, Utah, reported long-term follow-up of an original cohort of 15 patients who underwent extended aortoplasty for supravalvular AS with follow-up obtained in 14 patients. An echocardiogram, chest x-ray, and electrocardiogram were obtained for each surviving patient with a median length of follow-up of 141 months (range, 36 to 238). The median preoperative gradient was 90 mm Hg (range, 55 to 150). The median immediate postoperative gradient was 20 mm Hg (range, 0 to 50) and the median long-term gradient was 32 mm Hg (range, 6 to 96). There were 2 deaths, 1 from LV failure after subsequent AVR and 1 from chronic LV failure. Estimated survival at 218 months for all patients was 77% (70% confidence limits 62% to 93%). Estimated freedom from reoperation for all patients was 69% at 218 months (70% confidence limits 56% to 82%). Univariate analysis revealed that the presence of a bicuspid valve was a significant risk factor for reoperation but not for death. The estimate of freedom from reoperation for a patient with a bicuspid valve was 43% at 141 months (70% confidence limits 21% to 65%). Extended aortoplasty provides effective long-term relief of the pressure gradient across the supravalvular ridge. These authors show excellent results for relief of the discrete type of supravalvular AS in all but 1 of their patients. One patient had diffuse stenosis which is much more difficult to treat effectively long-term.

Aortic Valve Atresia and Other Hypoplastic Left-Sided Cardiac Syndromes

Remmell-Dow and associates[42] from Columbus, Ohio, and Oaklawn, Illinois, examined the eustachian valve and the limbus of the foramen ovale in 42 hearts with hypoplastic left heart syndrome and 16 normal hearts. In hypoplastic left heart, only 5% of valves were moderately to well developed, whereas the remaining 95% were abnormal: 93% were absent or markedly hypoplastic, and 2% had an abnormally redundant and enlarged eustachian valve. The valve was well developed in 88% of normal hearts. In addition, the lesser development of the valve seemed to correlate with lesser development of the left side of the heart. The limbus of the fossa of the foramen ovale was well developed in 100% of the normal hearts and moderately well developed in only 33% of the hypoplastic group. This interesting study suggests there may be anatomical abnormalities in a small area of the heart which can lead to hypoplastic left heart syndrome with further development of the fetus.

Bu'Lock and associates[43] from Birmingham, United Kingdom, reported prospective results for 17 infants who underwent a Norwood type repair in early infancy for hypoplastic systemic ventricle and severe outflow obstruction. Operation was performed using a new modification of the Norwood-type arch repair, without the use of exogenous material and a 3.5mm Gore-tex shunt between the innominate and right PAs. The Gore-tex shunt was replaced with a cavopulmonary shunt between 3 and 5 months after the initial operation. There were

10 survivors (59%) of the initial surgery, and all proceeded to cavopulmonary shunt without further loss. Significant AV valve regurgitation was the main risk factor for poor outcome, and with this risk factor excluded, the morphology of the dominant ventricle seemed to have little effect on the outcome of initial surgery. These investigators show good early results for this most difficult group of patients with survival characteristics approaching those of centers with the best results previously reported. The construction of a neoaorta without the use of exogenous material may allow improved later growth of this vessel.

Mosca and associates[44] from Ann Arbor, Michigan, reviewed the postoperative course of 25 consecutive infants undergoing first stage palliation for hypoplastic left heart syndrome. There was 1 operative death and 2 patients died within 2 days, but 22 were extubated at a mean of 5 days after surgery. Hospital mortality was 25%. Mean pH was ≥ 7.5 for the first 9 hours after surgery and was ≥ 7.45 for the entire period. The mean FiO_2 was $\geq 50\%$ for the first 18 hours. The PaO_2 was appropriate (37 ± 6 mm Hg at 1 hour after surgery, increasing to 45 ± 5 mm Hg by about hour 73). Only modest inotropic support was needed to maintain appropriate blood pressure. These data suggest that neither alkalosis nor relatively high inspired oxygen necessarily cause hemodynamic instability in these patients. To what extent these results are generalizable is unclear but they suggest that there is nothing inherent with hypoplastic left heart syndrome that mandates postoperative hemodynamic instability or unacceptable mortality. These results for initial palliation are impressive and hopefully can be duplicated in many different centers.

Weldner and associates[45] from Hershey, Pennsylvania, reported 60 infants who underwent a Norwood operation for complex congenital heart disease including hypoplastic left heart syndrome in 41, VSD and subaortic stenosis with aortic arch interruption or severe coarctation in 7, complex single right ventricle with subaortic stenosis in 8, critical AS with endocardial fibroelastosis in 2, and malaligned primum ASD with coarctation in 2. Age at operation ranged from 1 day to 4 months with a mean of 9 days and a median of 3.5 days. The operative morality was 33%, and late mortality was 17%. Early operative deaths occurred in 9 of 20 during the first 2 days after surgery as a result of sudden hemodynamic instability. Since 1992, 7 operative deaths have occurred in 36 patients (19%); in the past 2 years no operative deaths have occurred in 22 patients. Overall there are 30 long-term survivors, with 21 having undergone a 2-stage repair with modified Fontan operation at 7 to 28 months of age (mean, 18 months) with no mortality. A 3-stage repair strategy was used in 6 patients undergoing a hemi-Fontan procedure at 7 to 23 months with no mortality and 2 of these patients have now had their modified Fontan at 23 to 47 months of age with no mortality. A 2-ventricle repair with a Rastelli procedure was performed in 2 patients with no mortality at 7 and 14 months. Early in the experience infants undergoing Norwood operation had a high early mortality most often related to sudden hemodynamic instability. The authors indicate that adding carbon dioxide to the inspired gas during the postoperative mechanical ventilation period has resulted in a more stable postoperative course.

Forbess and associates[46] from Boston, Massachusetts, reviewed 212 consecutive patients who underwent stage I palliative surgery for hypoplastic left heart syndrome. Six surgeons participated in the care of these patients and follow-up was 97% complete. Hospital mortality was not significantly lower during the second half of the study period and was 46%. Multivariate analysis revealed improved stage I operative survival in patients with MS and AS. Additional risk factors for stage I mortality were lower preoperative, pH and weight <3 kg. Overall first year actuarial survival for MS/AS was 59% and 33% for all others. Among stage I survivors, patients with MS/AS were more likely to survive to stage II palliation. Analysis of actuarial survival of stage I survivors showed that a smaller ascending aorta, aortic atresia, and mitral atresia were all risk factors for intermediate death. Preoperative anatomic and physiological state are predictors of stage I mortality in hypoplastic left heart syndrome. Although these mortality figures are discouraging for this group of patients, subsequent reports indicate that improved results are feasible, although the learning curve can be somewhat prolonged.

Aortic Isthmic Coarctation

Engvall and associates[47] from Linkoping, Sweden, studied 22 patients ages 17 to 66 years (mean age, 33 years) who were suspected of having hemodynamically significant coarctation. Previous coarctation surgery had been performed in 8 of the patients. Arm and ankle blood pressure (BP) was measured with a cuff at rest and 1–10 minutes after treadmill exercise. Invasive pressures and cardiac output were recorded during catheterization while patients were at rest and during and after supine bicycle exercise. Twelve health volunteers provided reference values for cuff pressures after exercise. All patients with a difference in cuff pressure at rest of ≥35 mm Hg had a difference in invasive pressure of ≥35 mm Hg. Increasing severity of coarctation on angiography correlated with larger pressure gradient at rest and during exercise. A pressure gradient between arm and ankle developed in normal subjects after maximal but not after submaximal exercise. In most patients with suspected coarctation, the difference in cuff pressure between arm and ankle at rest is sufficient to select patients for further evaluation. The use of the same cuff used to measure arm BP applied to the lower leg, just above the ankle, combined with pencil Doppler determination of systolic BP can be an excellent way to determine significant pressure gradients in the office. I have used this method for over 20 years and agree with the authors on the usefulness of this simple noninvasive measurement.

Fletcher and associates[48] from Houston, Texas, reviewed results from balloon angioplasty for 102 patients ages 3 days to 29 years (mean age, 5 years). Follow-up data were available from 2 to 117 months (mean, 36 months) in 92 patients. Immediate success was achieved in 93 of 102 patients, and 71 patients with intermediate follow-up ranging from 12 to 117 months were asymptomatic and normotensive with insignificant arm to leg BP gradient (≤20 mm Hg). After initial successful results, 21 patients (23%) developed an increase in gradient 2 to 86 months after angioplasty; reintervention was required in 18. Follow-up >72 months was available in 17 patients, 16 of whom were normotensive and have not required additional reintervention. No additional intervention was needed in 88% of older children and infants >7 months old. Reangioplasty or operation 14 days to 10 months (median, 5 months) after angioplasty was required in 10 of 13 surviving neonates who initially had a successful dilatation. Transverse arch hypoplasia had minimal effect on follow-up blood pressure gradient, whereas isthmic hypoplasia was associated with reintervention in

50%. A small aneurysm was noted in 2 of 102 patients, but surgery was not required and there has been no progression of these aneurysms during the 3 to 91 months of follow-up. Late aneurysm development has not been observed in the 32 patients who have had a second catheterization or the 26 patients who have had an MRI study. This form of therapy is a definite alternative to surgery in the hands of an experienced physician.

Rao and Koscik[49] from Madison, Wisconsin, report 37 infants and children aged 2 days to 15 years who underwent balloon angioplasty for native coarctation with resultant reduction in gradient from 45 ± 17 to 12 ± 9 mm Hg. At 4 to 48 months' follow-up, recoarctation had developed in 8 (27%). The younger the age, the narrower the aortic isthmus, and the smaller the coarcted segment both before and after angioplasty, the greater the chance for recoarctation. In this study, although the prevalence of recoarctation was high, especially in neonates and infants, the recoarctation could easily be ballooned dilated. Knowledge of these factors should be used to select patients for angioplasty in native coarctation.

Parks and associates[50] from Atlanta, Georgia, reported MRI results in 44 patients who had Dacron patch aortoplasty of coarctation of the aorta. There were 20 patients who developed aneurysms, of which 9 were detected in patients studied by MRI. Aortic rupture occurred in 8 female patients, 3 of whom were pregnant. Surface renderings accurately defined the aortic anatomy or aneurysms in all patients. On follow-up no aneurysms have been detected in patients with negative MRI results. Precise anatomic correlation with operative findings was reported. These authors show that only 11% of 9 patients developed aneurysms <2 years after surgery, whereas 63% of 30 patients developed aneurysms >2 years after surgery. MRI angiography provides an excellent noninvasive method for evaluation of this potentially lethal complication in patients who have previously had this type of surgery.

Bogaert and associates[51] from Leuven, Belgium, reported MRI in 73 of 85 patients with patch angioplasty for coarctation of the aorta. Imaging was performed in all 33 patients with an aneurysm at the patch site. The results were compared with 13 patients without aneurysm and 10 normal subjects. Mean time between surgery and study was 12 ± 2 years. Aneurysm was defined as the ratio of the diameter of the aorta at the repair site to the diaphragmatic aorta ≥ 1.5. Hypoplasia of the transverse arch and recoarctation at the repair site were defined as a ratio of <0.9. All 33 patients with an aneurysm had a hypoplastic transverse arch. The 13 patients with a normal ratio at the repair site had a normal transverse arch ratio. A significant pressure difference between the patient's right and left arm was found in patients with an aneurysm compared with those without. No significant difference was found between transverse arch ratios on preoperative cineangiography and postoperative MRI. Aneurysm formation at the repair site is highly related to hypoplasia of the transverse arch, and sufficient catch-up growth of a hypoplastic transverse arch is rare after patch angioplasty. The actual incidence of aneurysm formation in this series was 46% and is higher than that which was found previously. Dynamic phenomena such as flow acceleration and turbulence originating in a narrow transverse arch can contribute to aneurysm formation at the repair site after patch angioplasty.

Ralph-Edwards and associates[52] from Toronto, Canada, reported 43 patients who underwent surgical intervention for recurrent coarctation. Other congenital anomalies were present in 70%; 86% of patients initially treated by subclavian flap aortoplasty or end-to-end anastomosis were managed at reoperation by patch angioplasty, and 26% also required augmentation of a hypoplastic transverse arch under hypothermic circulatory arrest. Three patients underwent a second reoperation, and all were treated with tube graft interposition. No ischemic spinal injury occurred in patients managed with either simple proximal aortic cross-clamping or cardiopulmonary bypass. No patient treated with transverse arch augmentation has required further intervention. Mortality at reoperation was 7%, and at follow-up at a mean duration of 4.5 years, 57% of patients were normotensive, with no measurable arm–leg gradient. These authors present excellent results for the difficult problem of recurrent coarctation. Many of these patients also can be treated successfully with balloon angioplasty.

Conte and associates[53] from Le Plessis Robinson, France, reported 307 consecutive neonates who underwent coarctation repair by a single surgical technique by means of extended end-to-end anastomosis. Mean age at operation was 13±8 days. Isolated coarctation was present in 95 (group 1), associated VSD was present in 102 (group 2), and 110 patients had associated complex lesions (group 3). Aortic arch hypoplasia was present in 81% of patients, 62% of group 1, 85% in group 2, and 93% in group 3. In 271 patients, the arch reconstruction was performed via a left thoracotomy with normothermia: 100% of group 1, 95% of group 2, and 72% of group 3. In the other 36 patients undergoing a 1-stage repair or palliation of the associated lesions, it was performed via a midline sternotomy during a short period of deep hypothermia and circulatory arrest, and represented 5% of group 2 and 28% of group 3. PA banding was performed in 94 patients. Spontaneous VSD closure was observed in 39% of the patients in group 2 who were operated on via thoracotomy. Early mortality rates in groups 1 (2%) and 2 (2%) were significantly less than in group 3 (17%). There were 29 late deaths, all related to associated cardiac lesions or their subsequent repair. The overall total mortality was 17%. In group 3 the rate was significantly higher in patients undergoing 2-stage repair (47%) than those undergoing 1-stage repair (23%). All but 14 survivors were followed up, for a mean of 61±36 months. Actuarial survivals at 10 years were 98% in group 1, 94% in group 2, and 60% in group 3. The recoarctation rate was 10% leading to 21 reoperations and 3 angioplasties without mortality. Patients with a more extended or severe form of aortic arch hypoplasia had a significantly higher risk of reoperation. Actuarial freedom from reoperation for recoarctation at 10 years was 93%. These data suggest that extended end-to-end anastomosis provides adequate and safe repair of neonatal coarctation with a low recoarctation rate due to effective relief of the obstruction created by arch hypoplasia and to complete resection of ductal tissue.

Anomalous Pulmonary Venous Connection

Papa and associates[54] from Milan, Italy, described 4 cases in which fetal echocardiographic findings obtained during the third trimester of pregnancy were highly suggestive of anomalous pulmonary venous connection. The findings that led to this diagnosis were RV and atrial dominance associated with an enlarged coronary sinus or dilated superior vena cava. These findings were confirmed after birth, but the infants had normal pulmonary venous connections postnatally and cardiac chambers and vessels were completely normal by 6 months of age. Despite improvements in prenatal detection of congenital heart disease, important conditions such as ASD, aortic coarctation, total anomalous pulmonary venous connection, and muscular VSDs can be difficult to diagnose. Indirect signs of coarctation or total anomalous pulmonary venous connection have been suggested by RV dominance; enlargement of the right atrium and coronary sinus or superior vena cava also have been associated with anomalous pulmonary venous connection. These authors have shown the danger of using indirect signs to make fetal diagnoses.

Gaynor and associates[55] from London, United Kingdom, reported results for repair of anomalous pulmonary venous connection to the superior vena cava by a new technique. There were 3 patients with total venous connection, and partial connection was present in 8 patients. All patients were alive and asymptomatic at a mean follow-up of 2 ± 1 years. This new technique for an unusual anomaly deserves wider application and further long-term study to determine its ultimate usefulness.

Coronary Arterial Anomaly

Post and colleagues[56] in Amsterdam, the Netherlands, postulated that fast magnetic resonance angiography would allow accurate detection of anomalous coronary artery origins and delineation of their proximal course. They studied 38 patients, 19 of whom had an anomalously originating coronary artery. Blinded analysis of randomly ordered magnetic resonance coronary angiography studies was performed independently by two observers. Both origin and proximal course of the coronary arteries were defined. Two cardiologists reviewed all x-ray coronary angiograms. After separate analyses, a final consensus result was defined for each patient. In 37 patients, successful magnetic resonance coronary angiography could be performed. Interobserver agreement for determining both origin and proximal course for the arteries was 100%. An x-ray coronary angiogram was available in 36 patients. In 3 patients with an anomalous origin for the left main coronary artery in which it originated from the right aortic sinus, there was disagreement about the proximal course between the results of magnetic resonance coronary angiography and x-ray coronary angiography. Review of these cases demonstrated that magnetic resonance angiography had visualized a proximal coronary artery course correctly, whereas the results of x-ray angiography had been equivocal. Thus, in this study, the sensitivity and specificity for detecting an anomalous origin for coronary arteries and delineating their proximal course were 100%. These data indicate that fast magnetic resonance angiography is a highly accurate technique for determining the origin and identifying the proximal course of anomalous coronary arteries.

McConnell and colleagues[57] in Boston, Massachusetts, studied 16 patients with anomalous aortic origins of their coronary arteries using magnetic resonance coronary angiography and hypothesized that the magnetic resonance coronary angiography may be useful in the identification of anomalous coronary arteries and their anatomic course. Multiple images of the major epicardial coronary arteries were obtained by use of a breathhold, fat-suppressed, seg-mented-k space, gradient-echo technique by investigators blinded to all patient data. Anomalous coronary artery pathology, by x-ray angiography, included right sided left main coronary artery in 3 cases, a right-sided LC artery in 6 cases, separate left-sided LAD and LC arteries in 2 patients, left-sided right coronary artery in 4 patients, and an anteriorly displaced right coronary artery in 1 patient. The magnetic resonance coronary angiography correctly identified the anomalous coronary arteries in 14 of 15 patients. In 1 patient, the anomalous origin for the artery was incorrectly identified, and in 2 patients, the course of the anomalous artery was not clearly seen. One of these anomalous origins for a coronary artery not clearly seen was a nondominant, anomalous origin for a right coronary artery. These data suggest that magnetic resonance coronary angiography is a useful technique for the noninvasive identification of anoma-lous origin for coronary arteries and their anatomic course.

Tanel and associates[58] from Boston, Massachusetts, reviewed the cineangio-grams and hemodynamic data in 366 patients who underwent postoperative catheterization after arterial switch operation for TGA. Of these, 13 (3%) had previously unsuspected coronary abnormalities diagnosed angiographically. No patient had noninvasive evidence of resting systolic dysfunction. Findings included left main coronary artery stenosis in 3 or occlusion in 2 anterior descending coronary artery stenosis in 1 or occlusion in 2, right coronary artery stenosis in 1 or occlusion in 1, and small coronary artery fistulas in 3. One patient died suddenly 3 years after surgery, and 1 patient was lost to follow-up. The remaining 10 patients were alive and asymptomatic up to 11 years after repair. Resting end-diastolic pressure was elevated to 12 mm Hg or more in 4 of 12 patients. These authors show a very small number of abnormalities in patients with coronary anastomosis in early infancy. Obvious compensation for coronary abnormalities was provided by collateral flow in most of these patients. The small number of abnormalities provide a continued testament to the skill of the cardiac surgeons who perform this operation.

Laks and associates[59] form Los Angeles, California, used direct implantation of the anomalous left coronary artery into the aorta to provide a 2–coronary artery system using a modification of previous technique to allow anastomosis with the excised button of PA from within the lumen of the aorta. This procedure was instituted in 6 infants and 1 adult with favorable outcome in all, including improvement in ventricular function in 3 of 5 with impaired preoperative EF. The potential benefits of this technique are improved operative exposure, ability to implant the anomalous coronary in the appropriate sinus, avoidance of aortic valve damage or distortion because of improved exposure, and applicability to patients of all ages.

Turley and associates[60] form San Francisco, California, reported 11 patients (age, 6 months to 8 years) who underwent repair of anomalous origin of the left coronary artery from the PA. Coronary artery origin from the PA included left sinus in 3, posterior in 2, right sinus in 2, intramural aorta with its orifice at the bifurcation of the main and right PA in 1, high left main PA in 1, high at the bifurcation of main and right PA in 1, and anterior in 1. Findings included angina in 4, prior infarctions in 3, ischemia in 7, LV dysfunction in 6, MR in 5, ASD in 2, and echocardiograms suggestive of endocardial fibrosis in 4. One patient had prior ligation with ventricular dysfunction, collateralization, and recanalization. A single patient was asymptomatic. Repair was accomplished by direct transfer using the PA sinus as a button in only 6; tubular reconstruction was used in 4 when the distance was too great to avoid tension; 2 short tubes were constructed with PA wall in 2 of the 3 left sinus origins, whereas 2 long tubes of PA wall were used in 2. Division of the PA, mobilization of the distal PA, division of the ductus, and direct reanastomosis of the PA was performed in 3 tubular reconstructions, as well as all 6 direct coronary transfers. There were no operative or late deaths and follow-up was 2 to 100 months, with a mean of 46 months. There was no new angina or infarctions, and improved function and decreased MR was present in all. Echocardiographic and angiographic studies demonstrated patency in all the new coronary systems. These authors show excellent results from this difficult group of patients with establishment of a 2-coronary system possible in all of these who are 6 months of age or greater. Whether similar results can be duplicated in patients who present in the first several months of life is unclear.

Mitral Valve Disease

Uva and associates[61] from Paris, France, reported 20 patients >1 year of age who underwent surgery for congenital mitral valve disease. MR was predominant in 10 and MS in 10. Mean age was 7 ± 3 months and mean weight was 6 ± 2 kg. AV canal defects, univentricular heart, hypoplastic left heart syndrome, discordant AV and ventriculoarterial connections, and acquired mitral valve disease were excluded. Indications for surgery were intractable heart failure or severe pulmonary hypertension, or both. Associated lesions present in 90% of patients had been corrected by previous operation in 7. In congenital MR there was normal leaflet motion in 3, leaflet prolapse in 2, and restricted leaflet motion in 5. In congenital MS anatomic abnormalities were parachute mitral valve in 4, typical MS in 3, hammock mitral valve in 2, and supramitral ring in 1. Mitral valve repair was initially performed in 19 patients and valve replacement in 1 with hammock valve. Concurrent repair of associated lesions was performed in 12 patients with no operative mortality. In 5 patients there were 6 early reoperations for MVR in 4, a second repair in 1, and prosthetic valve thrombectomy in 1. There was 1 late death 9 months after MVR. Late reoperations for MVR occurred in 2, AVR in 1, mitral valve repair in 2, subaortic stenosis resection in 1, and second MVR in 1. Freedom from reoperation was $58\pm11\%$ (70% confidence limits, 47% to 69%) at 7 years. After a mean follow-up of 68 ± 43 months, 94% of living patients are asymptomatic. Doppler studies among the 13 patients with a native mitral valve show MR of less than moderate degree in 1 patient and no significant residual MS. Overall, 6 patients have mitral prosthetic valves with a mean transprosthetic gradient of 6 ± 4 mm Hg. These authors show that surgical treatment for congenital mitral valve disease during the first year of life can be performed with a low mortality with valve repair a realistic goal in about 70% of patients. The reoperation rate is high and is related to complexity of mitral lesions and associated anomalies. Late functional results continue to be encouraging.

Tulloh and associates[62] from London, United Kingdom, studied 23 consecutive children who underwent resection of supravalvar MS with follow-up (mean, 58 months; range, 0.5 to 167 months). Recurrent MS occurred in 4 patients and was recognized 14 to 108 months after resection and confirmed at repeat operation. Successful reoperation was performed in 3, but 1 died. There were 5 other deaths and on multivariate analysis the only variable associated with survival free or recurrent MS was older age (18 months or more) at time of surgery. Actuarial survival free of recurrent obstruction at 5 years, for cases in which MS was resected at <18 months, was 39% compared with 73% in older patients. Supravalvar MS is part of a spectrum of obstructive lesions affecting the left side of the heart. Recurrent MS can develop after surgical resection. The prognosis in those who require resection within the first 18 months of life is poor. Echocardiographic studies are important in long-term follow-up of these patients.

Arrhythmias and Conduction Defects

Dodo and associates[63] from Toronto, Canada, studied 9 children with chaotic atrial rhythm whose age at presentation ranged from 1 day to 30 months; 6 patients were age or younger. Tachycardia was present in 6, and 3 of those had CHF. The atrial rate was 200 to 500 beats per minute (mean, 369) and the ventricular rate was 150 to 300 (mean, 251). Cardiac abnormalities were present in 8 patients. Intravenous drug therapy was not successful in converting to sinus rhythm. Three to 5 drugs were used in each patient; amiodarone and propafenone alone or in combination proved most successful. There were 2 deaths in neonates with HC, and 7 of 9 patients were discharged from the hospital with full control achieved in 3, good control in 3, and ventricular rate control in 1. Long-term follow-up showed that chaotic atrial rhythm had resolved in 5 patients but persisted in 2. This rhythm disorder remains difficult to control despite the use of new antiarrhythmic agents but may resolve during long-term follow-up.

Bauersfeld and associates[64] from Toronto, Canada, reported 19 infants <6 months old who had atrial ectopic tachycardia treated with antiarrhythmic drugs. The arrhythmia was controlled with digoxin in 1 patient, propafenone in 2, digoxin with propafenone in 9, digoxin with amiodarone in 4, and digoxin with propafenone and amiodarone in 2. Radiofrequency ablation was performed in 1 drug-resistant case. Atrial ectopic tachycardia resolved in 14 of 15 infants within 1 year. Twelve of the infants had a structurally normal heart, and 7 had congenital cardiac defects. CHF was present in 5 of 12 with structurally normally hearts and 6 of 7 with associated congenital heart disease. Heart failure and echocardiographically detected decreased ventricular function resolved in all cases under treatment. These authors recommend a systematic 3-step approach to therapy with radiofrequency ablation reserved for those infants who do not respond to medical therapy.

Rhodes and associates[65] from Boston, Massachusetts, used transesophageal atrial pacing to terminate atrial reentry tachycardia in 102 pediatric patients who had 158 episodes. Patients ranged in age from 1 hour to 42 years, and conversion was successful in 71% of 158 episodes. An infusion of procainamide after initial attempts at pacing led to AF in 6 of 112 episodes. There were no significant differences between the ages of patients or the duration of tachycardia in comparing successful versus unsuccessful conversions. In contrast, the atrial cycle lengths for the successfully converted tachycardia were significantly greater than for unsuccessful attempts. Transesophageal pacing is a safe and effective means of terminating atrial flutter in the pediatric population. The technique can be performed in an outpatient setting and may occasionally be facilitated by infusion of intravenous procainamide.

O'Sullivan and associates[66] from Newcastle-upon-Tyne, United Kingdom, retrospectively reviewed the records of all infants with SVT caused by AV reentry. There were 39 infants (age, 1–330 days; median, 12 days. Intravenous flecainide was required to maintain immediate control in 6 who were then treated with oral flecainide. The other 33 patients were treated with oral digoxin. There was no recurrence of tachycardia in 14 of the 33 patients (42%). In the other 19 patients, digoxin was replaced by oral flecainide because of multiple recurrence of tachycardia. Full control was achieved in all 19 of these patients and in 5 of the 6 patients treated with both intravenous and oral flecainide. Thus, overall, flecainide was effective in 24 of 25 patients (96%). Comparison with previous natural history studies suggests that flecainide may be more effective than digoxin in the prophylaxis of SVT. This study should be interpreted with caution because of the small number of patients and because of the question of possible proarrhythmic effects with flecainide.

Pfammatter and associates[67] from Hanover, Germany, reported 6 consecutive infants with postoperative junctional ectopic tachycardia who presented at a mean age at surgery of 14 weeks and were treated with surface cooling. The decision to start treatment was based on the definition of a critical heart rate from 180–200 beats per minute in the presence of junctional ectopic tachycardia diagnosed established criteria. Moderate hypothermia with rectal temperature between 32° and 34°C was achieved by surface ice bags, sedation, mechanical ventilation, and paralysis. Mean interval between diagnosis of tachycardia and initiation of hypothermia was 4 hours and rectal temperature was rapidly lowered within 1 hour in all 6 patients. This significantly lowered the tachycardia rate from 219±27 to 165±25. Three patients with low cardiac output had restoration of stable hemodynamics once the heart rate decreased. Cooling was maintained for a period of 24–88 hours (mean, 59 hours), and no serious side effects were observed. Early institution of moderate hypothermia can be useful to control ventricular rates with postoperative junctional ectopic tachycardia.

Triedman and associates[68] from Boston, Massachusetts, reported 10 consecutive patients referred for treatment of recurrent intra-atrial reentrant tachycardia after surgery for congenital heart disease. Median age was 18 years and the median duration of arrhythmia was 6 years. Previous surgical procedures were Fontan in 6, Mustard/Senning in 2, and biventricular repair in 2. Intracardiac electrophysiological study demonstrated 30 distinct intra-atrial reentrant tachycardia circuits, defined by activation sequence and cycle length. Cycle length was significantly longer in circuits that were successfully ablated compared with those that were not (381 vs. 248 msec). Ablation was attempted in 22 of these circuits, and ablation sites were targeted to presumed exit points from zones of slow conduction. Of 22 circuit ablations attempted, 77% resulted in acute termination of the tachycardia. In 8 of 10 patients in whom at least 1 circuit was successfully ablated, 4 were free of clinical tachycardia and 3 were improved over short-term follow-up. No complications were encountered. These authors show encouraging results in this common and potentially lethal complication of surgical repair of congenital heart disease.

Leenhardt and associates[69] from Paris, France, reported 21 children (mean age, 10 ± 4 years) who had catecholaminergic polymorphic VT, no structural heart disease, and a normal QT interval. They were referred for stress or emotion induced syncope related to VT which consisted of isolated polymorphic ventricular extra-systoles followed by salvoes of bidirectional and polymorphic tachycardia susceptible to degeneration into VF. There was a family history of syncope or sudden death in 30% of the patients. On receiving therapy with the appropriate beta blocker, the patients' symptoms and VT disappeared. During a mean follow-up period of 7 years, there were 3 syncopal events and 2 sudden deaths, probably because of treatment interruption. This entity may form a variant of the congenital long QT syndrome in which the electrocardiographic marker is lacking. This type of VT must be guarded against in a pediatric patient with stress- or emotion-induced syncope because only β-blocker therapy apparently can prevent sudden death.

Fenrich and associates[70] from Houston, Texas, studied the safety and efficacy of combined flecainide and amiodarone therapy in controlling refractory tachyarrhythmias in infancy. These authors performed a retrospective analysis of 9 infants (median age, 2 months) who received combined therapy. Trough drug levels of flecainide were monitored and 24-hour ambulatory electrocardiographic monitoring was used to determine efficacy. Single-drug treatment with either drug failed in all of the infants studied. An average of 4 drugs (range, 1 to 6) failed before administration of combined therapy. During combined therapy, the flecainide dose was 70–110 mg/m^2 per day and that for amiodarone was 7.5–13.5 mg/kg per day for a mean of 9 days to load and 5–12 mg/kg per day as maintenance. Successful control of arrhythmias was demonstrated in 78% of 9 infants (3 of 3 with congenital junctional ectopic tachycardia, 3 of 3 with SVT, and 1 of 3 with VT). During combined therapy corrected QT intervals varied from .440 to .448 msec and no proarrhythmia occurred. None required a pacemaker, and all had normal LV size and fractional shortening and 8 of 9 had a structurally normal heart. This therapy appears to be safe and effective in a small number of infants with refractory tachyarrhythmias. It may allow delay in the need for interventional therapy or obviate the need for such in small infants.

Pfammatter and associates[71] from Hanover, Germany, reported 71 pediatric patients (mean age, 7 years) with various supraventricular and ventricular tachyarrhythmias who were treated with oral sotalol. Sotalol was either completely effective (27 of 41 patients, or 66%), partially effective (11 of 41 patients, or 27%) in 38 of 41 patients with supraventricular reentrant tachycardia. In patients with atrial flutter, sotalol was effective in 84% of patients (completely in 9 of 19 and partially in 7 of 19). Ventricular tachycardia was effectively controlled in 64% of children (completely in 3 of 11 and partially in 4 of 11). Proarrhythmia occurred in 7 patients (10%) and consisted of symptomatic bradycardia from sinoatrial block and high-grade AV block, respectively, in 2 children; asymptomatic high-grade AV block in 1, torsade de pointes in 1, and increased ventricular ectopic activity in 3. Proarrhythmia required drug discontinuation in 4 patients. Mean duration of treatment for all patients was 18 months (range, 1–40 months). Sotalol is an effective antiarrhythmic drug for a wide range of pediatric tachyarrhythmias, but proarrhythmic effects indicate the need for monitoring of drug effects.

Michaelsson and associates[72] from Uppsala, Sweden, performed a retrospective review of all patients having complete congenital heart block. There were 102 patients, including 61 women and 41 men. The time of observation, after the age of 15 years, was between 7 and 30 years. The mean age at follow-up or death was 38 years (median, 37 years, range, 16–55 years. Stokes-Adams attacks occurred in 27 patients, with a fatal outcome in 8. The first attack was fatal in 6 of these 8 patients. There were 19 survivors and a pacemaker was implanted thereafter. Another 8 patients received a pacemaker because of repeated fainting spells and 27 others have had a pacemaker implanted for fatigue, effort dyspnea, dizziness, ectopy during exercise, MR, and/or a low ventricular rate. Ventricular rate decreased with age with a mean rate at 15 years of 46 beats per minute, at 16 to 20 years of 43 beats per minute, at 21 to 30 years of 41 beats per minute, at 31 to 40 years of 40 beats per minute, and after 40 years of 39 beats per minute. Stokes-Adams attacks occurred in all 7 patients with prolonged QT_c time. Low ventricular rate at rest or at work, presence of BBB pattern, low working capacity, and ectopy at rest and/or during effort were not statistically significant risk factors. Stokes-Adams attacks occurred in 6 patients without any of these signs. MR developed in 16 patients and 4 died. A pacemaker reduced the risk of death. Prophylactic pacemaker treatment is recommended even for symptom-free adults with congenital heart block because of a high prevalence of unpredictable Stokes-Adams attack with considerable mortality, a gradually decreasing ventricular rate, significant morbidity, and a high incidence of MR. These authors make a strong argument for pacemaker implantation when these patients reach adulthood. The prevalence of MR in these patients is a relatively new finding and the pathogenesis remains unproven.

Transhepatic Cardiac Catheterization

Sommer and associates[73] from New York, New York, studied 12 children (age, 3–52 months) in whom a percutaneous transhepatic approach was required for catheterization. Indication for the procedure included bilateral femoral vein and superior vena cava obstruction in 4, bilateral femoral vein obstruction with bidirectional Glenn shunt in 2, and bilateral femoral vein obstruction and the need for catheter intervention in 1, an interventional procedure in a small infant posing a significant risk to femoral or internal jugular vessels in 1, and need for catheterization as well as chronic venous access in a patient who would require multiple interventional catheterizations. Central venous access was obtained in all patients and complete right-heart catheterization was performed. Complete transseptal left-heart catheterization was accomplished in 4 patients. There were no complications associated with transhepatic sheath placement, catheterization, or interventional procedures. Broviac catheter placement for chronic central venous access was accomplished in 10 of the 11 cases attempted after catheterization. These catheters were left in place for 18–290 days (median, 35 days), and no catheter became occluded or infected while in place. No clinical compromise occurred during catheter removal in any patient. This procedure can be a valuable tool for experienced interventional cardiologists and will be required in a number of patients with chronic access problems and complex congenital defects.

Shim and associates[74] from Ann Arbor, Michigan, presented data using percutaneous transhepatic puncture for performing cardiac catheterization. The procedure was performed successfully in 17 of 18 children (mean age, 30 ± 8 months; range, 1 day to 9 years) with a weight of 3–28 kg. Time from initial needle puncture to RA entry was 6 ± 1 minutes; diagnostic catheterization was performed successfully in all 17 children, and additional interventional procedures were performed in 5 children. Total catheterization time was 2.0 ± 0.2 hours. Ultrasound was performed 24 hours after catheterization, and no evidence was found in any patient of hemorrhage or subcapsular hematoma. This novel transhepatic approach provides an effective and relatively safe route for diagnostic and interventional cardiac catheterization for children in whom other routes are not possible. It is a procedure that should be learned by interventional pediatric cardiologists who are involved with a large number of preoperative and postoperative patients in whom venous access frequently becomes a serious problem.

Intravascular Stents

Ward and associates[75] from Houston, Texas, reported the use of balloon-expandable intravascular stents for systemic venous and systemic venous baffle obstructions in 12 patients who had 21 stents implanted in 13 systemic venous obstructions. In the baffle group, 4 of 13 obstructions were at the superior vena cava/right atrial junction after atrial baffling for TGA. One of 4 patients had complete obstruction requiring transseptal needle perforation before stent implantation. There was an immediate gradient reduction from 12 ± 8 to 1.3 ± 1.0 mm Hg. The obstructed segment diameter increased from 3.5 ± 3.9 to 16 ± 2.7 mm. In the central vein group, 9 of 13 obstructions were in large central veins and 3 of those 9 had complete obstruction requiring needle perforation before stent implantation. There was an immediate gradient reduction from 10 ± 9 to 0.8 ± 1.0 mm Hg, and the obstructed segment increased from 1.3 ± 1.1 to 9.4 ± 1.7 mm. There were no acute complications in either group. Patients then had follow-up studies at 3, 6, and 12 months with echocardiography or MRI and repeat catheterization at 12 months. All stents were patent by echocardiography or MRI when studied at follow-up. At repeat cardiac catheterization in 6 of 12 patients, all stents remained patent without compression or fracture. Follow-up and immediate poststent gradients were not significantly different. Neointimal hyperplasia reduced the stent lumen only from 12.5 ± 4.7 to 10.6 ± 4.7 mm. No stents required redilatation. Balloon-expandable intravascular stents can be safely and effectively used to relieve systemic venous obstruction even when the obstruction is complete or nearly complete. This treatment should become the treatment of choice for the relief of selected venous obstructions in pediatric patients.

Fogelman and associates[76] from Toronto, Canada, reported the use of 55 balloon-expanded stents that were implanted in 42 patients (age, 6 ± 5 years) with PA stenosis. Patients were followed prospectively for a median of 15 months and recatheterized 1 year after implantation. Implants were positioned percutaneously in 49 patients whereas 4 patients had 6 implants during surgery. There was a diameter increase in the stenotic area of $109\pm79\%$ and a gradient reduction of $74\pm26\%$. There were 12 stents that straddled the orifice of side-branch PAs and reduced flow to the branch vessel acutely in 7 patients. Recatheterization was carried out in 29 patients and various degrees and locations of acquired intraluminal narrowings were observed in all cases, particularly in areas of diameter mismatch between the stented and nonstented vessels. Further dilation with diameter improvement was performed in 11 patients. Of the 38 patients who underwent percutaneous implantation, planned surgery for PA stenosis was avoided in 33 and deferred in 4. One patient who was considered inoperable had stent implantation as a palliative procedure. Symptomatic improvement was reported in 27 patients, and 15 patients remained asymptomatic. Stent redilation remains an important part of the management of these patients with severe PA anomalies that are extremely difficult to treat surgically.

Ing and associates[77] from Houston, Texas, evaluated the prevalence of restenosis and demonstration of the safety and efficacy of repeat dilation of stents in patients with congenital and acquired branch PS. Of 94 patients with 163 implanted stents, 43 patients with 73 stents underwent recatheterization. Only 2 of 73 restudied stents developed significant restenosis. In 20 patients, 30 stents were redilated. At stent implantation, the mean age of the subgroup was 14 years, the mean intraluminal diameter increased from 5 to 11 mm, and the systolic gradient across the stent decreased from 52 to 11 mm Hg. At recatheterization at a mean of 13 months later, all stents were patent; the mean diameter decreased by 1.2 mm, but the increase in the gradient of 3 mm Hg mean was not significant. After repeat dilation, the diameter increased from 10 to 12 mm and the gradient decreased from 14 to 8 mm Hg. The 2 stents with restenosis were redilated successfully. There were 2 patients who underwent successful redilation of 3 stents at 18 and 26 months. There were no complications. These authors show outstanding results in the use of stents for PA stenosis and the ability to redilate stents with growth of the patient or with a mild decrease in the stent diameter. This is an important new treatment modality for patients with congenital and acquired PA stenosis.

Coles and associates[78] from Toronto, Canada, reported intraoperative implantation of pulmonary arterial stents from 5–15 mm in diameter in patients with pulmonary atresia with VSD (4), TF (2), truncus arteriosus (1), hypoplastic left heart (2), and miscellaneous PA stenoses (3). In addition, 3 patients with pulmonary venous obstruction and 1 patient with combined pulmonary arterial (PA) and venous obstruction were stented. The stents were effective at achieving immediate patency in all patients; there were 2 early deaths, 1 related to acute thrombosis of a small diameter left PA stent. Reintervention because of stent related stenosis was frequently necessary and in 5 of 7 patients who survived more than 1 month after implantation of a stent 8 mm or smaller, severe PA obstruction developed. In 4 of the 5 pulmonary vein stents, intractable obstruction developed resulting in death in all 3 patients who had bilateral stent implantation. These authors conclude that recurring intraluminal obstruction as a result of neointimal hyperplasia is a frequent problem in currently designed small diameter endovascular stents. A number of investigators, however, have found residual patency of most PA stents, particularly when the stent is dilated to >10 mm. Pulmonary venous obstruction still appears to be a very difficult condition to treat despite multiple strategies to alleviate obstruction.

Powell and associates[79] from Boston, Massachusetts, reported a retrospective study in which 44 patients underwent placement of 48 stents in obstructed right ventricle-PA conduits. Median patient age was 7 years (range, 7 months to 30 years), and median follow-up time was 14 months (range, 0 to 48 months). Stent implantation initially decreased the RV-PA pressure gradient from 61±17 to 30±12 mm Hg and the RV-to-systemic pressure ratio from 0.9±0.2 to 0.6±0.2. The diameter of the stenotic region expanded from 9±4 to 12±3 mm in one view and from 7±3 to 11±3 in the orthogonal view. During the follow-up period, two patients had their stents redilated, 7 had additional conduit stents deployed, and 14 underwent surgical replacement of their conduits. Actuarial freedom from conduit reoperation was 65% at 30 months after the procedure. On follow-up, 7 patients were found to have fractured stents, suggesting an important role for external compressive forces in conduit failure. Recatheterization in 16 patients at a median of 12 months after the procedure demonstrated hemodynamic evidence of recurrent obstruction despite sustained enlargement at the previously stented sites. Complications included stent displacement in 1, bacterial endocarditis in 1, and false aneurysm formation in 1. One patient died awaiting conduit replacement surgery. Both high pressure balloon dilatation and stent implantation may be useful to prolong conduit life in patients with difficult situations for reoperation.

Cavopulmonary Anastomotic Procedures

Reddy and associates[80] from San Francisco, California, reported the performance of a primary bidirectional superior cavopulmonary shunt in 9 patients (age, 1–4 months, with 5 patients <2 months). Associated lesions of immediate surgical importance were total anomalous pulmonary veins in 2, a restrictive ASD in 4, bilateral superior venae cavae in 5, and PDA in 5. Surgery consisted of unilateral in 4 or bilateral in 5 bidirectional superior cavopulmonary shunt and the repair of associated lesions. A very limited additional source of pulmonary blood flow was provided in 4 of the first 5 patients because of a low arterial oxygen tension immediately after bypass. Pleural effusions developed in 2 of these 4 patients. In subsequent patients cardiopulmonary bypass was not used whenever possible or, if it was needed, an extra source of pulmonary blood flow was avoided. There were no early deaths. The bidirectional shunt was taken down to a classic Glenn shunt in 1 patient in whom viral pneumonia developed. There were 2 late deaths at a median follow-up of 11 months. The cause of death was extensive pulmonary arteriovenous fistulae in 1 patient and unknown in the other. These authors have demonstrated the usefulness of this shunt in younger patients. Further data are needed to determine when this is the preferred procedure for both early and long-term palliation in the young.

Stumper and associates[81] from Birmingham, United Kingdom, reported detailed follow-up of 6 children who underwent creation of a total cavopulmonary shunt but had interrupted inferior vena cava such that the hepatic vein continued to enter the atrial chambers and provide desaturated blood to the systemic circulation. There were no early or late deaths. Oxygen saturations at discharge ranged from 89–92%. At last follow-up at a mean of 5 years, saturations at rest ranged from 73–81% (mean, 71%). At peak exercise, oxygen saturations ranged from 62–87% (mean, 72%). Cardiac catheterization was performed in 5 patients with saturations of <80% at rest or peak exercise. No patient had pulmonary arteriovenous fistula, but systemic venous to hepatic venous collaterals were documented in 4 patients. They were localized below the diaphragm in 3 and above the diaphragm in 1 patient. The collateral vessel was successfully embolized in 3 of these patients with a rise in resting oxygen saturations from 6–10%. Although other authors have found pulmonary arterio-venous fistulas in patients with this anatomy, these authors have shown systemic venous to hepatic venous collaterals that can be embolized with transcatheter therapy and provide relief of cyanosis that appears prominent in these patients.

Uemura and associates[82] from Osaka, Japan, and London, United Kingdom, reported 27 patients who underwent a bidirectional Glenn procedure in the presence of forward flow from the ventricle to the PA with the flow maintained through the pulmonary trunk in 22 or systemic to pulmonary shunt in 5. There was 1 surgical death due to AV valve regurgitation. Subsequently, 9 patients have successfully undergone a total cavopulmonary connection 3 ± 2 years after the initial procedure. Pre and postoperative catheterizations revealed changes in arterial oxygen saturation from 75 ± 11 to $83\pm7\%$ and end diastolic volumes of the systemic ventricles from 238 ± 92 to $188\pm97\%$ of the expected normal. There was no difference detected in the mean cross-sectional area of the right PA compared with the expected normal value ($76\pm21\%$ to $81\pm20\%$) or in the ventricular EF ($53\pm8\%$ to $50\pm14\%$). The relative regression or growth of the pulmonary arterial size was statistically related to the size of the channel for forward flow. Maintenance of forward flow from the ventricle provides a feasible means when performing a bidirectional Glenn procedure, protecting against regression of pulmonary arterial size as well as off-loading the ventricles and improving arterial oxygen saturation.

Frommelt and associates[83] from Milwaukee, Wisconsin, reviewed the medical and surgical records of all patients who underwent a bidirectional cavopulmonary shunt from 1991 to 1993. A total of 43 patients were identified, including 14 patients with double inlet left ventricle, 8 with tricuspid atresia, 6 with pulmonary atresia and intact septum, 5 with single right ventricle, 3 with hypoplastic left heart, 3 with unbalanced AVSD, and 4 with other complex lesions. Patients were divided into 2 groups, including 22 in group 1 who had only the cavopulmonary shunt as a source of pulmonary blood flow and 21 in group 2 who had an additional source of pulmonary flow. Patient age at the time of shunt ranged from 6 months to 12 years with group 1 patients being younger: 31 vs. 45 months. Group 2 patients had higher postoperative central venous pressures (18 versus 14 mmHg) and oxygen saturations (86 versus 81%) than did group 1 patients. There was no statistical difference between groups in the number of chest tube days or hospital days. There was 1 early death in group 1 related to ventricular dysfunction and 1 late death in group 2 related to sepsis. There were 5 patients requiring readmission in group 2 for drainage of a large chylothorax vs. none in group 1. These authors conclude that patients with an additional source of pulmonary blood flow after bidirectional cavopulmonary shunt have higher postoperative central venous pressures, higher oxygen saturations, and are at high risk for the late development of a chylothorax.

Webber and associates[84] from South Hampton, United Kingdom; Vancouver, Canada; and Prague, Czech Republic, reviewed early- and medium-term clinical and hemodynamic findings in 108 consecutive patients 3 weeks to 25 years old undergoing bidirectional cavopulmonary shunt at 3 institutions. Preoperatively, pulmonary blood flow was dependent on antegrade ventricular flow in 50, systemic-to-pulmonary shunts in 33, or mixed sources in 25. Competitive sources of pulmonary blood flow were left open in 43 of 108 patients. There were 4 early and 4 late deaths, none related to persistence of competitive flow. After bidirectional cavopulmonary anastomosis, patients with competitive flow had significantly higher systemic oxygen saturations at 1 hour, 24 hours, and at hospital discharge and required a shorter period of artificial ventilation and intensive care. Oxygen saturations at late follow-up at a median of 3 years did not differ (83% vs. 82%). No patient developed pulmonary arteriovenous malformations. Competitive flow is well tolerated in the short- and medium-term after bicavopulmonary anastomosis and results in higher early postoperative systemic oxygen saturations.

Mainwaring and associates[85] from San Diego, California, reported 92 patients with complex cyanotic congenital heart disease who underwent a bidirectional Glenn with 40 patients having either a systemic to PA shunt or patent RV outflow tract as an additional source of pulmonary flow. There were 3 operative deaths, and 4 procedures have failed and required subsequent revision. Thus, there were 85 patients who underwent successful operation. Effusion (defined as chest tube drainage exceeding 7 days duration) occurred in 8 of 85 patients; this complication was seen in 7 of 36 patients (19%) with accessory pulmonary blood flow and in 1 of 49 (2%) in patients without accessory pulmonary blood flow. There were 11 deaths, including 6 of 36 patients (17%) with accessory pulmonary flow, 2 of 49 patients (4%) without accessory pulmonary flow, and 3 of 4 patients (75%) who had a failed Glenn shunt. These data suggest that morbidity and mortality are lower in patients in whom accessory pulmonary blood flow is eliminated at the time of the bidirectional Glenn shunt.

Kavey and associates[86] from Syracuse, New York, compared electrocardiographic findings after total cavopulmonary connection and Fontan operation to evaluate the impact of cavopulmonary connection on sinus rhythm postoperatively. The Fontan group consisted of 17 patients repaired at 8±3 years and the total cavopulmonary connection consisted of 19 patients repaired at 5±3 years. Mean follow-up after Fontan was 8±3 years versus 3±2 years for total cavopulmonary connection. Preoperative electrocardiograms on all total cavopulmonary connection patients showed sinus rhythm, whereas 16 of 17 Fontan patients had sinus rhythm and one had nonsinus atrial rhythm. On the first postdischarge electrocardiogram, 12 of 19 total cavopulmonary connection patients (63%) were in sinus rhythm, 4 were in junctional rhythm, and 3 were in nonsinus atrial rhythm. In comparison, 15 of 17 Fontan patients (88%) were in sinus rhythm, 1 of 17 was in nonsinus atrial rhythm, and 1 was in SVT. By 2 years postoperatively, only 6 of 15 total cavopulmonary connection patients available for follow-up (40%) were in sinus rhythm with 7 of 15 in junctional rhythm and 2 of 15 in nonsinus atrial rhythm. By contrast, 13 of 17 Fontan patients (76%) remained in sinus rhythm. This significant prevalence of loss of sinus rhythm temporally related to surgery suggests that operative compromise of the sinus node area is common with total cavopulmonary connections.

Bernstein and associates[87] from San Francisco, California, compared 29 patients with cavopulmonary shunts or total caval exclusion with 53 control subjects using contrast echocardiography. The primary cardiac lesion, age at the time of surgery, type of right-sided heart bypass procedures, provision of auxiliary pulmonary blood flow, and changes in oxygen saturation over time were compared. The prevalence of pulmonary arteriovenous fistulae in children after cavopulmonary anastomosis is 60%, higher than previously reported. The prevalence is significantly higher in infants <6 month of age and in those with heterotaxy syndrome. The provision of an additional source of pulsatile pulmonary blood flow appears to have little effect on the development of fistulae. Patients who developed fistulae had arterial oxygen saturations at the time of discharge from surgery similar to those who did not develop them. In addition, those with fistulae had significantly lower arterial and pulmonary venous oxygen saturation at follow-up as a result of their intrapulmonary shunt. Contrast echocardiography provides a sensitive method for the detection of pulmonary arteriovenous fistulae.

Pulmonary artery distortion is a risk factor among candidates for the Fontan procedure. In 57 patients evaluated by catheterization after successful cavopulmonary anastomosis, 8 had proximal left PA stenosis, either discrete (4 patients) or long segment (4 patients).[88] Median age was 27 months (range, 19–60 months). Median weight was 11 kg (range, 9.1–20). Mean diameter at left PA stenosis was 4.4±0.4 mm. Proximal right PA mean diameter was 10±1.0 mm. After angiographic and hemodynamic assessment, short 11F sheaths were placed in the right internal jugular (6 patients) or subclavian veins (2 patients). PA angioplasty and stent placement were performed. Left PA stenoses were enlarged using 10 Palmaz stents dilated to 10 mm (7 patients) or to 12 mm (3 patients). Poststent angiograms showed that narrowest left PA dimensions were significantly enlarged to 9.9±1.0 mm. There were no complications. Follow-up studies (catheterizations in 4 patients, echocardiograms in 8 patients) were performed 4 to 9 months after stent implantation. No restenosis was observed. Five patients had completion of their Fontan procedures; 3 are pending Fontan completion. This study demonstrates the efficacy and safety of the percutaneous use of Palmaz stents to correct PA stenosis in young children after cavopulmonary anastomosis.

Homograft or Allograft

Bando and associates[89] from Rochester, Minnesota, reported late patient outcome and homograft durability in 326 patients who received aortic (n=230) or pulmonary (n=118) cryopreserved homografts for RV outflow tract reconstruction. Patient survival, including operative mortality, 5 years after the operation was similar between the 2 groups (pulmonary homograft, 86%: aortic homograft, 80%). However, 5-year freedom from homograft failure was significantly better for pulmonary homografts (94% vs. 70%). Late calcification was evaluated by chest roentgenography and echocardiography. Overall, 20% of aortic homografts became moderately or severely calcified compared with 4% of pulmonary homografts. Moderate or severe obstruction associated with calcification occurred in 26% of aortic homografts in children 4 years of age or younger, whereas only 11% of aortic homografts in patients over 4 years of age had calcification obstruction. There were no late deaths among patients receiving pulmonary homografts that were related to graft failure; 2 late deaths in the aortic group were homograft related. Risk factors for patient mortality and homograft failure were identified as aortic type of homograft for homograft failure but type of homograft was not correlated with patient mortality. Age 4 years or younger was a significant risk factor for both mortality and homograft failure in aortic homograft recipients but not in pulmonary homograft recipients. These results indicate that both aortic and pulmonary homografts provided excellent intermediate patient survival after RV outflow tract reconstruction, but pulmonary homografts are more durable than aortic homografts with less calcification and obstruction, especially among children 4 years old or younger.

Yankah and associates[90] from Berlin, Germany, reported 53 patients who received cryopreserved aortic and pulmonary allografts for reconstruction of the pulmonary circuit in the first 2 years of life with body weight ranging from 2–18 kg (mean, 8 kg). The implanted allografts ranged in internal diameter from 9 to 23 mm (mean, 16 mm). Of the 38 survivors who regularly had postoperative echocardiographic examinations, 40% underwent cardiac catheterization 1 to 31 months after surgery. Allograft dysfunction, defined as gradient ≥50 mm Hg with or without pulmonary insufficiency, was confirmed in 9 patients leading to reoperation in 5 and valvulo-angioplasty in 4. At 48, months actuarial survival was 64%. In the aortic and pulmonary allografts, freedom from wall calcification at 20 months was 19% and 100%, respectively. Freedom from valve dysfunction in patients with aortic and pulmonary allografts was 53% and 88%, respectively, and was 49% in allografts with an internal diameter of 17 mm or smaller. Freedom from reoperation in all patients was 78%. Young age, ABO compatibility, and type of allograft seemed to be independent risk factors for early allograft conduit degeneration and late valve dysfunction. Pulmonary allografts seemed to be more resistant to early wall calcification and valve dysfunction than aortic allografts when placed in the pulmonary position.

Fontan Procedure

Laks and associates[91] from Los Angeles, California, reported the use of a modification of the Fontan procedure in which the superior vena cava is connected to the left PA and the inferior vena cava connected to the right PA via a lateral tunnel. This allows matching of the superior and inferior venae caval flows with the lung of appropriate size. The authors applied this technique in 18 patients (median age, 4 years; range of 13 months to 36 years). A previous bidirectional Glenn shunt had been present in 6 patients. Preoperative PA pressures were 13 ± 2 mm Hg and a transpulmonary gradient of 5 ± 3 mm Hg was present. Ventricular function was satisfactory in all patients. At the completion of bypass the pressures in the superior and inferior cavae were 16 ± 4 and 10 ± 3 mm Hg, respectively. The left atrial pressures was 6 ± 3 mm Hg and the arterial oxygen saturation on 100% oxygen was 93 ± 3%. There was 1 death as a result of intractable atrial arrhythmias, and the remaining 17 patients had a mean hospital stay of 10 days (range, 6 to 18 days). The length of pleural drainage was 7 ± 3 days. An adjustable ASD was made smaller in 11 patients before discharge. Oxygen saturation at discharge was 85 ± 4%. The ASD was completely closed in 6 patients an average of 2.5 months after surgery (range, 3 weeks to 5 months). After ASD closure the arterial saturation was 96 ± 3% and the cavae pressures were both 13 ± 3 mm Hg. This modified Fontan approach appears to be a valuable technique in certain patients whose anatomy would favor its use.

Kuhn and associates[92] from Los Angeles, California, reported the effect of late ASD closure on cardiac output and oxygen delivery in patients who have undergone the Fontan procedure. Evaluation of closure of ASD was performed in 12 patients (age, 20 months to 12 years), with a mean interval of 4 months after Fontan procedure. The study included 6 patients with a high transpulmonary gradient or poor ventricular function preoperatively or both, and 6 who had only borderline increased pulmonary vascular resistance (low-risk group). Patients in both groups had a mean RA pressure >15 mm Hg when the ASD was test occluded in the first week after the Fontan procedure. Ventricular end-diastolic pressure was significantly lower with the ASD open in low-risk than in high-risk patients, and low-risk patients had a significantly higher cardiac index than the high-risk group. There was no significant difference in cardiac index between the two groups with occlusion of the ASD. Oxygen delivery was also significantly higher with the ASD open in the low risk patients than in the high risk group but there was no significant difference in oxygen delivery after ASD occlusion. In all patients there was a significant decrease in ventricular end-diastolic volume with ASD occlusion from 58 ± 17 to 47 ± 13 ml/m^2 with EF decreasing from 0.7 to 0.65. Oxygen delivery decreased in all but oxygen saturation increased to a mean of 95%. An intraatrial communication results in increased postoperative systemic perfusion and oxygen delivery in patients with good diastolic ventricular function after the Fontan procedure. Guidelines as to when to close these defects are not available.

Kelley and associates[93] from New Haven, Connecticut, studied 6 subjects who had undergone the Fontan operation and compared them to 6 healthy age-, sex-, height-, and weight-matched control subjects. Resting blood volume was similar for Fontan and control subjects while central venous pressure was elevated in Fontan subjects. Forearm venous capacitance at a distending pressure of 40 mm Hg was lower in Fontan subjects than in control subjects, whereas resting plasma norepinephrine level was elevated in Fontan subjects. The increase in calf volume and decrease in central venous pressure during a lower body negative pressure of −30 mm Hg were smaller for Fontan than control subjects. Reduced forearm venous capacitance and diminished pooling of blood into capacitance vessels of the leg during orthostatic stress indicated higher venous tone in Fontan than control subjects. These data suggest that increased venous resting tone in Fontan subjects may limit their ability to mobilize blood from capacitance vessels during exercise and may contribute to their impaired cardiac output response.

Uemura and associates[94] from Osaka, Japan, and London, United Kingdom, used catheterization data to assess ventricular performance in 57 patients at a mean of 15 months after Fontan operation for a univentricular heart. End-diastolic volume, end-systolic volume, EF, and end-diastolic pressure of the systemic ventricle were analyzed together with an estimation of the systemic flow index. These parameters were influenced significantly by the presence of AV valve insufficiency. The morphological left ventricle showed a better EF than did the morphological right ventricle, whereas the systemic flow index was greater in patients undergoing total cavopulmonary connection than in those receiving an atriopulmonary connection. Young age was significantly associated with better postoperative contractility, whereas the potential for impaired ventricular compliance was suggested in several patients undergoing the operation after 4 years of age. These data indicate that total cavopulmonary connection performed at a young age should be the surgical procedure of choice and that AV insufficiency should be treated at the initial definitive repair. The paper does not address the question of using the intermediate step of a bidirectional Glenn shunt and then later cavopulmonary connection as an alternative approach. This management option may yield similar or improved results.

Cecchin and associates[95] from Houston, Texas, reported a retrospective review of 151 consecutive patients ranging in age from 1 to 49 years who underwent a Fontan procedure between 1987 and 1993. Risk factors were identified for early and intermediate arrhythmias. Age at the time of the procedure was an independent predictor of early atrial arrhythmias, ventricular arrhythmias, and junctional ectopic tachycardia. The older the patient at surgery, the higher the incidence of atrial arrhythmias, whereas the younger the patient, the higher the incidence of junctional ectopic tachycardia. The risk of intermediate atrial arrhythmias after lateral tunnel modification was 1/3 that after atriopulmonary connection.

Harrison and associates[96] from Toronto, Canada, reported follow-up of 47 adults seen after the Fontan operation with an age at follow-up of 26 ± 6 years. These patients were seen an average of 7 ± 4 years after the Fontan operation performed at a mean age of 19 ± 8 years. The underlying anatomy was tricuspid atresia in 20, double inlet left ventricle in 9, and complex single ventricle or transposition complexes in the remainder. Clinically, 93% were in functional class I or II. The Fontan patients had a significantly lower maximal workload, anaerobic threshold, and maximal oxygen consumption using bicycle ergometry than normal control subjects. Systemic ventricular EF was lower at rest ($38 \pm 12\%$ vs. $58 \pm 7\%$) and during exercise ($40 \pm 15\%$ vs. $70 \pm 8\%$). Despite a clinical impression of good function, by objective measures adult patients continue to have significant cardiovascular limitations late after the Fontan operation.

Rosenthal and associates[97] from New Haven, Connecticut, identified 70 patients who underwent a Fontan operation and divided them into 3 groups: total cavopulmonary connection, atriopulmonary connection, and conduit interposition. A thromboembolic complication occurred in 14 patients (20%) during a mean follow-up of 5 ± 5 years. The rate of thrombosis was similar in each group. The time from the Fontan operation to thrombosis averaged 6 ± 5 years. The overall rate of thromboembolic events was 4 per 100 patient-years. The location of thrombi were within the venous circulation in 12 of 14 patients, in the left ventricle in 1, and undetermined in 1. Six of the patients (43%) were asymptomatic, 3 (21%) presented with cerebrovascular events, and 5 (36%) presented with other symptoms. Thromboembolic events occurred from the perioperative period to 15 years after surgery. These complications appear more common than was previously recognized. The benefit of Coumadin or other therapy is not clear.

Rychik and associates[98] from Philadelphia, Pennsylvania, reviewed the results of echocardiography performed before and 8 ± 7 days after Fontan operation for tricuspid atresia in 9, hemi-Fontan operation for tricuspid atresia in 10, and closure of VSD in 13. Wall thickness increased in all groups with the greatest degree of increase after the Fontan operation. Cavity size decreased most dramatically after the Fontan operation, with less dramatic and equivalent changes noted after the hemi-Fontan operation and VSD closure. Posterior wall thickness to cavity diameter ratios were equivalent in all before operation, increased after operation, and were greatest after the Fontan operation. Changes in ventricular geometry identified as an increase in wall thickness and a decrease in cavity dimension are most dramatic after the Fontan operation. Changes seen after the hemi-Fontan operation are of a milder degree, which may partially explain the relatively benign clinical course after this operation in most infants.

Hsu and associates[99] from Toronto, Canada, reported 8 patients assessed for persistent cyanosis after a modified Fontan procedure who were found to have unusual venous right-to-left shunts and were treated successfully by transcatheter occlusion therapy with either a double umbrella or coil. There were 3 types of communications. The first consisted of thin tortuous channels originating from the RA wall and draining into the left atrium through a capillary network. The second type was in the superior anterior portion of the atrial baffle, incorporating the pectinate muscles of the right atrium, draining into the neoleft atrium. The third communication originated from the inferior vena cava, connecting inferior phrenic veins to pericardial veins and subsequently to the left atrium. Before device occlusion, the room air oxygen saturation was $88\pm4\%$ and increased to $95\pm3\%$ following occlusion. The mean RA pressure was 14 mm Hg and did not change. There was complete shunt obliteration in 6 patients and small residual shunts in 2 patients. Persistent cyanosis after successful Fontan that is not caused by a planned fenestration can be difficult to trace in some patients. These authors show excellent results with catheter intervention therapy for such patients.

Day and associates[100] from Salt Lake City, Utah, reviewed the results of 68 consecutive Fontan procedures and found 2 surviving patients who had transient neurologic symptoms or signs with no evidence of brain injury by MRI, whereas 6 surviving patients had strokes defined by sustained neurological symptoms or signs with areas of brain injury identified by MRI. Collectively, patients with neurological symptoms had normal hemoglobin values, platelet counts, partial thromboplastin times, and prothrombin times at the onset of clinical neurological findings. Two patients were taking antiplatelet agents, and 1 patient was taking Coumadin. One of the patients with transient neurological findings and all of the stroke patients had residual right-to-left shunts. These authors show a 9% incidence of strokes after a Fontan procedure, usually associated with right-to-left shunts. Whether antiplatelet drugs decrease this complication is unclear.

Miscellaneous Topics

Single-Stage Repair of Aortic Arch Obstruction and Associated Defects

Sandhu and associates[101] from Ann Arbor, Michigan, reported experience in 60 neonates (median age, 8 days; range, 1 to 28 days) who underwent a single stage repair of aortic arch obstruction and associated intracardiac defects. Coarctation plus VSD was present in 19 (32%), interrupted arch with VSD in 18 (30%), and coarctation or interrupted arch with complex intracardiac anatomy in 23 (38%). The arch obstruction was repaired using resection and primary anastomosis in 54 patients, synthetic patch aortoplasty in 3, subclavian flap aortoplasty in 2, and interposition graft in 1. Total circulatory arrest time was

48±3 minutes, and there were 7 early postoperative deaths (12%; 70% confidence limits 8 to 17%). The 53 survivors were followed for a mean of 23 months (range, 1 to 78 months). Recurrent arch obstruction has occurred in 2 of 53 (4%). Both underwent successful balloon angioplasty. There were 2 late deaths, 1 of which was noncardiac. The authors conclude that repair of arch obstruction and intracardiac defects by a single-stage approach through a median sternotomy can be accomplished with low mortality in infants, even with complex intracardiac anatomy, including truncus arteriosus and transposition.

Systemic Obstruction in Univentricular Heart

Brawn and associates[102] from Birmingham, United Kingdom, reported 19 consecutive infants (age, 1 to 170 days; median, 6 days), who underwent a modified Damus operation without the use of exogenous material for treatment of complex single ventricle physiology and systemic outflow obstruction. There 9 early deaths, and all 15 survivors (median follow-up, 7 months) were clinically well without major systemic ventricular dysfunction or AV or arterial valve regurgitation. A superior vena cava–PA shunt was performed in 10 infants (1 death), and 1 has required patch angioplasty of the aortic arch and innominate artery with revision of the aortopulmonary shunt. The other 4 survivors are awaiting a cavopulmonary shunt. Univariate analysis yielded the chronological rank for an individual procedure revealed presence of aortic arch atresia or absence of TGA as predictors of death. This aggressive surgical approach provides excellent early palliation and ameliorates abnormal ventricular hypertrophy from pressure or volume overload with conservation of systemic ventricular function for future Fontan operation. These authors show good results for this complex group of patients by using a modified Damus procedure, which has some resemblance to the Norwood procedure. Further follow-up with a larger group will be necessary to determine if this type of palliation provides a good long-term result.

Serraf and associates[103] from Le Plessis-Robinson, France, reported 27 of 96 patients with univentricular heart and unobstructed pulmonary blood flow who were referred for surgical palliation and had systemic obstruction. There were 26 neonates with coarctation and 21 with subaortic stenosis. In 8 other patients, subaortic stenosis developed after initial PA banding. There were 4 different palliative procedures performed: coarctation repair with PA banding in 15, Norwood or Damus-Kaye-Stansel or arterial switch operation in 9, coarctation repair with PA banding and bulboventricular foramen enlargement in 2, and orthotopic heart transplantation with coarctation repair in 1. The mortality rate was 34% for all patients, 53% in patients with coarctation plus PA banding, and 50% in patients with coarctation, PA banding, and bulboventricular foramen enlargement. There were 9 patients who had development of subaortic stenosis and underwent a subsequent procedure: Damus-Kaye-Stansel in 5, arterial switch operation in 3, and bulboventricular foramen enlargement in 1. In addition, 3 had a concomitant or subsequent Fontan procedure and 2 a bidirectional Glenn procedure. In patients with subaortic stenosis after initial PA banding, a second stage consisted of a Damus-Kaye-Stansel procedure in 3, bulboventricular foramen enlargement in 2, and creation of aortico-pulmonary window in 1. Actuarial 4-year survival was 66±8% for all patients but 40% in patients with coarctation and PA banding alone. These authors suggest initial management of patients with univentricular heart and systemic obstruction by Norwood-like procedures provide a better outcome. Whether this can be translated to large groups of patients is unclear. It is clear, however, that subaortic obstruction must be treated early to avoid severe hypertrophy and myocardial diastolic dysfunction.

Norwood Procedure For Nonhypoplastic Left-Sided Anomalies

Jacob and associates[104] from Philadelphia, Pennsylvania, reported 60 neonates with malformations other than hypoplastic left heart syndrome who underwent initial palliation by the Norwood procedure. Diagnoses included single left ventricle with left-sided TGA (12), critical AS (8), complex double outlet right ventricle (8), interrupted aortic arch with VSD and subaortic stenosis (7), VSD, subaortic stenosis, and coarctation (7), aortic atresia with large VSD (6), tricuspid atresia with TGA (6), heterotaxy syndrome with subaortic obstruction (3), and miscellaneous (3). There were 10 hospital deaths, with 83% survival. Mortality was independent of diagnosis and essentially the same as that for hypoplastic left heart syndrome. Depending on the nature of the underlying anomaly and subsequent postoperative course, patients have undergone either biventricular or Fontan repair at a later date.

Extracorporeal Membrane Oxygenation

Black and associates[105] from Toronto, Ontario, gathered information on 31 consecutive children with myocardial failure who could not be resuscitated with other means and underwent extracorporeal membrane oxygenation. Of the children who underwent extracorporeal membrane oxygenation as a means of cardiac rescue, 14 of 31 (45%) were weaned successfully. There were 2 distinct groups based on initial indications for extracorporeal membrane oxygenation: 25 who had postcardiotomy myocardial dysfunction and 6 with cardiomyopathy or myocarditis. Children with residual defects after cardiotomy did not survive extracorporeal membrane oxygenation (n=10), whereas 4 of 6 children with cardiomyopathy and myocarditis were weaned successfully. In either group of patients, extracorporeal membrane oxygenation support beyond 6 days failed to resuscitate the myocardium; all attempts to violate this time barrier failed. Postcardiotomy residual defects are a contraindication to extracorporeal membrane oxygenation. If children with residual defects are excluded, successful weaning from extracorporeal membrane oxygenation can be achieved in almost 70% with almost all recovery occurring within the first 6 days of treatment. Residual lesions that led to unsuccessful extracorporeal membrane oxygenation included 2 VSDs, 4 cases of residual RV outflow obstruction with and without PR, 2 cases of residual LV outflow obstruction, and 3 cases of residual left-sided valvular regurgitation.

Walters and associates[106] from Detroit, Michigan, retrospectively reviewed the records of 73 pediatric patients with congenital heart disease who were placed on extracorporeal membrane oxygenation. The patients were grouped by timing of extracorporeal membrane oxygenation cannulation: group 1 patients (10%) were placed on extracorporeal membrane oxygenation preoperatively, and group 2 patients (90%) were placed on extracorporeal membrane oxygenation at any interval after cardiac repair. A subgroup of postoperative patients consisted of 26% who could not be weaned from bypass and were converted directly to extracorporeal membrane oxygenation after repair. The remainder of the postoperative patients were cannulated postoperatively after an initial period of clinical stability. Hospital survival for all patients was 58% and did not differ between groups 1 and 2. Only 4 of 17 patients who could not be weaned from cardiopulmonary bypass survived their hospitalization compared with 70% of those patients who had an initial period of stabilization and then were cannulated postoperatively. Multivariate analysis identified elevated RA pressure after extracorporeal membrane oxygenation decannulation and inability to wean from cardiopulmonary bypass as independent risk factors for hospital death. Extracorporeal membrane oxygenation is most effective in salvaging pediatric cardiac surgical patients who demonstrate medically refractory deterioration at some interval after being successfully weaned from cardiopulmonary bypass.

Neurological Status After Hypothermic Cardiac Arrest or Low-Flow Cardiopulmonary Bypass

Bellinger and associates[107] from Boston, Massachusetts, compared developmental and neurological sequelae of total circulatory arrest or low-flow cardiopulmonary bypass in 171 patients with left-sided TGA who underwent an arterial switch operation. After adjustment for the presence or absence of a VSD, the infants assigned to circulatory arrest had a lower mean score on the Psychomotor Development Index of Infant Development and a higher proportion had scores ≤80 (i.e., 2 SDs or more below the population mean). The score was inversely related to the duration of circulatory arrest and the risk of neurological abnormalities increased with the duration of arrest. The method of support was not associated with the prevalence of abnormalities on MRI scans of the brain, scores on the Mental Development Index of the Bayley Scale, or scores on a test of visual recognition memory. Perioperative seizure activity was associated with lower scores on the Psychomotor Development Index and an increased likelihood of abnormalities on magnetic resonance imaging scans of the brain. Heart surgery performed with circulatory arrest as the predominant support strategy is associated with a slightly higher risk of delayed motor development and neurological abnormalities at the age of 1 year than is surgery with low-flow bypass as the predominant support strategy.

Modified Blalock-Taussig Shunt

Odim and associates[108] from Boston, Massachusetts, reported 104 primary modified Blalock-Taussig shunts with 52 constructed by thoracotomy approach and 52 by sternotomy approach. Fifteen of the thoracotomy patients were <1 month of age (8 were <7 days old). Of the sternotomy patients, 36 were <1 month of age (20 were <7 days old). There were 10 shunt failures and 3 hospital deaths in the thoracotomy group and 4 shunt failures with 6 hospital deaths in the sternotomy group. The overall hospital mortality rate was 9% and operative route was not a predictor of mortality. There was a significant difference between the two operative approaches in shunt failure, with shunts created by thoracotomy 4 times more likely to fail than those created by the sternotomy route. The side of the shunt was also a significant predictor of failure with left-sided shunts 4 times more prone to failure. The sternotomy route is technically less challenging and is associated with fewer shunt failures than the classic thoracotomy approach. The theoretical disadvantage of this method for future sternal reentry was not apparent but requires prospective analysis.

Coronary Sinus Atresia

Adatia and Gittenberger-DeGroot[109] from Freiburg, Germany, and Leiden, the Netherlands, studied 26 heart-lung specimens without a coronary sinus draining to the right atrium. They were classified into specimens with an unroofed coronary sinus and those with atresia of the coronary sinus orifice. In 14 of 26 specimens there was an unroofed coronary sinus associated with persistence of the left superior caval vein. An inferior-posterior location of an ASD was detected in 2 of 14 and atrial appendage anomalies were seen in 13 of 14, exemplified by both right and left atrial isomerism. Isomerism was associated with an AV septal defect in 12 of 14. An atretic coronary sinus orifice was seen in 12 of 26 and atrial appendage anomalies were rare in these cases, seen in only 2 of 12. The drainage was then by way of a left superior vena caval vein or, in its absence, a coronary sinus to left atrial window. Ventricular hypoplasia was seen in both categories of coronary sinus abnormalities (12 of 26). These findings emphasize the need to study coronary sinus drainage before procedures such as ligation or transcatheter coil embolization of a left superior caval vein, venous redirection, or closure of a dorsal ASD are contemplated. Such procedures might inadvertently lead to impairment of coronary venous return or persistence of an intracardiac shunt. Two-dimensional echocardiographic imaging and Doppler interrogation of directional flow in the superior vena caval vein would be extremely important when a left superior caval vein is found in patients in whom surgery is contemplated.

Thoracoscopic Surgery

Burke and associates[110] from Boston, Massachusetts, used video assisted endoscopic techniques for neonates and infants in 48 thoracic operations in 46 pediatric patients ranging in age from 2 hours to 14 years with a median of 9 months. Patients weighed from 575 g to 54 kg (median, 9 kg). Clinical applications included PDA interruption in infants (n=26) and premature neonates (n=5), vascular ring division (n=8), pericardial drainage and resection (n=3), arterial and venous collateral interruption (n=2), thoracic duct ligation (n=2), epicardial pacemaker lead insertion (n=1), and diagnostic thoracoscopy (n=1). There was no operative mortality and technical success, defined as a video-assisted procedure completed without incising chest wall muscle or spreading the ribs, was achieved in 39 of 48 procedures (82%), with thoracotomy required to complete 9 procedures. Most patients (22 of 25, 88%) undergoing elective ductus ligation were extubated in the operating room and discharged from the hospital within 48 hours of the operation. Discharge on the first postoperative day was possible in the last 8 of 10 patients undergoing ductal ligation. Residual ductal flow was 0 of 25 in the operating room, 1 of 30 by discharge auscultation, and 3 of 25 by follow-up Doppler echocardiography. These authors feel video-assisted thoracoscopy techniques can be safely applied to pediatric patients with PDAs.

With the current successful of coil occlusion for PDA, it is unlikely that this procedure is going to be used for the small PDA in those patients who are approximately 3 kg or greater in size. The use of this technique for other procedures may gain advocacy, but physicians will need considerable training and expertise in order to carry out these procedures safely. It is unlikely that many centers will have enough patients where this will be possible.

Intra-Aortic Spring Coil Loops

Verma and associates[111] from New York, New York, and Boston, Massachusetts, reviewed the cineangiograms of all patients who had at least one aortopulmonary collateral vessel or PDA closed between January 1, 1988, and August 31, 1993. From this group, 53 patients had multiple-plane angiographic evidence of intra-aortic coil loops. All subsequent cineangiograms were reviewed to determine coil position or movement and evidence of recanalization or endothelial coverage of the coil loop. Of the 53 patients with intra-aortic coil loops, 49 patients had closure of 1 or more aortopulmonary (59) collateral vessels and 4 had closure of a PDA (4 vessels). Patient follow-up ranged from 1 day to 66 months (median, 20 months); follow-up was not available in 6 patients. Five of the 53 patients (9%) died at operation or of end-stage heart failure. Patients with late angiography had no residual flow in 31 of 35 aortopulmonary collateral vessels (89%), and 0.5 mm separated the coil and aortic contrast column in all 12 coils with adequate angiography, suggesting endothelial coverage of the intra-aortic coil loop. No episode of stroke, embolic events, endocarditis, or coil migration were reported. Although coil occlusion of aortopulmonary collaterals or PDA may produce an intra-aortic loop, endothelialization appears routine and no late complications have been observed in this group of patients.

Renal Replacement Therapy After Operation

Fleming and associates[112] from Toronto, Canada, reported the use of renal replacement therapy in 42 children over a 5-year period; 17 were managed with peritoneal dialysis, 8 with continuous arteriovenous hemofiltration, and 9 with continuous venovenous hemofiltration. A negative fluid balance was achieved in only 35% of patients treated with peritoneal dialysis compared with 50% of those treated with continuous arteriovenous hemofiltration and 89% of those treated with continuous venovenous hemofiltration. Caloric intake increased by 43% after peritoneal dialysis was started compared with 515% and 409% in the arteriovenous and venovenous groups. The serum urea levels fell by 36% and 39% compared with pretherapy levels with arteriovenous and venovenous hemofiltration, respectively, and the creatinine content was reduced by 19% and 33%. Neither parameter was reduced in the peritoneal dialysis group. Hemofiltration is a highly effective renal replacement therapy after surgical repair of congenital heart disease and offers significant advantages over peritoneal dialysis. Unfortunately, in this small group of patients an improvement in mortality was not achieved with this therapy.

Right Ventricular Function

Helbing and associates[113] from Leiden, the Netherlands, performed MRI for assessment of RV size and function in 22 healthy children, 7 after Senning correction of TGA, 7 after TF correction, and 6 with ASD. Close correlation between RV vs. LV stroke volumes and RV stroke volume vs. great artery flow were observed with small interobserver and intraobserver variability. Results of healthy children were end-diastolic volume 70 ± 9 ml/m^2 and EF $70\pm4\%$. There were small decreases in EF in the Senning and TF patients and increased RV end-diastolic volume in ASD patients. Although extremely time consuming, these studies provide probably the most accurate methods for quantifying RV size and function in patients with abnormal RV shapes.

Associated Pulmonary Arteriovenous Malformation

Srivastava and associates[114] from Boston, Massachusetts, reported 10 patients with congenital heart disease who were found to have developed pulmonary arteriovenous malformations as diagnosed by cardiac catheterizations. Diagnoses include heterotaxy syndrome/polsyplenia, with interrupted inferior vena cava and hepatic veins draining to the right atrium in 6, heterotaxy/asplenia in 1, corrected TGA with PS in 1, and biliary atresia and associated congenital heart disease in 2. Pulmonary malformations were diagnosed 0.1 to 7 years after creation of a cavopulmonary anastomosis that resulted in exclusion of the hepatic venous flow from 1 or both lungs in 8 of the 10 patients; the remaining 2 patients have normal drainage of hepatic veins to the lungs but had biliary atresia. In all, the common anatomic feature was the exclusion of normal hepatic venous return from the affected pulmonary circulation. The cases of all patients with interrupted inferior vena cava who had hepatic veins draining to the right atrium were reviewed to determine the incidence of pulmonary arteriovenous malformation in those with cavopulmonary anastomosis. There were 6 of 28 (21%) of those with vs. 1 of 56 (2%) of those without cavopulmonary anastomosis who developed pulmonary arteriovenous malformations. The 1 patient without cavopulmonary anastomosis who had pulmonary malformations also had biliary atresia. Among patients with cavopulmonary anastomosis, the probability of developing pulmonary arteriovenous malformations was 15% and 28% at 3 and 5 years, respectively, after cavopulmonary anastomosis. These authors postulate that pulmonary arteriovenous malformations after cavopulmonary anastomosis are related to the abnormal hepatic venous flow away from the pulmonary circulation. Redirection of hepatic flow to the pulmonary circulation in some patients with pulmonary arteriovenous malformation may lead to reversibility of this condition.

Cardiac Isomerism

Horooka and associates[115] from Osaka, Japan, reported surgical results in 93 patients with cardiac isomerism. There were 3 patients among the 93 with right and 14 with left isomerism who underwent biventricular repair at ages ranging from 4 months to 41 years (mean, 5 years). Anatomic repair was accomplished in 14 patients and functional repair with the right ventricle used as a systemic ventricle in 2 patients. Methods of atrial septation to separate pulmonary venous flow from systemic venous flow included atrial partition with a straight patch in 7 patients, interatrial rerouting with a tailored baffle in 5, and a Mustard-type atrial switch in 5. There was 1 hospital death (6%) and 2 late deaths (12%). Two patients required reoperation: 1 had reconstruction of a stenotic venous connection and 1 had mitral valve replacement because of incompetence. Surgically induced complete AV block was not observed in any patients. Optimal atrial septation offers the possibility of biventricular repair for some patients with cardiac isomerism with acceptable intraventricular structure. These data should be studied by all cardiologists who deal with this difficult group of patients. Most of them are relegated to Fontan repair, but these authors have indicated that biventricular repair is another possibility to consider.

Prenatal Echocardiography in Left-Sided Obstruction

Hornberger and associates[116] from Boston, Massachusetts, reviewed the prenatal and postnatal echocardiograms of 21 fetuses with left heart obstructive lesions, including 15 with serial study, to attempt to elucidate the prenatal natural history of disease and identify features indicative of postnatal disease severity. Ventricular, AV valve, and great artery dimensions were measured and growth curves developed with comparisons to 40 normal fetuses. Fetuses were divided into groups according to whether postnatally the left heart was capable (group 1, n=10) or incapable (group 2, n=7) of supporting the systemic circulation in the presence of a patent aortic valve. Group 3 (n=4) included fetuses with aortic atresia. At initial examination at 22±3 weeks' gestation, left heart dimensions were normal or reduced, with the most diminutive measurements in group 3. There were 3 fetuses in group 2 and most in group 1 who had normal initial left heart dimensions. Subsequent growth of left heart structures either paralleled normal growth or was reduced, the latter resulting in the development or progression of left heart hypoplasia. All left heart dimensions grew more slowly in groups 2 and 3 than in group 1, and other prenatal features observed only in groups 2 and 3 included reversed or bidirectional foramen ovale flow and retrograde distal arch flow. Initial midtrimester mitral valve and ascending aorta Z scores and the growth rates of all left heart structures correlated strongly with postnatal LV end-diastolic dimension. Only 1 fetus in group 1 developed severe AS late in gestation. These data should prove useful in predicting the severity of LV obstruction postnatally and in allowing appropriate planning for delivery of severe affected fetuses at perinatal centers with facilities for performing neonatal cardiac surgery.

Intravascular Ultrasonic Imaging

Berger and associates[117] from Rotterdam, the Netherlands, performed intravascular ultrasound imaging in 11 pediatric patients with congenital heart disease. Luminal diameter, area, and pulsatility were determined at 2 to 5 sites in the pulmonary branches and pulmonary vascular reaction to 100% oxygen inhalation was studied. Luminal size and pulsatility could be determined reproducibly in arteries with diameters from 1.6 to 9.3 mm. Pulsatility was directly related to vessel size, and after 100% oxygen inhalation, pulsatility increased in all arteries from 20% to 26%. These methods could prove extremely useful if they could be adapted to provide flow velocity and total flow to individual lungs and lung segments to aid in direct determination of pulmonary vascular resistance.

In-Hospital Mortality and Hospital Case Volume

Jenkins and associates[118] from Boston, Massachusetts, reviewed the impact of hospital caseload on in-hospital mortality for pediatric patients undergoing congenital heart surgery in acute care hospitals in California and Massachusetts during 1988 and 1989. Cases were grouped into 4 categories based on the complexity of the procedure, and an adjusted OR for in-hospital death was estimated using generalized estimating equations that account for the intra-institution correlation among patients. A total of 2833 cases at 37 centers were identified. Compared with centers handling more than 300 cases per year and after controlling for patient characteristics, centers performing <10 surgeries per year had an OR for in-hospital death of 8; 10 to 100 cases, OR=3; and 101 to 300, OR=3. Independent risk factors for mortality included procedure complexity category, use of cardiopulmonary bypass, young age at surgery, and transfer from another acute care hospital. Few differences were found by hospital caseload in length of stay or total hospital charges. For children with congenital heart disease who underwent surgery in California in 1988 or Massachusetts in 1989, the risk of dying in-hospital was much lower if the surgery was performed at an institution performing more than 300 cases annually.

Fetal Cardiac Neoplasms

Holley and associates[119] from Washington, D.C.; Baltimore, Maryland; Charleston, South Carolina; Philadelphia, Pennsylvania, New Haven, Connecticut; and San Francisco, California, presented a retrospective review over an 8-year period at 7 centers regarding prevalence and natural history of cardiac tumors in patients referred for fetal echocardiography. Cardiac tumors were present in 19 pregnancies with gestational age at diagnosis ranging from 21–38 weeks. The most common indication for referral was a mass on an obstetric ultrasound study. The tumors were singular in 10 and multiple in 9 patients. Tumor size ranged from 0.4×0.4 to 3.5×4 cm; the majority of the tumors were not hemodynamically significant. There were 17 patients with rhabdomyomas, 1 with a fibroma, and 1 with an atrial hemangioma. Tuberous sclerosis complex was diagnosed in 10 patients. Partial or complete tumor regression was seen in 8 patients; tumors were unchanged in 5 and 3 required operations. Although these are rare conditions, they are almost always benign. The majority are rhabdomyomas which rarely need surgery and usually have marked regression and even resolution postnatally.

Tuberous Sclerosis and Cardiac Rhabdomyoma

Nir and associates[120] from Rochester, Minnesota, provide a retrospective review over 13 years of 109 patients with tuberous sclerosis complex who underwent echocardiography. There were 47 patients (43%) with cardiac rhabdomyoma on echocardiographic examination, and 3 patients had questionable rhabdomyoma. Visible tumors were located in the left ventricle in 68%, in the LV septum in 38%, LV apex in 38%, LV lateral wall in 37%, LV outflow tract in 13%, and LV papillary muscle in 11%. The tumor was located in the right ventricle in 31 patients (61%); these were in the RV septum in 38%, RV apex in 32%, RV lateral wall in 8%, and RV outflow tract in 21%. Tumors were located in the left ventricle only in 38%, whereas 30% had tumors in the right ventricle only and 32% had tumors in both ventricles. RA tumors were present in 6%, and 1 patient had a tumor in the main PA. Ninety-eight percent of 44 patients who had an EF measured, and 98% were normal. Congenital heart disease was present in 2 patients or 4%; 1 patient had coarctation of the aorta and 1 had AS. Arrhythmias were reported in 8, including premature ventricular contractions and preexcitation. There were no cases of thromboembolic events, and no patient had cardiac surgery for tumor removal. Follow-up was complete in 40 of 47 patients; in 58% the tumors decreased in size and number or both, and in 42% there was no change in tumor size or number. Echocardiographically detected cardiac rhabdomyomas are common in patients with tuberous sclerosis complex and more prevalent and prominent in younger patients. Tumors regressed in size, number, or both in most patients ages <4 years and less so in older patients. These tumors are associated with a relatively high prevalence of preexcitation which may increase the risk for arrhythmias.

Kawasaki Disease

Paridon and associates[121] from Detroit, Michigan; Washington, DC; and Houston, Texas, studied exercise performance and myocardial perfusion after Kawasaki disease. There were 46 patients classified into 3 groups on the basis of coronary artery status: group 1 (n=27) had no objective evidence of coronary artery lesions, group 2 (n=11) had resolved aneurysms, and group 3 (n=8) had persistent coronary aneurysms. All patients underwent exercise testing and single-photon emission computed tomographic imaging was performed at rest and during peak exercise using technetium-99m sestamibi. Maximal oxygen consumption was within normal limits and was similar in all 3 groups; ST segment changes at peak exercise were present in 5 patients and 2 of these 5 had stress induced perfusion defects. Myocardial perfusion defects were present in 37% of patients in group 1, 63% in group 2, and 100% in group 3. These defects corresponded to the coronary artery lesion site in all but 3 patients. Stress-induced perfusion defects are frequent even in the absence of coronary abnormalities and are common even in the absence of ST segment changes suggestive of ischemia. These studies suggest caution in using exercise or perfusion data to evaluate coronary ischemia in patients with Kawasaki disease. There may be problems with the ability of these arteries to dilate even in the absence of obstructive CAD. There are rare instances of symptomatic ischemic CAD late after Kawasaki disease and further long-term investigations of such patients is warranted.

Knowledge of Infective Endocarditis Prophylaxis

To determine whether adults with congenital heart disease have adequate knowledge of infective endocarditis and its prophylaxis and to ascertain whether an educational program effectively improves patient knowledge and compliance, Cetta and Warnes[122] from Rochester, Minnesota, asked 102 consecutive patients to complete a 12-question survey to assess their knowledge of heart disease, infective endocarditis, and its prophylaxis. Of 102 patients, 100 (98%) completed the questionnaire. Sixty-eight patients knew the name of their heart disease. Fifty patients correctly defined endocarditis, but only 43 knew hygiene measures that could prevent endocarditis. Ninety-six patients knew that they needed to take "a medicine" before dental procedures, and 76 of those patients (79%) knew that an antibiotic was necessary. Patient use of cardiac medications and a history of endocarditis correlated significantly with knowledge of endocarditis. Patients who had been to the Adult Congenital Heart Disease Clinic at least once knew endocarditis prevention measures and the importance of regular dental and cardiology follow-up significantly more frequently than did first-time attendees. Despite educational counseling, however, patient recall of endocarditis and its prevention is disappointing many adults with congenital heart disease have inadequate knowledge of their cardiac lesion, endocarditis, and endocarditis prophylaxis. Educational efforts for adults with congenital heart disease need to be updated and reinforced regularly.

Superior Vena Caval Flow in Normal Children

Salim and associates[123] from Memphis, Tennessee, used 2-dimensional and Doppler echocardiography to measure the diameter and mean flow velocities in the superior vena cava and the PAs of 145 healthy children. Cardiac output and superior vena caval flow increased with increasing age and body surface area and superior vena caval flow accounted for 49% of output in newborn infants. This contribution increased to a maximum of 55% at the age of 2.5 years. Afterward, there was a slow decline in the ratio of superior vena caval–PA flow; it reached the adult value of 35% by 6.6 years of age. This maturational change in the superior vena caval contribution to total output may explain the higher systemic saturation in infants as compared with older children after cavopulmonary anastomosis.

1. Konstantinides S, Geibel A, Olschewski M, Gornandt L, Roskamm H, Spillner G, Just H, Kasper W: A comparison of surgical and medical therapy for atrial septal defect in adults. N Eng J Med 1995 (August 24);333:469–473.
2. Marx GR, Fulton DR, Pandian NG, Vogel M, Cao Q-L, Ludomirsky A, Delabays A, Sugeng L, Klas B: Delineation of site, relative size and dynamic geometry of atrial septal defects by real-time three-dimensional echocardiography. J Am Coll Cardiol 1995 (February);25:482–90.
3. Holmvang G, Palacios IF, Vlahakes GJ, Dinsmore RE, Miller SW, Liberthson RR, Block PC, Ballen B, Brady TJ, Kantor HL: Imaging and sizing of atrial septal defects by magnetic resonance. Circulation 1995 (December);92:3473–3480.
4. Sigfusson G, Ettedgul JA, Silverman NH, Anderson RH: Is a cleft in the anterior leaflet of an otherwise normal mitral valve an atrioventricular canal malformation? J Am Coll Cardiol 1995 (August);26:508–515.
5. van Arsdell GS, Williams WG, Boutin C, Trusler GA, Coles JG, Rebeyka IM, Freedom RM: Subaortic stenosis in the spectrum of atrioventricular septal defects. J Thorac Cardiovasc Surg 1995 (November);110:1534–1542.
6. Backer CL, Mavroudis C, Alboliras ET, Zales VR: Repair of complete atrioventricular canal defects: Results with the two-patch technique. Ann Thorac Surg 1995 (September);60:530–537.
7. Bando K, Turrentine MW, Sun K, Sharp TG, Ensing GJ, Miller AP, Kesler KA, Binford RS, Carlos GN, Hurwitz RA, Caldwell RL, Darragh RK, Hubbard J, Cordes TM, Girod DA, King H, Brown JW: Surgical management of complete atrioventricular septal defects. J Thorac Cardiovasc Surg 1995 (November);110:1543–1545.

8. Wu M-H, Wang J-K, Chang C-I, Chiu I-S, Lue H-C: Implication of anterior septal malalignment in isolated VSD. Br Heart J 1995 (August);74:180–185.

9. Ramaciotti C, Vetter JM, Bornemeier RA, Chin AJ: Prevalence, relation to spontaneous closure, and association of muscular ventricular septal defects with other cardiac defects. Am J Cardiol 1995 (January 1);75:61–65.

10. Roguin N, Du Z-D, Barak M, Nasser N, Hershkowitz S, Milgram E: High prevalence of muscular ventricular septal defects in neonates. J Am Coll Cardiol 1995 (November 15);26:1545–1548.

11. Donofrio MT, Jacobs ML, Norwood WI, Rychik J: Early changes in ventriuclar septal defect size and ventricular geometry in the single left ventricle after volume-unloading surgery. J Am Coll Cardiol 1995 (October);26:1008–1015.

12. Zhou Q, Lai Y, Wei H, Song R, Wu Y, Zhang H: Unidirectional valve patch for repair of cardiac septal defects with pulmonary hypertension. Ann Thorac Surg 1995 (November);60:1245–1249.

13. Fedderly RT, Lloyd TR, Mendelsohn AM, Beekman RH: Determinants of successful balloon valvotomy in infants with critical pulmonary stenosis or membranous pulmonary atresia with intact ventricular septum. J Am Coll Cardiol 1995 (February);25:460–465.

14. Horngerger LK, Sanders SP, Sahn DJ, Rice MJ, Spevak PJ, Benaceraff BR, McDonald RW, Colan SD: In utero pulmonary artery and aortic growth and potential for progression of pulmonary outflow tract obstruction in tetralogy of fallot. J Am Coll cardiol 1995 (March 1);25:739–745.

15. Geva T, Ayers NA, Pac FA, Pignatelli R: Quantitative morphometric analysis of progressive infundibular obstruction in tetralogy of fallot. Circulation 1995 (August 15);92:886–892.

16. Sluysmans T, Neven B, Rubay J, Lintermans J, Ovaert C, Mcumbitsi J, Shango P, Stijns M, Vilers A: Early balloon dilatation of the pulmonary valve in infants with tetralogy of Fallot: Risks and benefits. Circulation 1995 (March 1);91:1506–1511.

17. Hennein HA, Mosca RS, Urcelay G, Crowley DC, Bove EL: Intermediate results after complete repair of tetralogy of Fallot in neonates. J Thorac Cardiovasc Surg 1995 (February);109:332–344.

18. Gatzoulls MA, Clark AL, Cullen S, Newman CGH, Redington AN: Right ventricular diastolic function 15 to 35 years after repair of tetralogy of Fallot. Circulation 1995 (March 15);91:1775–1781.

19. Cullen S, Shor D, Redington A: Characterization of right ventricular diastolic performance after complete repair of tetralogy of fallot. Circulation 1995 (March 15);91:1782–1789.

20. Jonasson H, Ivert T, Jonasson R, Holmgren A, Bjork VO: Work capacity and central hemodynamics thirteen to twenty-six years after repair of tetralogy of Fallot. J Thorac Cardiovasc Surg 1995 (August);110–416–426.

21. Okita Y, Miki S, Ueda Y, Tahata T, Sakai T, Matsuyama K, Matsumura M, Tamura T: Early and late results of repair of tetralogy of Fallot with subarterial ventricular septal defect. J Thorac Cardiovasc Surg 1995 (July);110:180–185.

22. Meijboom F, Szatmari A, Deckers JW, Uten EMWJ, Roelandt JRTC, Bos E, Hess J: Cardiac status and health-related quality of life in the long term after surgical repair of tetralogy of Fallot in infancy and childhood. J Thorac Cardiovasc Surg 1995 (October);110:883–891.

23. Kondo C, Nakazawa M, Kusakabe K, Momma K: Left ventricular dysfunction on exercise long-term after total repair of tetralogy of Fallot. Circulation 1995 (November 1);92 (suppl II):II-250–II-255.

24. Reddy VM, Liddicoat JR, Hanley FL: Midline one-stage complete unifocalization and repair of pulmonary atresia with ventricular septal defect and major aortopulmonary collaterals. J Thorac Cardiovasc Surg 1995 (April);109:832–845.

25. Pagani FD, Cheatham JP, Beekman RH, Lloyd TR, Mosca RS, Bove EL: The management of tetralogy of Fallot with pulmonary atresia and diminutive pulmonary arteries. J Thorac Cardiovasc Surg 1995 (November);110:1521–1533.

26. Gournay V, Piéchaud J-F, Delogu A, Sidi D, Kachaner J: Balloon valvotomy for critical stenosis of atresia of pulmonary valve in newborns. J Am Coll Cardiol 1995 (December);26:1725–1731.

27. Dinarevic S, Redington A, Rigby M, Shinebourne EA: Outcome of pulmonary atresia and ventricular septal defect during infancy. Pediatr Cardiol 1995 (November/December);16:276–282.
28. Wernovsky G, Mayer JE Jr, Jonas RA, Hanley FL, Blackstone EH, Kirklin JW, Castaneda AR: Factors influencing early and late outcome of the arterial switch operation for transposition of the great arteries. J Thorac Cardiovasc Surg 1995 (February);109:289–302.
29. Colan SD, Boutin C, Castaneda AR, Wernovsky G: Status of the left ventricle after arterial switch operation for transposition of the great arteries. J Thorac Cardiovasc Surg 1995 (February);109:311–321.
30. Rhodes LA, Wernovsky GT, Keane JF, Mayer JE Jr, Shuren A, Dindy C, Colan SD, Walsh EP: Arrhythmias and Intracardiac conduction after the arterial switch operation. J Thorac Cardiovasc Surg 1995 (February);109:303–310.
31. Turley K, Verrier ED, Congenital Heart Surgeons Society Database: Intermediate results from the period of the congenital heart surgeons transposition study: 1985 to 1989. Ann Thorac Surg 1995 (September);60:505–510.
32. Wernovsky G, Wypij D, Jonas RA, Mayer Jr JE, Hanley FL, Hickey Pr, Walsh AZ, Chang AC, Castaneda AR, Newburger JW, Wessel DL: Postoperative course and hemodynamic profile after the arterial switch operation in neonates and infants. Circulation 1995 (October 15);92:2226–2235.
33. Seraff A, Roux D, Lacour-Gayet F, Touchot A, Bruniaux J, Sousa-Uva M, Planche C: Reoperation after the arterial switch operation for transposition of the great arteries. J Thorac Cardiovasc Surg 1995 (October);110–892–899.
34. Lorenz CH, Walker ES, Graham Jr TP, Powers TA: Right ventricular performance and mass by use of cine MRI late after atrial repair of transposition of the great arteries. Circulation 1995 (November 1);92(suppl II):II-233–II-239.
35. Presbitero P, Somerville J, Rabajoli F, Stone S, Conte MR: Corrected transposition of the great arteries without associated defects in adult patients: Clinical profile and follow up. Br Heart J 1995 (July);74:57–59.
36. Sano T, Riesenfeld T, Karl TR, Wilkinson JL: Intermediate-term outcome after intracardiac repair of associated cardiac defects in patients with atrioventricular and ventriculoarterial discordance. Circulation 1995 (November 1);92 (suppl II):II-272–II-278.
37. Stumper O, Wright JGC, De Giovanni JV, Silove ED, Sethia B, Brawn WJ: Combined atrial and arterial switch procedure for congenital corrected transposition with ventricular septal defect. Br Heart J 1995 (May);73:479–482.
38. van Son JAM, Danielson GK, Huhta JC, Warnes CA, Edwards WD, Schaff HV, Puga FJ, Ilstrup DM: Late results of systemic atrioventricular valve replacement in corrected transposition. J Thorac Cardiovasc Surg 1995 (April);109:642–653.
39. Behrendt DM and Dick M III: Truncus repair with a valveless conduit in neonates. J Thorac Cardiovasc Surg 1995 (October);110:1148–1150.
40. Gaynor JW, Bull C, Sullivan ID, Armstrong BE, Deanfield JE, Taylor JFN, Rees PH, Ungerieider RM, de Laval MR, Stark J, Elliott MJ: Late outcome of survivors of intervention for neonatal aortic valve stenosis. Ann Thorac Surg 1995 (July);60:122–126.
41. Delius RE, Steinberg JB, L'Ecuyer T, Doty DB, Behrendt DM: Long-term follow-up of extended aortoplasty for supravalvular aortic stenosis. J Thorac Cardiovasc Surg 1995 (January);109:155–163.
42. Remmell-Dow DR, Bharati S, David JT, Lev M, Allen HD: Hypoplasia of the eustachian valve and abnormal orientation of the limbus of the foramen ovale in hypoplastic left heart syndrome. Am Heart J 1995 (July);130:148–152.
43. Bu'Lock FA, Stumper O, Jagtap R, Silove ED, De Giovanni JV, Wright JGC, Sethia B, Brawn WJ: Surgery for infants with a hypoplastic systemic ventricle and severe outflow obstruction: Early results with a modified Norwood procedure. Br Heart J 1995 (May);73:456–461.
44. Mosca RS, Bove EL, Crowley DC, Sandhu SK, Schork MA, Kulik TJ: Hemodynamic characteristics of neonates following first stage palliation for hypoplastic left heart syndrome. Circulation 1995 (November 1);92 (suppl II)II-267–II-271.

45. Wediner PW, Myers JL, Gleason MM, Cyran SE, Weber HS, White MG, Baylen BG: The Norwood operation and subsequent Fontan operation in infants with complex congenital heart disease. J Thorac Cardiovasc Surg 1995 (April);109:654–662.

46. Forbess JM, Cook N, Roth SJ, Seraff A, Mayer Jr JE, Jonas RA: Ten-year institutional experience with palliative surgery for hypoplastic left heart syndrome: Risk factors related to stage I mortality. Circulation 1995 (November 1);92 (suppl II):II-262–II-266.

47. Engvall J, Sonnhag C, Nylander E, Stenport G, Karlsson E, Wranne B: Arm-ankle systolic blood pressure difference at rest and after exercise in the assessment of aortic coarctation. Br Heart J 1995 (March);73:270–276.

48. Fletcher SC, Nihill MR, Grifka RG, O'Laughlin MP, Mullins CE: Balloon angioplasty of native coarctation of the aorta: Midterm follow-up and prognostic factors. J Am Coll Cardiol 1995 (March 1);25:730–734.

49. Rao PS and Koscik R: Validation of risk factors in predicting recoarctation after initially successful balloon angioplasty for native aortic coarctation. Am Heart J 1995 (July);130:116–121.

50. Parks WJ, Ngo GD, Plauth WH, Bank ER, Sheppard SK, Pettigrew RI, Williams WH: Incidence of aneurysm formation after dacron patch aortoplasty repair for coarctation of the aorta: Long-term results and assessment utilizing magnetic resonance angiography with three-dimensional surface rendering. J Am Coll Cardiol 1995 (August);26:266–271.

51. Bogaert J, Gewillig M, Rademakers F, Bosmans H, Verschakelen J, Daenen W, Baert AL: Transverse arch hypoplasia predisposes to aneurysm formation at the repair site after patch angioplasty for coarctation of the aorta. J Am Coll Cardiol 1995 (August);26:521–527.

52. Ralph-Edwards AC, Williams WG, Coles JC, Rebeyka IM, Trusler GA, Freedom RM: Reoperation for recurrent aortic coarctation. Ann Thorac Surg 1995 (November);60:1303–1307.

53. Conte S, Lacour-Gayet F, Seraff A, Sousa-Uva M, Bruniauz J, Touchot A, Planche C: Surgical management of neonatal coarctation. J Thorac Cardiovasc Surg 1995 (April);109:663–675.

54. Papa M, Camesasca C, Santoro F, Zoia E, Fragasso G, Giannico S, Chierchia SL: Fetal echocardiography in detecting anomalous pulmonary venous connection: Four false positive cases. Br Heart J 1995 (April);73:355–358.

55. Gaynor JW, Burch M, Dollery C, Sullivan ID, Deanfield JE, Elliott MJ: repair of anomalous pulmonary venous connection to the superior vena cava. Ann Thorac Surg 1995 (June);59:1471–1475.

56. Post JC, van Rossum AC, Bronzwaer JGF, de Cock CC, Hofman MBM, Valk J, Visser CA: Magnetic resonance angiography of anomalous coronary arteries: A new gold standard for delineating the proximal course? Circulation 1995 (December);92:3163–3171.

57. McConnell MV, Ganz P, Selwyn AP, Li W, Edelman RR, Manning WJ: Identification of anomalous coronary arteries and their anatomic course by magnetic resonance coronary angiography. Circulation 1995 (December);92:3158–3162.

58. Tanel RE, Wernovsky G, Landzberg MJ, Perry SB, Burke RP: Coronary artery abnormalities detected at cardiac catheterization following the arterial switch operation for transposition of the great arteries. Am J Cardiol 1995 (July 15);76:153–157.

59. Laks H, Ardehall A, Grant PW, Allada V: Aortic implantation of anomalous left coronary artery: An improved surgical approach. J Thorac Cardiovasc Surg 1995 (March);109:519–523.

60. Turley K, Szarnicki RJ, Flachsbart KD, Richter RC, Popper RW, Tarnoff H: Aortic implantation is possible in all cases of anomalous origin of the left coronary artery from the pulmonary artery. Ann Thorac Surg 1995 (July);60:84–89.

61. Uva MS, Galletti L, Gayet FL, Plot D, Seraff A, Bruniaux J, Comas J, Roussin R, Touchot A, Binet JP, Planche C: Surgery for congenital mitral valve disease in the first year of life. J Thorac Cardiovasc Surg 1995 (January);109:164–176.

62. Tulloh RMR, Buff C, Elliott MJ, Sullivan ID: Supravalvar mitral stenosis: risk factors for recurrence or death after resection. Br Heart J 1995 (February);73:164–168.

63. Dodo H, Gow RM, Hamilton RM, Freedom RM: Chaotic atrial rhythm in children. Am Heart J 1995 (May);129:990–995.
64. Bauersfeld U, Gow RM, Hamilton RM, Izukawa T: Treatment of atrial ectopic tachycardia in infants <6 months old. Am Heart J (June) 1995;129:1145–1148.
65. Rhodes LA, Walsh EP, Saul JP: Conversion of atrial flutter in pediatric patients by transesophageal atrial pacing: A safe, effective, minimally invasive procedure. Am Heart J 1995 (August);130:323–327.
66. O'Sullivan JJ, Gardiner HM, Wren C: Digoxin or flecainide for prophylaxis of supraventricular tachycardia in infants? J Am Coll Cardiol 1995 (October); 26:991–994.
67. Pfammatter J-P, Paul T, Ziemer G, Kallfelz HC: Successful management of junctional tachycardia by hypothermia after cardiac operations in infants. Ann Thorac Surg 1995 (September);60:556–560.
68. Triedman JK, Saul JP, Weindling SN, Walsh EP: Radiofrequency ablation of intra-atrial reentrant tachycardia after surgical palliation of congenital heart disease. Circulation 1995 (February 1);91:707–714.
69. Leenhardt A, Lucet V, Denjoy I, Grau F, Ngoc DD, Coumel P: Catecholaminergic polymorphic ventricular tachycardia in children: A 7-year follow-up of 21 patients. Circulation 1995 (March 1);91:1512–1519.
70. Fenrich AL, Perry JC, Friedman RA: Flecainide and amiodarone: combined therapy for refractory tachyarrhythmias in infancy. J Am Coll Cardiol 1995 (April); 25:1195–1198.
71. Pfammatter JP, Paul T, Lehman C, Kallfelz HC: Efficacy and proarrhythmia of oral sotalol in pediatric patients. J Am Coll Cardiol 1995 (October);26:1002–1007.
72. Michaelsson M, Jonzon A, Riesenfeld T: Isolated congenital complete atrioventricular block in adult life. Circulation 1995 (August 1);92:442–449.
73. Sommer RJ, Golinko RJ, Mitty HA: Initial experience with percutaneous transhepatic cardiac catheterization in infants and children. Am J Cardiol 1995 (June 15);75:1289–1291.
74. Shim D, Lloyd TR, Cho KJ, Moorehead CP, Beekman III RH: Transhepatic cardiac catheterization in children. Evaluation of efficacy and safety. Circulation 1995 (September 15);92:1526–1530.
75. Ward CJB, Mullins CE, Nihill MR, Grifka RF, Vick GW III: Use of intravascular stents in systemic venous and systemic venous baffle obstructions. Circulation 1995 (June 15);91:2948–2954.
76. Fogelman R, Nykanen D, Small JF, McCrindle BW, Freedom RM, Benson LN: Endovascular stents in the pulmonary circulation. Circulation 1995 (August 15);92:881–885.
77. Ing FF, Grifka RG, Nihill MR, Mullins CE: Repeat dilation of intravascular stents in congenital heart defects. Circulation 1995 (August 15);92:893–897.
78. Coles JH, Yemets I, Najm HK, Lukanich JM, Perron J, Wilson GJ, Rabinovitch IM, Nykanen DG, Benson LN, Rebeyka IM, Trusler GA, Freedom RM, Williams WG: Experience with repair of congenital heart defects using adjunctive endovascular devices. J Thorac Cardiovasc Surg 1995 (November);110:1513–1520.
79. Powell AJ, Lock JE, Keane JF, Perry SB: Prolongation of RV-PA conduit life span by percutaneous stent implantation: Intermediate-term results. Circulation 1995 (December 1);92:3282–3288.
80. Reddy VM, Liddicoat JR, Hanely FL: Primary bidirectional superior cavopulmonary shunt in infants between 1 and 4 months of age. Ann Thorac Surg 1995 (May);59:1120–1126.
81. Stumper O, Wright JGC, Sadiq M, De Giovanni JV: Late systemic desaturation after total cavopulmonary shunt operations. Br Heart J 1995 (September);74:282–286.
82. Uemura H, Yagihara T, Kawashima Y, Okada K, Kamiya T, Anderson RH: Use of bidirectional Glenn procedure in the presence of forward flow from the ventricles to the pulmonary arteries. Circulation 1995 (November 1);92 (suppl II):II-228–II-232.
83. Frommelt MA, Frommelt PC, Berger S, Pelech AN, Lewis DA, Tweddell JS, Litwin SB: Does an additional source of pulmonary blood flow alter outcome after a

bidirectional cavopulmonary shunt? Circulation 1995 (November 1);92 (suppl II):II-240–II-244.

84. Webber SA, Horvath P, LeBlanc JG, Slavik Z, Lamb RK, Monro JL, Reich O, Hruda J, Sandor GGS, Keeton BR, Salmon AP: Influence of competitive pulmonary blood flow on the bidirectional superior cavopulmonary shunt: A multi-institutional study. Circulation 1995 (November 1);92 (suppl II)II-279–II-286.

85. Mainwaring RD, Lamberti JJ, Uzark K, Spicer RL: Bidirectional Glenn: Is accessory pulmonary blood flow good or bad? Circulation 1995 (November 1);92 (suppl II):II-294–II-297.

86. Kavey R-EW, Gaum WE, Byrum CJ, Smith FC, Kveselis DA: Loss of sinus rhythm after total cavopulmonary connection. Circulation 1995 (November 1);92 (suppl II):II-304–II-308.

87. Bernstein HS, Brook MM, Silverman NH, Bristow J: Development of pulmonary arteriovenous fistulae in children after cavopulmonary shunt. Circulation 1995 (November 1);92 (suppl II):II-309–II-314.

88. Moore JW, Spicer RL, Perry JC, Mathewson JW, Kirkpatrick SE, George L, Uzark K, Mainwaring RL, Lamberti JJ: Percutaneous use of stents to correct pulmonary artery stenosis in young children after cavopulmonary anastomosis. Am Heart J 1995 (December);130:1245–1249.

89. Bando K, Danielson GK, Schaff HV, Mair DD, Julsrud PR, Puga FJ: Outcome of pulmonary and aortic homografts for right ventricular outflow tract obstruction. J Thorac Cardiovasc Surg 1995 (March);109:509–518.

90. Yankah AC, Alexi-Meskhishvili V, Weng Y, Schorn K, Lange PE, Hetzer R: Accelerated degeneration of allografts in the first two years of life. Ann Thorac Surg 1995 (August);60:571–577.

91. Laks H, Ardehall A, Grant PW, Permut L, Aharon A, Kuhn M, Isabel-Jones J, Galindo A: Modification of the Fontan procedure. Circulation 1995 (June 15);91:2943–2947.

92. Kuhn MA, Jarmakani JM, Laks H, Alejos JC, Permut LC, Galindo A, Isabel-Jones JB: Effect of late postoperative atrial septal defect closure on hemodynamic function in patients with a lateral tunnel Fontan procedure. J Am Coll Cardiol 1995 (July);26:259–265.

93. Kelley JR, Mack GW, Fahey JT: Diminished venous vascular capacitance in patients with univentricular hearts after the Fontan operation. Am J Cardiol 1995 (July 15);76:158–163.

94. Uemura H, Yagihara T, Kawashima Y, Yamamoto F, Nishigaki K, Matsuki O, Okada K, Kamiya T, Anderson RH: What factors affect ventricular performance after a Fontan-type operation. J Thorac Cardiovasc Surg 1995 (August);110:405–415.

95. Cecchin F, Johnsrude CL, Perry JC, Friedman RA: Effect of age and surgical technique on symptomatic arrhythmias after the Fontan procedure. Am J Cardiol 1995 (August 15);76:386–391.

96. Harrison DA, Liu P, Walters JE, Goodman JM, Siu SC, Webb GD, Williams WG, McLaughiln PR: Cardiopulmonary function in adult patients late after Fontan repair. J Am Coll Cardiol 1995 (October);26:1016–1021.

97. Rosenthal DN, Friendman AH, Kleinman CS, Kopf GS, Rosenfeld LE, Hellenbrand WE: Thromboembolic complications after Fontan operations. Circulation 1995 (November 1);92: (suppl II):II-287–II-293.

98. Rychik J, Jacobs ML, Norwood WI Jr: Acute changes in left ventricular geometry after volume reduction operation. Ann Thorac Surg 1995 (November);60:1267–1274.

99. Hsu H, Nykanen DG, Williams WG, Freedom RM, Benson LN: Right to left interatrial communications after the modified Fontan procedure: Identification and management with transcather occlusion. Br Heart J 1995 (November);74:548–552.

100. Day RW, Boyer RS, Tait VF, Ruttenberg HD: Factors associated with stroke following the Fontan procedure. Pediatr Cardiol 1995 (November/December);16:270–275.

101. Sandhu SK, Beekman RH, Mosca RS, Bove EL: Single-stage repair of aortic arch obstruction and associated intracardiac defects in the neonate. Am J Cardiol 1995 (February 15);75:370–373.

102. Brawn WJ, Sethia B, Jagtap R, Stumper OFW, Wright JGC, De Giovanni JV, Silove ED, Jackson M, Sreeram N: Univentricular heart with systemic outflow obstruction: Palliation by primary Damus procedure. Ann Thorac Surg 1995 (June);59:1441–1447.

103. Serraf A, Conte S, Lacour-Gayet F, Bruniauz J, Sousa-Uva M, Roussin R, Planché: Systemic obstruction in univentricular hearts: Surgical options for neonates. Ann Thorac Surg 1995 (October);60:970–977.

104. Jacobs ML, Rychik J, Murphy JD, Nicolson SC, Steven JM, Norwood WI: Results of Norwood's operation for lesions other than hypoplastic left heart syndrome. J Thorac Cardiovasc Surg 1995 (November);110:1555–1562.

105. Black MD, Coles JH, Williams WG, Rebeyka IM, Trusler GA, Bohn D, Gruenwald C, Freedom RM: Determinants of success in pediatric cardiac patients undergoing extracorporeal membrane oxygenation. Ann Thorac Surg 1995 (July);60:133–138.

106. Walter HL III, Hakimi M, Rice MD, Lyons JM, Whittlesey GC, Klein MD: Pediatric cardiac surgical ECMO: Multivariate analysis of risk factors for hospital death. Ann Thorac Surg 1995 (August);60:329–337.

107. Bellinger DC, Jonas RA, Rappaport LA, Wypu D, Wernovsky G, Kuban KCK, Barnes PD, Holmes FL, Hickey PR, Stand RD, Walsh AZ, Helmer SL, Constantinou JE, Carrazan EJ, Mayer JE, Hanley FL, Castaneda AR, Ware JH, Newburger JW: Developmental and neurological status of children after heart surgery with hypothermic circulatory arrest or low-flow cardiopulmonary bypass. N Engl J Med 1995 (March 2);332:549–555.

108. Odim J, Portzky M, Zurakowski D, Wernovsky G, Burke RP, Mayer Jr JE, Castaneda AR, Jonas RA: Sternotomy approach for the modified Blalock-Taussig shunt. Circulation 1995 (November 1);92 (suppl II):II-256–II-261.

109. Adatla I, Gittenberger-DeGroot AC: Unroofed coronary sinus and coronary sinus orifice atresia: Implications of management of complex congenital heart disease. J Am Coll Cardiol 1995 (March 15);25:948–953.

110. Burke RP, Wernovsky G, van der Velde M, Hansey D, Castaneda AR: Video-assisted thoracoscopic surgery for congenital heart disease. J Thorac Cardiovasc Surg 1995 (March);109:499–508.

111. Verma R, Lock BG, Perry SB, Moore P, Keane JF, Lock JE: Intraaortic spring coil loops: Early and late results. J Am Coll Cardiol 1995 (May);25:1416–1419.

112. Fleming F, Bohn D, Edwards E, Cox P, Geary D, McCrindle BW, Williams WG: Renal replacement therapy after repair of congenital heart disease. J Thorac Cardiovasc Surg 1995 (February);1099:322–331.

113. Helbing WA, Rebergen SA, Maliepaard C, Hansen B, Ottenkamp J, Reiber JHC, de Roos A: Quantification of right ventricular function with magnetic resonance imaging in children with normal hearts and with congenital heart disease. Am Heart J 1995 (October);130:828–837.

114. Srivastava D, Preminger T, Lock JE, Mandell V, Keane JF, Mayer JE, Kozakewich H, Spevak PJ: Hepatic venous blood and the development of pulmonary arteriovenous malformations in congenital heart disease. Circulation 1995 (September 1);92:1217–1222.

115. Hirooka K, Yagihara T, Kishimoto H, Isobe F, Yamamoto F, Nishigaki K, Matuski O, Uemura H, Kawashima Y: Biventriuclar repair of cardiac isomerism. J Thorac Cardiovasc Surg 1995 (March);109:530–535.

116. Hornberger LK, Sanders SP, Rein AJJT, Spevak PJ, Parness IA, Colan SD: Left heart obstructive lesions and left ventricular growth in the midtrimester fetus. Circulation 1995 (September 15);92:1531–1583.

117. Berger RMF, Cromme-Dijkhuis AH, van Vilet AM, Hess J: Evaluation of the pulmonary vasculature and dynamics with intravascular ultrasound imaging in children and infants. Pediatr Res 1995 (July);38:36–41.

118. Jenkins KJ, Newburger JW, Lock JE, Davis RG, Coffman GA, Iezonni LI: In-hospital mortality for surgical repair of congenital heart defects: Preliminary observations of variation by hospital caseload. Pediatrics 1995 (March);95:323–330.

119. Holley DG, Martin GR, Brenner JI, Fyfe DA, Huhta JC, Kleinman CS, Ritter SB, Silverman NH: Diagnosis and management of fetal cardiac tumors: A multicenter

experience and review of published reports. J Am Coll Cardiol 1995 (August);26:516–520.

120. Nir A, Tajik AJ, Freeman WK, Seward JB, Offord KP, Edwards WD, Mair DD, Gomez MR: Tuberous sclerosis and cardiac rhabdomyoma. Am J Cardiol 1995 (August 15);76:419–421.

121. Paridon SM, Galioto FM, Vincent JA, Tomassoni TL, Sullivan NM, Bricker JT: Exercise capacity and incidence of myocardial perfusion defects after Kawasaki disease in children and adolescents. J Am Coll Cardiol 1995 (May);25:1420–1424.

122. Cetta F, Warnes CA: Adults with congenital heart disease: Patient knowledge of endocarditis prophylaxis. Mayo Clin Proc 1995 (January);70:5–54.

123. Salim MA, DiSessa TG, Arheart KL, Alpert BS: Contribution of superior vena caval flow to total cardiac output in children. Circulation 1995 (October 1);92:1860–1865.

9

Congestive Heart Failure

General Topics

Rate of Hospitalization

To determine whether the higher rate of hospitalization among African Americans for CHF could be explained by racial differences in the prevalence of clinical risk factors for CHF, Alexander and associates[1] from San Francisco and Oakland, California, examined 64 877 enrollees (27% African Americans and 73% white persons) of the Northern California Kaiser Permanente Medical Care Program who took at least 1 multiphasic medical checkup at or after the age of 40 years and were free of CHF at the time. Among cohort members younger than 60 years at baseline multiphasic health checkup, the age-adjusted RR was 1.48 for both sexes. Cox proportional hazards models were used to adjust for risk factors and length of follow-up. In persons aged 60 years and older, the race difference was explained by greater prevalence of hypertension and diabetes in African Americans (RR, 1.2, 0.94–1.34 after adjustment for hypertension and diabetes). In those younger than 60 years, findings differed by sex. For men, African-American race was no longer a significant predictor of CHF after adjusting for hypertension, diabetes, LF hypertrophy on electrocardiogram, and body mass index (RR, 1.16). However, among younger women, African Americans continued at increased risk despite adjustment for these variables as well as smoking, plasma cholesterol, renal function, alcohol use, and AMI (adjusted RR, 1.4). In this HMO population, the race differences in first hospitalization for CHF are largely explained by known clinical and behavioral risk factors, although in younger women these risk factors do not completely explain the excess risk among African Americans. These findings highlight the role of hypertension and diabetes in the development of CHF, particularly among African Americans.

Preventing Readmission

CHF is the most common indication for admission to the hospital among persons ≥70 years of age. Behavioral modifications, such as full compliance with treatment, frequently contribute to exacerbation of CHF, a fact suggesting that many admissions could be prevented. Rich and associates[2] from St. Louis, Missouri, conducted a prospective, randomized trial of the effect of a nurse-directed, multidisciplinary intervention on rates of readmission within 90 days of hospital discharge, quality of life, and costs of care for high-risk patients 70 years of age or older who are hospitalized with CHF. The intervention consisted of comprehensive education of the patient and family, a prescribed diet, social-service consultation and planning for an early discharge, a review of medications, and intensive follow-up. Survival for 90 days without readmission, the primary outcome measure, was achieved in 91 of the 142 patients in the treatment group compared with 75 of the 140 patients in the control group, who received conventional care. There were 94 readmissions in the control group and 53 in the treatment group. The number of readmissions for CHF was reduced by 56.2% in the treatment group (54 vs. 24 in the control group), whereas the number of readmissions for other causes was reduced by 28.5% (40 vs. 29). In the control group, 23 patients (16.4%) had more than 1 readmission compared with 9 patients (6.3%) in the treatment group. In a subgroup of 126 patients, quality-of-life scores at 90 days improved more from base line for patients in the treatment group. Because of the reduction in hospital admissions, the overall cost of care was $460 less per patient in the treatment group. A nurse-directed, multidisciplinary intervention can improve quality of life and reduce hospital use and medical costs for elderly patients with CHF.

Home Care

Kornowski and associates[3] from Tel Aviv, Israel, examined the impact of intensive home-care surveillance on morbidity rates of elderly patients with severe CHF. Forty-two patients aged 78±8 years who had severe CHF (New York Heart Association functional classes III through IV, mean EF 27±6%) were examined at least once a week at home by internists from the district hospital and by a trained paramedical team. The year before entry to the home-care program was compared with the first year of home surveillance. The mean total hospitalization rate was reduced from 3.2±1.5 hosp per year to 1.2±1.6 hosp per year and duration from 26±14 days per year to 6±7 days per year. Cardiovascular admissions decreased from 2.9±1.5 to 0.8±1.1 per year and duration from 23±13 to 4±4 days per year. The vital status (ability to perform daily activities, expressed in a 1 to 4 scale) was improved from 1.4±0.9 to 2.3±0.7. In conclusion, an intensive home-care program was associated with a marked decrease in the need for hospitalization and improved the functional status of elderly patient with severe CHF. Such a service might also have a cost-effective advantage and a major impact on health expenditure.

Survival While Awaiting Transplantation

Recent trials have suggested that ACE inhibitors might benefit patients with mild to moderate CHF. Stevenson and colleagues[4] from Boston, Massachusetts, and Los Angeles, California reviewed their experience in the treatment of patients with CHF to determine whether survival and risk of sudden death have improved for patients with advanced CHF who are referred for consideration of heart transplantation. One-year mortality and sudden death were determined in 737 consecutive patients referred for heart transplantation and discharged home on medical therapy over 8 years. The total 1-year mortality rate decreased from 33% before 1989 to 16% after 1990. Sudden death rate decreased from 20% to 8%. These authors concluded that the large reduction in mortality, particularly in sudden death, may reflect an enhanced impact of therapeutic advances shown in large clinical trials.

Cheyne-Stokes Respirations

Cheyne-Stokes respirations have frequently been noted in certain groups of patients with CHF, but their prevalence in an unselected population with CHF is undefined. Blackshear and associates[5] from Jacksonville, Florida, and Rochester, Minnesota, screened 100 unselected outpatients or stable inpatients with CHF encountered by 3 cardiologists in a 6-month period and screened the patients for Cheyne-Stokes respirations with overnight oximetry. The mean age of the patients was 70±9 years. Of the patients, 33% had had previous CABG, 77% were men, 57% had hypertension, and 32% had AF. The mean EF (±SD) was 34±13%. Periodic breathing was assessed qualitatively as Cheyne-Stokes respirations in 27% of patients, nonspecific sleep-disordered breathing (apneas and/or hypopneas) in 43%, and normal in 30%. For patients with Cheyne-Stokes respirations, patients with nonspecific sleep-disordered breathing, and normal subjects, the mean numbers of oxyhemoglobin desaturation events per hour were 24, 10, and 2, and the total numbers of desaturations of 4% or more that lasted less than 3 minutes were 172, 74, and 13. Independent predictors of Cheyne-Stokes respirations vs. non–Cheyne-Stokes respirations included a history of nocturnal dyspnea (OR, 4.00) and AF (OR, 3.24). Cheyne-Stokes respirations and nonspecific sleep-disordered breathing are common in unselected patients with CHF, and Cheyne-Stokes respirations are predicted by a history of nocturnal dyspnea and the presence of AF. Techniques designed to modify the nocturnal breathing pattern of patients with CHF may be applicable to a large portion of the CHF population.

Sleep-Disordered Breathing

To determine the prevalence and effect of sleep-disordered breathing in ambulatory patients with stable, optimally treated CHF, Javaheri and associates[6] from Cincinnati, Ohio, studied 42 patients with stable CHF and LVEF ≤45%. The patients were divided into 2 groups. Group 1 (n=23) had an hourly rate of apnea and hypopnea (apnea-hypopnea index) of 20 episodes per hour or less; group 2 (n=19) had an index of 20 episodes/hour. In group 2, the index varied from 26.5 to 82.2 episodes per hour (mean±SD, 44±13 episodes per hour, 38–51 episodes per hour). Group 2 had significantly more arousals (24±12 compared with 3±3 in group 1) that were directly attributable to episodes of apnea and hypopnea, longer periods of time with an arterial oxyhemoglobin saturation of less than 90% (23±24% of total sleep time compared with 2±4%), lower arterial oxyhemoglobin saturation during sleep (74±13% compared with 87±4%), lower LVEF (22±9% compared with 30±10%), and a significantly increased number of episodes of nocturnal ventricular arrhythmias. Multiple regression analyses showed that LV systolic dysfunction was an independent risk factor for sleep apnea in patients with CHF. The prevalence of severe occult sleep-disordered breathing is high in ambulatory patients with stable, optimally treated chronic CHF. The breathing episodes are associated with severe nocturnal arterial blood oxyhemoglobin desaturation and excessive arousals. Severe untreated sleep-disordered breathing may adversely affect LV function, resulting in a vicious cycle that could contribute to death in patients with CHF. Prospective, longitudinal studies on survival are needed.

Right Ventricular Ejection Fraction as Prognostic Factor

A number of prognostic variables have been identified in patients with advanced CHF. DiSalvo and colleagues[7] from Boston, Massachusetts, evaluated the results of maximum symptom limited cardiopulmonary exercise testing and first-pass radionuclide ventriculography in 67 patients with advanced CHF who were referred for evaluation for cardiac transplantation. They found that RV EF >.35 at rest and exercise is a better predictor of survival in advanced CHF than VO_2. Thus, RV function is an important determinant of prognosis in patients with severe CHF.

Skeletal Muscle Oxygenation

Patients with chronic CHF are frequently limited by muscle fatigue resulting from impaired skeletal muscle blood flow. Accordingly, Matsui and associates[8] from Ishikawa, Japan, assessed working skeletal muscle oxygenation in such patients using near-infrared spectroscopy. Nine normal subjects (mean age, 52 years) and 12 patients with CHF (mean age, 60 years) were studied. Near-infrared spectroscopy was used to monitor relative changes in oxygenated hemoglobin and myoglobin, deoxygenated hemoglobin and myoglobin, and total hemoglobin and myoglobin contents in the vastus lateralis muscle at rest, during warm-up (0 W, 30 cycles per minute for 3 minute), incremental maximal supine bicycle exercise (ramp protocol, 15 W/min, 50 cycles per minute), and recovery. At peak exercise the patients exhibited reduced heart rate, systolic BP, peak exercise oxygen consumption (15 ± 3.0 mL/kg per minute vs. 32 ± 8.5 mL/kg per minute), and workload (99 ± 23.4 W vs. 183 ± 68.4 W) compared with the normal individuals. The respiratory quotient was comparable in both groups. In the normal subjects, oxygenated hemoglobin and myoglobin was increased from the warm-up period to the early phase of exercise, followed by a progressive decrease to peak exercise. In the recovery phase of exercise, oxygenated hemoglobin and myoglobin was increased abruptly. For these patients, change in oxygenated hemoglobin and myoglobin followed a pattern similar to that seen in normal individuals, and oxygenated hemoglobin and myoglobin was decreased earlier in contrast to that in the normal individuals. There was a significant difference in the change of oxygenated hemoglobin and myoglobin during warm-up, early-phase exercise, and recovery between the 2 groups. Changes in deoxygenated hemoglobin and myoglobin and oxygenated hemoglobin and myoglobin were inversely proportionate in both groups. In the recovery phase, the change in total hemoglobin and myoglobin was smaller than that in the normal individuals. These data suggest that oxygen delivery to working skeletal muscle is impaired throughout exercise and a reactive hyperemic response to strenuous exercise is blunted in patients with CHF.

Wilson and colleagues[9] in Nashville, Tennessee, investigated the relation between exertional symptoms, ventilatory and skeletal muscle dysfunction, and circulatory function in patients with CHF. Fifty-two ambulatory patients with CHF had hemodynamic monitoring during maximal treadmill exercise testing. During exercise, the severity of dyspnea and fatigue was evaluated on a Borg scale. The level of perceived exercise intolerance during daily activities was evaluated with a Minnesota Living With Heart Failure Questionnaire and the Yale Dyspnea-Fatigue Index. Maximal treadmill exercise increased myocardial oxygen consumption, the dyspnea score, the fatigue score, the pulmonary capillary wedge pressure to 28 mm Hg, and the pulmonary artery lactate concentration to 35 mg/dL while decreasing the pulmonary artery hemoglobin oxygen saturation to 30%. The level of perceived dyspnea had no relation to the pulmonary capillary wedge pressure and correlated only weakly with the level of excessive ventilation. The level of perceived fatigue correlated weakly with blood lactate concentrations. Eleven patients had a normal cardiac output and wedge pressure during exercise, 22 had a normal cardiac output but wedge pressure >20 mm Hg during exercise, and 19 had reduced cardiac output and elevated wedge pressure >20 mm Hg during exercise. Despite the markedly different hemodynamic responses, all three groups of patients had similar levels of fatigue and dyspnea at comparable workloads and comparable total scores for the Minnesota Living With Heart Failure Questionnaire and the Yale Dyspnea-Fatigue Index. There was no relation between the Living With Heart Failure Questionnaire and peak exercise oxygen consumption and a weak correlation between the Dyspnea-Fatigue Index and peak oxygen consumption. Thus, the level of exercise intolerance in ambulatory patients with heart failure had little or no relation to objective measurements of circulatory, ventilatory, or metabolic dysfunction during exercise.

Neurohumoral Variability

Kirlin and colleagues[10] in Ontario, Canada, measured the immediate and longer term variability of selected vasoactive- and volume-regulating neurohormones in patients entering a substudy of the Studies of Left Ventricular Dysfunction, a randomized clinical trial in patients with LVEF ≤35%. The variability of these hormones has not been determined in a large cohort of patients. Immediate variability was assessed by systematically comparing levels after 15 and 30 minutes of supine rest at the initial visit, and longer term variability was assessed by comparing 30-minute supine rest values at the initial visit with corresponding values taken at 30 minutes after 16 to 24 days of stable therapy. Initial values obtained at the first visit after 30-minute supine rest for all 209 patients were 512 pg/mL for plasma norepinephrine, 1.9 ng/mL per hour for plasma renin activity, 3.0 pg/mL for plasma arginine vasopressin, and 129 pg/mL for plasma atrial natriuretic peptide. All variables were moderately increased relative to established normal values. There was a small but significant decrease from 15- to 30-minute supine posture in all neurohormones, except arginine vasopressin. In the presence of stable background therapy, no significant differences were found between measurements obtained after 30 minutes supine rest at the initial visit and 16 to 24 days later. Spearman correlation coefficients corresponding to immediate and longer term variability were high. The investigators concluded that plasma neurohormone levels are relatively constant over several weeks in patients with chronic LV dysfunction who have received stable background therapy throughout this 3-week period. This suggests that major variations in plasma neurohormone levels may therefore be a possible marker of disease progression or may reflect treatment effects in this population.

Signal-Averaged Electrocardiogram and Prolonged QRS

Studies of electrocardiographic predictors of mortality in patients with CHF have reached varying conclusions. Differences in the characteristics of the patients studies may explain the conflicting results regarding both a prolonged QRS and an abnormal signal-averaged electrocardiogram. Silverman and colleagues[11] in Baltimore, Maryland, investigated the impact of the etiology of heart failure on the prognostic importance of a prolonged QRS and an abnormal signal-averaged electrocardiogram in 200 patients with heart failure. Patients were categorized according to etiology of heart failure and electrocardiographic parameters. The mortality of patients with a prolonged QRS was compared with mortality in those with both abnormal and normal signal-averaged electrocardiograms. This was done for the entire group, and separately for those with ischemic and those with nonischemic cardiomyopathy. The mean follow-up was 19 months. Nonischemic patients with a prolonged QRS had significantly worse survival than other patients. However, nonischemic patients with an abnormal signal-averaged electrocardiogram did not have a worse prognosis than patients with a normal signal-averaged electrocardiogram. One-year survival of patients with a prolonged QRS was 71% compared with 98% in patients with a normal and 87% in patients with an abnormal signal-averaged electrocardiogram. In contrast, a prolonged QRS was not a predictor of poor prognosis in patients with ischemic cardiomyopathy (81% 1-year mortality). Patients with ischemic cardiomyopathy and an abnormal signal-averaged electrocardiogram tended to have a poorer survival than patients with a normal signal-averaged electrocardiogram (73% and 81% 1-year mortality, respectively). Thus, the etiology of CHF affects the prognostic importance of both a prolonged QRS and an abnormal signal-averaged electrocardiogram.

Endothelial Cell Dysfunction

CHF is commonly associated with high plasma concentrations of endothelin-1, a powerful vasoconstrictor produced by endothelium. The role of endogenously released endothelin-1 in the maintenance of vascular tone in CHF was assessed by Kiowski et al[12] from Zurich and Basel, Switzerland, by acute administration of an endothelium resector antagonist, *bosentan*. Twenty-four patients with CHF received randomly and in a double-blind manner 2 intravenous infusions of either placebo or bosentan (100 mg followed after 60 minutes by 200 mg). Systemic hemodynamics and plasma endothelin-1 and big-endothelin-1 concentrations were determined before and repeatedly during the 120 minute observation period. Baseline endothelin-1 and big-endothelin-1 concentrations, which were above the normal range in all patients, correlated directly with the extent of pulmonary hypertension, with left- and right-sided heart filling pressures, and with pulmonary vascular resistance and inversely with cardiac index. Compared with placebo, bosentan reduced mean arterial pressure by 7.7%, PA pressure by 13.7%, RA pressure by 13.7%, and PA wedge pressure by 8.6%; it increased vascular resistance by 16.5%, and decreased pulmonary vascular resistance by 33.2%. Heart rate did not change. Plasma endothelin-1 concentrations rose >2-fold from baseline in bosentan recipients while big-endothelin-1 concentrations were unchanged. These findings indicate that, in patients with chronic CHF who have high circulatory endothelin-1 concentrations, this peptide contributes to maintenance of vascular tone. The acute hemodynamic effects of bosentan suggest that chronic endothelin antagonism could be beneficial in such patients.

Ramsey and colleagues[13] in Cardiff, United Kingdom, attempted to establish whether an endothelium-derived relaxing factor influences the distensibility of conduit arteries and whether endothelium-mediated increases in distensibility are impaired in patients with chronic CHF. Conduit artery distensibility was measured by two methods in healthy subjects and in nine patients with CHF caused by dilated cardiomyopathy. In the first method, pulse-wave velocity was measured in the right common iliac artery at rest and during local infusions of acetylcholine or adenosine with correction for systemic effects. Acetylcholine-induced concentration-dependent local reductions of pulse wave velocity in healthy subjects, but not in patients with CHF. Adenosine induced similar reductions in pulse wave velocity in both healthy subjects and patients with CHF. In the second method, brachial artery diameter, blood flow, and BP were measured noninvasively by high-resolution ultrasound, continuous-wave Doppler, and photo-plethysmography during reactive hyperemia in the hand and after sublingual glyceryl trinitrate. Hyperemic flow was similar in healthy subjects and those with CHF and was associated with increases in diameter and distensibility in healthy subjects, but not in patients with CHF. Glyceryl trinitrate induced similar effects in both healthy subjects and patients with CHF. These data demonstrate that conduit artery distensibility is increased by acetylcholine and increased blood flow in healthy subjects, but not in patients with CHF, whereas the effects of adenosine and glyceryl trinitrate on distensibility are preserved in patients with CHF. These data suggest that endothelium-derived relaxing factor-mediated increases in distensibility are impaired in patients with CHF.

Tumor Necrosis Factor Soluble Receptors

Ferrari and colleagues[14] in Brescia, Italy, examined the concentration of soluble tumor necrosis factor receptors and of bioactive and antigenic tumor necrosis factor-α in 37 consecutive patients with various degrees of CHF compared with that of 26 age-matched healthy subjects. The antigenic tumor necrosis factor-α increased 14 to 34 pg/mL in preterminal patients with severe CHF (New York Heart Association class IV). In these patients, soluble tumor necrosis factor receptors were also increased from 1 to 4 ng/mL and soluble tumor necrosis factor receptors from 2 to 8 ng/mL. When measured by cytolytic bioassay, tumor necrosis factor-α was undetectable. Addition of 625 pg/mL recombinant human tumor necrosis factor-α corresponding in the bioassay to 60% of the lethal dose to the serum of healthy subjects resulted in a significant increase of the expected cytotoxicity. Addition of the same dose of recombinant human tumor necrosis factor-α to the serum of patients with mild to moderate CHF (New York Heart Association classes II and III) increased the cytotoxicity. In 4 patients with severe CHF, the expected cytotoxicity was inhibited, or reduced from 625 to 263 pg/mL in the remaining 8 patients. Ten patients died within 1 month of entry into the study. These patients had the highest levels of soluble tumor necrosis factor soluble receptors. Soluble tumor necrosis factor receptor II was a more powerful independent predictor of mortality than tumor necrosis factor-α, soluble tumor necrosis factor–receptor I, New York Heart Association class, norepinephrine levels and atrial natriuretic peptide. Thus, measurement of soluble tumor necrosis factor receptors is useful in evaluating prognosis in patients with severe CHF.

Implantable Defibrillators

Saxon and associates[15] from Los Angeles, California, assessed the operative risk and efficacy of implantable defibrillators for preventing sudden death in patients with heart failure awaiting transplantation. The average waiting time for elective cardiac transplantation is 6 months to 1 year. Sudden cardiac death is the major source of mortality in outpatients in stable condition awaiting cardiac transplantation. The efficacy of implantable defibrillator therapy in this population is not established. The investigators analyzed the operative risk, time to appropriate shock and sudden death in 15 patients determined to be at high risk of sudden death who were accepted onto the outpatient cardiac transplant waiting list. Nonfatal postoperative complications occurred in 2 (13%) subjects with epicardial defibrillating lead systems and in none with transvenous lead systems. Sudden death–free survival until transplantation was 93%. Most of the patients (60%) had an appropriate shock during a mean follow-up of 11±12 months. The mean time to an appropriate shock was 3±3 months. Hospital readmission was required in 3 (20%) individuals to await transplantation on an urgent basis. However, 2 of these individuals had received appropriate shocks before readmission. In selected patients at high risk for sudden death while on the outpatient cardiac transplant waiting list, the operative risk is low and adequate defibrillation energies can be obtained to allow implantable defibrillator placement. Most individuals will have an appropriate shock as outpatients before transplantation, and sudden death–free survival is excellent. Even in patients eventually requiring readmission to await transplantation on an urgent basis, there is a high likelihood of appropriate device discharge before decompensation.

Treatment

ACE Inhibitors—Trials

To evaluate the effect of ACE inhibitors on mortality and morbidity in patients with symptomatic CHF, Garg and associates[16] for the Collaborative Group on ACE Inhibitor Trials obtained data for all completed, published or unpublished, randomized, placebo-controlled trials of ACE inhibitors that were at least 8 weeks in duration and had determined total mortality by intention to treat, regardless of sample size. Trials were identified based on literature review and correspondence with investigators and pharmaceutical firms. Using standard tables, data were extracted by one author and confirmed where necessary by the other author or the principal investigator of the trial. Unpublished data were obtained by direct correspondence with the principal investigator of each study or pharmaceutical firm. The data for each outcome were combined using the Yusuf-Peto adaptation of the Mantel-Haenszel method. Overall, there was a statistically significant reduction in total mortality (OR, 0.77) and in the combined endpoint of mortality or hospitalization for CHF (OR, 0.65). Similar benefits were observed with several different ACE inhibitors, although the data were largely based on enalapril maleate, captopril, ramipril, quinapril hydrochloride, and lisinopril. Reductions for total mortality and the combined endpoint were similar for various subgroups examined (age, sex, etiology, and New York Heart Association class). However, patients with the lowest ejection fraction appeared to have the greatest benefit. The greater effect was seen during the first 3 months, but additional benefit was observed during further treatment. The reduction in mortality was primarily due to fewer deaths from progressive heart failure (OR, 0.69); point estimates for effects on sudden or presumed arrhythmic deaths (OR, 09.91) and fatal AMI (OR, 0.82) were <1 but were not significant. Total mortality and hospitalization for CHF are significantly reduced by ACE inhibitors with consistent effects in a broad range of patients.

Captopril vs. Digoxin

Heck and associates[17] from Bonn, Germany, studied 116 patients (mean age, 58 years) with mild-to-moderate chronic CHF who were in sinus rhythm and randomly assigned some patients to receive captopril 25 mg twice daily initially (and up to 50 mg twice daily if needed) plus hydrochlorothiazide (group 1) or 0.1 mg of digoxin twice daily plus hydrochlorothiazide (group 2) for 12 months. During a 3- to 4-week pretreatment stabilization period, group 1 received a mean of 37.7 mg of hydrochlorothiazide daily and group 2 received 34.9 mg daily. After 6 weeks and 12 months of treatment, improvement was noted in both treatment groups on 5 measures of cardiac function: exercise tolerance, LV end-diastolic diameter, ejection fraction, BP, and heart rate. At 12 months, significantly greater improvement was noted in group 1 than in group 2 in exercise tolerance (from 329 seconds at baseline to 445 seconds at 12 months in group 1 and from 353 to 427 seconds in group 2); LV end-diastolic diameter (from 60.5 to 56.5 mm in group 1 and from 60.3 to 57.9 mm in group 2); and BP (from 103.5 to 95.6 mm Hg in group 1 and from 101.9 to 97.0 mm Hg in group 2). Clinical severity (New York Heart Association class) improved in both groups; 52% of the patients in group 1 and 41% in group 2 dropped an average of 1 functional class. The results indicate that captopril combined with a diuretic is an effective initial treatment for patients with mild-to-moderate CHF.

Enalapril

Greenberg and colleagues[18] for the SOLVD Investigators evaluated changes in LV structure and function to test the hypothesis that enalapril, an angiotensin-converting enzyme inhibitor, attenuates remodeling in patients with LV dysfunction. Patients entering both the prevention and treatment arms of SOLVD from 5 of the 23 clinical centers were recruited for this substudy. The 301 patients who participated underwent Doppler-echocardiographic evaluation according to standard protocol before randomization to either enalapril or placebo and again after 4 and 12 months of therapy. Recorded data were analyzed in a blinded fashion at a central core laboratory. Analysis of baseline clinical characteristics showed that patients enrolled in the substudy were generally representative of the SOLVD population, although prevention arm patients were slightly overrepresented in the substudy group. The enalapril group demonstrated significant reductions in the mitral annular E-to-A–wave velocity ratio, and this response was different from that seen in the placebo group. Changes in the E-to-A ratio in the enalapril group correlated significantly with changes in plasma atrial natriuretic peptide. LV end-diastolic and end-systolic volumes increased in placebo but not enalapril-treated patients, and the differences in response between the treatment groups were significant. LV mass increased in placebo patients and tended to be reduced in enalapril-treated patients and the difference in response between the groups was highly significant. Thus, these data demonstrate that enalapril attenuates progressive increases in LV dilatation and hypertrophy in patients with LV dysfunction and alters the remodeling phenomenon in a favorable way.

Losartin

Crozier and colleagues[19] in Christchurch, New Zealand, assessed the short- and long-term effects of multiple doses of the angiotensin II–receptor antagonist losartan in patients in CHF. A multicenter, placebo-controlled, oral, multidose (2.5, 10, 25, and 50 mg losartan once daily) double-blind comparison in patients with symptomatic CHF and impaired LVEF (LVEF <40%) was performed. Invasive 24-hour hemodynamic measurements were made after the first dose and after 12 weeks of therapy. Clinical status and tolerability of treatment with losartan over the 12-week period were evaluated. One hundred fifty-four patients were enrolled, among which 134 met the protocol criterion of baseline pulmonary capillary wedge pressure ≥13 mm Hg. The short-term administration, systemic vascular resistance and blood pressure fell significantly with 50 mg and lesser decreases were seen with 25 mg. There were no discernible effects with 2.5 and 10 mg. After 12 weeks of therapy, similar effects were seen on systemic vascular resistance and BP. Pulmonary capillary wedge pressure fell with 2.5, 25, and 50 mg with the largest reduction against placebo at 6 hours with 50 mg. Cardiac index rose with 25 and 50 mg, and heart rate was lower with all active treatment groups. Active treatment was well tolerated. No excess coughing was reported. Thus, these data indicate that oral losartan administered to patients with symptomatic CHF results in beneficial hemodynamic effects with short-term administration, with additional beneficial hemodynamic effects found after 12 weeks of therapy. Definite beneficial hemodynamic effects were seen with both 25 and 50 mg with the greatest effect noted with 50 mg.

Losartin vs. Enalapril

Dickstein and colleagues[20] studied the feasibility of an efficacy trial comparing ACE inhibition and angiotensin II–receptor antagonism in CHF; 166 patients with stable CHF in New York Heart Association functional class III or IV and with an ejection fraction <35% were included in a multicenter, double-blind, parallel, enalapril-controlled trial. After a 3-week stabilization period with optimal therapy, including digitalis, diuretics, and a converting enzyme inhibitor, patients were randomly assigned to 8 weeks of therapy with losartan, 25 mg/d (n=52); losartan, 50 mg/d (n=56); or enalapril, 20 mg/d (n=58). Results showed no significant differences between groups in terms of changes in exercise capacity, clinical status, neurohumoral activation, or incidence of adverse experiences. These authors concluded that losartan and enalapril are of comparable efficacy and tolerability in the short-term treatment of moderate or severe CHF. Thus, a trial designed to compare the efficacy, tolerability and effect on mortality of long-term angiotensin II–receptor blockade with converting enzyme inhibition is both feasible and ethically responsible.

Fosinopril

Brown and coinvestigators[21] in East Meadow, New York, entered a total of 241 men and women with mild to moderately severe CHF (New York Heart Association functional class II [90%] or III) and a mean LVEF of 25% in a 24-week, prospective, double-blind, placebo-controlled trial of 10 or 20 mg/d of fosinopril, a phosphinic acid ACE inhibitor. Patients received concomitant diuretic therapy but not digitalis. Primary end points were mean change in maximal treadmill exercise time and occurrence of prospectively defined clinical events indicative or worsening CHF (most to least severe): death, withdrawal for worsening heart failure, hospitalization for worsening heart failure, need for supplemental diuretic or emergency room visit for worsening heart failure, and no event. At study end point, treadmill exercise time had improved in the fosinopril versus the placebo group (+28 vs. –14 seconds). The New York Heart Association functional class had improved at end point more frequently (24% vs. 13%) and deteriorated less frequently (18% vs. 32%) in the fosinopril group. More patients treated with fosinopril (66% vs. 50%) remained free of clinical events indicative of worsening CHF, and fosinopril-treated patients had less severe clinical events. Dyspnea, fatigue, and paroxysmal nocturnal dyspnea improved more often and worsened less often in this group and edema showed a trend toward improvement. These clinical benefits did not require concomitant digitalis therapy. Fosinopril was associated with an acceptable safety profile.

Digoxin + Diuretic + ACE Inhibitor

Gheorghiade and colleagues[22] in Chicago, Illinois, studied 22 patients with CHF who were receiving constant daily doses of digoxin, diuretics, and ACE inhibitors. In 18 patients, the oral daily dose of digoxin was increased from a mean of 0.20 to 0.39 mg/d corresponding to an increase in the serum digoxin concentration from 0.7 to 1.2 ng/mL. Radionuclide and echocardiographic LVEF; maximal treadmill time; CHF score; serum concentrations of norepinephrine, aldosterone, atrial natriuretic factor, and antidiuretic hormone; and plasma renin activity were obtained before and after the increase in digoxin dose. Subsequently, 9 patients were randomly assigned to receive digoxin and 9 to receive placebo and radionuclide LVEF measurements were obtained 12 weeks later. With the higher dose of digoxin compared with the lower dose, there was a significant increase in LVEF from 24% to 27% (Figure 9-1). No significant changes were found in CHF score, exercise tolerance, serum concentrations of norepinephrine, atrial natriuretic factor, and antidiuretic hormone, and plasma renin activity. There was, however, an increase in serum aldosterone concentration. Twelve weeks after the patients were randomized to receive digoxin or placebo, there was a significant decrease in LVEF from 29% to 24% in the placebo group, but not in patients who continued to receive digoxin. The increase in maintenance digoxin dose, while preserving serum concentrations

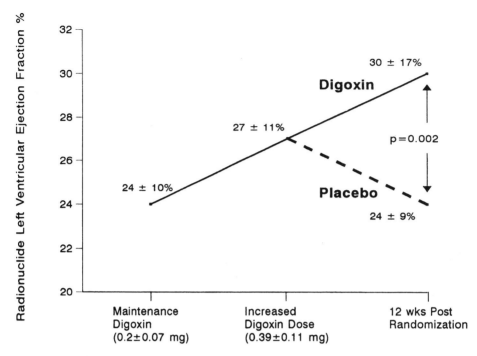

Figure 9-1. Plot of radionuclide LV ejection fraction in 18 patients in whom maintenance digoxin dose was increased and in patients randomly assigned to digoxin (9 patients) or placebo (9 patients). Reproduced with permission from Gheorghiade et al.[22]

within a therapeutic level, resulted in a significant increase in LVEF that was not associated with significant changes in heart failure score, exercise tolerance, and neurohumoral profile.

Ibopamine + Digoxin

There is increasing evidence that clinical deterioration in manifest CHF is related to both hemodynamic and neurohumoral factors. Only few data are available, however, on the progression of disease in its early stages, when treatment has not yet been initiated. Van Veldhuisen and colleagues[23] in Groningen, the Netherlands, designed a study to examine the changes in clinical and neurohumoral variables that occur over 6 months in patients with clinically stable and untreated CHF, and to evaluate the influence of drugs that may affect these variables. Accordingly, the investigators studied 64 patients with CHF who were in New York Heart Association functional class II (88%) and III (12%). They were randomly assigned to double-blind treatment with the oral dopamine agonist ibopamine (100 mg 3 times daily), digoxin (0.25 mg once daily) or placebo. Their mean age was 60 years, and mean LV EF was 0.33. Of the 64 patients, 56 (88%) completed the 6-month study period. Exercise time decreased in patients treated with placebo after 6 months (median −62 seconds), but it increased with ibopamine (+48 seconds) and digoxin (+17 seconds). Plasma norepinephrine increased in the placebo group after 6 months, but decreased in patients receiving active drug treatment, either ibopamine or digoxin. Plasma renin and aldosterone levels were unchanged after 6 months in the placebo group, but digoxin therapy slightly reduced plasma renin concentration. In conclusion, even in stable, untreated CHF, a small but significant progression of disease occurs during 6 months, as reflected by both clinical and neurohumoral changes. Both ibopamine and digoxin monotherapy may favorably affect these changes, and may thus be of value in this patient group.

Carvedilol

Carvedilol is a mildly β-selective β-adrenergic blocking agent with vasodilator properties. This combination of effects might be especially beneficial in patients with CHF. Olsen and colleagues[24] from Salt Lake City, Utah, evaluated 60 patients with CHF and LVEF <0.35. All patients tolerated a challenge with carvedilol (3.125 mg twice a day) and were randomized to receive either carvedilol or placebo. Study medication was titrated over 1 month from 6.25 mg to 25 mg or 50 mg twice a day. Carvedilol therapy resulted in a significant reduction in heart rate, mean PA and pulmonary capillary wedge pressure and a significant increase in supraventricular and LV stroke work. LVEF increased from .21 to .32 in the carvedilol group. Carvedilol-treated patients also reported a significant lessening of CHF symptoms. These authors concluded that long-term carvedilol therapy improved rest cardiac function and lessened symptoms in patients with CHF.

The Australia-New Zealand Heart Failure Research Collaborative Group[25] investigated the effects of carvedilol, a β-blocker with α_1-adrenergic blocking properties, on LV size and function, maximal and submaximal exercise performance, and symptoms in 415 patients with stable CHF associated with CAD and with LVEF <45%. After a 2–3 week run-in phase on open-label low-dose carvedilol, patients were randomly assigned to continue treatment with carvedilol up to 25 mg twice a day or to matching placebo. After 6 months, LVEF measured by radionuclide ventriculography had increased by 5% in the carvedilol group compared with the placebo group and LV end-systolic and end-diastolic dimensions measured by 2-dimensional M-mode echocardiography had decreased by 2.6 mm and 1.3 mm, respectively. There were no significant changes in either treadmill exercise duration or a 6-minute walk distance between the carvedilol and placebo groups. However, in the carvedilol group, exercise performance was maintained with a 23% lower rate-pressure product. Symptoms assessed by New York Heart Association scale and the Specific Activity Scale were unchanged in two thirds of patients in both groups, but there was a small excess of patients whose symptoms worsened and a deficit of patients whose symptoms improved among those assigned to carvedilol. Thus, in patients with CHF of CAD etiology, 6-month treatment with carvedilol improved LV function and maintained exercise performance at a lower heart rate–BP product, but symptoms assessed by functional class were slightly worsened. The authors recommend a large-scale trial to evaluate the efficacy of carvedilol in reducing morbidity and mortality in patients with CHF.

Krum and colleagues[26] in New York City, New York, enrolled 56 patients with severe CHF into a double-blind, placebo-controlled study of the vasodilating β-blocker, carvedilol. All patients had advanced CHF as evidenced by a mean LVEF of 0.16 and a mean maximal oxygen consumption of 14 mL/kg per minute despite digitalis, and an angiotensin-converting enzyme inhibitor if tolerated.

After a 3-week, open-label, up-titration period, 49 of the 56 patients were assigned to receive either carvedilol 25 mg twice a day (n=33) or matching placebo (n=16) for 14 weeks while background therapy remained constant. Hemodynamic and functional variables were measured at the start and end of the study. Compared with the placebo group, patients in the carvedilol group showed improved cardiac performance as reflected by an increase in LVEF and stroke volume index and a decrease in pulmonary capillary wedge pressure, mean RA pressure, and systemic vascular resistance, respectively. When compared with placebo, patients treated with carvedilol benefited clinically as shown by an improvement in symptom scores, functional class, and submaximal exercise tolerance. The combined risk of death, worsening CHF, and life-threatening ventricular arrhythmias was lower in the carvedilol than placebo group, but carvedilol-treated patients had more dizziness and advanced heart block. These data indicate that carvedilol produces clinical and hemodynamic improvement in patients who have severe CHF despite treatment with ACE inhibitors.

Metoprolol

Previous studies have shown that beta-adrenergic blocking agents when administered long-term improve ventricular function in patients with CHF. Hall et al[27] from Dallas, Texas, evaluated the time course of this improvement on ventricular mass and geometry. Twenty-six men with dilated cardiomyopathy underwent serial echocardiography up to an average of 18 months on metoprolol therapy. Patients treated with metoprolol had an initial decline in ventricular function on day 1. Ventricular function improved between months 1 and 3 and LV mass regressed at 18 months. These authors concluded that patients with CHF treated with metoprolol do not demonstrate any improvement in systolic performance until after 1 month of therapy and may have a mild reduction in function initially. Long-term therapy with metoprolol resulted in a reversal of maladaptive remodeling with reduction in LV volumes, regression of LV mass, and improved ventricular geometry by 18 months.

Candoxatrilat

Candoxatrilat, a neutral endopeptidase inhibitor, reduces degradation of atrial natriuretic peptide and provokes diuresis in patients with mild CHF. Good and colleagues[28] from London and Sandwich, United Kingdom, evaluated its renal effects in patients with moderately severe CHF in a placebo-controlled trial. In a double-blind crossover trial, the effects of intravenous boluses of saline vehicle (placebo) and 50, 100 and 200 mg candoxatrilat were compared on separate days in 12 patients with CHF. All doses of candoxatrilat increased urinary volume (263 to 490 mL saline solution and 200 mg dose, respectively). Plasma atrial natriuretic peptide increased (140 to 279 pg/mL) whereas aldosterone decreased (178 to 125 pg/mL) and renin activity was unchanged. These authors concluded that candoxatrilat given acutely causes diuresis, even in patients with moderately severe CHF.

Nitrate + Hydralazine

Early development of nitrate tolerance leads to significant attenuation of nitrate-mediated hemodynamic and anti-ischemic effects. In recent animal experiments, prevention of nitrate-induced hemodynamic tolerance was demonstrated with the concomitant use of hydralazine. To evaluate this finding in patients, Gogia and colleagues[29] from Los Angeles, California, evaluated 28 patients with CHF who were randomly assigned to receive either a continuous infusion of nitroglycerin alone or concomitantly with oral hydralazine 75 mg 4 times a day. In the group receiving nitroglycerin alone, there was a significant attentuation of the hemodynamic effects at 24 hours. Conversely, in the group that received oral hydralazine in addition, there was a persistent effect on mean pulmonary artery and wedge pressures throughout the study period. These authors concluded that in patients with CHF due to LV systolic dysfunction, the concomitant use of oral hydralazine prevents the early development of nitrate tolerance. This data may help explain the benefit effects of the combination of nitrates and hydralazine in the V-Heft I study.

Amiodarone

Asymptomatic ventricular arrhythmias in patients with CHF are associated with increased rates of overall mortality and sudden death. Amiodarone is now used widely to prevent VT and VF. Singh and associates[30] for the Survival Trial of Antiarrhythmic Therapy in Congestive Heart Failure conducted a trial to determine whether amiodarone can reduce overall mortality in patients with CHF and asymptomatic ventricular arrhythmias. The authors used a double-blind, placebo-controlled protocol in which 674 patients with symptoms of CHF, cardiac enlargement, 10 or more VPCs/hour and LVEF of 40% or less were randomly assigned to receive amiodarone (336 patients) or placebo (338 patients). The primary end point was overall mortality, and the medial follow-up was 45 months. There was no significant difference in overall mortality between the 2 treatment groups. The 2-year actuarial survival rate was 69.4% for the patients in the amiodarone group and 70.8% for those in the placebo group. At 2 years, the rate of sudden death was 15% in the amiodarone group and 19% in the placebo group. There was a trend toward reduction in overall mortality among the patients with nonischemic cardiomyopathy who received amiodarone. Amiodarone was significantly more effective in suppressing ventricular arrhythmias and increased the LVEF by 42% at 2 years. Although amiodarone was effective in suppressing ventricular arrhythmias and improving ventricular function, it did not reduce the incidence of sudden death or prolong survival among patients with CHF, except for a trend toward reduced mortality among those with nonischemic cardiomyopathy.

Thiamine

Thiamine deficiency previously has been found in patients with CHF who had received long-term furosemide therapy. In the present study, Shimon and associates[31] from Tel-Hashomer, Israel, assessed the effect of thiamine depletion on thiamine status, functional capacity and LVEF in patients with moderate to severe CHF who had received furosemide in doses of 80 mg/d or more for at least 3 months. Thirty patients were randomized to 1 week of double-blind impatient therapy with either intravenous thiamine 200 mg/d or placebo (n=15 each). All previous drugs were continued. Following discharge, all 30 patients received oral thiamine 200 mg/d as outpatients for 6 weeks. Thiamine status was determined by the erythrocyte thiamine-pyrophosphate effect. LVEF was determined by echocardiography. Thiamine-pyrophosphate effect, diuresis, and LVEF were unchanged with intravenous placebo. After intravenous thiamine, thiamine-pyrophosphate effect decreased (11.7±6.5% to 5.4±3.2%). LVEF increased (0.28±0.11 to 0.32±0.09), as did diuresis (1731±800 mL/d to 2389±752 mL/d), and sodium excretion (84±52 mEq/d to 116±83 mEq/d). In the 27 patients completing the full 7-week intervention, LVEF rose by 22% (0.27±0.10 to 0.33±0.11). Thiamine repletion can improve left ventricular function and biochemical evidence of thiamine deficiency in some patients with moderate-to-severe CHF who are receiving long-term furosemide therapy.

L-Arginine

Endothelium-dependent vasodilation is impaired in patients with CHF, perhaps by decreased synthesis of nitric oxide from L-arginine. Koifman and colleagues[32] from Tel Aviv, Israel, evaluated the effects of an L-arginine infusion in patients with CHF. Twelve patients with a decreased EF were given 20 grams of L-arginine by intravenous infusion over 1 hour at a constant rate. Stroke volume increased from 68 to 76 and cardiac output from 4.07 to 4.7 without a change in heart rate. Mean arterial BP decreased from 102 to 89. Clearance of NO_2/NO_3 increased significantly during L-arginine administration. These authors concluded that infusion of L-arginine in patients with CHF resulted in increased production of nitric oxide, peripheral vasodilation, and increased cardiac output. This suggests the possibility of a therapeutic role L-arginine in patients with CHF.

Respiratory Muscle Training

Mancini and colleagues[33] in Philadelphia, Pennsylvania, studied 14 patients with chronic CHF and man LVEFs of 22% and determined whether selective respiratory muscle training reduces dyspnea and improves exercise performance. The exercise regimen used consisted of three weekly sessions of isocapnic hyperpnea at maximal sustainable ventilatory capacity, resistive breathing, and strength training. Maximum sustainable ventilatory capacity, maximum voluntary ventilation, maximal inspiratory and expiratory pressures, peak oxygen consumption, and the 6 minute walk test were measured before and 3 months after training. Eight patients completed the training program. Respiratory muscle endurance was improved with training, as evidenced by increases in maximal sustainable ventilatory capacity and in maximal voluntary ventilation. Respiratory muscle strength was also increased with training as maximal respiratory and expiratory pressures rose. Submaximal and maximal exercise capacity were significantly improved with selective respiratory muscle training as evidenced by significant increases in the 6-minute walk and peak exercise achieved. Dyspnea during activities of daily living seemed improved in the patients in the exercise regimen. Dyspnea quantified objectively was significantly reduced during progressive isocapnic hyperpnea but not during bicycle exercise. No significant improvement was found in the 6 patients who did not complete the training program. Thus, selective respiratory muscle training improves respiratory muscle endurance and strength with an enhancement of submaximal and maximal exercise capacity in patients with chronic CHF.

Dual-Chamber Pacing

Recently, dual-chamber pacing was proposed as a therapeutic alternative for relief of symptoms in patients with dilated cardiomyopathy and severe CHF unresponsive to optimal medical therapy. Nishimura and associates[34] from Rochester, Minnesota, evaluated dual-chamber pacing in 15 patients with severe LV systolic dysfunction. AV sequential pacing was conducted at AV intervals of 60, 100, 120, 140, 180, and 240 msec. Neither cardiac output nor mean LA pressure was significantly different comparing the baseline state with AV sequential pacing at the various intervals. In 8 patients with PR intervals >200 msec on the rest 12-lead electrocardiogram, however, cardiac output was significantly increased when AV sequential pacing at the optimal AV interval was compared to the baseline (3.0 vs. 3.9 L/min). In addition, LV end-diastolic pressure and duration of diastolic filling were increased, and diastolic MR was abolished. No such improvement was seen in the 7 patients who had normal A-V conduction at rest. These authors concluded that dual-chamber pacing may improve acute hemodynamic variables in selected patients with dilated cardiomyopathy who have resting PR intervals >200 msec on the rest 12-lead electrocardiogram by optimizing the timing of mechanical atrial and ventricular synchrony.

Some recent data has suggested that a short atrioventricular delay in patients with CHF may improve hemodynamics. Gold and colleagues[35] from Baltimore, Maryland, evaluated dual-chamber pacing in a double-blind, randomized, crossover trial in 12 subjects with chronic heart failure despite optimal medical therapy. Patients were in sinus rhythm with no bradyarrhythmias. On the day after implantation, AV delays were varied between 100 and 200 msec. Patients were then randomized to either dual-chamber pacing with a 100 msec AV delay or backup mode. After 4 to 6 weeks, crossover to the other pacing mode was programmed. Hemodynamic measurements on the day after implantation showed no benefit with any AV delay compared with intrinsic conduction. Over the 6-week period, no patient had an increase in ejection fraction nor did any patient improve in New York Heart Association functional class. Also, there were no significant reductions in body weight or diuretic requirements during the pacing. These authors concluded that dual-chamber pacing with a short AV delay does not improve hemodynamics, clinical status, or ejection fraction either acutely or in a follow-up period at 4 to 6 weeks in patients with CHF.

Left Ventricular Assist Device

Levin and colleagues[36] in New York, New York, determined whether ventricular dilation occurring in patients with end-stage heart failure might be reversed with sufficient hemodynamic unloading, such as that provided by an LV assist device. The LV end diastolic pressure-volume relation in hearts from 7 patients with end-stage idiopathic cardiomyopathy and comparable baseline hemodynamics were measured ex vivo at the time of heart transplantation, and compared with the end-diastolic pressure-volume relation in three normal hearts that were technically unsuitable for transplantation. Four of the patients received optimal medical therapy; 3 of the patients who deteriorated on optimal therapy had LV assist devices inserted, and they were supported for approximately 4 months. Compared with the normal hearts, the end-diastolic pressure-volume relations of hearts from medically treated patients were shifted toward markedly larger volumes, but the end-diastolic pressure-volume relations of hearts from patients supported with an LV assist device were similar to those of the normal hearts. These data demonstrate that chronic hemodynamic unloading of sufficient magnitude and duration may result in reversal of chamber enlargement and normalization of cardiac structure as evaluated by the LV end-diastolic pressure-volume relation.

1. Alexander M, Grumbach K, Selby J, Brown AF, Washington E: Hospitalization for congestive heart failure. JAMA 1995 (October 4);274:1037–1042.
2. Rich MW, Beckham V, Wittenberg C, Leven CL, Freedland KE, Carney RM: A multidisciplinary intervention to prevent the readmission of elderly patients with congestive heart failure. N Engl J Med 1995 (November 2);333:1190–1195.
3. Kornowski R, Zeeli D, Averbuch M, Finkelstein A, Schwartz D, Moshkovitz M, Weinreb B, Hershkovitz R, Eyal D, Miller M, Levo Y, Pines A: Intensive home-care surveillance prevents hospitalization and improves morbidity rates among elderly patients with severe congestive heart failure. Am Heart J 1995 (April);129:762–766.
4. Stevenson WG, Stevenson LW, Middlekauff HR, Fonarow GC, Hamilton MA, Woo MA, Saxon LA, Natterson PD, Steimle A, Walden JA, Tillisch JH: Improving survival for patients with advanced heart failure: A study of 737 consecutive patients. J Am Coll Cardiol 1995 (November 15);26:1417–1423.
5. Blackshear JL, Kaplan J, Thompson RC, Safford RE, Atkinson EJ: Nocturnal dyspnea and atrial fibrillation predict Cheyne-Stokes respirations in patients with congestive heart failure. Arch Intern Med 1995 (June 26);155:1297–1302.
6. Javaheri S, Parker TJ, Wexler L, Michaels SE, Stanberry E, Nishyama H, Rosell GA: Occult sleep-disordered breathing in stable congestive heart failure. Ann Intern Med 1995 (April 1);122:487–492.
7. DiSalvo TG, Mathier M, Semigran MJ, Dec GW: Preserved right ventricular ejection fraction predicts exercise capacity and survival in advanced heart failure. J Am Coll Cardiol 1995 (April);25:1143–1153.
8. Matsui S, Tamura N, Hirakawa T, Kobayashi S, Takekoshi N, Murakami E: Assessment of working skeletal muscle oxygenation in patients with chronic heart failure. Am Heart J 1995 (April);129:690–695.
9. Wilson JR, Rayos G, Yeoh TK, Gothard P, Bak K: Dissociation between exertional symptoms and circulatory function in patients with heart failure. Circulation 1995 (July);92:47–53.
10. Kirlin PC, Benedict C, Shelton BJ, Francis G, Nicklas J, Liang CS, Kubo S, Johnstone D, Probstfield J, Yusuf S, for the SOLVD Investigators: Neurohumoral variability in left ventricular dysfunction. Am J Cardiol 1995 (February 15);75:354–359.
11. Silverman ME, Pressel MD, Brackett JC, Lauria SS, Gold MR, Gottlieb SS: Prognostic value of the signal-averaged electrocardiogram and a prolonged QRS in ischemic and nonischemic cardiomyopathy. Am J Cardiol 1995 (March 1);75:460–464.
12. Kiowski W, Sutsch G, Hunziker P, Muller P, Kim J, Oechslin E, Schmitt R, Jones R, Bertel O: Evidence for endothelin-1-mediated vasoconstriction in severe chronic heart failure. Lancet 1995;346:732–736.
13. Ramsey MW, Goodfellow J, Jones CJH, Luddington LA, Lewis MJ, Henderson AH: Endothelial control of arterial distensibility is impaired in chronic heart failure. Circulation 1995 (December);92:3212–3219.
14. Ferrari R, Bachetti T, Confortini R, Opasich C, Febo O, Corti A, Cassani G, Visioli O: Tumor necrosis factor soluble receptors in patients with various degrees of congestive heart failure. Circulation 1995 (September);92:1479–1486.
15. Saxon LA, Wiener I, DeLurgio DB, Natterson PD, Laks H, Drinkwater DC, Stevenson WG: Implantable defibrillators for high-risk patients with heart failure who are awaiting cardiac transplantation. Am Heart J 1995 (September);130:501–506.
16. Garg R, Yusuf S, Collaborative Group on ACE Inhibitor Trials: Overview of randomized trials of angiotensin-converting enzyme inhibitors on mortality and morbidity in patients with heart failure. JAMA 1995 (May 10);273:18:1450–1456.

17. Heck I, Luderitz B, Muller HM, Esser H: A comparison of captoril and digoxin in the treatment of patients with mild-to-moderate chronic congestive heart failure. Clin Ther 1995;17:2:270–279.

18. Greenberg B, Quinones MA, Koilpillai C, Limacher M, Shindler D, Benedict C, Shelton B, for the SOLVD Investigators: Effects of long-term enalapril therapy on cardiac structure and function in patients with left ventricular dysfunction. Results of the SOLVD echocardiography substudy. Circulation 1995 (May);91:2573–2581.

19. Crozier I, Ikram H, Awan N, Cleland J, Stephen N, Dickstein K, Frey M, Young J, Klinger G, Makris L, Rucinska E, for the Losartan Hemodynamic Study Group: Losartan in heart failure: Hemodynamic effects and tolerability. Circulation 1995 (February);91:691–697.

20. Dickstein K, Chang P, Willenheimer R, Haunso S, Remes J, Hall C, Kjekshus J: Comparison of the effects of losartan and enalapril on clinical status and exercise performance in patients with moderate or severe chronic heart failure. J Am Coll Cardiol 1995 (August);26:438–445.

21. Brown EJ Jr, Chew PH, MacLean A, Gelperin K, Ilgenfritz JP, Blumenthal M, for the Fosinopril Heart Failure Study Group: Effects of fosinopril on exercise tolerance and clinical deterioration in patients with chronic congestive heart failure not taking digitalis. Am J Cardiol 1995 (March 15);75:596–600.

22. Gheorghiade M, Hall VB, Jacobsen G, Alam M, Rosman H, Goldstein S: Effects of increasing maintenance dose of digoxin on left ventricular function and neurohormones in patients with chronic heart failure treated with diuretics and angiotensin-converting enzyme inhibitors. Circulation 1995 (October);92:1801–1807.

23. van Veldhuisen DJ, Brouwer J, Man in 't Veld AJ, Dunselman PHJM, Boomsma F, Lie KI, for the DIMT Study Group: Progression of mild untreated heart failure during six months follow-up and clinical and neurohumoral effects of ibopamine and digoxin as monotherapy. Am J Cardiol (April 15);75:796–800.

24. Olsen SL, Gilbert EM, Renlund DG, Taylor DO, Yanowitz FD, Bristow MR: Carvedilol improves left ventricular function and symptoms in chronic heart failure: A double-blind randomized study. J Am Coll Cardiol 1995 (May);25:1225–1231.

25. Australia-New Zealand Heart Failure Research Collaborative Group: Effects of carvedilol, a vasodilator β-blocker, in patients with congestive heart failure due to ischemic heart disease. Circulation 1995 (July);92:212–218.

26. Krum H, Sackner-Bernstein JD, Goldsmith RL, Kukin ML, Schwartz B, Penn J, Medina N, Yushak M, Horn E, Katz SD, Levin HR, Neuberg GW, DeLong G, Packer M: Double-blind, placebo-controlled study of the long-term efficacy of carvedilol in patients with severe chronic heart failure. Circulation 1995 (September);92:1499–1506.

27. Hall SA, Cigarroa CG, Marcoux L, Risser RC, Grayburn PA, Eichhorn EJ: Time course of improvement in left ventricular function, mass and geometry in patients with congestive heart failure treated with beta-adrenergic blockade. J Am Coll Cardiol 1995 (April);25:1154–1161.

28. Good JM, Peters M, Wilkins M, Jackson N, Oakley CM, Cleland JGF: Renal response to candoxatrilat in patients with heart failure. J Am Coll Cardiol 1995 (May);25:1273–1281.

29. Gogia H, Mehra A, Parikh S, Raman M, Ajit-Uppal J, Johnson JV, Elkayam U: Prevention of tolerance to hemodynamic effects of nitrates with concomitant use of hydralazine in patients with chronic heart failure. J Am Coll Cardiol 1995 (November 15);26:1575–1580.

30. Singh SN, Fletcher RD, Fisher SG, Singh BN, Lewis HD, Deedwania PC, Massie BM, Colling C, Lazzeri D, Survival Trial of Antiarrhythmic Therapy in Congestive Heart Failure Group: Amiodarone in patients with congestive heart failure and asymptomatic ventricular arrhythmia. N Engl J Med 1995 (July 13);333:77–82.

31. Shimon I, Almog S, Vered Z, Seligmann H, Shefi M, Peleg E, Rosenthal T, Motro M, Halkin H, Ezra D: Improved left ventricular function after thiamine supplementation in patients with congestive heart failure receiving long-term furosemide therapy. Am J Med 1995 (May);98:485–490.

32. Koifman B, Wollman Y, Bogomolny N, Chernichowsky T, Finkelstein A, Peer G, Scherez J, Blum M, Laniado S, Iaina A, Keren G: Improvement of cardiac performance

by intravenous infusion of L-arginine in patients with moderate congestive heart failure. J Am Coll Cardiol 1995 (November 1);26:1251–1256.

33. Mancini DM, Henson D, La Manca J, Donchez L, Levine S: Benefit of selective respiratory muscle training on exercise capacity in patients with chronic congestive heart failure. Circulation 1995 (January);91:320–329.

34. Nishimura RA, Hayes DL, Holmes DR, Tajik AJ: Mechanism of hemodynamic improvement by dual-chamber pacing for severe left ventricular dysfunction: An acute Doppler and catheterization hemodynamic study. J Am Coll Cardiol 1995 (February);25:281–288.

35. Gold MR, Feliciano Z, Gottlieb SS, Fisher ML: Dual-chamber pacing with a short atrioventricular delay in congestive heart failure: A randomized study. J Am Coll Cardiol 1995 (October);26:967–973.

36. Levin HR, Oz MC, Chen JM, Packer M, Rose EA, Burkhoff D: Reversal of chronic ventricular dilation in patients with end-stage cardiomyopathy by prolonged mechanical unloading. Circulation 1995 (June);91:2717–2720.

10
Miscellaneous Topics

Cardiac and/or Pulmonary Transplantation

Swenson and associates[1] from Pittsburgh, Pennsylvania, studied rejection, allograft function and side effects in 7 patients switched from cyclosporine-based triple-drug immunosuppression to FK 506. Patients were deemed corticosteroid dependent prior to being switched and the switch was performed using an established protocol. Follow-up has ranged from 15 to 41 months, and serial right heart catheterization and endomyocardial biopsies were performed after each reduction of corticosteriod dosing. Catheterization showed no significant change in pulmonary wedge pressure, RA pressure, or cardiac index. Serial echocardiographic variables of allograft function were also stable. At present, all 7 patients are free of the corticosteriod portion of their immune suppression and there have been only 2 episodes of significant acute rejection requiring treatment with intravenous corticosteroids. Antihypertensive medications have been discontinued in 5 of 6 patients previously treated with these drugs. Plasma cholesterol, LDL and triglyceride levels were decreased, and renal function was stable. These preliminary studies suggest that FK 506 may be an alternative immunosuppressive agent for pediatric and adolescent patients experiencing ongoing rejection or significant morbidity from cyclosporine and corticosteroids.

Fullerton and associates[2] from Denver, Colorado, studied 30 patients (age, 8 months to 24 years) with end-stage heart failure who underwent cardiac transplantation: 12 for postoperative end-stage heart failure, 9 as primary treatment for congenital heart disease, 5 for dilated cardiomyopathy, and 4 for restrictive/HC. Prior operations were performed in 19 patients (63%), and 4 patients received transplants for failed Fontan procedures. Operative mortality was 1 of 30 (3%) and post-transplantation follow-up ranged from 3 to 78 months. No patients have been diagnosed with either accelerated atherosclerosis or posttransplant lympho-proliferative disease.

Hsu and associates[3] from New York, New York, report 37 children (mean age, 9 years) with congenital heart disease who underwent cardiac transplantation; 86% had undergone 1 or more previous operations. Repair of extracardiac defects at transplantation was necessary in 23 patients and causes of death after transplantation were donor failure in 2, surgical bleeding in 2, pulmonary hemorrhage in 1, infection in 4, rejection in 3, and graft atherosclerosis in 1. There was no difference in 1- and 5-year survival rates (70% vs. 77% and 65% vs 65%, respectively), rejection frequency or length of hospital stay between children with and without congenital heart disease. Cardiopulmonary bypass and donor ischemia time were significantly longer in patients with congenital heart disease. Serious infections were more common in children with than without congenital heart disease. Despite the more complex cardiac surgery required at implantation and longer ischemic time, heart transplantation can be performed in children with complex congenital heart disease with success similar to that in patients with acquired disease.

Wechsler and colleagues[4] in New York, New York, evaluated factors that explain sex differences affecting mortality after cardiac transplantation. A retrospective analysis of adult patients undergoing orthotopic cardiac transplantation was undertaken at the Columbia-Presbyterian Medical Center in 379 patients, including 75 women and 304 men ≥18 years of age who survived for ≥48 hours after the procedure between March 1985 and March 1992. The following were analyzed: incidence of death and treated rejection episodes, donor and recipient cytomegalovirus matches, use of OKT3 induction therapy, and donor and recipient HLA mismatches. Women with a mean age of 49 years and men with a mean age of 47 years were characterized by differences in race and diagnosis. Women were more likely to be nonwhite and have idiopathic cardiomyopathy than were men. A trend toward an increase in first rejection frequency was seen in women compared with men. Actuarial survival was significantly reduced in women after transplantation. At 36 months, female actuarial survival was 64% vs. 76% for men. The majority of patients in this study did not receive prophylaxis against cytomegalovirus. Univariate analysis revealed that only cytomegalovirus-positive donor status and use of OKT3 induction therapy affected survival in women. Multivariate analysis revealed a marked reduction in survival in female recipients of cytomegalovirus-positive donors given OKT3 induction therapy. At 36 months, only 25% of women were still alive compared with 86% of women with neither risk factor. Even without OKT3 induction, there was a markedly reduced survival in women with mismatched cytomegalovirus status, i.e., cytomegalovirus-negative recipients of positive donor. Thus, women are at risk for reduced survival up to 3 years after cardiac transplantation, especially those women receiving hearts from cytomegalovirus-positive donors and after receiving OKT3 induction therapy when they are themselves negative.

Of patients awaiting cardiac transplantation, 10% to 20% die before a donor heart becomes available. Embolization of LV thrombus is a source of morbidity and mortality in this population. To define the incidence and possible risk factors for systemic arterial embolization, Natterson and associates[5] from Los Angeles, California, examined the frequency of arterial embolic events and their relation to clinical, hemodynamic, and echocardiographic variables in 224 consecutive outpatients awaiting cardiac transplantation (LVEF 0.20±0.07 and LV end-diastolic dimension 76±11 mm). Over a follow-up period of 301±371 days, during which 82 (37%) patients received warfarin, arterial embolization occurred in 6 (3%) patients, 1 of whom was receiving and 5 of whom were not receiving warfarin. The risk of embolization was not statistically different in patients with AF, previous embolization, or LV thrombus on transthoracic echocardiogram, regardless of warfarin therapy. Cumulative risk of sudden death was similar for patients with or without echocardiographically documented LV thrombus. Nonfatal bleeding complications associated with warfarin therapy occurred in 2 (2%) patients. Thus in patients who are awaiting cardiac transplantation and who receive anticoagulation therapy for LV thrombus, AF, or previous arterial embolization, the incidence of clinically detectable arterial embolization is low despite severe ventricular dilatation. Embolization is not likely a major cause of sudden death or morbidity in this population.

To identify the preoperative factors that influence hospital survival after cardiac transplantation, Ibrahim and associates[6] from Ottawa, Canada, analyzed their consecutive experience of 183 transplantations in 179 patients over a 10-year period. There were 151 male and 29 female transplant recipients ranging in age from 10 days to 70 years (mean, 48±1 years). Diagnoses included CAD in 110 patients, cardiomyopathy in 55 patients, valvular disease in 6 patients, and congenital heart disease in 9 patients. Seventy-seven had undergone a previous cardiac operation, and 30 patients required preoperative mechanical support. Forty patients received hearts from donors who were 40 years old or older (range, 40–62 years). Ischemic time was >240 minutes in 32 cases, and pulmonary vascular resistance was >3 Wood units in 40 patients (range, 3.1–10.0 Wood units). Cyclosporine induction was used in 52 patients, whereas 128 recipients received polyclonal antibody prophylaxis. There were 25 hospital deaths. Recipient diagnosis, use of mechanical support, donor age, and the immune suppression protocol were related to hospital survival according to univariate analysis. Using multiple logistic regression only the method of immune suppression induction and the use of mechanical assists were significant independent determinants of survival. In conclusion, the authors believe that extended ischemic times and donor age do not adversely affect the early success of transplantation, whereas induction with immune globulin may reduce early mortality. Patients requiring mechanical support before transplantation continue to be a challenge.

The clinical status and quality of life of 40 patients who lived or are still alive more than 10 years after cardiac transplantation at Stanford University were reviewed by DeCampli and associates[7] from Stanford, California. Patient-perceived health status was determined with use of the Nottingham Health Profile and General Well Being examinations. Factors associated with longevity were determined by a Cox proportional hazards model. Twenty-six patients are alive, and 14 have died. The mean age at transplant was 32±12 years, and the current age (or age at death) is 46±13 years. Actuarial freedom from rejection was similar to that of patients surviving less than 10 years (P=0.8), but freedom from all types of infection was less (P=0.005). Immunosuppressive drugs include cyclosporine (11 of 26 patients), azathioprine (24 of 26 patients), and prednisone (26 of 26; mean dose 12.7 mg/d). Catheterization hemodynamic data show well-preserved graft function at a mean follow-up of 12±3 years. Graft coronary artery disease prevalence is 51±8%. Exercise test results are as follows: duration, 9±4 minutes (range, 2–16 minutes); maximum heart rate/expected rate, 77.3±11% (50% to 92%); maximum systolic BP, 171±23 mm Hg (140–208 mm Hg); and metabolic equivalents, 9.2±2.3 units (5.5 to 12.9 units), or about 84% of predicted. Mean score on the General Well Being examination was 75±22 (normal). Nottingham Health Profile scores were nearly normal, except for in the 50- to 64-year-old age group in categories of mobility, pain, sleep quality, and energy level. Causes of death were coronary artery disease in 7 of 14, infection in 4 of 14, lymphoma in 1 of 14, and nonlymphoid cancer in 2 of 14. In the Cox regression, variables most associated with survival were age at transplantation, preoperative duration of illness, postoperative cytomegalovirus infection and EF at 12 months after operation.

Keogh and associates[8] from Darlinghurst, Australia, randomly assigned 43 patients at the time of cardiac transplantation to receive ketoconazole

(200 mg/d) (23 patients) or no ketoconazole (20 patients). The main end points were the dose of cyclosporine required and the incidence of cardiac rejection and infection. Ketoconazole reduced the dose of cyclosporine needed to maintain target levels by 62% at 1 week and by 80% at 1 year. The cost savings per patient (in US dollars, inclusive of the cost of ketoconazole) was about $5200 in the first year and about $3920 in each subsequent year. The mean ($\pm$SD) rate of rejection in the first month was lower in the ketoconazole group than in the control group (4.2$\pm$0.8 vs. 5.7$\pm$1.0 episodes per 100 patient-days), and the average number of days to the first rejection was higher (30$\pm$29 vs. 15$\pm$8). In the first year, 22% of the ketoconazole group required cytolytic therapy compared with 35% of the control group and 9% of the ketoconazole group required total lymphoid irradiation compared with 15% of the control group. The incidence of infection was lower in ketoconazole-treated patients than in the control group in the second month (1.4$\pm$0.5 vs. 2.8$\pm$0.7 episodes per 100 patient-days) and in the third month (0.8$\pm$0.3 vs. 2.3$\pm$0.6 episodes per 100 patient-days). Transient asymptomatic cholestasis was observed in the ketoconazole group. After cardiac transplantation, ketoconazole greatly reduced the need for cyclosporine, resulting in substantial cost savings. Ketoconazole also reduced the rates of rejection and infection, without persistent toxic effects. The authors now use ketoconazole routinely in cardiac-transplant recipients.

Hypercholesterolemia is common after cardiac transplantation and almost certainly contributes to the development of CAD after transplantation. Kobashigawa and associates[9] early after transplantation randomly assigned 47 consecutive patients to receive either pravastatin (47 patients) or no statin drug (50 patients). Twelve months after transplantation, the pravastatin group had lower mean ($\pm$SD) cholesterol levels than the control group (193$\pm$36 vs. 248$\pm$49 mg/dL) (Figure 10-1) less frequent cardiac rejection accompanied by hemodynamic compromise (3 vs. 14 patients), better survival (94% vs. 78%) (Figure 10-2), and a lower incidence of coronary vasculopathy in the transplant as determined by angiography and at autopsy (3 vs. 10 patients). There was no difference between the 2 groups in the incidence of mild or moderate episodes of cardiac rejection. In a subgroup of study patients, intracoronary ultrasound measure-

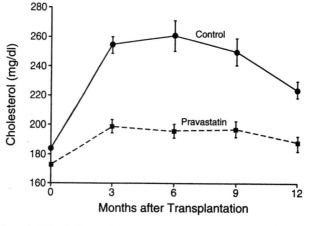

Figure 10-1. Mean ($\pm$SE) cholesterol levels during the first year after cardiac transplantation in the study patients. Reproduced with permission from Kobashigawa et al.[9]

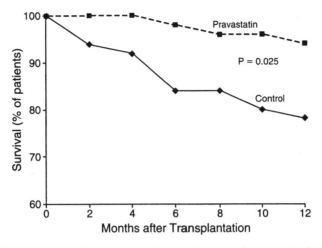

Figure 10-2. Survival during the first year after cardiac transplantation in the study patients. Reproduced with permission from Kobashigawa et al.[9]

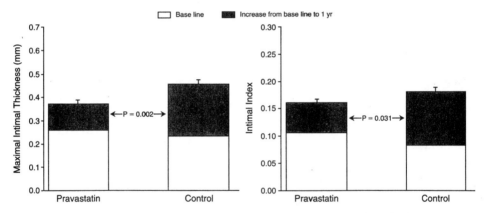

Figure 10-3. Results of intracoronary ultrasonography. As compared with the pravastatin group, the control group had significantly greater increases in maximal intimal thickness (*P*= 0.002) and the intimal index (*P*=0.031) during the first year after cardiac transplantation. Maximal intimal thickness represents the thickness of the most severely atherosclerotic area, and the intimal index the ratio of the area of plaque to the total vessel area. Values obtained at 1 year are expressed as means ±SE. Reproduced with permission from Kobashigawa et al.[9]

ments at baseline and 1 year after transplantation showed less progression in the pravastatin group in maximal intimal thickness (0.11±0.09 mm vs. 0.23±0.16 mm in the control group) and in the intimal index (0.05±0.03 vs. 0.10±0.10) (Figure 10-3). In a subgroup of patients, the cytotoxicity of natural killer cells was lower in the pravastatin group than in the control group (10% vs. 22% specific lysis). After cardiac transplantation pravastatin had beneficial effects on cholesterol levels, the incidence of rejection causing hemodynamic compromise, 1-year survival, and the incidence of coronary vasculopathy.

HLA matching in cardiac transplants is perceived as being logistically difficult. Smith and associates[10] from Middlesex, United Kingdom, studied 1135 consecutive primary cardiac allografts between 1980 and 1994 to assess the effect of HLA mismatching on long-term graft survival and cellular rejection episodes within 3 months of transplantation. The authors found a significant association between HLA-DR mismatching and the number of episodes of rejection (no mismatch, 0.80 [SE 0.13]; 1 mismatch, 1.22 [0.06]; 2 mismatches, 1.42 [0.06]). The authors found a similar correlation between the total number of biopsy specimens showing evidence of cellular rejection and HLA-DR mismatch. The time between operation and the first rejection episode shortened with increasing HLA-DR mismatch (no mismatch, 85.5 [37.3] days; 1 mismatch, 43.1 [8.1]; 2 mismatches, 24.1 [2.9]). Furthermore, the proportion of patients with no evidence of rejection correlated with HLA-DR incompatibility. A significant association between improved graft survival and HLA-DR mismatching was found over 1, 5, and 10 years after transplantation (no mismatch: 1 year, 92%; 5 years, 83%; 10 years, 76%; 1 mismatch: 1 year, 81%; 5 years, 73%; 10 years, 59%; and 10 years, 52%). Increased efforts to prospectively HLA match patients has resulted in 25% of patients transplanted between January and May 1995 (n=13 of 52) receiving grafts matched for HLA-DR. HLA matching reduces the frequency and severity of acute cardiac allograft rejection and improves graft survival for up to 10 years. The preliminary results suggest that it is possible to use HLA matching prospectively for selection of recipients.

Winters and colleagues[11] in Boston, Massachusetts determined whether isolated foci of moderate acute rejection on endomyocardial biopsy requires special treatment. Recipients with endomyocardial biopsies having focal moderate acute rejection defined as 1 or 2 isolated foci of cellular infiltrates with associated myocyte damage do not routinely receive intensified immunosuppression at some centers. To determine the outcome of such individuals, Winters et al. reviewed 4398 endomyocardial biopsies obtained after orthotopic heart transplantation in 208 consecutive recipients maintained on triple immunosuppressive therapy. The incidence of progression vs. resolution of focal myocardial rejection, the time interval after transplantation when focal myocardial rejection was identified, and the relation of untreated focal myocardial rejection to recipient survival were analyzed. Focal myocardial rejection was categorized as one or two foci present in 401 endomyocardial biopsies obtained 10 days to 8 years after transplantation in 149 recipients. Endomyocardial biopsies with focal myocardial rejection resolved without treatment in 341 of 401 and only 60 of 401 progressed to higher grade rejection. Endomyocardial biopsies that progressed occurred 8 months after transplantation compared with 14 months after transplantation for those that resolved. Of the 60 endomyocardial biopsies that progressed, 55% occurred within the first 6 months, 78% within the first year, and 97% within the first 2 years after transplantation. Endomyocardial biopsies with two foci of focal myocardial rejection were no more likely to progress than those with one focus. Thirty-nine recipients experienced 1, 2, 3, or 4 episodes of focal myocardial necrosis that progressed. One or more episodes of focal myocardial necrosis that did not progress occurred in 110 recipients. Survival at 1 and 5 years was similar in patients with and those without focal myocardial necrosis progression. Thus, these data suggest that untreated focal myocardial necrosis consisting of either 1 or 2 foci has a low rate of progression. Progression of focal myocardial necrosis decreases with increasing postoperative interval and becomes rare after 2 years. It did not identify patients with decreased survival.

De Marco and associates[12] from San Francisco, California, studied whether cardiac sympathetic reinnervation occurs late after orthotopic heart transplantation. Iodine-123 MIBG cardiac uptake reflects intact myocardial sympathetic innervation of the heart. Cardiac transplant recipients do not demonstrate MIBG cardiac uptake when studied less than 6 months from transplantation. Serial cardial MIBG imaging was studied in 23 cardiac transplant recipients early (<1 year) and late (>1 year) after the operation. No subject had visible MIBG uptake on imaging <1 year after transplantation. However, 48% developed visible MIBG uptake 1–2 years after transplantation. Only 25% of patients with a pretransplant diagnosis of idiopathic cardiomyopathy demonstrated MIBG uptake compared with 73% of patients with a pretransplant diagnosis of ischemic or valvular heart disease. These authors concluded that sympathetic reinnervation of the transplanted human heart can occur more than 1 year after operation as assessed by iodine-123 MIBG imaging and the transmyocardial release of norepinephrine. Reinnervation is less likely to occur in patients with a pretransplant diagnosis of idiopathic cardiomyopathy than in those with other etiologies of CHF.

Prolonged nonspecific immunosuppression after solid-organ transplantation is associated with an increased risk of certain cancers. Pham and associates[13] from Pittsburgh, Pennsylvania, identified 38 solid tumors after cardiac transplantation in 36 (6%) of 608 cardiac transplant recipients who survived more than 30 days. Two patients had 2 types of skin tumors (basal cell and squamous cell). The tumors included the following types: skin (15), lung (10), breast (1), bladder (2), larynx (2), liver (1), parotid (1), testicle (1), uterus (2), melanoma (2), and Merkel's cell (1). Four immunosuppression regimens based on cyclosporin A or FK 506 were used during this period. There was no association between the incidence of solid tumors and the use of lympholytic therapy. After the diagnosis of tumor was made, the actuarial 2-year survival rates of recipients with skin, lung, and other solid tumors were 71%, 22%, and 23%, respectively. Eight of 10 patients with lung cancer were in stage IIIA or higher at the time of diagnosis. Skin and lung tumors are the most frequent solid tumors in heart transplant recipients. Skin tumors (except Merkel's cell carcinoma and melanoma) usually have a benign course, whereas lung and other tumors developing in cardiac transplant recipients carry a poor prognosis. Advanced disease at the time of diagnosis is responsible for the dismal outcome of recipients in whom solid tumors develop. Close postoperative tumor surveillance after cardiac transplantation is warranted.

Riou and colleagues[14] in Paris, France, prospectively measured circulating cardiac troponin T in 100 brain-dead patients and measured the LVEF using transesophageal echocardiography. Sixty-one patients had normal LVEFs, 25 had moderate decrease in LVEF (30% to 50%), and 14 had severe decrease in LVEFs (≤30%). Circulating cardiac troponin T concentration was significantly higher in patients, with a severe decrease in LVEF compared with the other two groups. There was a significant correlation between LVEF and cardiac troponin T concentrations. An elevated circulating cardiac troponin T concentration was more accurate in predicting a severe decrease in LVEF than an elevated creatine kinase–MB or an increased the ratio of creatine kinase—MB to creatine kinase. Thus, elevated circulating cardiac troponin T was associated with severe decrease in LVEF in brain-dead patients suggesting that severe and potentially irreversible myocardial cell damage had occurred. The creatine kinase–MB determinations were not as useful in this study. Measurement of circulating cardiac troponin T concentration may be useful to heart transplantation teams in selecting ideal hearts for transplantation.

The etiology of TR and MR after heart transplantation is controversial. De Simone and associates[15] from Heidelberg, Germany, studied 25 patients undergoing cardiac transplantation and intraoperative transesophageal echocardiography to evaluate the incidence, degree, and the cause of TR and MR. The degree of valve regurgitation was assessed by color Doppler echocardiography. Cross-sectional areas of the recipient and donor portions of the atria and their ratio were measured to assess the distortion of atrial geometry. Tricuspid and mitral valve annuli, their systolic shortening, and hemodynamic indices were measured preoperatively and perioperatively. TR was found in 21 of 25 patients (84%) and MR in 12 of 25 (48%). The degree of MR was mild, whereas TR was mild to moderate. MR did not show any correlation with the studied indices; TR showed no correlation with the hemodynamic indices but a significant correlation with the recipient-to-donor ratio. An inverse correlation was found between the degree of TR and systolic shortening of tricuspid annulus and between recipient-to-donor ratio and systolic shortening of tricuspid annulus. TR has a higher incidence than MR and occurs immediately after transplantation; MR is mild and correlates with neither hemodynamic indices nor atrial distortion. An increased recipient-to-donor ratio, and hence distortion of RA geometry, may lead to a reduction in systolic annulus shortening which in turn causes TR. Surgical attempts to reduce the recipient-to-donor ratio may decrease the incidence and the degree of TR after heart transplantation.

Burke and colleagues[16] from Minneapolis, Minnesota, determined directly the presence or absence of functional sympathetic reinnervation and measured LV or coronary hemodynamics in 11 patients ≤4 months after heart transplantation, in 45 patients ≥1 year after transplantation, and in 13 untransplanted, normally innervated patients. Sympathetic neurons were stimulated with left coronary injection of tyramine, which causes norepinephrine release from intact sympathetic nerve terminals. Reinnervation was defined as a measure of cardiac norepinephrine release after intracoronary tyramine injection. LV pressure was measured before and at 1-minute intervals after tyramine with a micromanometer-tipped catheter. Coronary blood flow velocity was measured with a 3F Doppler catheter and coronary artery cross-sectional area was calculated using quantitative coronary angiography. In both early patients and patients studied ≥4 months after transplantation without reinnervation, there was no change in LV function in response to tyramine. In transplant patients with reinnervation, LV dP/dt rose significantly, but less than in healthy patients. In both early and late denervated patients, there was no change in coronary blood flow in response to tyramine. In late reinnervated patients, coronary blood flow velocity fell significantly. In healthy patients, coronary blood flow velocity fell even more than in the transplant patients. These data suggest that stimulation of reinnervating sympathetic neurons with tyramine in transplant recipients causes a significant, but subnormal increase in dP/dt and a transient decrease in coronary blood flow velocity demonstrating that reinnervating sympathetic neurons may produce physiologically meaningful changes in LV function and coronary artery tone.

Transplant CAD has emerged as the major cause of morbidity and mortality in long-term heart transplant survivors. In the Stanford series, the prevalence of angiographically detectable transplant CAD at 1, 3, and 5 years after transplantation in cyclosporin treated patients was 14%, 37%, and 50%. Rickenbacher and associates[17] from Stanford, California, evaluated lesion characteristics early and up to 15 years after heart transplantation using intracoronary ultrasound. A total of 304 intracoronary ultrasound studies were performed in 174 heart transplant recipients at baseline and up to 15 years after transplantation. Mean intimal thickness, intimal index, and mean severity class were significantly higher 1 year after transplantation. Calcification of lesions was detected in 2% to 12% of studies up to 5 years after transplantation with a significant increase to 24% at 6–10 years. These authors concluded that the severity of transplant CAD appeared to progress with time after transplantation in this cross-sectional study. This was most prominent during the first 2 years after transplantation whereas calcification of plaques occurred to a significant extent only later in the process.

Deng and colleagues[18] at Stanford, California, hypothesized that alterations of microvascular cell surface makers mirror changes in the epicardial vessels that may be important in the pathophysiology of intimal proliferation in cardiac allograft vascular disease. They used 43 heart transplant patients examined by intracoronary ultrasound more than 1 year after transplantation, and these images were analyzed to obtain mean intimal thickness and intimal thickness class calculated from mean thickness and circumferential involvement. Right ventricular endomyocardial biopsies obtained at the time of intracoronary ultrasound were examined by immunohistochemistry to detect microvascular expression of histocompatibility leukocyte antigen HLA classes I and II. Endothelial-specific antigen detected by monoclonal antibody; intercellular adhesion molecules; CD4 and CD8 lymphocytes and macrophages (CD14+) were also sought. Microvascular antigen expression was graded 1 through 5 on the basis of the diffuseness of positive staining. The number of each inflammatory cell phenotype present per high-power field was counted. Scores for HLA DR, HLA DQ, and E1.5 expression were lower in intimal thickness classes II, III, and IV compared with class I. This inverse relationship was significant by linear regression analysis of mean intimal thickness. Inflammatory cells were not significantly correlated with intimal thickening. Rejection incidence was higher and time since transplantation longer in intimal thickness classes II, III, and IV compared with class I. Thus, transplant coronary artery intimal proliferation is associated with alterations of microvascular endothelial cell surface markers. These changes in cell surface antigen expression could provide the substrate for coronary artery intimal proliferation and narrowing.

Tuzcu and colleagues[19] in Cleveland, Ohio, determined the potential contribution of coronary atherosclerosis in the donor heart to cardiac allograft vasculopathy. They performed quantitative coronary angiography and intravascular ultrasound imaging in 50 of 62 consecutive heart transplant recipients 4.6 ± 2.6 weeks after transplantation. The donor population consisted of 30 men and 20 women (mean age, 32 years). Ultrasound imaging visualized all 3 coronary arteries in 22 patients, 2 coronary arteries in 23, and 1 coronary artery in 5. Ultrasound imaging detected coronary atherosclerosis as evidenced by an intimal thickness ≥0.5 mm in 28 patients (56%) (Figures 10-4 and 10-5). However, the angiography was abnormal in only 13 patients (26%). The sensitivity and specificity of coronary angiography were 43% and 95%, respectively. With

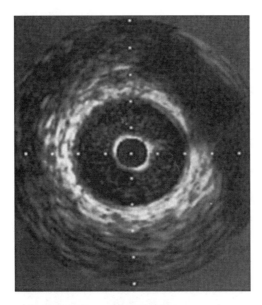

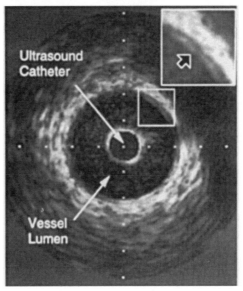

Figure 10-4. Ultrasound image of a normal coronary artery. Inset shows the three layers of the vessel wall (black arrow). The thin echogenic inner layer corresponds to the intima, the thin echolucent middle layer to the media, and the echogenic outer layer to the adventitia. Reproduced with permission from Tuzcu et al.[19]

ultrasound, the average atherosclerotic plaque thickness was 1.3±0.6 mm and the cross-sectional area narrowing was 34±16%. Atherosclerotic involvement frequently was focal (85%), eccentric and near arterial bifurcations. Donors of the transplant recipients with coronary atherosclerosis were older than those without atherosclerosis (37 vs. 25 years on average). Mean intimal thickness correlated with donor age and multivariate analysis demonstrated that donor age, male sex of donor, and recipient age were independent predictors of atherosclerosis. Thus, coronary atherosclerosis is frequently but inadvertently trans-

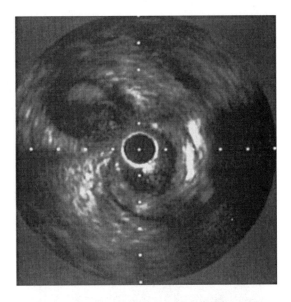

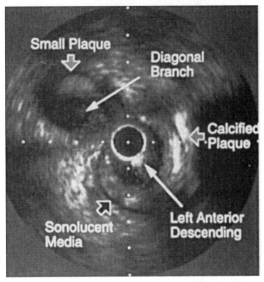

Figure 10-5. Ultrasound image of an eccentric, partially calcified atherosclerotic plaque in the left anterior descending artery at the bifurcation site of the major diagonal branch. A small eccentric plaque is seen in the diagonal branch opposite the flow-dividing wall. Reproduced with permission from Tuzcu et al.[19]

mitted by means of cardiac transplantation from the donor to the recipient. Long-term outcomes of donor-transmitted CAD will need to be studied.

CAD after cardiac transplantation is a major obstacle to long-term survival. McGiffin and associates[20] from Birmingham, Alabama, analyzed the development and progression of CAD after cardiac transplantation in 217 consecutive patients undergoing transplantation. The actuarial freedom from any CAD (by angiography or autopsy) was 81% at 2 years and 20% at 8 years after transplantation. CAD was more prevalent in male than female patients (30% vs. 50% free of CAD at 5 years). By multivariable analysis, pretransplantation risk factors identified for CAD included pretransplantation positive cytomegalovirus sero-logic status of the recipient and older donor age. Progression of CAD was variable in both time of onset and rate. Earlier detection did not result in more rapid progression. Coronary events severe enough for retransplantation (n=8) and/or death from CAD (n=9) occurred in 15 patients, of whom 4 underwent retransplantation. The actuarial freedom from coronary events was 88% at 5 years and 79% at 8 years. By multivariable analysis, only male recipient (*P*= 0.05) was a risk factor for coronary events. Seven of the 15 patients (47%) with coronary events died suddenly of CAD without prior angiographic evidence of severe CAD. CAD is progressive. Improved surveillance methods are required to detect the disease and institute timely intervention to prevent the occurrence of unanticipated death.

Hosenpud and colleagues[21] in Portland, Oregon, determined whether car-diac allograft vasculopathy is a manifestation of chronic allograft rejection as a consequence of humoral or cell-mediated alloreactivity. Human aortic endothelial cells were isolated from donor aortas obtained at the time of organ acquisition for 52 cardiac allograft recipients. Serum and peripheral blood mononuclear cells were obtained from 52 allograft recipients at several time points during the first year after transplantation. Lymphocyte proliferation in response to donor-specific human aortic endothelial cells as determined and alloantibody binding to interferon-γ–treated donor-specific human aortic endo-thelial cells was documented and correlated with clinical variables, including HLA matching, acute cellular rejection, and CAD as determined by arteriogra-phy. Ten of the 52 patients studied had angiographic or autopsy evidence of CAD in the first posttransplantation year. The CAV+ group had higher lymphocyte proliferation responses to their donor human aortic endothelial cells at 1 week, 3 months, and 6 months after transplantation compared with the cardiac allograft vasculopathy negative group. Only 8 of the 52 patients had donor-specific alloantibodies, and there was no relation between antibody presence and car-diac allograft vasculopathy. Other clinical variables that correlated with cardiac allograft vasculopathy included the level of HLA-DR mismatch and the presence of late acute rejection. Thus, cardiac allograft vasculopathy is associated with donor-specific cell-mediated alloreactivity to vascular endothelium. The data obtained in this study do not suggest that humoral immunity plays an important role in cardiac allograft vasculopathy.

Accelerated CAD is the leading cause of death in heart transplant recipients by the first year after transplantation. The prevalence of allograft CAD reaches 40–50% by 5 years after transplantation. Halle and colleagues[22] from Richmond, Virginia, evaluated the outcomes of revascularization procedures in the treat-ment of allograft CAD. In 13 medical centers, 66 patients underwent PTCA of 162 lesions. Sixty-one percent of patients are alive without retransplantation at a mean of 19 months after PTCA. CABG was performed in 12 patients with 4 perioperative mortalities. Seven patients are alive without re-transplantation at an average of 9 months after operation. These authors concluded that CABG may be an effective palliative therapy in suitable cardiac transplant recipients. They further concluded that PTCA has an acceptable survival in patients with-out angiographic distal arteriopathy.

An aggressive and potentially fatal form of CAD may develop after cardiac transplantation. Labarrere and associates[23] from Indianapolis, Indiana, studied the role of vascular t-PA, the primary mediator of fibrinolysis in the development of this problem. The authors studied 78 consecutive recipients of cardiac allografts over a 5-year period and collected follow-up data over a mean of 32 ± 2 months. The patients were studied with ventricular function tests, serial endomyocardial biopsies (16.6 ± 0.5 per patient), and annual coronary angiography. Measurements of t-PA and its inhibitor were performed immunocytochemically on unfixed cryostat sections of endomyocardial-biopsy specimens with the use of monoclonal antibodies to t-PA and its inhibitor. In biopsy specimens obtained during the first 3 months of follow-up, 38 allografts had a normal distribution of t-PA in arteriolar smooth-muscle cells, whereas in 40 allografts there was depletion of t-PA that persisted in subsequent follow-up. CAD developed during follow-up in 31 of 40 allografts (78%) with depletion of t-PA but the disease developed in only 9 of the 38 allografts (24%) with normal t-PA levels. Allografts with depletion of t-PA also had the t-PA inhibitor and were at greater risk for earlier and more severe disease than were allografts with normal arteriolar t-PA levels. Twelve patients whose allografts were depleted of t-PA either received a second transplant or died, whereas only 1 of the patients whose allografts had persistently normal t-PA levels died. These findings reveal an association between the depletion of t-PA from arteriolar smooth-muscle cells and the subsequent development of CAD and decreased graft survival. Although the authors cannot be certain about a cause-and-effect relation, the authors' data suggest a possible role for deficient fibrinolysis in the development of CAD in transplanted human hearts.

Bridges and associates[24] from St. Louis, Mo., reported results of 20 patients (average age, 6 years; range, 3 months to 24 years) who had single or bilateral lung transplantation. All were severely symptomatic and 6 were hospitalized and receiving intensive support before transplantation. Hospital survival was 70% (14 of 20) with 3 additional deaths at 7, 11, and 27 months. A prior thoracic operation contributed to 3 of 6 hospital deaths from hemorrhage. All late deaths were due directly or indirectly to obliterative bronchiolitis. At a mean follow-up of 19 months (range, 2 to 48 months) 10 of 11 survivors without symptoms. Survival after hospital discharge and incidence of obliterative bronchiolitis are similar in a contemporary group of 41 patients of comparable age who underwent lung transplantation for pulmonary disease. Single or bilateral lung transplantation is an acceptable therapy for children with pulmonary hypertension, congenital heart disease, or both. Further data are needed to develop optimal decision-making strategies for patients with end-stage cardiopulmonary disease.

Pericardial Heart Disease

Tamponade

Cardiac tamponade causes elevation and equalization of cardiac filling pressures, sodium and water retention, and a paradoxically low plasma atrial natriuretic factor concentration despite increased intraatrial pressures. Recent reports suggest that plasma atrial natriuretic factor concentrations rise after relief of tamponade. The purposes of the present study by Panayiotou and associates[25] from Mobile, Alabama; Nashville, Tennessee; and Denver, Colorado, were 1) to determine the time course and extent of atrial natriuretic factor release on relief of cardiac tamponade; 2) to measure the atrial transmural wall pressures, atrial sizes, and atrial wall tension changes associated with relief of tamponade; and 3) to determine the biological activity of elevated plasma atrial natriuretic factor during and after relief of tamponade. These investigators sampled blood for atrial natriuretic factor and cyclic guanosine monophosphate immediately before and up to 24 hours after relief of cardiac tamponade in 10 patients. Atrial and pericardial pressures were measured immediately before and shortly after pericardiocentesis, and atrial dimensions were determined by 2-dimensional echocardiography before and within 1 hour after the tap. Urine volumes were measured in 8-hour increments before and after the procedure. Relief of cardiac tamponade was associated with a prompt and massive increase in plasma atrial natriuretic factor concentrations, reaching pharmacologically active levels. The rise in atrial natriuretic factor was negatively correlated with atrial pressures but positively correlated with atrial transmural pressures, atrial size, and calculated wall tension. Plasma atrial natriuretic factor levels peaked at 515 ± 95 pg/mL 40 minutes after relief of tamponade and leveled off at 140% to 180% of the pretap concentrations. Plasma cyclic guanosine monophosphate exhibited a slightly delayed but similar time course to the rise in atrial natriuretic factor levels, and urine flow rate increased fourfold in the 8 hours after relief of tamponade. It was concluded that 1) the relief of cardiac tamponade stimulates the release of atrial natriuretic factor by increasing atrial transmural wall pressures, atrial size, and calculated wall tensions; 2) evidence for the biologic activity of the increased plasma atrial natriuretic factor concentrations is provided by the temporal association of increased cyclic guanosine monophosphate levels and increased urine flow rate; and 3) that the release of atrial natriuretic factor is governed by changes in atrial transmural wall pressures and calculated atrial wall tensions.

Bommer and associates[26] from Sacramento, California, evaluated the sensitivity of current echocardiographic criteria in detecting cardiac tamponade in the patient who has undergone cardiovascular surgery. Because the current echocardiographic criteria for tamponade were initially developed and studied predominantly in patients with medical problems, relatively less information is available in patients who have undergone cardiac surgery. Of 848 consecutive patients who underwent cardiovascular surgery, patients were selected for the study if they had clinical or hemodynamic deterioration and had undergone an echocardiogram just before a successful pericardiocentesis or a surgical evacuation of pericardial blood or clot. The echocardiograms were evaluated for evidence of chamber collapse, cardiac motion, Doppler flow variations, and the location and width of pericardial separation. Fourteen patients were identified who met the inclusion criteria (clinical or hemodynamic deterioration, recent echocardiogram, and successful intervention) for cardiac tamponade. The clinical and hemodynamic findings were hypotension (13 patients), low cardiac output (7), low urine output (3), cardiopulmonary arrest (1), elevated central venous pressure (1), and shortness of breath (1). In these patients current echocardiographic criteria were seen infrequently: chamber collapse in the right atrium (6 of 14 patients) and right ventricle (4 of 14), Doppler flow variation (2 of 5), and swinging heart (0 of 15), whereas increased pericardial separation ($\geq$10 mm) was seen in all (14 of 14) of the patients. Although the sensitivity of current echocardiographic criteria for tamponade was not high

(0% to 43%), the sensitivity of a combined index (unexplained clinical or hemodynamic deterioration and pericardial echo separation width ≥10 mm) was high (100%) in this group of patients who had undergone surgery. In this study standard echocardiographic criteria were found to be relatively unreliable in detecting cardiac tamponade in patients who had undergone cardiac surgery. However, the presence of ≥10 mm of pericardial separation (fluid/clot) and unexplained clinical or hemodynamic deterioration appeared to be sensitive in detecting tamponade.

In AIDS

Heidenreich and colleagues[27] in San Francisco, California, determined the incidence of pericardial effusion and its relation to survival in patients infected with HIV. The incidence of pericardial effusion and its relation to mortality in HIV-positive subjects was evaluated in 601 echocardiograms obtained from 231 subjects recruited over a 5-year period. Among these patients, 59 subjects had asymptomatic HIV, 62 patients had AIDS-related complex, and there were 74 patients with AIDS. Twenty-one HIV-negative healthy gay men and 15 subjects with non-HIV end-stage medical illness were also evaluated. Echocardiograms were performed every 3 to 6 months with an 82% follow-up evaluation. Sixteen subjects were recognized as having pericardial effusions yielding a prevalence for pericardial effusion in AIDS patients entering the study of 5%. Thirteen subjects developed pericardial effusions during follow-up; 12 of these were patients with AIDS. The majority of the pericardial effusions were small and asymptomatic. The survival of patients with AIDS with effusions was significantly shorter than survival for patients with AIDS without effusions. This shortened survival remains significant after adjustment for lead time bias and was independent of CD4 count and serum albumin level. Thus, there is a relatively high incidence of pericardial effusion in patients with AIDS and the presence of an effusion is associated with shortened survival. The development of an effusion in the setting of HIV infection suggests end-stage HIV disease.

Venous Thrombosis and/or Pulmonary Embolism

A large portion of hospitalized patients who are at high risk for venous thromboembolism do not receive prophylaxis. Reluctance to use the venous thromboembolism prophylaxis in surgical patients may be due to fear of perioperative bleeding when anticoagulants are given preoperatively. Kearon and Hirsh[28] from Hamilton, Canada, performed a literature review to determine whether prophylaxis for venous thromboembolism is effective when started postoperatively and the relative efficacy of preoperatively and postoperatively initiated prophylaxis. Randomized, controlled trials establish that pharmacological and nonpharmacological methods of prophylaxis that are effective when started preoperatively are also effective when they are started postoperatively, with relative risks for venous thromboembolism of 0.16 to 0.49. Low rates of venous thromboembolism in noncontrolled randomized trials that included postoperatively initiated prophylactic regimens support this finding. The relative efficacy of preoperatively and postoperatively initiated venous thromboembolism prophylaxis could not be determined definitely, because direct comparisons of the same regimens have not been performed. Indirect comparisons suggest that any loss of efficacy resulting from deferring venous thromboembolism prophylaxis until after surgery is unlikely to be marked. Randomized trials are required to resolve this question. This comparison may be of greatest clinical importance when twice-daily, low molecular-weight heparin is used to prevent venous thromboembolism after major orthopedic surgery.

The optimal duration of oral anticoagulant therapy after a first episode of venous embolism is still a matter of debate. Schulman and associates[29] of the Duration of Anticoagulation Trial study group performed a multicenter trial comparing 6 weeks of oral anticoagulant treatment with 6 months of such therapy in patients who had a first episode of venous thromboembolism. Anticoagulant therapy consisted of warfarin or dicumarol. Of the 902 patients enrolled, 5 were later excluded because they had congenital protein C deficiency; 443 were randomly assigned to receive 6 weeks of oral anticoagulant therapy with a targeted INR of 2.0 to 2.85, and 454 were randomly assigned to receive 6 months of such therapy. The initial diagnoses were confirmed by means of venography in cases of deep-vein thromboses (n=790) and with perfusion-ventilation scanning or angiography in cases of pulmonary embolism (n=107); recurrences were confirmed in the same way. After 2 years of follow-up, there had been 123 recurrences of venous thromboembolism that met the diagnostic criteria, 80 in the 6-week group (18.1%) and 43 in the 6-month group (9.5%). The OR for recurrence in the 6-week group was 2.1. There was no difference in mortality or the rate of major hemorrhage between the 6-week and 6-month groups. Six months of prophylactic oral anticoagulation after a first episode of venous thromboembolism led to a lower recurrence rate than did treatment lasting for 6 weeks. The difference between the 2 groups occurred between 6 weeks and 6 months after the start of treatment, and the rates of recurrence remained nearly parallel for 1 1/2 years thereafter.

Definite diagnosis of pulmonary embolism by conventional methods such as angiography is frequently difficult. If residual thromboemboli incorporated into the pulmonary arterial wall or in the distal small segments are visible, differential diagnosis of pulmonary embolism vs. primary pulmonary hypertension can be made without open-chest pulmonary biopsy. Six patients suspected of having acute pulmonary embolism, 6 suspected of having chronic pulmonary embolism, and 4 with primary pulmonary hypertension diagnosed by pulmonary biopsy underwent percutaneous pulmonary angioscopy in this investigation by Uchida and associates[30] from Tokyo and Funabashi, Japan. In patients suspected of having pulmonary embolism, globular and mural thromboemboli were detected by both angioscopy and angiography in 4 and 1 patients, respectively. By angioscopy, emboli incorporated into the arterial wall were detected in 7 and microemboli obstructing the distal small segments were detected in 6. However, these emboli were detected by angiography in none. In patients with primary pulmonary hypertension, no embolus was detected by angioscopy and angiography. Angioscopically, however, stenoses were observed in the distal small segments in all patients. The results indicate that residual pulmonary thromboemboli in pulmonary embolism and stenoses of distal pulmonary arteries in primary pulmonary hypertension are detectable by percutaneous angioscopy, and therefore this method is feasible for differential diagnosis of pulmonary embolism.

Aortic Disease

The Marfan Syndrome

Finkbohner and colleagues[31] in Houston, Texas, reviewed medical records on 192 patients with the Marfan syndrome who underwent aortic aneurysm repair during the prior 26 years. One hundred three patients were interviewed and complete preoperative and postoperative medical information was obtained. Survival curves were generated and data were analyzed. The median cumulative probability of survival was 61 years, which was significantly increased compared with a median survival of 47 years for patients with Marfan syndrome determined 30 years ago (Figure 10-6). Most patients (53%) had second surgeries to repair subsequent aneurysms or dissections at other sites, most of which involved the aorta. The most common pattern of aneurysm repair was proximal ascending aortic aneurysm repair followed by descending thoracic aneurysm surgery. The following variables predicted patients requiring second vascular surgeries: presence of acute or chronic dissection at the time of the first surgery, hypertension after the first surgery, and a history of smoking. Thus, the life expectancy of Marfan patients undergoing surgical repair of aortic aneurysms has improved. However, many patients have subsequent surgeries at other sites throughout the aorta indicating the diffuse nature of the aorta in the Marfan patient and their ongoing risks.

Gott and associates[32] from Baltimore, Maryland, reported results of aortic root replacement at their institution in 270 patients having the operation be-

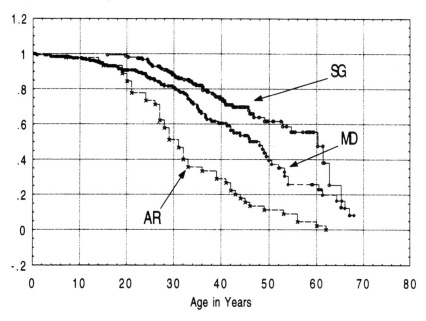

Figure 10-6. Comparison of cumulative probability of survival of patients with Marfan syndrome. Patients who underwent surgical repair of aortic aneurysms are shown in the open circles (SG). Affected relatives who died before diagnosis or the availability of surgical techniques to repair aortic aneurysms are indicated by X (AR). The original survival data by Murdoch et al. are shown in the closed circles (MD). Reproduced with permission from Finkbohner et al.[31]

tween September 1976 and September 1993. Two-hundred fifty-two patients underwent a Bentall composite graft repair, and 18 patients received a cryopreserved homograft aortic root. One hundred eighty-seven patients had a Marfan aneurysm of the ascending aorta (41 with dissection), and 53 patients had an aneurysm resulting from nonspecific medial degeneration (17 with dissection). These 240 patients were considered to have annuloaortic ectasia. Thirty patients were operated on for miscellaneous lesions of the aortic root. Thirty-day mortality for the overall series of 270 patients was 4.8% (13 of 270). There was no 30-day mortality among 182 patients undergoing elective root replacement for annuloaortic ectasia without dissection. Thirty-six of the 270 patients having root replacement also had mitral valve operations. There was no hospital mortality for aortic root replacement in these 36 patients, but there were 7 late deaths. Twenty-two patients received a cryopreserved homograft aortic root; 18 of these were primary root replacements and 4 were repeat root replacements for late endocarditis. One early death and 2 late deaths occurred in this group. Actuarial survival for the overall group of 270 patients was 73% at 10 years. In a multivariate analysis, only poor New Year Heart Association class (III and IV), non-Marfan status, preoperative dissection, and male gender emerged as significant predictors of early or late death. Endocarditis was the most common late complication (14 of 256 hospital survivors) and was optimally treated by root replacement with a cryopreserved aortic homograft. Late problems with the part of the aorta not operated on occur with moderate frequency; careful follow-up of the distal aorta is critical to long-term survival.

To review the available information on the diagnostic, prognostic, and therapeutic aspects of cardiac complications in women with the Marfan Syndrome during the peripartum period and to develop guidelines for the approach to these patients on the basis of this information, Elkayam and associates[33] from Los Angeles, California, did a MEDLINE search for articles that reported on pregnancy in patients with the Marfan Syndrome or that potentially discussed relevant aspects of the syndrome. Pregnancy in the Marfan syndrome is associated with 2 primary problems: potential catastrophic aortic dissection and the risk for having a child with the syndrome. The risk for peripartum aortic dissection is especially high in women in whom aortic root dilatation is diagnosed before pregnancy. Gestation seems to be safer in women without preexisting cardiovascular disease; however, an event-free pregnancy cannot be guaranteed. The Marfan syndrome is inherited in an autosomal dominant manner, and the fetus has a 50% risk for inheriting the mutant gene. Women with the syndrome should be counseled before conception about the risks of pregnancy to both mother and fetus. Because preconceptual dilatation of the ascending aorta seems to be an important predictor for aortic dissection, it should be excluded before pregnancy. Transesophageal echocardiography seems to be preferable for noninvasive assessment of aortic dilatation before and during pregnancy. Prophylactic use of β-blockers may be useful in preventing aortic dilatation. Surgery should be considered during gestation in patients with progressive aortic dilatation when or before the aortic root reaches 5.5 cm. Because of the potential risk of ionizing radiation to the fetus, noninvasive methods such as transesophageal echocardiography and magnetic resonance imaging are preferred to contrast aortography for the diagnosis of aortic dissection during pregnancy. Vaginal delivery can be done in patients with the Marfan syndrome who do not have cardiovascular system abnormalities. In patients with aortic dilatation, aortic dissection, or other important cardiac abnormalities, cesarean section should be the preferred method of delivery.

Protruding Plaque

Protruding aortic arch atheromas are associated with otherwise unexplained strokes and transient ischemic attacks. Therefore aortic atheromas also may be important in patients with carotid artery disease. Forty-five patients with ≥50% carotid stenosis and stroke or transient ischemic attack within 6 weeks underwent transesophageal echocardiographic examination by Demoupoulos and associates[34] from New York, New York. The patients were matched for age, sex, and hypertension with 45 control subjects who had also had a recent cerebral event but in whom significant carotid stenosis was absent. Protruding aortic arch atheromas were present in 17 (38%) of 45 patients with carotid disease and only 7 (16%) of 45 of control individuals. Mobile atheromas (with the greatest embolic potential) were present almost exclusively in case patients, 6 (13%) of 45 vs. 1 (2%) of 45 control individuals. Case patients with mobile atheromas had the most severe carotid stenosis (≥80%). Cerebral symptoms were discordant with the side of the carotid stenosis in 10 case patients, and 4 had atheromas. In conclusion, protruding atheromas of the aortic arch are present in significant numbers of symptomatic patients with carotid artery disease. These atheromas may represent an additional cause of symptoms in patients with carotid stenosis. Transesophageal echocardiography to look for protruding aortic atheromas may be considered in patients with neurological events despite the presence of significant carotid stenosis, especially if the symptoms are discordant with the side of carotid stenosis.

Atherosclerotic plaque ulcers ≥2 mm in depth and width in the thoracic aorta have been implicated by autopsy study as a cause of unexplained or cryptogenic ischemic strokes. Transesophageal echocardiography allows visualization of complex atherosclerotic lesions of the thoracic aorta. Stone and associates[35] from Baltimore, Maryland, compared the prevalence of thoracic aorta ulcerated plaques (ulcers ≥2 mm in both depth and width) in 3 age-matched groups undergoing multiplane transesophageal echocardiography: group 1, 23 patients with cryptogenic ischemic stroke; group 2, 26 patients with known-cause strokes; and group 3, 57 control patients without strokes. Transesophageal echocardiograms were interpreted in a blinded fashion. Ulcerated plaques were found in 9 (39%) group 1 patients but in only 2 (8%) group 2 patients and in only 4 (7%) group 3 patients. There was an association between advancing age and the presence of ulcerated plaques. It was concluded that ulcerated atherosclerotic plaques in the thoracic aorta are associated with cryptogenic ischemic stroke and should be considered a potential source of cerebral emboli.

Abdominal Aortic Aneurysm

There is evidence that the risk of abdominal aortic aneurysm is greater in first-degree relatives of patients with the disorder than in the same age group of the general population. Baird and associates[36] from Vancouver and Ottawa, Canada, conducted a 3-year study of siblings of abdominal aortic aneurysm

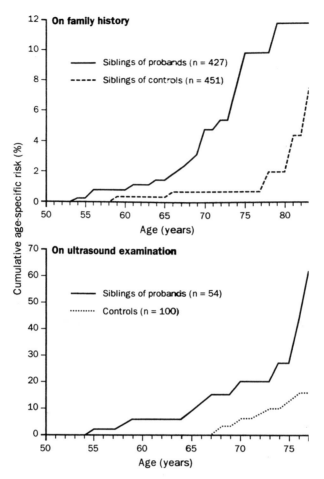

Figure 10-7. Cumulative age-specific risk of abdominal aortic aneurysm among siblings of abdominal aortic aneurysm probands and siblings of controls. Tables giving SDs of risks are available from *The Lancet* on request. Reproduced with permission from Baird et al.[36]

probands and siblings of a control group (cataract surgery patients) of the same age. Genetic information was obtained by interview from 126 probands and 100 control subjects; another family member was present at the interview. Medical records were obtained and further information verified before a sibling (over age 50) was assigned affected status. Of 427 siblings of probands, 19 (4%) had probable or definite abdominal aortic aneurysm compared with 5 (1%) of 451 siblings of control subjects (Figure 10-7). The lifetime cumulative risks of abdominal aortic aneurysm at age 83 were 12% (SD, 3) and 8% (SD, 4), respectively. The risk of abdominal aortic aneurysm began at an earlier age and increased more rapidly for probands' siblings than for controls' siblings. A risk comparison, based on the results of ultrasound screening of 54 geographically accessible siblings of probands and the 100 controls showed a similar pattern. Ten (19%) siblings and 8 (8% 0 control subjects had an abdominal aortic aneurysm on ultrasound (lifetime cumulative risk, 61% [19] vs. 15% [5]). These results show that familial factors influence the age of onset of abdominal aortic aneurysm. The authors recommend routine ultrasound examination of siblings of patients with abdominal aortic aneurysm.

Bayazit and associates[37] from Ankara, Turkey, performed coronary arteriography before elective repair of abdominal aortic aneurysm in 125 patients operated on between 1986–1994. All cases with critical LAD narrowings underwent CABG either simultaneously or shortly before AAA repair. In addition, PTCA was performed for symptomatic and critical stenosis of arteries other than the LAD or if noncritical but symptomatic stenosis of the LAD existed. Coronary artery narrowings were found in 66 patients (53%) (Figure 10-8). In 24 patients, abdominal aortic aneurysm repairs were performed a mean of 2.3 months after CABG whereas in 4 patients both procedures were performed simultaneously. PTCA was performed in 4 patients 3–4 days before the abdominal surgery. Even though the coronary artery narrowings were found preoperatively in 7 cases, these patients underwent repair of abdominal aortic aneurysm because of rapidly-expanding aneurysms or painful aneurysms. Early mortality rate was 4% (5 patients) and 3 of those were from the group inoperable for CABG. The follow-up range from 3–87 months and cumulative survival rates for 6 months and 1, 2, 3, and 6 years were 99%, 99%, 95%, 93%, and 89%, respectively.

To estimate elective perioperative mortality, Steyerberg and associates[38] from Rotterdam and Leiden, the Netherlands, developed a clinical prediction rule based on several well-established risk factors including age, gender, a history of AMI, CHF, myocardial ischemia on the electrocardiogram, pulmonary impairment, and renal impairment in patients undergoing elective abdominal aortic aneurysms surgery. Two sources of data were used: individual patient data from 246 patients operated on at the University Hospital of Leiden, and published studies between 1980–1994. The strongest adverse risk factors were CHF and myocardial ischemia on the electrocardiogram followed by renal impairment, history of AMI, pulmonary impairment, and female gender. A 10-year increase in age more than doubled surgical risk.

Dissection

The use of preoperative coronary arteriography in patients with type A dissection of the aorta is controversial. To determine the prevalence of arteriosclerotic CAD in patients with type A dissection of the aorta, Creswell and associates[39] from St. Louis, Missouri, reviewed their experience in 62 patients

Results of Coronary Arteriographies in Patients With Abdominal Aortic Aneurysm

Result	No. of Cases	PTCA	CABG
Normal coronary arteries	59 (47%)	–	–
Mild to moderate coronary artery lesions	31 (25%)	4*	–
Severe operable coronary artery lesions	28 (22%)	–	28†
Inoperable coronary artery disease	7 (6%)	–	–

Figure 10-8. Results of coronary arteriographies in patients with abdominal aortic aneurysm. Procedures were performed 2 or 3 days before surgery for AAA. In four cases CABG was performed simultaneously with AAA repair. In the remaining 24 cases, CABG was performed a mean of 2.3 months before AAA repair. PTCA indicates percutaneous transluminal coronary angioplasty; CABG, coronary artery bypass grafting; AAA, abdominal aortic aneurysm. Reproduced with permission from Bayazit et al.[37]

(42 with acute dissection and 20 with chronic dissection) who underwent operation between January 1, 1986, and December 31, 1993. Among 23 patients with acute dissection who underwent coronary arteriography, 8 (34.8%) had one or more coronary artery lesions causing a >50% narrowing. There were no fatal complications associated with coronary arteriography. Four patients with acute dissection and 6 patients with chronic dissection underwent coronary artery bypass grafting at the time of operative repair of the aortic dissection, with no operative deaths. On the basis of these findings and the success of combined coronary artery bypass grafting and aortic repair, we recommend that patients with an acute type A dissection who are in stable condition and all patients with a chronic type A dissection of the aorta should undergo preoperative coronary arteriography.

Peripherial Arterial Disease

Carotid Arteries

LV hypertrophy is a known risk factor for subsequent cardiovascular morbidity and mortality. Roman and associates[40] from New York, New York, evaluated the prevalence of carotid atherosclerosis in a large group of asymptomatic hypertensive and normotensive adults to examine its relation to the presence of LV hypertrophy. Two hundred, seventy-seven normotensive and 209 untreated hypertensive adults who were free of cardiovascular disease were studied prospectively with echocardiography to determine left ventricular mass, and carotid ultrasound to detect atherosclerosis. Carotid atherosclerosis was present in 16% of normotensive and 23% of hypertensive patients and it was associated with older age, higher systolic and pulse pressures, and larger left ventricular mass index. Subjects with LV hypertrophy were twice as likely to have carotid atheromas (35% vs. 18%) than those without LV hypertrophy. These authors concluded that higher LV mass as detected by echocardiography is associated with the presence of carotid plaque. This association may contribute to the pathogenesis of the high incidence of vascular events seen in patients with LV hypertrophy.

Screening and carotid endarterectomy have been advocated for asymptomatic carotid artery stenosis. The risk of stroke without treatment, however, has not been adequately defined. The European Carotid Surgery Trialists Collaborative Group[41] investigated the risks of stroke in the distribution of symptomatic carotid artery in 2295 patients randomized in the European Carotid Surgery Trial. During a mean follow-up of 4.5 years, there were 69 carotid territory strokes, 9 of which were fatal, giving 3-year Kaplan-Meier risks of stroke and fatal stroke of 2.1% and 0.3%, respectively. The stroke risk in the 127 patients with severe (70–99%) carotid stenosis was 5.7% (Figure 10-9). Given these low stroke risks, the potential benefit of endarterectomy for asymptomatic carotid stenosis is small. Population screening is not justified and endarterectomy for asymptomatic carotid stenosis should only be performed in the context of well organized randomized controlled trials.

Salenius and associates[42] from Tampere and Kuopio, Finland, assessed long term efficacy of guar gum in 40 patients with moderate hypercholesteremia during a 24-month period. All 40 patients had hemodynamic measurable carotid arterial stenosis. Postoperatively after carotid endarterectomy the patients re-

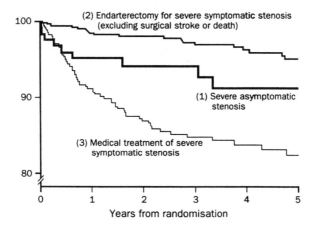

Figure 10-9. Actuarial analysis of survival free from stroke in the distribution of a severe (70–99%) carotid stenosis. 1) patients with asymptomatic stenosis including all carotid territory strokes ipsilateral to the asymptomatic stenosis; 2) patients with symptomatic stenosis randomised to carotid endarterectomy, excluding all surgery-related strokes and deaths, i.e., the background ipsilateral stroke risk after successful surgery; 3) patients with symptomatic stenosis randomised to medical treatment, including all carotid territory ischaemic strokes ipsilateral to the symptomatic stenosis. Reproduced with permission of the European Trialists Collaborative Group.[41]

ceived 5 g of granulated guar gum or placebo 3 times a day. Significant differences between treatment and placebo group were found in concentration of both total and LDL cholesterol at 24 months. The authors concluded that 15 g guar gum daily considerably reduced serum concentration of total and LDL cholesterol without attenuation over 2 years' treatment.

Epidemiological studies have identified hyperhomocysteinemia as a possible risk factor for atherosclerosis. Selhub and associates[43] from Boston and Framingham, Massachusetts, determined the risk of carotid-artery atherosclerosis in relation to both plasma homocysteines concentrations and nutritional determinants of hyperhomocysteinemia. The authors performed a cross-sectional study of 1041 elderly subjects (418 men and 623 women; age range, 67–96 years) from the Framingham Heart Study. The authors examined the relation between the maximal degree of stenosis of the extracranial carotid arteries (as assessed by ultrasonography) and plasma homocysteine concentrations, as well as plasma concentrations and intakes of vitamins involved in homocysteine metabolism, including folate, vitamin B_{12} and vitamin B_6 The subjects were classified into 2 categories according to the findings in the more diseased of the 2 carotid vessels: stenosis of 0–24% and stenosis of 25–100%. The prevalence of carotid stenosis of ≥25% was 43% in the men and 34% in the women. The odds ratio for stenosis of ≥25% was 2.0 for subjects with the highest plasma homocysteine concentrations (≥14.4 μmol/L) as compared with those with the lowest concentrations (≥9.1 μmol/L), after adjustment for sex, age, plasma HDL cholesterol concentration, systolic BP, and smoking status. Plasma concentrations of folate and pyridoxal-5'-phosphate (the coenzyme form of vitamin B_6) and the level of folate intake were inversely associated with carotid-artery stenosis after adjustment for age, sex, and other risk factors. High plasma homocysteine concentrations and low concentrations of folate and vitamin B_6, through their role in homocysteines metabolism, are associated with an increased risk of extracranial carotid-artery stenosis in the elderly.

Crouse and coinvestigators[44] in Winston-Salem, North Carolina, randomly assigned 151 coronary patients to placebo or pravastatin and treated them for 3 years. B-mode ultrasound quantification of carotid artery intimal-medial thickness was obtained at baseline and sequentially during this period. The primary outcome was the change in the mean of the maximal intimal-medial thickness measurements across time. Effects on individual carotid artery segments (common, bifurcation, and internal carotid) and on clinical events were also investigated. Plasma concentrations of total cholesterol were lower with active treatment than with placebo (4.8 vs. 6.1 mmol/L [186 vs. 235 mg/dl], respectively) as were concentrations of LDL cholesterol (3.1 vs. 4.3 mmol/L [120 vs. 167 mg/dl], respectively). Plasma concentrations of HDL_2 cholesterol were higher with active treatment (0.2 vs. 0.1 mmol/L [6.1 vs. 5.5 mg/dl], respectively). Active treatment resulted in a nonsignificant 12% reduction in progression of the mean-maximum intimal-medial thickness (from 0.07 to 0.06 mm/year) and a statistically significant 35% reduction in intimal-medial thickness progression in the common carotid. Active treatment was also associated with a reduction in fatal and nonfatal AMI ($P=0.09$) and of any fatal event plus nonfatal AMI ($P=0.04$).

To determine whether the addition of carotid endarterectomy to aggressive medical management can reduce the incidence of cerebral infarction in patients with asymptomatic carotid artery stenosis, a prospective randomized multicenter trial was performed involving 39 clinical sites in the United States and Canada, and the results were reported by the executive Committee for the Asymptomatic Carotid Atherosclerosis Study.[45] Between December 1987 and December 1993, a total of 1662 patients with asymptomatic carotid artery stenosis of 60% or greater in diameter were randomized. At baseline, recognized risk factors for stroke were similar between the 2 treatment groups. Daily aspirin administration and medical risk factor management for all patients; carotid endarterectomy for patients randomly assigned to receive surgery. Initially, transient ischemic attack or cerebral infarction occurring in the distribution of the study artery and any transient ischemic attack, stroke, or death occurring in the perioperative period. In March 1993, the primary outcome measures were changed to cerebral infarction occurring in the distribution of the study artery or any stroke or death occurring in the perioperative period. After a median follow-up of 2.7 years, with 4657 patient-years of observation, the aggregate risk over 5 years for ipsilateral stroke and any perioperative stroke or death was estimated to be 5.1% for surgical patients and 11.0% for patients treated medically (aggregate risk reduction of 53%). Patients with asymptomatic carotid artery stenosis of 60% or greater reduction in diameter and whose general health makes them good candidates for elective surgery will have a reduced 5-year risk of ipsilateral stroke if carotid endarterectomy performed with less than 3% perioperative morbidity and mortality is added to aggressive management of modifiable risk factors.

To assess the cost-effectiveness of 4 diagnostic strategies for the preoperative evaluation of symptomatic patients who are potential candidates for carotid endarterectomy (70–99% diameter stenosis): 1) duplex sonography, 2) magnetic resonance angiography, 3) contrast angiography, and 4) the combination of duplex sonography and magnetic resonance angiography supplemented by contrast angiography for disparate results, Kent and associates[46] from Boston, Massachusetts, performed a cost-effectiveness analysis based largely on published clinical trial data from 81 patients undergoing prospective evaluation with duplex sonography, magnetic resonance angiography, and contrast angiography. For a hypothetical cohort of symptomatic patients undergoing evaluation for carotid endarterectomy, the combination of tests resulted in the greatest quality-adjusted life expectancy of the 4 options considered. After incorporating the costs of testing, surgery, and stroke, we found that neither magnetic resonance angiography nor contrast angiography was cost effective. The combination of tests was more effective but more costly than duplex sonography, resulting in an additional cost of $22 400 per quality-adjusted year of life gained. For centers that do not have adequate magnetic resonance angiography, contrast angiography resulted in an additional cost of $99 200 per quality-adjusted year of life saved compared with duplex sonography. The authors' results suggest that for the preoperative detection of a 70–99% carotid stenosis, the combination of duplex sonography and magnetic resonance angiography, supplemented by contrast angiography for disparate results, is associated with the lowest long-term morbidity and mortality and has a favorable cost-effectiveness ratio. The combination of tests, or duplex sonography alone when magnetic resonance angiography is not available, could potentially replace the current practice of using contrast angiography alone in the preoperative evaluation of patients with symptomatic carotid stenosis.

To determine the effectiveness of aspirin in preventing ischemic events in patients with asymptomatic carotid artery stenosis, Côté and associates[47] for the Asymptomatic Cervical Bruit Study Group performed a double-blind, placebo-controlled trial involving 372 neurologically asymptomatic patients with carotid narrowing of 50% of more in diameter in at least 1 artery as determined by duplex ultrasonography. Patients were randomly assigned to receive either enteric coated aspirin, 325 mg/d, or identically appearing placebo. The duration of therapy was 2.0 years for the aspirin recipients and 1.9 years for the placebo recipients. At baseline, the 188 patients receiving aspirin and the 184 patients receiving placebo had similar demographic, ultrasonographic, and laboratory characteristics. The median duration of follow-up was 2.3 years. The annual rate of all ischemic events and death from any cause was 12.3% for the placebo group and 11.0% for the aspirin group. The Cox proportional hazards analysis yielded an adjusted hazard ratio (aspirin-placebo) of 0.99. The annual rates for vascular events only were 11% for the placebo group and 10.7% for the aspirin group. The multivariate analysis yielded a hazard ratio of 1.08. Aspirin did not have a significant long-term protective effect in asymptomatic patients with high-grade ($\geq$50%) carotid stenosis.

Leg Arteries

To assess the value of magnetic resonance angiography in presurgical evaluation of patients with severe lower limb atherosclerotic occlusive disease, Baum and associates[48] for the American College of Radiology Rapid Technology Assessment Group imaged 15 arterial segments of the leg and foot with magnetic resonance angiography and contrast arteriography. The sensitivity in distinguishing patent segments from completely occluded segments was 83% for contrast angiography and 85% for magnetic resonance angiography; both had

81% specificity. For distinguishing near-normal segments (suitable as bypassed graft termini), contrast angiography was less sensitive than magnetic resonance angiography (77% vs. 82%) but more specific (92% vs. 84%). The authors concluded that magnetic resonance angiography and contrast angiography are approximately equivalent in diagnostic accuracy, but that the addition of magnetic resonance angiography to treatment plans based only on contrast angiography and other diagnostic information clearly improved the plans.

Vanderschueren and colleagues[49] in Leuven, Belgium, evaluated the thrombolytic efficacy, safety, fibrin specificity, and immunogenicity in patients with peripheral arterial occlusive disease. Recombinant staphylokinase has been shown to be a fibrin-specific and potent thrombolytic intervention. Thirty patients (age range, 37–86 years) with angiographically documented thromboembolic peripheral arterial occlusion of recent origin were treated with heparin and intra-arterial staphylokinase given as a 1-mg bolus followed by a 0.5-mg/hour infusion in 20 patients or as a 2-mg bolus followed by a 1-mg/hour infusion in 10 subsequent patients. With 7 mg staphylokinase infused over 9 hours, recanalization was complete in 25 patients, partial in 2, and absent in 3. Two major hemorrhagic complications occurred, including one fatal hemorrhagic cerebrovascular accident and hypovolemic shock occurring in another patient caused by bleeding at the angiographic puncture site. Administration of staphylokinase did not induce fibrinogen breakdown or a significant prolongation in bleeding time. Staphylokinase neutralizing activity and antibodies to staphylokinase were low at baseline, but they increased markedly from the second week on and remained elevated for several months. These data indicate that the intra-arterial administration of staphylokinase restores vessel patency in patients with peripheral arterial occlusion in the absence of fibrinogen degradation, but it is antigenic and antibodies develop against it within 2 weeks of its administration.

Previous human and animal studies have suggested that proprionyl-L-carnitine increases carnitine content and improves energy metabolism in ischemic skeletal muscle. Brevetti and colleagues[50] from Naples and Bari, Italy, conducted a double-blind, placebo-controlled, dose titration, multicenter trial to assess the efficacy and safety of proprionyl-L-carnitine in intermittent claudication. Two hundred forty-five patients were randomly assigned to receive the drug or placebo. The initial oral dose of 500 mg twice daily was increased at 2-month intervals to 2 g/d and then to 3 g/d in patients showing improvement in treadmill performance. There was a statistically significant improvement of 73% in maximal walking distance with proprionyl-L-carnitine as compared to 46% with placebo (P=0.03). These authors concluded that although the precise mode of therapeutic action of proprionyl-L-carnitine remains to be clarified, at a dose of 1 to 2 g/d it appears to be well tolerated and effective in patients with intermittent claudication.

Odds and Ends

Left Atrial Size and Stroke

Benjamin and colleagues[51] for the Framingham Heart Study determined the relation of LA size to risk of stroke and death in the general population in subjects 50 years of age and older included in the Framingham Heart Study.

During 8 years of follow-up, 64 of 1371 (5%) men and 73 of 1728 (4%) women had a cerebrovascular accident and 296 (22%) men and 271 (16%) women died. Cox proportional-hazards models were adjusted for age, hypertension, diabetes, AF, smoking, electrocardiographic evidence of LV hypertrophy, and CHF or AMI. After multivariable adjustment, every 10-mm increase in LA size, the RR of stroke was 2.4 in men and 1.4 in women. The relative risk of death was 1.3 in men and 1.4 in women. Adjusting for electrocardiographic LA enlargement is a significant predictor of stroke in men and death in both sexes. The relation of LA enlargement to stroke and death appears to be partially mediated by LV mass.

Diagnosing Left Atrial Thrombi

To determine the ability of transesophageal echocardiography to accurately identify or exclude LA thrombi, Manning and associates[52] from Boston, Massachusetts, examined 231 consecutive patients having transesophageal echocardiography before elective repair or replacement of the mitral valve or excision of a LA tumor. Fifty-six percent of patients had a history of AF, and 17% had a history of thromboembolism. Transesophageal echocardiography identified 14 LA thrombi in 14 patients (6%). Thrombus size ranged from 3–80 mm. Surgery confirmed 12 of 14 thrombi (86%), including 9 thrombi confined to the LA appendage. No additional thrombi were found on direct inspection of the atria (sensitivity, 100%; specificity, 99%; positive predictive value, 86%; negative predictive value, 100%; for a population that had a 5.2% prevalence of thrombi). All 12 surgically confirmed thrombi were identified by 2 independent observers. Neither thrombus seen by only a single observer on transesophageal echocardiography was confirmed during direct inspection of the atria at surgery. Transesophageal echocardiography is highly accurate for identifying LA thrombi and can be used clinically to exclude LA thrombi.

Atrial Septal Aneurysm

Mügge and colleagues[53] in a multicenter study defined morphologic characteristics of atrial septal aneurysms by transesophageal echocardiography to elucidate the incidence of atrial septal aneurysm-associated abnormalities and to investigate whether certain morphologic characteristics of these aneurysms are different in patients with and without previous events compatible with systemic embolism from a cardiac source. Patients with atrial septal aneurysms were enrolled from 11 centers. Each patient had to undergo transthoracic and transesophageal echocardiography within 24 hours of one another. Atrial septal aneurysms were defined as a protrusion of the aneurysm >10 mm beyond the plane of the atrial septum as measured by transesophageal echocardiography (Figure 10-10). Patient with mitral stenosis or prosthesis or after cardiothoracic surgery involving the atrial septum were excluded. Based on these criteria, 195 patients (mean age, 55 years) were included in the study. Atrial septal aneurysm defined by transesophageal echocardiography was missed by transthoracic echocardiography in 92 patients (47%). As judged from the transesophageal echocardiogram, atrial septal aneurysm involved the entire septum in 100 patients and were limited to the fossa ovalis in 95. Atrial septal aneurysm was an isolated structural defect in 62 patients. In 106 patients, atrial septal aneu-

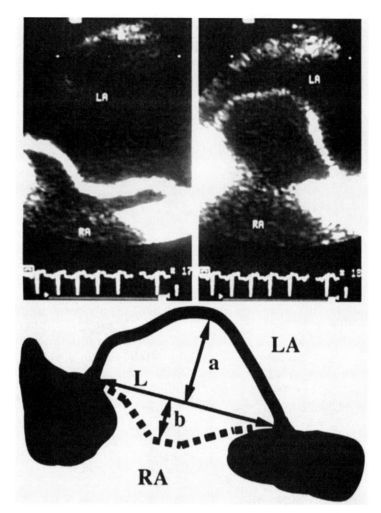

Figure 10-10. Original transesophageal echocardiogram demonstrating a mobile atrial septal aneurysm (top); bottom, schematic showing the various measurements. L indicates length of the aneurysm; a and b, maximal extent of oscillation; LA, left atrium; and RA, right atrium. Reproduced with permission from Mügge et al.[53]

rysm was associated with interatrial shunting in the form of an atrial septal defect in 38 patients, a patent foramen ovale in 65 patients, and a sinus venosus defect in 3 patients. In only 2 patients (1%) were thrombi attached to the region of the atrial septal aneurysm. Prior clinical events compatible with systemic embolization from a cardiac source were found in 87 patients with atrial septal aneurysms. In 21 patients with prior presumed systemic embolism, no other potential cardiac sources of embolism were present. The length of the atrial septal aneurysm, the extent of bulging, and the incidence of spontaneous oscillations were similar in patients with and without previous systemic embolism from a cardiac source. However, associated abnormalities, such as atrial shunts were significantly more frequent in patients with possible embolism. Thus, transesophageal echocardiography is superior to the transthoracic approach in the diagnosis of atrial septal aneurysm. The most common abnormalities associated

with the atrial septal aneurysms were interatrial shunts, especially patent foramen ovale. Patients with atrial septal aneurysms with shunts showed a high frequency of previous clinical events compatible with systemic embolism from a
cardiac source. These data are consistent with the atrial septal aneurysm being a
risk factor for systemic embolization, even though thrombi attached to atrial septal aneurysms are infrequently detected by transesophageal echocardiography.

Energy of Heavy Snow Shoveling

To assess the physiologic responses to manual (shoveling) vs. automated
(electric snow thrower) snow removal in healthy, untrained men was assessed
by Franklin and associates[54] from Royal Oak, Michigan, in 10 apparently health,
untrained men (mean age 32.4±2 years). Each subject cleared two 10±2-cm
high, 15-m-long tracts of heavy, wet snow in the cold (2° C) temperature, using
self-paced manual and automated methods, in random order, with 10- to 15-
minute rest periods between each 10-minute bout of work. Mean heart rate
during shoveling was 154 and 173 beats per minute at 2 and 10 minutes,
respectively, corresponding to 86% and 97% of maximal heart rate. Relative
heart rate (percentage of maximal heart rat) during shoveling was inversely
related to aerobic fitness (r=0.65). The highest heart rate and perceived exertion
responses during shoveling, armergometer, and treadmill testing were comparable. Systolic BP during snow shoveling (198±17 mm Hg) was significantly
greater than during arm ergometry or automated snow removal and slightly
greater than during maximal treadmill testing (181±25 mm Hg). Oxygen uptake
during shoveling was similar to that for arm ergometry (5.7 vs. 6.3 metabolic
equivalents), but lower than for treadmill testing (9.3 metabolic equivalents).
Cardiorespiratory and perceived exertion responses were reduced during automated snow removal. Heavy snow shoveling elicits myocardial and aerobic
demands that rival maximal treadmill and arm-ergometer testing in sedentary
men. These responses may contribute to cardiovascular events reported after
heavy snowfalls.

Carcinoid Heart Disease

Robiolio and colleagues[55] in Durham, North Carolina, reviewed the experience with 604 patients in the Duke Carcinoid Database. Nineteen patients with
proven carcinoid heart disease by cardiac catheterization and/or echocardiograms were compared with the remaining 585 noncardiac patients in the database
with regard to circulating serotonin and its principal metabolite, 5-hydroxyin-
dole acetic acid. No significant demographic differences existed between the cardiac and noncardiac groups, but typical carcinoid syndrome symptoms, including flushing and diarrhea, were almost threefold more common in the cardiac
group. Compared with the noncardiac group, heart disease patients demonstrated
strikingly higher mean serum concentration from the serotonin, platelet serotonin, and urine serotonin metabolite concentrations (Figure 10-11). The spectrum
of heart disease among the 19 patients showed a strong right-sided valvular predominance with tricuspid regurgitation being the most common valvular lesion.
These data suggest that serotonin may play a role in the pathogenesis of cardiac
plaque formation observed in patients with carcinoid heart disease.

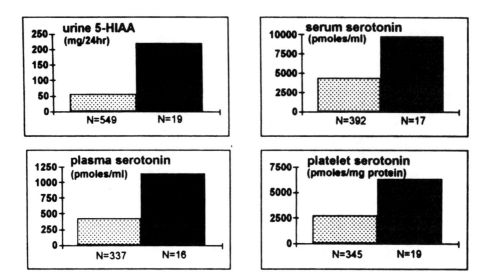

Figure 10-11. Bar graphs comparing cardiac and noncardiac patients. Cardiac patients demonstrated higher (*P*<0.0001) mean levels of urine 5-hydroxyindole acetic acid (5-HIAA; 219±124 vs. 55.3±141 mg/24 hr), serum serotonin (9750±4130 vs. 4350±6460 pmol/mL), plasma serotonin (1130±1210 vs. 426±1130 pmol/mL), and platelet serotonin (6240±4030 vs. 2700±2880 pmol/mg protein). Stippled box indicates no heart disease; solid box, heart disease. Reproduced with permission from Robiolio et al.[55]

Primary Pulmonary Hypertension

Sandoval and associates[56] from Mexico City, Mexico, reported 18 children (mean age, 10±3 years) with primary pulmonary hypertension. Survival estimates were compared with those of 42 adult patients with primary pulmonary hypertension (mean age, 28±9 years). Baseline mean PA pressure was similar in children and adults (66±15 vs. 65±18 mm Hg), but a higher cardiac index resulted in a lower mean pulmonary vascular resistance index in children (18±7 vs. 26±12 U/m^2). The proportion of patients who had a positive hemodynamic response to vasodilator treatment was higher in children than in adults (41% vs. 25%) and estimated median survival in children was 4 years and 3 years in adults. Elevated RA pressure and decreased stroke volume index were the only significant indicators of mortality. Children with primary pulmonary hypertension have a poor survival expectancy, despite a more common positive response to vasodilator therapy. More data are needed to determine which patients need urgent placement on the lung transplant list.

Pulmonary hypertension is characterized by abnormal thickening of the pulmonary arteries and increased pulmonary vascular resistance. Nitric oxide is a potent endothelium-derived vasorelaxant substance and an inhibitor of smooth-muscle-cell growth. Nitric oxide is produced in various cell types by the action of an enzyme, nitric oxide synthase. Giaid and Saleh[57] from Montreal, Canada, compared the expression of endothelial cell nitric oxide synthase in the lungs of control subjects with that in the lungs of patients with primary pulmonary hypertension, 22 patients with primary pulmonary hypertension, 24 patients with secondary pulmonary hypertension, and 23 control subjects. In the lungs of the control subjects, nitric oxide synthase was expressed at a high level in the vascular endothelium of all types of vessels and in the pulmonary epithelium. In contrast, little or no expression of the enzyme was found in the vascular endothelium of pulmonary arteries with severe histological abnormalities (i.e., plexiform lesions) in patients with pulmonary hypertension. The intensity of the enzyme immunoreactivity correlated inversely with the severity of histological changes. There was an inverse correlation between the arterial expression of the enzyme and total pulmonary resistance in patients with plexogenic pulmonary arteriopathy. Pulmonary hypertension is associated with diminished expression of endothelial nitric oxide synthase. It is possible that decreased expression of nitric oxide synthase may contribute to pulmonary vasoconstriction and to the excessive growth of the tunica media observed in this disease.

Herve and associates[58] from Paris, France, used radioenzymatic assays to measure serotonin in platelets and plasma and serotonin release during in vitro platelet aggregation in 16 patients with primary pulmonary hypertension, and in 16 normal control subjects matched for age and sex. The patients had decreased platelet serotonin concentration and increased plasma serotonin concentration compared with the control subjects. Serotonin released during in vitro platelet aggregation was higher in patients than in the control group. Thus, abnormal handling of serotonin by platelets leading to an increase in plasma serotonin occurs in primary pulmonary hypertension.

Raynaud's Disease

Freedman and colleagues[59] in Detroit, Michigan, studied 23 patients with idiopathic Raynaud's disease screened using conservative criteria and randomly assigned to receive brachial artery infusions of an α_1-antagonist, prazosin; an α_2-adrenergic antagonist, yohimbine; or both, while vasospastic attacks were induced by cooling in the laboratory. Previous research has shown that peripheral vascular α_2-adrenergic receptors are hypersensitive to local cooling in these patients, but the role of α_1-adrenergic receptors has not been elucidated. Each patient's hands were photographed and the number of attacks in the infused hand was compared with the number in the contralateral hand. The number of fingers with attacks in the infused hands during the various therapies were: 1) 0.3 with the yohimbine treatment; 2) 2.3 attacks with prazosin treatment; and 0.6 when both drugs were administered. The difference between prazosin and the other two drug groups was significant. These data indicate that activation of α_2- but not α_1-adrenergic receptors is associated with vasospastic attacks in patients with idiopathic Raynaud's disease.

Necropsy Findings in Octogenarians

Shirani and colleagues[60] in Bethesda, Maryland, examined the hearts of 366 octogenarians (184 women [50%] and 264 white [72%]; mean age, 84 years). The cause of death was cardiac in 195, noncardiac but vascular in 47, and noncardiac and nonvascular in 124 patients. Of the 195 patients with fatal cardiac disease, atherosclerotic CAD was the cause of death in 127 patients (65%): AMI in 87 (69%), sudden cardiac arrest outside the hospital in 19 (15%), chronic CHF with healed myocardial infarction in 15 (12%), and complications of CABG in 6 (4%). At least 1 of the 4 major (left main, LAD, LC, and right) epicardial coronary arteries was narrowed >75% in cross-sectional area by atherosclerotic plaque in 218 patients (60%). The mean number of significantly narrowed major epicardial coronary arteries was 1.7, 1.3, and 0.7 in those who died of cardiac, peripheral vascular, or noncardiovascular causes, respectively. Among the 87 patients with fatal AMI, the women more often had ruptured ventricles (21 of 54 [39%] vs. 3 of 33 [9%]), and fewer women had healed myocardial infarcts. Calcific deposits were present in the epicardial coronary arteries in 285 patients (78%), in the mitral annulus in 140 (38%), and in aortic valve cusps in 153 (42%). Most octogenarian women with fatal AMI had no previous nonfatal infarcts, but had a high frequency of cardiac rupture; in contrast most men with a fatal AMI had had a nonfatal infarct and a low frequency of cardiac rupture. Sudden death was uncommon in both sexes in this age group.

Good Books Appearing in 1995[61]

Major General Text

Chizner MA, editor. *Classic Teachings in Clinical Cardiology. A Tribute to W. Proctor Harvey, M.D.* Volume I and II. Cedar Grove, New Jersey: Laennec Publishing, Inc., 1996:1579, $145.00.

About 100 years ago it was not unusual for trainees of renowned professors of medicine, surgery, or pathology to compile a book in honor of their teacher. Not so in the last 50 years. Dr. Michael Chizner, however, has turned back the clock by gathering 52 of Dr. Proctor Harvey's former fellows to produce a well-rounded cardiology book in honor of their renowned teacher. The result is a fine book.

Smaller General Texts

Kloner RA, editor. *The Guide to Cardiology.* Third Edition. Greenwich, Connecticut: Le Jacq Communications. Inc., 1995:752, $68.00.

This edition is a quarter larger than the second edition. Good book at a good price.

Hillis LD, Lange RA, Winniford MD, Page RL. *Manual of Clinical Problems in Cardiology with Annotated Key References.* Fifth Edition. Boston: Little, Brown and Company, 1995:579, $34.95.

Very useful. Can keep it in the pocket of the white coat.

Crawford MH, editor. *Diagnosis and Treatment in Cardiology.* Norwalk, Connecticut: Appleton & Lange, 1995:498, $41.95.

Coronary Artery Disease and Atherosclerosis

Fuster V, Ross R, Topol EJ, editors. *Atherosclerosis and Coronary Artery Disease.* Volumes One and Two. Philadelphia: Lippincott-Raven Publishers, 1996:1701, $275.00.

Beautiful book. The best book in cardiology appearing in 1995!

Califf RM, Mark DB, Wagner GS, editors. *Acute Coronary Care.* Second Edition. St. Louis: Mosby, 1995:964, $95.00.

Francis GS, Alpert JS, editors. *Coronary Care.* Second Edition. Boston: Little, Brown and Company, 1995:804, $120.00.

Both the Califf and Francis-Alpert books are excellent. The Califf one is larger and less expensive.

Maseri A. *Ischemic Heart Disease. A Rational Basis for Clinical Practice and Clinical Research.* New York: Churchill Livingstone, 1995:713, $99.00.

Attillio Maseri, a major cardiologic investigator on the world scene for the last 2 decades, wrote every word of this fine book.

Ambrose JA, editor. *Complex Coronary Lesions in Acute Coronary Syndromes.* Armonk, New York: Futura Publishing Company, Inc., 1996:267, $65.00.

Koenig W, Hornbach V, Bond MG, Kramsch DM, editors. *Progression and Regression of Atherosclerosis.* Vienna: Blackwell Wissenschaft, 1995:510, $80.00.

This book contains papers presented at an International Symposium in Ulm, Germany, in May 1993. Discussed are imaging techniques and their applications and limitations in epidemiological studies and in clinical trials.

Interventional Cardiology

Ellis SG, Holmes DR Jr. editors. *Strategic Approaches in Coronary Intervention.* Baltimore: Williams & Wilkins, 1996:763, $95.00.

Vetrovec GW, Carabello BA, editors. *Invasive Cardiology, Current Diagnostic and Therapeutic Issues.* Armonk. New York: Futura Publishing Company, Inc., 1996:618, $115.00.

White CJ, Ramee SR, editors. *Interventional Cardiology, New Techniques and Strategies for Diagnosis and Treatment.* New York: Marcel Dekker, Inc., 1995:353, $120.00.

Topol EJ, Serruys PW, editors. *Current Review of Interventional Cardiology.* Second Edition. Philadelphia: Current Medicine, 1995;312, $149.95.

Lutz J, editor. *Complications of Interventional Procedures.* New York: Igaku-Shoin, 1995:248, $73.95.

Freed M, Grines C, Safian R, editors. *Manual of Interventional Cardiology.* Birmingham, Michigan: Physicians' Press, 1996:750, $75.00.

Heart Failure

McCall D, Rahimtoola SH, editors. *Heart Failure.* New York: Chapman & Hall, 1995:436, $79.95.

Dhalla NS, Beamish RE, Takeda N, Nagano M, editors. *The Failing Heart.* Philadelphia: Lippincott-Raven Publishers, 1995:524, $99.00.

Systemic Hypertension

Messerli FH, Aepfelbacher FC, editors. *Hypertension in Postmenopausal Women.* New York: Marcel Dekker, Inc., 1996:298, $79.80.

O'Brien E, Beevers DG, Marshall HJ. *ABC of Hypertension.* Third Edition. London: BMJ Publishing Group, 1995:79, $22.00.

A gem.

Electrocardiography

Levine GN, Podrid PJ. *The ECG Workbook. A Review and Discussion of ECG Findings and Abnormalities.* Armonk, New York: Futura Publishing Company, Inc., 1995:550, $74.00.

Arrhythmias and Conduction Defects

Mandel WJ, editor. *Cardiac Arrhythmias. Their Mechanisms, Diagnosis, and Management.* Third Edition. Philadelphia: JB Lippincott Company, 1995:1266, $165.00.

Saksena S, Lüderitz B, editors. *Interventional Electrophysiology. A Textbook.* Second Edition. Armonk, New York: Futura Publishing Company, Inc., 1996:634, $160.00.

Vlay SC, editor. *A Practical Approach to Cardiac Arrhythmias.* Second Edition, Boston: Little, Brown and Company, 1996:479, $49.95.

Fogoros RN. *Electrophysiologic Testing.* Second Edition. Cambridge, Massachusetts: Blackwell Science, 1995:270, $32.95.

DiMarco JP, Prystowsky EN, editors. *Atrial Arrhythmias. State of the Art.* Armonk, New York: Futura Publishing Company, Inc., 1995:432, $70.00.

Lüderitz B. *History of the Disorders of Cardiac Rhythm.* Armonk, New York: Futura Publishing Company, 1995:167, $75.00.

A splendid little book.

Echocardiography

D'Cruz IA. *Echocardiographic Anatomy. Understanding Normal and Abnormal Echocardiograms.* Stanford, Connecticut: Appleton & Lange, 1996:563, $95.00.

Chambers JB. *Clinical Echocardiography.* London: BMJ Publishing Group, 1995:260, $98.00.

Roelandt JRTC, Pandian NG, editors. *Multiplane Transesophageal Echocardiography.* New York: Churchill Livingstone, 1996:257, $99.00.

Rafferty TD. *Basics of Transesophageal Echocardiography.* New York: Churchill Livingstone, 1995:190, $85.00.

Stress Testing

Ellestad MH (main author), Selvester RHS, Mishkin FS, James FW, Mazumi K (contributors). *Stress Testing, Principles and Practice.* Edition 4. Philadelphia: F.A. Davis Company, 1996:593, $69.95.

This is it in stress testing.

Nuclear Cardiology

Iskandrian AS, Verani MS. *Nuclear Cardiac Imaging: Principles and Applications.* Second Edition, Philadelphia: F.A. Davis Company, 1996:451, $160.00.

Beller GA. *Clinical Nuclear Cardiology.* Philadelphia: W.B. Saunders Company, 1995:387, $95.00.

Both of these books are excellent. Neither is an edited book; one is double authored, the other single authored, both unusual these days. The Beller book is the better buy.

Other Imaging

Adachi H, Nagai J. *Three-Dimensional CT Angiography.* Boston: Little, Brown and Company, 1995:232, $149.95.
Beautiful.
Van Der Wall EE, Blanksma PK, Niemeyer MG, Paans AMJ, editors. *Positron Emission Tomography, Viability, Perfusion, Receptors and Cardiomyopathy.* Dordrecht Kluwer Academic Publishers, 1995:253, $120.00.
DePuey EG, Berman DS, Garcia EV, editors. *Cardiac SPECT Imaging.* New York: Raven Press, 1995:290, $130.00.
Beautiful but expensive. Each page costs 45¢.

Cardiac Catheterization

Baim DS, Grossman W, editors. *Cardiac Catheterization, Angiography and Intervention.* Fifth Edition. Baltimore: Williams & Wilkins, 1996:879, $85.00.
This classic is now an edited book.

Heart Rate Variability

Malik M, Camm AJ, editors. *Heart Rate Variability.* Armonk, New York: Futura Publishing Company, Inc., 1995:543, $98.00.
A needed reference.

Pharmacology and Drug Therapy

Opie IH. *Drugs for the Heart.* Fourth Edition. Philadelphia: W.B. Saunders Company, 1995:377, $29.95.
A jewel for the price.
Khan MG. *Cardiac Drug Therapy.* Fourth Edition. London: W.B. Saunders Company Ltd., 1995:426, $39.00.

Resuscitation

Paradis NA, Halperin HR, Nowak RM, editors. *Cardiac Arrest. The Science and Practice of Resuscitation Medicine.* Baltimore: Williams & Wilkins, 1996:981, $139.00.

Cardiovascular Rehabilitation

Fardy PS, Yanowitz FG, with assistance from Wilson PK. *Cardiac Rehabilitation, Adult Fitness, and Exercise Testing.* Third Edition. Baltimore: Williams & Wilkins, 1995:459, $62.50.

Pediatric Cardiology

Nichols DG, Cameron DE, Greeley WJ, Lappe DG, Ungerleider RM, Wetzel RC, editors. *Critical Heart Disease in Infants and Children.* St. Louis: Mosby, 1995:1069, $175.00.

A major text.

Gewitz MH, editor. *Primary Pediatric Cardiology,* Armonk, New York: Futura Publishing Company, Inc., 1995:482, $85.00.

Gillette PC, Zeigler VL, editors. *Pediatric Cardiac Pacing.* Armonk, New York: Futura Publishing Company, Inc., 1995:254, $45.00.

Guntheroth WG. *Crib Death. The Sudden Infant Death Syndrome.* Armonk, New York: Futura Publishing Company, Inc., 1995:439, $72.00.

Molecular Cardiology

Haber E, editor. *Scientific American Molecular Cardiovascular Medicine.* New York: Scientific American, Inc., 1995;338, $49.00.

Cardiovascular Surgery

Sabiston DC Jr, Spencer FC, editors. *Surgery of the Chest,* Sixth Edition. Volumes I and II. Philadelphia: W.B. Saunders Company, 1995;2174, $295.00.

Beautiful books. Packed full of the latest information.

Sabiston DC Jr, editor. *Atlas of Cardiothoracic Surgery.* Philadelphia: W.B. Saunders Company, 1995:598, $165.00.

Waldhausen JA, Pierce WS, Campbell DB, editors. *Surgery of the Chest.* Sixth Edition. St. Louis: Mosby, 1996:656, $125.00.

684 illustrations but lots of wasted space.

Harlan BJ, Starr A, Harwin FM. *Manual of Cardiac Surgery.* Second Edition. New York: Springer-Verlag, 1995:378, $185.00.

Three hundred sixty three color drawings.

Litwin SB. *Color Atlas of Congenital Heart Surgery.* St. Louis: Mosby, 1996:240, $225.00.

Six hundred twenty seven four-color intraoperative photographs. Some of the anomalies are difficult to discern.

Salerno TA, editor. *Warm Heart Surgery.* London: Arnold, 1995:230, $99.95.

Dean RH, Yao JST, Brewster DC, editors. *Diagnosis & Treatment in Vascular Surgery.* Norwalk, Connecticut: Appleton & Lange, 1995:461, $41.95.

Cardiac Transplantation

Frazier OH, editor, Macris MP and Radovančević, associate editors. *Support and Replacement of the Failing Heart.* Philadelphia: Lippincott-Raven Publishers, 1996:363, $149.95.

Helderman JH, Frist WH, editors. *Grand Rounds in Transplantation.* New York: Chapman & Hall, 1995:233, $69.95.

Basic Cardiovascular Pathophysiology and Electrophysiology

Sperelakis N, editor. *Physiology and Pathophysiology of the Heart.* Third Edition, Boston: Kluwer Academic Publishers, 1995:1173, $395.00.

This is a major reference work of basic cardiology focusing primarily on cardiac ultrastructure, electrophysiology, cardiac contractility, ion exchange, and coronary circulation. Each page costs 34¢.

Sperelakis N. *Electrogenesis of Biopotentials in the Cardiovascular System.* Boston: Kluwer Academic Publishers, 1995:364, $105.00.

Cardiovascular Pathology

Stehbens WE, Lie JT, editors. *Vascular Pathology.* London: Chapman & Hall Medical, 1995:797, $169.00.

Ho SY, Baker EJ, Rigby ML, Anderson RH. *Color Atlas of Congenital Heart Disease, Morphologic and Clinical Correlations.* London: Mosby-Wolfe, 1995:192, $115.00.

Cardiac Economics

Ott R, Tanner T, Henderson B, editors. *Managed Care and the Cardiac Patient.* Philadelphia: Hanley & Belfus, Inc., 1995:334, $45.00.

Miscellaneous

Daniel WG, Kronzon I, Mügge A, editors. *Cardiogenic Embolism.* Baltimore: Williams & Wilkins, 1996:380, $75.00.

Hurst JW. *Cardiac Puzzles.* London: Mosby-Wolfe Medical Communications, 1995:210, $32.95.

Part I of this neat book includes a discussion of the clues the physician must be able to collect from the patient, and Part II includes the presentation of 50 puzzles. The goal of the book appears simple—if one can solve the carefully selected puzzles, he/she will understand most of the principles of cardiovascular medicine. Each puzzle is shown on the right hand page and the discussion is on the back of the page.

Weber KT, editor. *Wound Healing in Cardiovascular Disease.* Armonk, New York: Futura Publishing Company, Inc., 1995:320, $88.00.

Boudoulas H, Toutouzas PK, Wooley CF, editors. *Functional Abnormalities of the Aorta.* Armonk, New York: Futura Publishing Company, Inc., 1996:384, $85.00.

National Diabetes Data Group. *Diabetes in America.* Second Edition. Bethesda, Maryland: National Institutes of Health (NIH Publication No 95-1468), 1995:782, $20.00.

This is a splendid reference volume. Because patients with diabetes mellitus tend to die from complications of atherosclerosis, this book will be of value to cardiovascular specialists. (This book can be obtained from The National Diabetes Information Clearinghouse, National Institute of Diabetes and Digestive and Kidney Diseases, 1 Information Way, Bethesda, Maryland 20892-3560, telephone 301-654-3327.)

DeJong JW, Ferrari R, editors. *The Carnitine System. A New Therapeutical Approach to Cardiovascular Diseases.* Dordrecht: Kluwer Academic Publishers, 1995:393, $250.00.

Cardiologic History

Neill C, Clark EB. *The Developing Heart: A "History" of Pediatric Cardiology.* Dordrecht: Kluwer Academic Publishers, 1995:169, $62.00.

A needed book.

Blackburn H. *On the Trail of Heart Attacks in Seven Countries.* Minneapolis: University of Minnesota, 1995:148, $20.00.

The Seven Countries study was the first to examine systematically the relation among lifestyle, diet, and the roles of heart attack and stroke in contrasting populations. It is the seminal study of cardiovascular disease epidemiology. Dr. Blackburn brings to life the adventures experienced while accumulating the data—both joys and tribulations—in these rural areas around the world.

Snellen HA. *Willhem Einthoven (1860–1927). Father of Electrocardiography, Life and Work, Ancestors and Contemporaries.* Dordrecht, Kluwer Academic Publishers, 1995:140, $40.00.

A splendid little book.

Annual Literature Reviews

Schlant RC, (editor-in-chief); Collins JJ Jr., Engle MA, Gersh BJ, Kaplan NM, Waldo AL, editors. *The 1995 Year Book of CARDIOLOGY.* St. Louis: Mosby, 1995 (October):525, $74.95.

Roberts WC, Rackley CE, Willerson JT, Mason DT, Parmley WW, Graham TP, Jr. *CARDIOLOGY 1995.* Armonk, New York: Futura Publishing Company, Inc., 1995 (June):499, $69.00.

The Schlant book summarizes 304 articles each appearing in either 1993 or 1994. Comments on each article are provided by the various editors. The Roberts book includes summaries of 723 articles, all published in 1994. Its advantage is the larger number of articles discussed and all articles on the same subject are grouped together to read as a chapter; its disadvantage is the opinions of each author are not always discernible. The higher price of the Schlant book and the fewer numbers of articles summarized translates into 25¢ per article; the Roberts book translates into 10¢ per article. I obviously prefer the Roberts book.

Comments

Of the 73 books mentioned herein; 20 (27%) have a 1996 publication date. The pages in the 73 books totalled 38,412, ranging from 79 *(ABC of Hypertension)* to 2,174 (Sabiston and Spencer, *Surgery of the Chest*) (mean 526 pages). The 73 books cost a total of $7,544.50, ranging from $20.00 to $395.00 (mean $103.00); 24 books (33%) cost more than $100.00. The 38,412 pages in the 73 books cost an average of 20¢ each. Of the 73 books, 47 (64%) were edited; 16 (22%) had a single author; 5 (7%) had 2 authors, and the remaining 5 books (7%) had 3 to 6 authors. Only 22 (30%) of the 73 books were published on acid-free (permanent) paper, the same percent as were published on acid-free paper last year. Authors need to stipulate acid-free paper in their contracts with publishers!

1. Swenson JM, Fricker FJ, Armitage JM: Immunosuppression switch in pediatric heart transplant recipients: cyclosporine to FK 506. J Am Coll Cardiol 1995 (April);25:1183–1188.
2. Fullerton DA, Campbell DN, Jones SD, Jaggers J, Brown JM, Wollmering MM, Grover FL, Mashburn C, Luna M, Sondheimer HM, Boucek MM: Heart transplantation in

children and young adults: Early and intermediate-term results. Ann Thorac Surg 1995 (April);59:804–812.

3. Hsu DT, Quaegebeur JM, Michler RE, Smith CR, Rose EA, Kichuk MR, Gersony WM, Douglas JF, Addonizio LJ: Heart transplantation in children with congenital heart disease. J Am Coll Cardiol 1995 (September);26:743–749.

4. Wechsler ME, Giardina EV, Sciacca RR, Rose EA, Barr ML: Increased early mortality in women undergoing cardiac transplantation. Circulation 1995 (February); 91:1029–1035.

5. Natterson PD, Stevenson WG, Saxon LA, Middlekauff HR, Stevenson LW: Risk of arterial embolization in 224 patients awaiting cardiac transplantation. Am Heart J 1995 (March);129:564–570.

6. Ibrahim M, Masters RG Hendry PJ, Davies RA, Smith S, Struthers C, Walley VM, Keon WJ: Determinants of hospital survival after cardiac transplantation. Ann Thor Surg 1995 (March);59:3:604–608.

7. DeCampli WM, Luikart H, Hunt S, Stinson EB: Characteristics of patients surviving more than ten years after cardiac transplantation. J Thorac Cardiovasc Surg 1995 (June);109:6:1103–1115.

8. Keogh A, Spratt P, McCosker C, MacDonald P, Mundy J, Kaan A: Ketoconazole to reduce the need for cyclosporine after cardiac transplantation. N Engl J Med 1995 (September 7);333:628–633.

9. Kobashigawa JA, Katznelson S, Laks H, Johnson JA, Yeatman L, Wang XM, Chia D, Terasaki PI, Sabad A, Cogert GA, Trosian K, Hamilton MA, Moriguchi JD, Kawata N, Hage AN, Drinkwater DC, Stevenson LW: Effect of pravastatin on outcomes after cardiac transplantation. N Engl J Med 1995 (September 7);333:621–627.

10. Smith JD, Rose ML, Pomerance A, Burke M, Yacoub MH: Reduction of cellular rejection and increase in longer-term survival after heart transplantation after HLA-DR matching. Lancet 1995 (November 18);346:1318–1322.

11. Winters GL, Loh E, Schoen FJ: Natural history of focal moderate cardiac allograft rejection. Is treatment warranted? Circulation 1995 (April);91:1975–1980.

12. De Marco T, Dae M, Yuen-Green MSF, Kumar S, Keith F, Amidon TM, Rifkin C, Klinski C, Lau D, Botvinick EH, Chatterjee K: Iodine-123 metaiodobenzylguanidine scintigraphic assessment of the transplanted human heart: Evidence for late reinnervation. J Am Coll Cardiol 1995 (March 15);25:927–931.

13. De Simone R, Lange R, Sack FU, Mehmanesh H, Hagl S: Atrioventricular valve insufficiency and atrial geometry after orthotopic heart transplantation. Ann Thorac Surg 1995 (December);60:1686–1693.

14. Riou B, Dreux S, Roche S, Arthaud M, Goarin J-P, Léger P, Saada M, Viars P: Circulating cardiac troponin T in potential heart transplant donors. Circulation 1995 (August);92:409–414.

15. Pham SM, Kormos RL, Landreneau RJ, Kawai A, Gonzalez-Cancel I, Hardesty RL, Hattler BG, Griffith BP. Solid tumors after heart transplantation: Lethality of lung cancer. Ann Thorac Surg 1995 (December);60:1623–1626.

16. Burke MN, McGinn AL, Homans DC, Christensen BV, Kubo SH, Wilson RF: Evidence for functional sympathetic reinnervation of left ventricle and coronary arteries after orthotopic cardiac transplantation in humans. Circulation 1995 (January);91:72–78.

17. Rickenbacher PT, Pinto FJ, Chenzbraun A, Botas J, Lewis NP, Alderman EL, Valantine JA, Hunt SA, Schroeder JS, Popp RL, Yeung AC: Incidence and severity of transplant coronary artery disease early and up to 15 years after transplantation as detected by intravascular ultrasound. J Am Coll Cardiol 1995 (January 17); 25:171–177.

18. Deng MC, Bell S, Huie P, Pinto F, Hunt SA, Stinson EB, Sibley R, Hall BM, Valantine HA: Cardiac allograft vascular disease. Relationship to microvascular cell surface markers and inflammatory cell phenotypes on endomyocardial biopsy. Circulation 1995 (March);91:1647–1654.

19. Tuzcu EM, Hobbs RE, Rincon G, Bott-Silverman C, De Franco AC, Robinson K, McCarthy PM, Stewart RW, Guyer S, Nissen SE: Occult and frequent transmission of atherosclerotic coronary disease with cardiac transplantation. Insights from intravascular ultrasound. Circulation 1995 (March);91:1706–1713.

20. McGiffin DC, Savunen T, Kirklin JK, Naftel DC, Bourge RC, Paine TD, White-Williams C, Sisto T, Early L: Cardiac transplant coronary artery disease. J Thorac Cardiovasc Surg 1995 (June);109:6:1081–1089.

21. Hosenpud JD, Everett JP, Morris TE, Mauck KA, Shipley GD, Wagner CR: Cardiac allograft vasculopathy: Association with cell-mediated but not humoral alloimmunity to donor-specific vascular endothelium. Circulation 1995 (July);92:205–211.

22. Halle AA, DiSciascio G, Massin EK, Wilson RF, Johnson MR, Sullivan HJ, Bourge RC, Kleiman NS, Miller LW, Aversano TR, Wray RB, Hunt SA, Weston MW, Davies RA, Rincon G, Crandall CC, Cowley MJ, Kubo SH, Fisher SG, Vetrovec GW: Coronary angioplasty, atherectomy and bypass surgery in cardiac transplant recipients. J Am Coll Cardiol 1995 (July);26:120–128.

23. Labarrere CA, Pitts D, Nelson DR, Faulk WP: Vascular tissue plasminogen activator and the development of coronary artery disease in heart-transplant recipients. N Engl J Med 1995 (October 36);333:1111–1116.

24. Bridges ND, Mallory GB Jr, Huddleston CB, Canter CE, Sweet SC, Spray TL: Lung transplantation in children and young adults with cardiovascular disease. Ann Thorac Surg 1995 (April);59:813–821.

25. Panayiotou H, Haitas B, Hollister AS: Atrial wall tension changes and the release of atrial natriuretic factor on relief of cardiac tamponade. Am Heart J 1995 (May);129:960–967.

26. Bommer WJ, Follette D, Pollock M, Arena F, Bognan M, Berkoff H: Tamponade in patients undergoing cardiac surgery: A clinical-echocardiographic diagnosis. Am Heart J 1995 (December);130:1216–1223.

27. Heidenreich PA, Eisenberg MJ, Kee LL, Somelofski CA, Hollander H, Schiller NB, Cheitlin MD: Pericardial effusion in AIDS: Incidence and survival. Circulation 1995 (December);92:3229–3234.

28. Kearon C, Hirsh J: Starting prophylaxis for venous thromboembolism postoperatively. Arch Intern Med 1995 (February 27);155:366–372.

29. Shulman S, Rhedin AS, Lindmarker P, Carlsson A, Larfars G, Nicol P, Loogna E, Svensson E, Ljungberg B, Walter H, Viering S, Nordlander S, Leijd B, Jonsson KA, Hjorth M, Linder O, Boberg J, and the Duration of Anticoagulation Trial Study Group: A comparison of six weeks with six months of oral anticoagulant therapy after a first episode of venous thromboembolism. N Engl J Med 1995 (June 22); 332:25:1661–1665.

30. Uchida Y, Oshima T, Hirose J, Sasaki T, Morizuki S, Morita T: Angioscopic detection of residual pulmonary thrombi in the differential diagnosis of pulmonary embolism. Am Heart J 1995 (October);130:854–859.

31. Finkbohner R, Johnston D, Crawford ES, Coselli J, Milewicz DM: Marfan syndrome. Long-term survival and complications after aortic aneurysm repair. Circulation 1995 (February);91:728–733.

32. Gott V L, Gillinov AM, Pyeritz RE, Cameron DE, Reitz BA, Greene PS, Stone CD, Ferris RL, Alejo DE, McKusick VA: Aortic root replacement. J Thorac Cardiovasc Surg 1995 (March);109:3:536–545.

33. Elkayam U, Ostrzega E, Shotan A, Mehra A: Cardiovascular problems in pregnant women with the Marfan syndrome. Ann Intern Med 1995 (July 15);123:117–122

34. Demopoulos LA, Tunick PA, Bernstein NE, Perez JL, Kronzon I: Protruding atheromas of the aortic arch in symptomatic patients with carotid artery disease. Am Heart J 1995 (January);129:40–44.

35. Stone DA, Hawke MW, LaMonte M, Kittner SJ, Acosta J, Corretti M, Sample C, Price TR, Plotnick GD: Ulcerated atherosclerotic plaques in the thoracic aorta are associated with cryptogenic stroke: A multiplane transesophageal echocardiographic study. Am Heart J 1995 (July);130:105–108.

36. Baird PA, Sadovnick AD, Yee IML, Cole CW, Cole L: Sibling risks of abdominal aortic aneurysm. Lancet 1995 (September 2);346:601–604.

37. Bayazit M, Gol MK, Battaloglu B, Tokmakoglu H, Tasdemir O, Bayazit K: Routine coronary arteriography before abdominal aortic aneurysm repair. Am J Surg 1995 (September);170:246–250.

38. Steyerberg EW, Kievit J, de Mol Van Otterloo A, van Bockel JH, Eijkemans MJC, Habbema JDF: Perioperative mortality of elective abdominal aortic aneurysm surgery. Arch Intern Med 1995 (October 9);155:1998–2004.

39. Creswell LL, Kouchoukos NT, Cox JL, Rosenbloom M: Coronary artery disease in patients with type A aortic dissection. Ann Thor Surg 1995 (March);59:3:585–590.
40. Roman MJ, Pickering TG, Schwartz JE, Pini R, Devereux RB: Association of carotid atherosclerosis and left ventricular hypertrophy. J Am Coll Cardiol 1995 (January);25:83–90.
41. The European Carotid Trialists Collaborative Group: Risk of stroke in the distribution of an asymptomatic carotid artery. Lancet 1995 (January 28);345:209–212.
42. Salenius JP, Harju E, Jokela H, Riekkinen H, and Silvasti M: Long term effects of guar gum on lipid metabolism after carotid endarterectomy. Br Med J 1995 (January 14);310:95–96.
43. Selhub J, Jacques PF, Bostom AG, D'Agostino RB, Wilson PWF, Belanger AJ, O'Leary DH, Wolf PA, Schaefer EJ, Roseberg IH: Association between plasma homocysteine concentrations and extracranial carotid-artery stenosis. N Engl J Med 1995 (February 2);322:5:286–297.
44. Crouse JR III, Byington RP, Bond MG, Espeland MA, Craven TE, Sprinkle JW, McGovern ME, Furberg CD: Pravastatin, Lipids, and Atherosclerosis in the Carotid Arteries (PLAC-II). Am J Cardiol 1995 (March 1);75:455–459.
45. Executive Committee for the Asymptomatic Carotid Atherosclerosis study: Endarterectomy for asymptomatic carotid artery stenosis. JAMA 1995 (May 10);273:1421–1428.
46. Kent KC, Kuntz KM, Patel MR, Kim D, Klufas RA, Whittemore AD, Polak JF, Skillman JJ, Edelman RR: Perioperative imaging strategies for carotid endarterectomy. JAMA 1995 (September 20);274:888–893.
47. Côté R, Battista RN, Abrahamowicz M, Langlois Y, Bourque F, Mackey A, and the Asymptomatic Cervical Bruit Study Group: Lack of effect of aspirin in asymptomatic patients with carotid bruits and substantial carotid narrowing. Ann Intern Med 1995 (November 1);123:469–655.
48. Baum RA, Rutter CM, Sunshine JH, Blebea JS, Blebea J, Carpenter JP, Dickey KW, Quinn SF, Gomes AS, Grist TM, McNeil BJ, the American College of Radiology Rapid Technology Assessment Group: Multicenter trial to evaluate vascular magnetic resonance angiography of the lower extremity. JAMA 1995 (September 20);274:875–880.
49. Vanderschueren S, Stockx L, Wilms G, Lacroix H, Verhaeghe R, Vermylen J, Collen D: Thrombolytic therapy of peripheral arterial occlusion with recombinant staphylokinase. Circulation 1995 (October);92:2050–2057.
50. Brevetti G, Perna S, Sabba C, Martone VD, Condorelli M: Proprionyl-L-carnitine in intermittent claudication: Double-blind, placebo-controlled, dose titration, multicenter study. J Am Coll Cardiol 1995 (November 15);26:1411–1416.
51. Benjamin EJ, D'Agostino RB, Belanger AJ, Wolf PA, Levy D: Left atrial size and the risk of stroke and death. The Framingham heart study. Circulation 1995 (August);92:835–841.
52. Manning WJ, Weintraub RM, Waksmonski CA, Haering JM, Rooney PS, Maslow AD, Johnson RG, Douglas PS: Accuracy of transesophageal echocardiography for identifying left atrial thrombi. Ann Intern Med 1995 (December 1);123:817–822.
53. Mügge A, Daniel WG, Angermann C, Spes C, Khandheria BK, Kronzon I, Freedberg RS, Keren A, Dennig K, Engberding R, Sutherland GR, Vered Z, Erbel R, Visser CA, Lindert O, Hausmann D, Wenzlaff P: Atrial septal aneurysm in adult patients: A multicenter study using transthoracic and transesophageal echocardiography. Circulation 1995 (June);91:2785–2792.
54. Franklin BA, Hogan P, Bonzheim K, Bakalyar D, Terrien E, Gordon S, Timmis GC: Cardiac demands of heavy snow shoveling. JAMA 1995 (March 15);273:11:880–882.
55. Robiolio PA, Rigolin VH, Wilson JS, Harrison JK, Sanders LL, Bashore TM, Feldman JM: Carcinoid heart disease. Correlation of high serotonin levels with valvular abnormalities detected by cardiac catheterization and echocardiography. Circulation 1995 (August);92:790–795.
56. Sandoval J, Bauerle O, Gomez A, Palomar A, Guerra MLM, Furuya ME: Primary pulmonary hypertension in children: clinical characterization and survival. J Am Coll Cardiol (February) 1995;25:466–474.

57. Giaid A, Saleh D: Reduced expression of endothelial nitric oxide synthase in the lungs of patients with pulmonary hypertension. N Engl J Med 1995 (July 27);333:214–221.

58. Herve P, Launay JM, Scrobohaci ML, Brenot F, Simonneau G, Petitpretz P, Poubeau P, Cerrina J, Duroux P, Drouet L: Increased plasma serotonin in primary pulmonary hypertension. Am J Med 1995 (September);99:249–254.

59. Freedman RR, Baer RP, Mayes MD: Blockade of vasospastic attacks by α_2-adrenergic but not α_1-adrenergic antagonists in idiopathic Raynaud's disease. Circulation 1995 (September);92:1448–1451.

60. Shirani J, Yousefi J, Roberts WC: Major cardiac findings at necropsy in 366 American octogenarians. Am J Cardiol 1995 (January 15);75:151–156.

61. Roberts WC. Good cardiologic books appearing in 1995. Am J Cardiol 1996 (January);77:111-114.

Author Index

Abdelmeguid, A.E., 121
Abrams, J., 98
Adatla, I., 410
Aguirre, F.V., 123, 253
Akins, C.W., 155
Alexander, M., 425
Alfonso, F., 75
Allen, J.K., 159
Allison, T.G., 63
Ambrosioni, E., 230
Ammar, A., 286
Anderson, J.W., 18
Anderson, T.J., 106
Arbustini, E., 136
Ardissino, D., 103
Ascherio, A., 52
Atger, V., 12
Atkison, P., 362
Australia-New Zealand Heart Failure Research Collaborative Group, 437
Avanzini, F., 222
Ayanian, J.Z., 161
Azizi, M., 332

Backer, C.L., 371
Baird, P.A., 463
Bando, K., 371, 402
Barbagelata, A., 251
Barbash, G.I., 238
Barsky, A.J., 309
Bartorelli, A.L., 145
Baudet, E.M., 342
Bauer, J.H., 329
Bauersfeld, U., 393
Baum, R.A., 470
Bauters, C., 135, 255
Bayazit, M., 465
Behar, S., 181, 195
Behrendt, D.M., 384
Belardinelli, R., 356
Bell, M.R., 120, 121
Bellinger, D.C., 409
Benditt, D.G., 296
Benjamin, E.J., 471
Berger, P.B., 153
Berger, R.M.F., 413
Bernstein, H.S., 401
Berntsen, R.F., 283, 286
Bertolet, B.D., 223
Bhatnagar, D., 5
Bittl, J.A., 124
Black, M.D., 408

Blackshear, J.L., 427
Blair, S.N., 34
Bogaert, J., 388
Bommer, W.J., 458
Bondestam, E., 258
Boushey, C.J., 48
Boylan, M.J., 152
Brand, D.A., 221
Brawn, W.J., 407
Bredie, S.J.H., 24
Brevetti, G., 470
Bridges, N.D., 457
Brink, P.A., 300
Brooks, R., 301
Brouwer, J., 102
Brown, E.J., Jr., 435
Bueno, H., 208
Bu'Lock, F.A., 385
Burchfiel, C.M., 7
Burke, M.N., 452
Burke, R.P., 410
Burnett, R.E., 200
Byington, R.P., 107

CABRI Trial Participants, 113
Calkins, H., 293, 295
Calvin, J.E., 79
Cameron, A.A.C., 159
Cane, M.E., 151
Cannan, C.R., 358
Cannegieter, S.C., 348
Cannistra, L.B., 259
Cannon, C.P., 199
Cantin, B., 11
Caracciolo, E.A., 76, 163
Carney, R.M., 63
Carroll, R.J., 65
Carstensen, S., 226
Casino, P.R., 42
Cecchin, F., 405
Cetta, F., 365, 415
Channer, K.S., 221
Chen, C.-R., 337
Chen, L., 81
Cheriex, E.C., 215
Chester, M.R., 89
Child, J.S., 363
Chinese Cardiac Study Collaborative Group, 223
Christakis, G.T., 157
Chung, M.K., 207
Cianflone, D., 80

Clark, R.E., 148
Clinical Quality Improvement Network Investigators, 61
Cohen, A., 151, 213
Cohen, D.J., 146
Cohen, M.B., 296
Col, N.F., 189
Colan, S.D., 380
Coles, J.H., 398
Collins, L.J., 273
Collins, P., 112
Colombo, A., 141
Conte, S., 389
Cook, N.R., 316
Coronary Angioplasty versus Bypass Revascularisation Investigation (CABRI) Trial Participants, 113
Corti, M.C., 9
Cosgrove, D.M., 347
Côte, R., 469
Cox, C., 21
Craver, J.M., 153
Creswell, L.L., 257, 466
Criqui, M.H., 51
Crouse, J.R., III, 468
Crozier, I., 434
Cullen, S., 376
Currie, P.F., 362
Curtis, A.B., 307
Czernin, J., 39

Dalery, K., 47
Danchin, N., 122
Daoud, E.G., 155, 308
David, T.E., 340
Davies, R.F., 104
Day, R.W., 406
The DCCT Research Group, 41
DeCampli, W.M., 447
de Feyter, P.J., 83
de Groote, P., 131
Delius, R.E., 385
Della Bella, P., 278
De Marco, T., 450
Demopoulos, L.A., 463
Deng, M.C., 453
Den Heijer, M., 47
Denke, M.A., 21, 29, 45
De Simone, R., 452
Desmarais, R.L., 133
Desmet, W., 132
Detre, K., 129
Devlin, W., 208
Devries, S., 69
de Winter, R.J., 198
Dhala, A., 293

The Diabetes Control and Complications Trial (DCCT) Research Group, 41
Dickstein, K., 434
Diekman, T., 16
Dinarevic, S., 379
Diodati, J.G., 104
DiSalvo, T.G., 428
Dodo, H., 393
Donofrio, M.T., 373
Dorogy, M.E., 197
Dubois-Rande, J.L., 43
Duflou, J., 290
Durand, J.-B., 357

Eeckhout, E., 148
Eisenberg, S.J., 283
Elkayam, U., 462
Ellenbogen, K.A., 276
Ellerbeck, E.F., 191
Elliot, W.J., 326
Elliott, J.M., 137
Ellis, S.G., 125
El-Tamimi, H., 91
Eltchaninoff, H., 215
Engvall, J., 387
Enriquez-Sarano, M., 338
Eriksen, U.H., 134
The European Atrial Fibrillation Trial Study Group, 274
The European Carotid Trialists Collaborative Group, 466
Executive Committee for Asymptomatic Carotid Atherosclerosis Study, 468
Ezekowitz, M.D., 271

Fall, C.H.D., 50
Fallen, E.L., 101
Farb, A., 139, 292
Faxon, D.P., 132
Fedderly, R.T., 374
Feinberg, W.M., 270
Fenrich, A.L., 395
Ferrari, R., 431
Ferrick, K.J., 287
Ferrieres, J., 65
Figueras, J., 216
Finkbohner, R., 461
Fischer, B., 278
Fitch, L.L., 217
Flack, J.M., 202
Flaker, G.C., 270
Flegal, K.M., 38
Flegel, K.M., 269
Fleming, F., 411
Fletcher, S.C., 387
Flickenger, A.L, 318
Fogelman, R., 397

Forbess, J.M., 386
Fourth International Study of Infarct
    Survival (ISIS-4) Collaborative
    Group, 224
Franklin, B.A., 473
Frasure-Smith, N., 209
Freedman, R.R., 475
Freedman, S.B., 99
Freis, E.D., 326
Frishman, W.H., 112
Frohwein, S., 72
Frommelt, M.A., 400
Fuchs, J., 88
Fujiwara, R., 14
Fullerton, D.A., 445

Gage, B.F., 275
Galerani, M., 15
Ganz, L.I., 281
Garcia-Dorado, D., 98
Garg, R., 432
Garguichevich, J.J., 287
Gatzoulls, M.A., 376
Gaynor, J.W., 384, 390
Ge, J., 66
Gebara, O.C.E., 45
Gersh, B.J., 257
Geva, T., 374
Gheorghiade, M., 435
Ghods, M., 158
Giaid, A., 475
Gibbons, L.W., 29
Giles, W.H., 181
Gilligan, D.M., 44
Glantz, S.A., 40
Glower, D.D., 345
Glueck, C.J., 46
Glynn, R.J., 316
Göbel, E.J.A.M., 86
Gogia, H., 439
Gold, M.R., 441
Goldberg, R.J., 1
Goldhaber, S.Z., 159
Goldstein, S., 282
Good, J.M., 438
Goode, G.K., 42
Gott, V.L., 461
Gould, K.L., 20
Gournay, V., 379
Greenberg, B., 433
Grines, C.L., 238
Grossman, E., 315
Grubb, N.R., 289
Grumbach, K., 150
Guadagnoli, E., 185
Gueret, P., 349
Gurfinkel, E., 84, 105

Haft, J.I., 140
Hall, S.A., 438
Halle, A.A., 456
Hamer, M.E., 281
Hamilton, V.H., 22
Hamm, C.W., 141
Han, T.S., 32
Hannan, E.L., 166
Harlan, W.R., III, 160
Harrington, R.A., 255
Harris, W.O., 121
Harrison, D.A., 405
Hartley, L.H., 224
Hartz, A.J., 162
Hasche, E.T., 202
He, G.W., 346
Hebert, P.R., 15
Heck, I., 433
Heidenreich, P.A., 459
Helbing, W.A., 411
Heller, R.F., 290
Henneln, H.A., 375
Heras, M., 345
Heric, B., 361
Hernández, M., 283
Herrmman, W., 110
Herve, P., 475
Hirooka, K., 412
Hirschl, M.M., 326
Hollander, J.E., 65, 196
Holley, D.G., 414
Holmes, D.R., 215
Holmes, D.R., Jr., 120, 121
Holmvang, G., 369
Hornberger, L.K., 374, 413
Hosenpud, J.D., 456
Hou, Z.-Y., 295
Houston, M.C., 315
Hsu, D.T., 445
Hsu, H., 406
Hueb, W.A., 118
Hundley, W.G., 338
Hunninghake, D.B., 27

Ibrahim, M., 447
Ikeda, H., 85
Imai, K., 55
Ing, F.F., 398
Iribarren, C., 5, 8, 15, 33
Isaacs, A.J., 46
ISIS-4 Collaborative Group, 224
Itoh, A., 132
Iwasaki, K., 250

Jacobs, M.L., 408
Jacobson, T.A., 23
Jadonath, R.L., 285
Jain, D., 93

Jamieson, W.R.E., 343
Javaheri, S., 427
Jenkins, K.J., 414
Jha, P., 30
Jiang, X., 13
Johnson, R.G., 152
Johnston, C.I., 329
Johnston, D.L., 71
Jones, J.K., 321
Jonsson, H., 376
Jordaens, L., 303
Jorenby, D.E., 37
Juillìere, Y, 64
Jukema, J.W., 107
Juliusson, G., 16

Kaikita, K., 96
Karetzky, M., 289
Karnash, S.L., 237
Kasiske, B.L., 324
Kaski, J.C., 81, 95
Katzel, L.I., 34
Kaufmann, R.B., 70
Kavey, R.-E.W., 401
Kawachi, I., 52, 292
Kawano, S., 358
Kawasuji, M., 154
Kearon, C., 459
Keil, J.E., 50
Kelley, J.R., 404
Kendall, M.J., 291
Kent, K.C., 469
Keogh, A., 447
Kessler, D.K., 309
Khosla, S., 101
Kiemeneij, F., 119, 143, 144
Kim, S.G., 307
Kimmel, S.E., 127
Kiowski, W., 430
Kirlin, P.C., 429
Kitazume, H., 129
Klein, M., 158
Klemperer, J.D., 162
Kloner, R.A., 238
Kobashigawa, J.A., 448
Køober, L., 228, 229
Koifman, B., 440
Kokkinos, P.F., 17, 319
Kondo, C., 378
Konstantinides, S., 369
Kornowski, R., 426
Kottkamp, H., 355
Kowey, P.R., 287
Koyama, J., 74
Krahn, A.D., 270
Kremastinos, D.Th., 364
Krittayaphong, R., 78
Krum, H., 437

Krumholz, H.M., 219
Kuhn, M.A., 404
Kullo, I.J., 364
Kurnik, P.B., 239
Kussmaul, W.G., 124

Laarman, G., 144
Labarrere, C.A., 456
Lacoste, L., 109
Lakkis, N.M., 164
Laks, H., 391, 403
Lamas, G.A., 223
Lane, D.M., 31
Laperche, T., 249
Lapinleimu, H., 19
Launer, L.J., 317
Lavie, C.J., 258
Lean, M.E.J., 32
Leclercq, C., 301
Lee, D.-Y., 74
Lee, I.M., 35
Lee, J.G., 62
Lee, K.L., 252
Leenhardt, A., 395
Lefkovits, J., 165
Legault, S.E., 93
Lemaitre, R.N., 35
Lenderink, T., 241
Levin, H.R., 441
Liao, Y., 49
Lichtlen, P.R., 96
Lieberman, E.B., 339
Limas, C.J., 357
Lincoff, A.M., 248
Lindpaintner, K., 54
Lipshultz, S.E., 362
Liu, M.W., 143
Lorenz, C.H., 382
Lystash, J.C., 214

Maes, A., 250
Maher, V.M.G., 28
Maheswaran, B., 75
Mainwaring, R.D., 401
Mairesse, G.H., 300
Maki, D.D., 325
Mancini, D.M., 440
Mangano, D.T., 61
Manning, W.J., 277, 280, 471
Manolio, T.A., 320
Manson, J.E., 32
Mark, D.B., 243
Marlmberg, K., 230
Maron, B.J., 357
Marsico, F., 140
Marx, G.R., 369
Mason, J.J., 61
Mason, J.W., 365

Materson, B.J., 321
Mathew, J., 342
Matsubara, K., 93
Matsui, S., 428
Matsumori, A., 366
Maynard, C., 243
McConnell, M.V., 390
McCully, R.B., 78
McGiffin, D.C., 455
McKendall, G.R., 256
McPherson, D.D., 64
Meijboom, F., 377
Mercando, A.D., 210
Michaelsson, M., 396
Mickley, H., 205
Middlekauff, H.R., 276
Miller, T.D., 210
Mintz, G.S., 73
Mittleman, M.A., 188
Mohr, F.W., 156
Moliterno, D.J., 123
Montalescot, G., 134
Morillo, C.A., 294
Morishima, I., 256
Mosca, R.S., 386
Moshkovitz, Y., 167
Moss, A.J., 299
Mueller, H.S., 251
Mugge, A., 471
Mullany, C.J., 340
Muller-Bardorff, M., 197
Murgatroyd, F.D., 277
Muscari, A., 190

Nadeau, C., 102
Nahser, P.J., 41
Nakagawa, Y., 205
Nakamura, S., 138
Natale, A., 294
Natterson, P.D., 446
Naylor, C.D., 150
Nease, R.J., Jr., 89
Neil, H.A.W., 21
Nĕskovic, A.N., 212
Niebauer, J., 92
Nieto, F.J., 1
Nihoyannopoulos, P., 94
Nir, A., 414
Nishi, H., 360
Nishimura, R.A., 441
Nunain, S.O., 306
Nwasokwa, O.N., 148
Nygard, O., 48

O'Connor, N.J., 187
Odim, J., 409
Okita, Y., 377
Olsen, S.L., 437

Omland, T., 209
O'Neill, W.W., 350
Orszulak, T.A., 343
Osswald, S., 304
O'Sullivan, J.J., 394
Ottani, F., 239
Ozaki, Y., 97, 145
Ozbek, C., 244

Pagani, F.D., 379
Palacios, I.F., 335
Pan, M., 142
Panayiotou, H., 457
Panza, J.A., 318
Papa, M., 389
Parish, S., 188
Parker, J.D., 98
Parker, J.O., 100
Parks, W.J., 388
Parldon, S.M., 415
Pasceri, V., 201
Patterson, R.E., 67
Paul, S.D., 186
Pellikka, P.A., 72
The PEPI Group, 43
Peters, R.W., 291
Petursson, M.K., 75
Pfammatter, J.P., 394, 395
Pham, S.M., 451
Picano, E., 212
Piehler, J.M., 351
Pilote, L., 216
Pinski, S.L., 301
Pocock, S.J., 114
Podrid, P.J., 310
Post, J.C., 390
Post, J.R., 336
The Postmenopausal Estrogen/Progestin
    Interventions   (PEPI) Group, 43
Poty, H., 279
Pouleur, H., 348
Powell, A.J., 399
Presbitero, P., 383
Prospective Studies Collaborators, 2
Psaty, B.M., 320
Pu, M., 337

Raitt, M.H., 304
Ralph-Edwards, A.C., 389
Ramaciotti, C., 372
Ramanathan, K.B., 62
Ramsey, M.W., 431
Randin, D., 332
Rao, P.S., 388
Rechavia, E., 142
Reddy, V.M., 378, 399
Reese, D.B., 284
Reimold, S.C., 269

Remmell-Dow, D.R., 385
Res, J.C.J, 199
Rhodes, L.A., 380, 393
Ribera, M., 12
Rich, M.W., 425
Rickenbacher, P.T., 453
Ricou, F.J., 82
Ridker, P.M., 53
Rihal, C.S., 154
Riou, B., 451
Robiolio, P.A., 473
Rodriguez, A.E., 141
Roger, V.L., 72
Rogers, W.J., 231
Roguin, N., 373
Roman, M.J., 466
Romeo, F., 248
Rosenthal, D.N., 405
Rubins, H.B., 14
Rumberger, J.A., 69
Rychik, J., 405

Sachs, D.P.L., 37
Sacks, F.M., 110
Salenius, J.P., 467
Salim, M.A., 416
Salomaa, V., 51
Salonen, J.T., 51
Sandhu, S.K., 406
Sandoval, J., 474
Sano, T., 383
Saumarez, R.C., 359
Saxon, L.A., 432
Scandinavian Simvastatin Survival
    Study Group, 110
Schaefer, E.J., 20
Schnohr, P., 188
Schreiber, T.L., 79
Schroder, R., 249
Schrott, H.G., 27
Schulman, S.P., 228
Schwartz, P.J., 299
Scully, H.E., 346
Selhub, J., 467
Seraff, A., 382
Serneri, G.G.N., 86
Serraf, A., 407
Serruys, P.W., 135
Shechter, M., 222
Shen, W.-K., 291
Shepherd, J., 23
Shim, D., 397
Shimon, I., 439
Shinozaki, K., 96
Shirani, J., 476
Shulman, S., 460
Sigfusson, G., 370
Sigurdsson, E., 191

Sigwart, U., 361
Silva, J.A., 83
Silverman, M.E., 430
Sim, I., 115
Simes, R.J., 252
Singh, B.N., 288
Singh, S.N., 439
Siscovick, D.S., 292
Sluysmans, T., 375
Smalling, R.W., 246
Smit, J.W., 24
Smith, J., 221
Smith, J.D., 449
Sohn, D.W., 72
Sommer, R.J., 396
Sowden, A.J., 149
Spence, J.D., 28
Spertus, J.A., 185
Srivastava, D., 412
Stanbridge, R.D.L., 166
Stauffer, J.-C., 145
Stein, B., 130
Steinberg, J.S., 279
Stengård, J.H., 11
Stevenson, W.G., 426
Steyerberg, E.W., 465
Stoddard, M.F., 277, 338
Stone, D.A., 463
Stone, G.W., 235, 251
Stratmann, H.G., 80
Strauss, W.E., 128
Straznicky, N.E., 23
Stroes, E.S.G., 46
Stumper, O., 383, 399
Sung, R.J., 282
Sweany, A.E., 26
Sweeney, M.O., 308
Swenson, J.M., 445
Szabo, B.M., 284

Tabata, H., 213
Taddei, S., 319
Tan, H.L., 296
Tanel, R.E., 391
Tçheng, J.E., 123
Theroux, P., 246
Thompson, G.R., 30
Thompson, S.G., 89
Thomson, S.P., 196
Tingleff, J., 341
Tokgozoglu, L.S., 363
Tornos, M.P., 340
Trappe, H.-J., 301
Treasure, C.B., 105
Triedman, J.K., 394
Tulloh, R.M.R., 393
Turley, K., 381, 391
Tuzcu, E.M., 453

Uchida, Y., 91, 460
Uemura, H., 400, 404
UK Propafenone PSVT Study Group, 281
Umans, V.A., 139
Unsworth-White, M.J., 162
Urban, P., 143
Urbano-Marquez, A., 355
Uva, Ms., 392

Vaarala, O., 53
Vacek, J.L., 236
Vallejo, J.L., 335
van Arsdell, G.S., 371
Van Bergen, P.F.M.M., 219
van der Lugt, A., 125
Vanderschueren, S., 247, 470
Van de Werf, F., 232
Vanhees, L., 212
Vanoli, E., 199
van Son, J.A.M., 384
van Veldhuisen, D.J., 436
Verma, R., 411
Verschuren, W.M.M., 6, 8
Villari, B., 339
Villella, A., 206
Violaris, A.G., 133
Viskin, S., 220

Waksman, R., 136
Wallen, N.H., 103
Walter, H.L., III, 408
Walton, C., 33
Wannamethee, G., 9
Ward, C.J.B., 397
Warner, J.G., Jr., 260

Waters, D., 106
Watkins, H., 360
Webber, S.A., 400
Weber, M.A., 329
Wechsler, M.E., 446
Wediner, P.W., 386
Weiner, D.A., 77, 94
Weintraub, W.S., 115
Welty, F.K., 256
Wernovsky, G., 380, 381
Wever, E.F.D., 305
Wilder, L.B., 13
Wilke, N.A., 67
Willett, W.C., 31
Williams, D.B., 151
Wilson, J.R., 428
Winters, G.L., 450
Wolfe, M.W., 126
Wood, M.A., 304
Wu, M.-H., 372

Yacoub, M., 348
Yamamoto, H., 136
Yankah, A.C., 403
Yokoshiki, H., 249
Young, D., 18
Young, T.K., 34

Zahger, D., 244
Zarembski, D.G., 280
Zeiher, A.M., 38
Zhang, H.P., 335
Zhou, Q., 373
Zhu, D.W.X., 288
Zipes, D.P., 307
Zuppiroli, A., 338

Subject Index

Abdominal aortic aneurysm, 463-465
  in bypass surgery, 156-157
Ablation, radiofrequency catheter
  in atrial fibrillation, 278-280
  in ventricular arrhythmias, 288
    with dilated cardiomyopathy, 355-356
Abrupt closure with coronary angioplasty, 122
Acetylcholine, hypertension and, 318-319
Acquired immunodeficiency syndrome, 459
Acute closure with coronary angioplasty, 122
Acute myocardial infarction, 181-268.
  See also Myocardial infarction
Adenosine in stress testing, 71
Aerobic exercise in coronary artery disease, 34
Age
  atrial fibrillation and, 270-272, 274
  bypass surgery and, 151
  hypertrophic cardiomyopathy and, 357-358
  lipids levels in, 9
  myocardial infarction and, 188-189, 205, 207-208
    cardiac procedure rates for, 182, 184
    mortality in, 183, 207
    rehabilitation for, 258
  necropsy and, 476
  unstable angina pectoris and, 82-83
AIDS, 459
Alcohol use and alcoholism
  in dilated cardiomyopathy, 355
  in hypertension, 332
Allografts in congenital heart disease, 402-403
Alteplase in thrombolysis, 233, 246, 247
Ambulatory electrocardiography, 309
Amiloride in hypertension, 323
Amiodarone, 310
  in atrial fibrillation, 276, 280
  in congestive heart failure, 439
  in ventricular arrhythmias, 286-288
  in ventricular tachycardia, 395
Amlodipine in myocardial ischemia, 104-105
Anastomotic procedures in congenital

heart disease, 399-402
Aneurysms
  abdominal aortic, 463-465
    in bypass surgery, 156-157
  in aortic isthmic coarctation, 388
  atrial septal, 471-473
  intravascular ultrasound in, 66-67
Angina pectoris
  after bypass surgery, 159
  diltiazem in, 102
  myocardial infarction and, 195, 205, 213
  rest, 119-120
  stable, 88-92
    nitroglycerin patch in, 98-99
  in syndrome X, 95-98
  thrombolysis and, 238-239
  unstable, 79-88
    angiography in, 80-83
    angioscopy in, 83-84
    aspirin in, 86
    atherectomy in, 136-137
    diltiazem in, 86, 87
    glyceryl trinitrate in, 86, 87
    heparin in, 86
    hirulog in, 88
    ischemic threshold in, 84-85
    management of, 79
    P-selectin in, 85
    risk stratification in, 79-80
    thrombotic reactant markers in, 84
    ultrasonography in, 83-84
Angiography
  in coronary artery disease, 67-68
  in coronary occlusion, 75
  in myocardial infarction, 181-185
  in unstable angina pectoris, 81-82
    of arterial narrowing, 80
    in octogenarians, 82-83
Angiopeptin after PTCA, 134
Angioplasty
  in aortic isthmic coarctation, 387-388
  atherectomy in, 136-148
    stenting with, 141-148
  bivalirudin after, 124
  bypass surgery and, 152-153, 165
  in coronary artery disease, 113-119
  costs of, 125-126, 127
  diabetes and, 130, 131
  follow-up for, 129-130
  hemostatic device in, 124-125
  hospital stay after, 126-128

in-laboratory closure in, 121-122
in men vs. women, 120-121
in myocardial infarction, 255-257
platelet inhibition in, 122-124
quality of life after, 128-129
in rest angina pectoris, 119-120
restenosis in, 131-136
for saphenous venous graft narrowing, 120
sixty-millimeter balloon in, 121
transradial approach to, 119
ultrasonography after, 125
Angioscopy
  of coronary arteries, 75-76
  after PTCA, 132
  in stable angina pectoris, 91
  in unstable angina pectoris, 83-84
Angiotensin-converting enzyme inhibitors
  in atherosclerosis, 54-55
  in congestive heart failure, 432-433, 435-436
  in hypertension, 320, 322
  in myocardial infarction, 193, 194, 221-222
Angiotensin-receptor antagonist in hypertension, 329
Anistreplase in thrombolysis, 233, 244
Anomalous pulmonary venous connection, 389-390
Antiarrhythmic drugs
  atrial fibrillation and, 269
  classification of, 297
  in myocardial infarction, 222-223
Antibodies in atherosclerosis, 53
Anticoagulants
  in aortic valve replacement, 348-349
  in atrial fibrillation, 273-275
  in coronary stenting, 141, 144-145
  in myocardial infarction, 219-222
  in PTCA, 122-124
  in venous embolism, 460
Antihypertensive agents, 319-320
  myocardial infarction from, 320-321
  renal function and, 325-326
Antioxidant vitamins in hyperlipidemia, 29-30
Antiphospholipid antibodies in atherosclerosis, 53
Aorta
  arch of, obstructed, 406-407
  atresia of, 385-387
  coarctation of, 387-389
Aortic disorders, 461-466
  aneurysms in, 463-465
    in bypass surgery, 156-157
  dissection in, 466
  Marfan syndrome in, 461-463

prosthetic replacement in
  homovital homografts for, 348
  in Marfan syndrome, 461-462
  pericardial, 347
  with small aortic root, 346-347
  protruding plaque in, 463
  regurgitation in, 340
  stenosis in, 339-340, 384-385
Aorto-ostial stents, 142-143
Apheresis, lipoprotein, 30-31
Apolipoprotein E in atherosclerosis, 11-12
Arbutamine in stress testing, 71
L-Arginine
  in congestive heart failure, 440
  endothelial function and, 43
Arrhythmias, 269-314
  ambulatory electrocardiography in, 309
  amiodarone in, 310
  bundle branch block and, 300
  cardiac arrest and, 289-293
  cardioverters-defibrillators in, 301-308
  in congenital heart disease, 393-396
  fibrillation in, 269-281. *See also* Atrial fibrillation
  genetics in, 299
  heart block and, 300
  long QT interval syndrome and, 296-298
  pacemakers for, 300-301
  palpitations in, 309
  supraventricular tachycardia in, 281-282
  syncope and, 293-296
  ventricular, 282-288
    amiodarone in, 286-288
    bretylium in, 287-288
    coronary narrowing in, 286
    origin of, 285
    procainamide in, 288
    prognostic predictors in, 282-285
    radiofrequency catheter ablation in, 288
    sotalol in, 288
Arterial disease
  atherosclerosis in, 1-60. *See also* Atherosclerosis
  coronary, 61-179. *See also* Coronary artery disease
  peripheral, 466-471
Arterial lumen
  after coronary stenting, 145
  after directional coronary atherectomy, 139
  after PTCA, 133-134
Arterial switch operation, 407

Arteriovenous malformation, pulmonary, 412
Aspirin
in atrial fibrillation, 275-276
in coronary stenting, 145
in myocardial infarction, 217-222
at discharge, 193, 194
effect of previous therapy with,
189-190
during hospitalization, 192, 194
in myocardial ischemia, 98, 99, 105
in unstable angina pectoris, 86
Atenolol
in hypertension, 322
in myocardial ischemia, 104-105
Atherectomy, 136-148
embolization in, 165
stenting with, 141-148
Atherosclerosis, 1-60. *See also* Coronary artery disease
antioxidant vitamins in, 29-30
arterial dilatation in, 53
body weight in, 31-34
after cardiac transplantation, 453-454
cholestyramine in, 29
cigarette smoking in, 36-41
colestipol in, 27-28
diabetes mellitus in, 41-42
diet in, 19-22
dilatation in, 64
endothelial-cell dysfunction in, 42-43
estrogen in, 43-46
fetal and infant growth in, 50
fluvastatin in, 24
gemfibrozil in, 24-27
homocysteine in, 46-49
hyperhomocysteinemia in, 467-469
left ventricular hypertrophy in, 49-50
lipids in, 5-19. *See also* Lipids
lovastatin in, 22-23, 27-29, 105
low-density lipoprotein apheresis in,
30-31
niacin in, 28-29
physical activity in, 34-36
pravastatin in, 23-26, 107
psyllium mucilloid in, 28-29
risk factors for, 1-5
in men, 50-55
simvastatin in, 24-27
Athletes, syncope in, 295
Atresia
aortic valve, 385-387
coronary sinus, 410
pulmonic valve, 378-380
Atrial fibrillation, 269-281
amiodarone in, 276
anticoagulants in, 273-275
aspirin in, 275-276

atrial thrombi in, 280-281
after bypass surgery, 158
cardioversion in, 277-278
cerebral infarction in, 271-273
Cheyne-Stokes respirations and, 427
diltiazem in, 276-277
history of, 269, 270-274
prevalence of, 270-272
quinidine in, 276
radiofrequency catheter ablation in,
278-280
resistant, 280
risk factors for, 269-270
in supraventricular tachycardia, 281
warfarin in, 275-276
Atrial natriuretic peptide
blood pressure and, 318
in hypertension, 318
Atrial septal aneurysm, 471-473
Atrial septal defect, 369-370
Fontan procedure in, 403-404
Atrial tachycardia, 393-394
Atrioventricular septal defect, 370-372
Atrium
stroke and, 471
thrombi of, 471
in atrial fibrillation, 273, 277, 280-
281
Augmentation of ST segment elevation,
249

Baldness in myocardial infarction, 188-
189
Balloon-expandable intravascular
stents, 397-399
Balloon in PTCA, 121
Balloon valvuloplasty, 335-337
Benazepril in hypertension, 322
Betaxolol in hypertension, 323
Bidirectional cavopulmonary shunt,
399-400
Bidirectional Glenn procedure, 400-401
Biochemical markers of reperfusion,
249-250
Bioprostheses, porcine, 342-345
Bivalirudin
after PTCA, 124
in thrombolysis, 246-247
in unstable angina pectoris, 88
Blalock-Taussig shunt, 409-410
Bleeding
after bypass surgery, 162
in PTCA, 123-124
β-Blockers
in cardiac arrest, 291-292
in hypertension, 320, 321-324
lipid levels and, 324-325
in myocardial infarction, 220-222

at discharge, 193, 194
myocardial infarction from, 321
Blood flow
in diabetes mellitus, 41
smoking and, 39-40
Blood glucose, myocardial infarction and, 195
Blood lipids. *See* Lipids
Blood pressure, 315-334. *See also* Hypertension
myocardial infarction and, 195, 202-204
Blood urea nitrogen in bypass grafting, 162
Body fat in atherosclerosis, 31-34
Body mass index
in bypass surgery, 157-158
in cardiovascular disease, 32
myocardial infarction and, 195
Body weight in atherosclerosis, 31-34
Bradykinin, hypertension and, 318-319
Breathing, sleep-disordered, 427
Bretylium in ventricular arrhythmias, 287-288
Bumetanide in hypertension, 323
Bundle branch block, 300
Bypass surgery, 148-168
abdominal aortic aneurysmal surgery and, 156-157
angina after, 159
angioplasty and, 152-153, 165
atherectomy and, 165
atrial fibrillation after, 158
bleeding in, 162
blood urea nitrogen in, 162
carotid endarterectomy and, 155-156
in chronic obstructive pulmonary disease, 151-152
in coronary artery disease, 113-119
deep vein thrombosis after, 159-160
in familial hypercholesterolemia, 154
in hypertrophic cardiomyopathy, 361-362
ileal, 231, 232
implantable cardioverter defibrillator and, 155
left ventricular function after, 158
minimal access, 166, 167
mortality in, 165-167
in myocardial infarction, 257
in octogenarians, 151
outcome of, 149-150
body size and, 157-158
patency in, 164-165
with peripheral vascular disease, 154-155
physical and psychological function after, 161, 162

regionalization of, 150
rehabilitation after, 160-161
review of, 148
risk factors after, 159, 160
Society of Thoracic Surgeons National Cardiac Database on, 148, 149
after stenting, 153-154
survival after, 163-166
thyroid hormone treatment after, 162-163
waiting for, 150-151
without cardiopulmonary bypass, 167-168

Calcium
in left atrial wall, 335
by ultrafast computed tomography, 69-71
Calcium antagonists
in hypertension, 320
lipid levels and, 324-325
in myocardial infarction, 221-222, 321
Candoxatrilat in congestive heart failure, 438
Captopril
in congestive heart failure, 433
in hypertension, 322, 323, 332
in myocardial infarction, 223-226, 227
Carcinoid heart disease, 473-474
Cardiac arrest, 289-293
neurological status after, 409
Cardiac catheterization, transhepatic, 396-397
Cardiac isomerism, 412-413
Cardiac neoplasms, 414
Cardiac pacing
atrial fibrillation and, 269-270
in congestive heart failure, 441
in syncope, 296
Cardiac rhabdomyoma, 414-415
Cardiac rupture, 215-216
Cardiac tamponade, 457-459
Cardiac transplantation, 445-457
in congenital heart disease, 445-446
in congestive heart failure, 426
coronary artery disease after, 452-457
in end-stage heart failure, 445
HLA matching in, 449-450
hypercholesterolemia after, 448-449
immunosuppression after, 451
ketoconazole in, 447-448
left ventricular ejection fraction after, 451-452
mitral regurgitation after, 452
mortality after, 446-447

Cardiac transplantation *(Continued)*
  quality of life after, 447
  reinnervation after, 451, 452
  rejection of, 445, 450
  tricuspid regurgitation after, 452
  troponin T in, 451-452
Cardiogenic shock after myocardial infarction, 215
Cardiologist in unstable angina pectoris, 79
Cardiomegaly, 195
Cardiomyopathy
  dilated, 355-357
  hypertrophic, 357-362
    genetic studies of, 360-361
    history of, 358
    isoproterenol in, 358-359
    nonsurgical treatment of, 361
    paced electrogram fractionation in, 359-360
    prevalence of, 357-358
    surgical treatment of, 361-362
    tacrolimus therapy in, 362
  restrictive, 365
Cardiopulmonary bypass
  bypass surgery without, 167-168
  neurological status after, 409
Cardiopulmonary resuscitation, 289-290
Cardioversion
  in atrial fibrillation, 277-278
  implantable cardioverter/defibrillators, 301-308
  in bypass surgery, 155
Carnitine
  in atherosclerosis, 470
  in myocardial infarction, 231
β-Carotene in hyperlipidemia, 29-30
Carotid artery stenosis, 466-469
Carotid endarterectomy
  in bypass surgery, 155-156
  in carotid artery stenosis, 466-469
Carpentier-Edwards bioprostheses, 343-344
  in aortic valve replacement, 347
  in tricuspid valve replacement, 345-346
Carvedilol in congestive heart failure, 437-438
Catheter ablation
  in atrial fibrillation, 278-280
  in ventricular arrhythmias, 288
    with dilated cardiomyopathy, 355-356
Catheterization, transhepatic cardiac, 396-397
Cavopulmonary anastomotic procedures, 399-402
Cerebral infarction, 271-273

Cheyne-Stokes respirations, 427
Chimeric monoclonal antibody c7E3 in PTCA, 123
Chiorthalidone in hypertension, 323
Cholesterol. *See also* Lipids
  atherosclerosis and, 19-22
  bypass surgery and, 159
  cardiac transplantation and, 448-449
  cholestyramine and, 29
  colestipol and, 27-28
  coronary events and, 111
  in familial hypercholesterolemia, 154
  fluvastatin and, 24
  hormone replacement therapy and, 45
  lovastatin and, 27-28, 29
  myocardial infarction and, 195, 259-260
  niacin and, 28
  pravastatin and, 23, 24
  psyllium mucilloid and, 28-29
  after PTCA, 133
  simvastatin and, 24-27
Cholestyramine
  in hyperlipidemia, 29
  in myocardial ischemia, 106-107
Chronic obstructive pulmonary disease, 151-152
Cigarette smoking
  atherosclerosis and, 36-41
  bypass surgery and, 159
  cardiac arrest and, 291
  myocardial infarction and, 188-190, 193-195
  thrombolysis and, 238
Cilazapril in restenosis, 132
Circadian variation in angina pectoris, 91, 92
Claudication, intermittent, 11
C3 levels in myocardial infarction, 190-191
Clinical depression
  after bypass surgery, 161
  in coronary artery disease, 63-64
  in myocardial infarction, 209
Clonidine in hypertension, 323
Coagulation factor V, 53-54
Coarctation, aortic, 387-389
Cocaine
  myocardial infarction and, 196
  myocardial ischemia and, 65
Cognition, hypertension and, 317
Cold pressure test, 43
Colestipol in hyperlipidemia, 27-29
Complex lesions, 140
Computed tomography
  graft patency by, 164-165
  single-photon emission

after bypass surgery, 164
  in coronary artery disease, 67-68
  ultrafast, coronary calcium by, 69-71
Congenital heart disease, 369-423
  allografts in, 402-403
  anastomotic procedures in, 399-402
  anomalous pulmonary venous connec-
    tion in, 389-390
  aortic atresia in, 385-387
  aortic coarctation in, 387-389
  aortic obstruction in, 406-407
  aortic stenosis in, 384-385
  arrhythmias in, 393-396
  atrial septal defect in, 369-370
  atrioventricular septal defect in, 370-
    372
  cardiopulmonary bypass in, 409
  coronary arterial anomaly in, 390-392
  coronary sinus atresia in, 410
  extracorporeal membrane oxygen-
    ation in, 408-409
  Fontan procedure in, 403-406
  homografts in, 402-403
  hypothermic cardiac arrest in, 409
  infective endocarditis in, 415-416
  in-hospital mortality in, 414
  intra-aortic spring coil loops in, 411
  isomerism in, 412-413
  Kawasaki disease in, 415
  left-sided anomalies in, 408
  mitral valve disease in, 392-393
  modified Blalock-Taussig shunt in,
    409-410
  neoplasms in, 414
  prenatal echocardiography in, 413
  pulmonary arteriovenous malforma-
    tion in, 412
  pulmonic atresia in, 378-380
  pulmonic stenosis in, 374-378
  renal replacement therapy in, 411
  rhabdomyoma in, 414-415
  right ventricular function in, 411-412
  stents in, 397-399
  superior vena caval flow in, 416
  supraventricular aortic stenosis in,
    385
  thoracoscopic surgery in, 410-411
  transhepatic cardiac catheterization
    in, 396-397
  transplantation in, 445-446
  transposition in
    complete, 380-383
    corrected, 383-384
  truncus arteriosus in, 384
  tuberous sclerosis in, 414-415
  ultrasonic imaging in, 413
  univentricular heart in, 407-408
  ventricular septal defect in, 372-374

Congestive heart failure, 425-444
  abdominal aortic aneurysmal surgery
    and, 157
  Cheyne-Stokes respirations in, 427
  electrocardiography in, 430
  endothelial cell dysfunction in, 430-
    431
  home care in, 426
  hospitalization in, 425-426
  implantable defibrillators in, 432
  after myocardial infarction, 214-215
  neurohumoral variability in, 429
  skeletal muscle oxygenation in, 428-
    429
  sleep-disordered breathing in, 427
  transplantation for, 426
  treatment of, 432-442
    ACE inhibitors in, 432-433, 435-
      436
    amiodarone in, 439
    L-arginine in, 440
    candoxatrilat in, 438
    captopril in, 433
    carvedilol in, 437-438
    digoxin in, 433, 435-437
    diuretics in, 435-436
    dual-chamber pacing in, 441
    enalapril in, 433-435
    fosinopril in, 435
    hydralazine in, 438-439
    ibopamine in, 436-437
    losartan in, 434-435
    metoprolol in, 438
    nitrate in, 438-439
    respiratory muscle training in, 440
    thiamine in, 439-440
    ventricular assist device in, 441-
      442
  tumor necrosis factor soluble recep-
    tors in, 431-432
  ventricular arrhythmias in, 284-285
  ventricular ejection fraction in, 428
Conjugated equine estrogen, 44
Converting enzyme inhibitors, 324-325
Coronary arteries
  aneurysms of, 66-67
  angioplasty of. *See* Angioplasty
  angioscopy of, 75-76
    after PTCA, 132
    in stable angina pectoris, 91
    in unstable angina pectoris, 83-84
  anomalies of, 390-392
  atherosclerosis of, 1-60. *See also* Ath-
    erosclerosis
  bypass grafting of, 148-168. *See also*
    Bypass surgery
  in cardiac arrest, 292-293
  in diabetes mellitus, 41

Coronary arteries *(Continued)*
  narrowing of
    after bypass surgery, 163
    in stable angina pectoris, 89-91
    in unstable angina pectoris, 80
  occlusion of, 75
  patency of
    in coronary artery disease, 78-79
    by thrombolytic therapy, 254
  in stable angina pectoris, 91, 92
  in ventricular arrhythmias, 286
Coronary artery disease, 61-179
  aneurysms in, 66-67
  angioplasty in
    versus bypass, 113-119
    percutaneous transluminal, 119-
      136. *See also* Percutaneous
      transluminal coronary angi-
      oplasty
  atherectomy in, 136-148
    stenting with, 141-148
  atherosclerosis in, 1-60. *See also* Ath-
    erosclerosis
  blood pressure in, 202-204
  bypass grafting in, 148-168. *See also*
    Bypass surgery
  after cardiac transplantation, 448,
    452-457
  cocaine-associated myocardial isch-
    emia in, 65
  detection of, 67-77
    angiography in, 75
    angioscopy in, 75-76
    computed tomography in, 69-71
    costs of, 67-68
    echocardiography in, 72-73
    left main equivalent disease in, 76-
      77
    stress testing in, 71-72
    ultrasonography in, 73-75
  echocardiography of, 212
  energy expenditure in, 67, 68
  exercise capacity in, 212
  in familial hypercholesterolemia, 65
  functional status in, 62
  heart rate in, 63
  hypertension in, 316
  lipids in, 14-15
  myocardial bridges in, 64
  myocardial ischemia in, 98-113. *See*
    also Myocardial ischemia
  preoperative assessment of, 61-62
  prognosis for, 77-79
  psychological distress in, 63-64
  risk factors in, 61
  stable angina pectoris in, 88-92
  survival in, 62-63
  syndrome X in, 95-98

  unstable angina pectoris in, 79-88.
    See also Unstable angina pectoris
  waiting times for procedures in, 65,
    66
  in young adults, 205
Coronary atherectomy, 136-148
  embolization in, 165
  stenting with, 141-148
Coronary calcium, 69-71
Coronary sinus atresia, 410
Coronary spasm
  in syndrome X, 96
  ultrasonography of, 74
Coronary stenting
  bypass surgery after, 153-154
  in coronary plaques, 140
  in directional coronary atherectomy,
    141-148
Cost considerations
  in coronary angioplasty, 125-126, 127
  in coronary artery disease
    of diagnostic tests, 67-68
    of psychological distress, 63
  in coronary stenting, 146-147
  in hyperlipidemia, 22-23
  in PTCA, 125-126, 127
Creatine kinase–MB isoenzyme, 196-
  199
Cyclosporine in cardiac transplantation,
  448

Damus-Kaye-Stansel procedure, 407-
  408
Death. *See also* Mortality
  cardiac, 290
  sudden, 89, 90
Deep vein thrombosis, 159-160
Defibrillators, implantable
  in bypass surgery, 155
  in congestive heart failure, 432
Depression
  after bypass surgery, 161
  in coronary artery disease, 63-64
  in myocardial infarction, 209
Dexamethasone in hypertension, 332
Dextran in coronary stenting, 145
Diabetes mellitus
  in atherosclerosis, 41-42
  in PTCA, 130, 131
Diastolic blood pressure, 202
Diet
  fish and mercury in, 51-52
  low-fat, 19-22
    in stable angina pectoris, 92
Digoxin
  in congestive heart failure, 433, 435-
    437
  myocardial infarction and, 195

in supraventricular tachycardia, 394
Dilatation in coronary artery disease, 64
Dilated cardiomyopathy, 355-357
Diltiazem
  in atrial fibrillation, 276-277
  in hypertension, 322
  in myocardial ischemia, 102-103
  in unstable angina pectoris, 86
Dipyridamole
  in coronary stenting, 145
  in stress testing, 71
  in valve replacement, 348-350
Directional coronary atherectomy, 136-148
  embolization in, 165
  stenting with, 141-148
Dissection in aortic disease, 466
Distal coronary atherectomy, 165
Diuretics
  in congestive heart failure, 435-436
  in hypertension, 320, 326
  lipids and, 324-325
  myocardial infarction and, 195, 321
Dobutamine in stress testing, 72
Doxazosin in hypertension, 323
Dual-chamber pacing
  atrial fibrillation and, 269-270
  in congestive heart failure, 441
Dysplasia, ventricular, 364-365
Dystrophy, myotonic, 363-364

Echocardiography
  in coronary artery disease, 72-73
  in left-sided obstruction, 413
  in mitral regurgitation, 337
  in myocardial infarction, 199, 211-212
Ectopic tachycardia, atrial, 393
Ejection fraction
  abdominal aortic aneurysmal surgery and, 156-157
  after cardiac transplantation, 451-452
  carvedilol and, 437
  in congestive heart failure, 20, 428
  digoxin and, 20
  losartan and, 434
  in mitral regurgitation, 338
  in myocardial infarction, 193, 208, 210
  in myocarditis, 365
  thiamine and, 439-440
  in ventricular arrhythmias, 283-284
Elderly
  bypass surgery in, 151
  lipid levels in, 9
  myocardial infarction in, 191
  necropsy in, 476
  unstable angina pectoris in, 82-83

Electrocardiography
  ambulatory, 309
  in congestive heart failure, 430
  in myocardial infarction, 210-211
  after PTCA, 132
Electroencephalography, 67-68
Electrogram fractionation, 359-360
Embolism
  in distal coronary atherectomy, 165
  pulmonary, 459-460
Enalapril
  in congestive heart failure, 433-435
  in hypertension, 322, 323, 326-329
  in myocardial infarction, 226-228
Endarterectomy, carotid, 466-469
Endocarditis, infective, 340-342
  prophylaxis for, 415-416
Endothelial function
  in atherosclerosis, 42-43
  in congestive heart failure, 430-431
  in hypertension, 318-319
  smoking and, 38-39
End-stage heart failure, 445
Energy expenditure from household tasks, 67, 68
Estradiol, atherosclerosis and, 44
Estrogen
  in atherosclerosis, 43-46
  in myocardial ischemia, 112, 113
Ethnic groups
  bypass surgery and, 160-161
  left ventricular hypertrophy and, 49-50
  myocardial infarction and, 181, 208, 209
  PTCA and, 120, 121
  syndrome X and, 95-96
Euthyroid state, 16
Exercise testing
  in coronary artery disease
    computed tomography in, 67-68
    diagnosis of, 67-68
    echocardiography in, 72
    pharmacologic agents in, 71-72
    prognosis for, 77-78
  in myocardial infarction, 206-207
  after PTCA, 132
  silent myocardial ischemia with, 93-94
Exercise training
  in atherosclerosis, 34-36
  in coronary artery disease, 34
  in dilated cardiomyopathy, 356-357
  in hypertension, 319
  lipid levels and, 17-18
  in myocardial infarction, 212-213
  respiratory muscle, 440
  in stable angina pectoris, 92

Exercise training *(Continued)*
  syncope during, 295
Extracorporeal membrane oxygenation,
  408-409

Facial wrinkling in myocardial infarction, 188-189
Fallot, tetralogy of, 374-378
Familial hypercholesterolemia
  bypass surgery after, 154
  coronary artery disease in, 65
Familial hypertrophic cardiomyopathy,
  360-361
Fasting in atherosclerosis, 13
Fat
  atherosclerosis and, 19-21
  body, 31-34
Fatty acids
  in cardiac arrest, 292
  in myocardial ischemia, 110-112
Felodipine in hypertension, 322
Fetus
  atherosclerosis and, 50
  cardiac neoplasms and, 414
Fibrillation
  atrial, 269-281
    amiodarone in, 276
    anticoagulants in, 273-275
    aspirin in, 275-276
    atrial thrombi in, 280-281
    after bypass surgery, 158
    cardioversion in, 277-278
    cerebral infarction in, 271-273
    Cheyne-Stokes respirations and,
      427
    diltiazem in, 276-277
    history of, 269, 270-274
    prevalence of, 270-272
    quinidine in, 276
    radiofrequency catheter ablation in,
      278-280
    resistant, 280
    risk factors for, 269-270
    in supraventricular tachycardia,
      281
    warfarin in, 275-276
  ventricular, 359
Fibrinogen after PTCA, 134
Fibrinolytic parameters, 51
Fish, dietary, 51-52, 110
Fitness
  in atherosclerosis, 34-36
  in coronary artery disease, 34
  in dilated cardiomyopathy, 356-357
  in hypertension, 319
  lipid levels and, 17-18
  in myocardial infarction, 212-213
  in stable angina pectoris, 92

  syncope and, 295
Flecainide
  in atrial fibrillation, 280
  in supraventricular tachycardia, 394
  in ventricular tachycardia, 395
Fluvastatin in hyperlipidemia, 24
Follow-up for angioplasty, 129-130
Fontan procedure
  in congenital heart disease, 403-406
  in pulmonary stenosis, 402
Fosinopril
  in congestive heart failure, 435
  in hypertension, 322
Fractionation in hypertrophic cardiomyopathy, 359-360
Fracture, mechanical valve strut, 349-
  351
French paradox of atherosclerosis, 51
Functional status of coronary artery disease, 62
Furosemide in hypertension, 323

Gemfibrozil in hyperlipidemia, 24-27
Gender
  bypass surgery and, 160-161
  left ventricular hypertrophy and, 49-
    50
  myocardial infarction and, 181, 208,
    209
  PTCA and, 120, 121
  syndrome X and, 95-96
Genetics
  in atherosclerosis, 53-54
  in conduction disturbances, 299
  in dilated cardiomyopathy, 357
  in hypertrophic cardiomyopathy,
    360-361
Gianturco-Roubin stent, 141
Glenn procedure, 400-401
Glomerular filtration rate, 325
Glucose, blood, 195
Glyceryl trinitrate in unstable angina
  pectoris, 86, 87
Gore-tex shunt, 385-386
Graying of hair, 188-189
Green tea in atherosclerosis, 55
Guanabenz in hypertension, 323
Guanfacine in hypertension, 323

Hair, graying of, 188-189
Hairy-cell leukemia, 16
Head-up tilt testing, 293-295
Heart
  anomalies of
    hypoplastic, 385-386
    nonhypoplastic, 408
  blockage of, 300
  disease of

carcinoid, 473-474
congenital, 369-423. *See also* Congenital heart disease
myocardial, 355-367. *See also* Myocardial heart disease
pericardial, 457-459
valvular, 335-353. *See also* Valvular heart disease
failure of
congestive, 425-444. *See also* Congestive heart failure
end-stage, 445
rate of
in cardiac arrest, 292
in coronary artery disease, 63
in mental stress, 78
in myocardial infarction, 199
transplantation of, 445-457
in congenital heart disease, 445-446
coronary artery disease after, 452-457
in end-stage heart failure, 445
HLA matching in, 449-450
hypercholesterolemia after, 448-449
immunosuppression after, 451
ketoconazole in, 447-448
left ventricular ejection fraction after, 451-452
mitral regurgitation after, 452
mortality after, 446-447
quality of life after, 447
reinnervation after, 451, 452
rejection of, 445, 450
tricuspid regurgitation after, 452
troponin T in, 451-452
univentricular, 407-408
Hemorrhage
after bypass surgery, 162
in PTCA, 123-124
Hemostatic device in PTCA, 124-125
Heparin
in bypass surgery, 159
in coronary stenting, 145
in myocardial infarction, 192, 194
in myocardial ischemia, 105
in thrombolysis, 246-247
in unstable angina pectoris, 86
Hepatitis C viral infection, 366
Hereditary dilated cardiomyopathy, 357
Heterozygous familial hypercholesterolemia, 65
High-density lipoproteins
atherosclerosis and, 7, 12-13, 19-21
bypass surgery and, 159
coronary events and, 111
gemfibrozil and, 24-27
hypercholesterolemia and, 154
myocardial infarction and, 260

psyllium mucilloid and, 28-29
PTCA and, 133
simvastatin and, 24-27
Hirudin after PTCA, 135
Hirulog
after PTCA, 124
in thrombolysis, 246-247
in unstable angina pectoris, 88
HIV, 362-363
HLA matching in cardiac transplantation, 449-450
Home care in congestive heart failure, 426
Homocysteine in atherosclerosis, 46-49, 467-468
Homografts
in aortic valve replacement, 348
in congenital heart disease, 402-403
Hospitalization
in congenital heart disease, 414
in congestive heart failure, 425-426
in PTCA, 126-128
Household tasks, 67, 68
Human immunodeficiency virus, 362-363
Hydralazine
in congestive heart failure, 438-439
in hypertension, 323
Hypercholesterolemia
in atherosclerosis, 1-3
bypass surgery after, 154
after cardiac transplantation, 448-449
cholestyramine in, 29
coronary artery disease in, 65
endothelial-cell dysfunction in, 42-43
lovastatin in, 29
pravastatin in, 23
vascular dysfunction in, 46
Hyperhomocysteinemia, 47
in atherosclerosis, 467-468
Hyperinsulinemia, 96
Hyperlipidemia, 22-31
antioxidant vitamins in, 29-30
cholestyramine in, 29
colestipol in, 27-28
fluvastatin in, 24
gemfibrozil in, 24-27
lipoprotein apheresis in, 30-31
lovastatin in, 22-23, 27-29
niacin in, 28-29
pravastatin in, 23-26
psyllium mucilloid in, 28-29
simvastatin in, 24-27
Hypertension, 315-334
in atherosclerosis, 1-3
atrial natriuretic peptide in, 318
drugs, poisons, and foods in, 315
endothelial function in, 318-319

Hypertension *(Continued)*
  late-life cognition and, 317
  mortality in, 316-317
  myocardial infarction and, 195
  nonsteroidal anti-inflammatory drugs
    and, 315-316
  pulmonary, 474-475
  small reductions in, 316
  treatment of, 319-332
    captopril in, 332
    change of, 321-324
    dexamethasone in, 332
    enalapril in, 326-329
    exercise in, 319
    losartan in, 329, 331, 332
    myocardial infarction in, 320-321
    pravastatin in, 23
    renal function in, 325-326
    serum lipids in, 324-325
    thiazides in, 326-328
    trends in, 319-320, 322-323
Hypertrophic cardiomyopathy, 357-362
  genetic studies of, 360-361
  history of, 358
  isoproterenol in, 358-359
  nonsurgical treatment of, 361
  paced electrogram fractionation in,
    359-360
  prevalence of, 357-358
  surgical treatment of, 361-362
  tacrolimus therapy in, 362
Hypertrophy, ventricular, 49-50
Hypocholesterolemia, 16
Hypoplastic anomalies, 385-386
Hypothermic cardiac arrest, 409
Hypothyroidism, 16-17

Ibopamine in congestive heart failure,
  436-437
Ibuprofen in hypertension, 315-316
Idiopathic cardiomyopathy
  dilated, 355-357
  restrictive, 365
Ileal bypass, 231, 232
Immunosuppression
  after cardiac transplantation, 451
  for myocarditis, 365-366
Implantable defibrillators
  in bypass surgery, 155
  in congestive heart failure, 432
Indapamide in hypertension, 323
Infarction
  cerebral, 271-273
  myocardial, 181-268. *See also* Myocardial infarction
  ventricular, 213-214
Infective endocarditis, 340-342
  prophylaxis for, 415-416

Injury, lipids in, 15
Insulin
  in atherosclerosis, 13
  in myocardial infarction, 230-231
  in vasospastic angina, 96
Insulin-dependent diabetes mellitus, 41
Integrelin in PTCA, 123
Interleukin-2 receptors in cardiomyopathy, 357
Intermittent claudication, 11
Internist management of angina pectoris, 79
Intra-aortic spring coil loops, 411
Intra-atrial reentrant tachycardia, 393
Intracoronary angioscopy, 83-84
Intravascular stents, 397-399
Intravascular ultrasonography
  in congenital heart disease, 413
  in coronary aneurysms, 66-67
  in coronary artery disease, 73-75
  after PTCA, 125
  in unstable angina pectoris, 83-84
Ischemia, myocardial, 98-113. *See also*
  Myocardial ischemia
Isomerism, cardiac, 412-413
Isoproterenol
  in hypertrophic cardiomyopathy,
    358-359
  in provocation maneuvers, 294
Isosorbide in myocardial ischemia, 100
Isradipine in hypertension, 322
Isthmic coarctation, 387-389

Kawasaki disease, 415
Ketoconazole in cardiac transplantation, 447-448

Left atrium, 471
Left coronary artery spasm, 96
Left main artery
  equivalent disease of, 76-77
  narrowing of, 163
Left-sided heart anomalies
  hypoplastic, 385-386
  nonhypoplastic, 408
Left-sided obstruction, 413
Left ventricle
  abdominal aortic aneurysmal surgery
    and, 156-157
  in aortic regurgitation, 340
  in aortic stenosis, 339
  after bypass surgery, 158
  after cardiac transplantation, 451-452
  in congestive heart failure, 433-434
    carvedilol and, 437
    digoxin and, 435
    losartan and, 434
    thiamine and, 439-440

in HIV, 362
in hypertrophic cardiomyopathy, 358
hypertrophy of, 49-50
in mitral regurgitation, 338
in myocardial infarction
    gender and, 208, 210
    on Holter monitoring, 205
    quality care and, 193
in myocarditis, 365
in β-thalassemia major, 364
in ventricular arrhythmias, 283-284
Left ventricular assist device, 441-442
Leukemia, 16
Leukocyte differential, 196-199
Liothyronine sodium after bypass surgery, 162-163
Lipids, 5-19
    apolipoprotein E in, 11-12
    atherosclerosis and, 19-21
        risk for, 5-9
    in coronary artery disease, 14-15
    coronary events and, 111
    in hairy-cell leukemia, 16
    high-density, 12-13
    hormone replacement therapy and, 45
    in hypertension, 324-325
    in hypothyroidism, 16-17
    insulin levels and, 13
    lipoprotein (a) in, 11
    low values of, 9-11
    nonsteroidal anti-inflammatory drugs and, 18-19
    running and, 17-18
    soy protein and, 18
    in stroke, 15
    in suicide, 15
Lipoproteins
    atherosclerosis and
        low-fat diet in, 19-21
        prediction of, 11
        risk for, 7
        subfractions of, 12-13
    bypass surgery and, 159
    cholestyramine and, 29
    colestipol and, 27-28
    coronary events and, 111
    in familial hypercholesterolemia, 154
    fluvastatin and, 24
    gemfibrozil and, 24-27
    hormone replacement therapy and, 45
    hypercholesterolemia and, 154
    in hyperlipidemia, 30-31
    lovastatin and, 27-29
    myocardial infarction and, 260
    niacin and, 28
    pravastatin and, 23, 24

psyllium mucilloid and, 28-29
PTCA and, 133
simvastatin and, 24-27
Lisinopril in hypertension, 322, 323
Long QT interval syndrome, 296-298
Long-term follow-up for PTCA, 129-130
Losartan
    in congestive heart failure, 434-435
    in hypertension, 329, 331, 332
Lovastatin
    in hyperlipidemia, 27-28
        cost effectiveness of, 22-23
    in myocardial ischemia, 105-107
Low-cholesterol diet, 19-22
Low-density lipoproteins
    atherosclerosis and, 19-21
    bypass surgery and, 159
    cholestyramine and, 29
    colestipol and, 27-28
    coronary events and, 111
    fluvastatin and, 24
    gemfibrozil and, 24-27
    hormone replacement therapy and, 45
    hypercholesterolemia and, 154
    in hyperlipidemia, 30-31
    lovastatin and, 27-28, 29
    niacin and, 28
    pravastatin and, 23, 24
    PTCA and, 133
    simvastatin and, 24-27
Low-fat diet
    in atherosclerosis, 19-22
    in stable angina pectoris, 92
Low-flow cardiopulmonary bypass, 409
Luminal diameter
    after coronary stenting, 145
    after directional coronary atherectomy, 139
    after PTCA, 133-134

Magnesium sulfate in myocardial infarction, 222, 224-226, 227
Magnetic resonance imaging in mitral regurgitation, 338
Malignant disorders, 16
Marfan syndrome, 461-463
Maximal exercise testing, 206-207
Mechanical valve strut fracture, 349-351
Mechanical valve thrombosis, 349
Medicare patient, 191-194
Medroxyprogesterone acetate, 44
Menstruation, thrombolysis during, 237-238
Mental health
    after bypass surgery, 161
    in coronary artery disease, 63-64

Mental health *(Continued)*
heart rate and, 78
in myocardial infarction, 209
silent myocardial ischemia and, 92-93
Mercury, dietary, 51-52
Methyldopa in hypertension, 323
Metoprolol
in congestive heart failure, 438
in hypertension, 322
in myocardial ischemia, 102-104
Microvascular angina, 95-98
Minimal access bypass, 166, 167
Mitral valve disorders, 392-393
prolapse in, 338-339
prosthetic replacement in, 361-362
regurgitation in, 337-338
after cardiac transplantation, 452
stenosis in, 335-337
Modified Blalock-Taussig shunt, 409-410
Mononitrate in myocardial infarction, 224-226, 227
Morbid obesity, 290
Mortality
body weight and, 33
in bypass surgery, 149-150
decline in, 166-167
gender and, 165-166
after left main narrowing, 163
in cardiac transplantation, 446-447
in congenital heart disease, 414
in congestive heart failure, 426
in coronary artery disease, 62-63
in directional coronary atherectomy, 139
in hypertension, 316-317
in myocardial infarction
age and, 183, 207
angiography and, 185-186
decrease of, 195-196
in prosthetic valve replacement, 343-344, 346
in pulmonary grafting, 402-403
in thrombolysis, 252-255
Mutation, gene, 53-54
Myectomy, septal, 361-362
Myeloid leukemia, 16
Myocardial blood flow, 39-40
Myocardial bridges, 64
Myocardial dysfunction, 94
Myocardial heart disease, 355-367
cardiomyopathy in
dilated, 355-357
hypertrophic, 357-362. *See also* Hypertrophic cardiomyopathy
restrictive, 365
hepatitis C viral infection in, 366

HIV involvement with, 362-363
myocarditis in, 365-366
myotonic dystrophy with, 363-364
β-thalassemia major with, 364
ventricular dysplasia in, 364-365
Myocardial infarction, 181-268
abdominal aortic aneurysmal surgery and, 157
ACE inhibitors in, 221-222
angina pectoris in, 205
antiarrhythmics in, 222-223
anticoagulants in, 219-222
from antihypertensive agents, 320-321
aspirin therapy in, 217-218, 221-222
effect of previous, 189-190
atherectomy in, 137-138
in atherosclerosis, 109
baldness in, 188-189
β-blockers in, 220-222
blood pressure in, 202-204
calcium antagonists in, 221-222
captopril in, 223-226, 227
cardiac arrest from, 290
after cardiac transplantation, 448
carnitine in, 231
carotid endarterectomy in, 155
C3 levels in, 190-191
with cocaine use, 196
complications of, 213-216
coronary angioplasty in, 255-257
coronary bypass in, 257
depression in, 209
diagnosis of, 196-202
echocardiography in, 211-212
electrocardiography in, 210-211
enalapril in, 226-228
exercise in, 212-213
exercise testing in, 206-207
facial wrinkling in, 188-189
gender and, 208, 209
gray hair in, 188-189
in hypertension, 320-321
infarct size in, 210, 211
insulin-glucose infusion in, 230-231
ischemic time in, 202
magnesium sulfate in, 222, 224-226, 227
management of, 216-217, 218
mononitrate in, 224-226, 227
mortality in, 195-196
neurohumoral factors in, 209-210
non–Q-wave, 199-200
in older age, 207-208
partial ileal bypass in, 231
physical activity and, 35-36
pravastatin in, 23
procedures in, 181-187

psychosocial factors in, 187-188
quality of care in, 191-194
rehabilitation in, 258-261
smoking in, 188, 189, 190
in stable angina pectoris, 89, 90
ST segment elevation in, 205-206
theophylline in, 223
thrombolysis in, 231-255. *See also*
    Thrombolysis
trandolapril in, 228-229
treatment algorithm for, 235
unrecognized, 191-195
in young adults, 205
zofenopril in, 229-230
Myocardial ischemia, 98-113
amlodipine in, 104-105
aspirin in, 98, 99, 105
atenolol in, 104-105
cholestyramine in, 106-107
cocaine-associated, 65
diltiazem in, 102-103
estrogen in, 112, 113
fatty acids in, 110-112
heparin in, 105
high-density lipoproteins in, 12
lovastatin in, 105-107
metoprolol in, 102-104
in myocardial infarction, 202
nifedipine in, 103
nitrates in, 98-101
nitroglycerin in, 104
nitroprusside in, 104
pravastatin in, 107-110
probucol in, 106-107
silent, 92-95
simvastatin in, 110, 111
after thrombolysis, 251-252
in unstable angina pectoris, 84-85
verapamil in, 103-104
zatebradine in, 112-113
Myocardial perfusion, 20
Myocarditis, 365-366
Myoglobin in myocardial infarction,
    196-199
Myotonic dystrophy, 363-364

Nabumetone, 18-19
Naproxen
in hypertension, 315-316
lipid levels and, 18-19
Narrowing, arterial
after bypass surgery, 163
in stable angina pectoris, 89-91
in unstable angina pectoris, 80
Necropsy, 476
Neoplasms, fetal cardiac, 414
Neurohumoral factors
in congestive heart failure, 429

in myocardial infarction, 209-210
Neurological status after cardiac arrest,
    409
Niacin in hyperlipidemia, 28-29
Nicardipine in hypertension, 322
Nicotine therapy, 36-38
Nifedipine
in hypertension, 322
in myocardial ischemia, 103
Nitrates
in congestive heart failure, 438-439
in myocardial ischemia, 98-101
Nitroglycerin
in myocardial infarction, 192, 194
in myocardial ischemia, 98-101, 104
thrombolysis and, 248-249
Nitroprusside in myocardial ischemia,
    104
Nonhypoplastic heart anomalies, 408
Non–Q-wave infarction, 199-200
Nonsteroidal anti-inflammatory drugs
hypertension and, 315-316
lipid levels and, 18-19
Norwood procedure
for hypoplastic anomalies, 385-386
for nonhypoplastic anomalies, 408
N-3 polyunsaturated fatty acids in car-
    diac arrest, 292

Obesity
in atherosclerosis, 31-34
cardiac arrest in, 290
Obstructive pulmonary disease, 151-152
Occlusion, coronary, 75
Octogenarians
bypass surgery in, 151
lipid levels in, 9
myocardial infarction in, 207-208
necropsy in, 476
unstable angina pectoris in, 82-83
Orifice area, 337
Ostial lesions, 138
Oxygenation
in congenital heart disease, 408-409
in congestive heart failure, 428-429

Paced electrogram fractionation, 359-
    360
Pacemakers, 300-301
Pacing
atrial fibrillation and, 269-270
in congestive heart failure, 441
in syncope, 296
Pain in myocardial infarction, 201-202
Palmaz-Schatz stent, 141-144
Palpitations, 309
Parasuicide, 15

Paroxysmal supraventricular tachycardia, 281
Partial ileal bypass, 231, 232
Passive smoking, 40-41
Patency
    in bypass surgery, 164-165
    in coronary artery disease, 78-79
    after thrombolysis, 247-248
Percutaneous balloon valvuloplasty, 335-337
Percutaneous coronary angioscopy, 91
Percutaneous transluminal coronary angioplasty, 119-136
    atherectomy versus, 137-138
    bivalirudin after, 124
    in coronary artery disease, 81-82
    costs of, 125-126, 127
    diabetes and, 130, 131
    follow-up for, 129-130
    hemostatic device in, 124-125
    hospital stay after, 126-128
    in-laboratory closure in, 121-122
    in men vs. women, 120-121
    platelet inhibition in, 122-124
    quality of life after, 128-129
    in rest angina pectoris, 119-120
    restenosis in, 131-136
    for saphenous venous graft narrowing, 120
    sixty-millimeter balloon in, 121
    transradial approach to, 119
    ultrasonography after, 125
Pericardial aortic valve, 347
Pericardial heart disease, 457-459
Peripheral vascular disease, 466-471
    bypass surgery after, 154-155
    of carotid arteries, 466-469
    in hypercholesterolemia, 46
    of leg arteries, 470-471
Personality, type A, 187-188
Pharmacological echocardiography, 211-212
Pharmacologic stress testing, 71-72
Physical activity
    in atherosclerosis, 34-36
    after bypass surgery, 161, 162
    in coronary artery disease, 34
    in dilated cardiomyopathy, 356-357
    in hypertension, 319
    lipid levels and, 17-18
    in myocardial infarction, 212-213
    in stable angina pectoris, 92
    syncope during, 295
Pindolol
    in hypertension, 323
    in syncope, 296
Plaque
    protruding, 463

ruptured, 140
Plasminogen activator
    recombinant urokinase type, 247
    tissue, 239-244
Platelet function, 103-104
Platelet inhibition therapy, 122-124
Polacrilex in nicotine therapy, 36-38
Polyunsaturated fatty acids, 292
Porcine bioprostheses, 342-345
Positron emission tomography, 67-68
Pravastatin
    in hypercholesterolemia, 448-449
    in hyperlipidemia, 23-26
    in myocardial ischemia, 107-110
Prazosin in hypertension, 323
Prenatal echocardiography, 413
Preoperative assessment of coronary artery disease, 61-62
P-R interval syndrome, 281-282
Probucol in myocardial ischemia, 106-107
Procainamide in ventricular arrhythmias, 288
Prolapse, mitral valve, 338-339
Propafenone in supraventricular tachycardia, 281
Prophylaxis, infective endocarditis, 415-416
Propranolol in hypertension, 322
Prosthetic heart valves, 342-351
    aortic
        homovital homografts for, 348
        pericardial, 347
        with small aortic root, 346-347
    dipyridamole and, 348-350
    porcine bioprostheses for, 342-345
    reoperations for, 351
    St. Jude medical prosthesis for, 342, 343
    strut fracture of, 349-351
    thrombosis of, 349
    tricuspid, 345-346
    warfarin and, 348-350
Protein, soy, 18
Proteinuria, 325
Protruding plaque, 463
Provocation maneuvers in syncope, 293-295
P-selectin
    in syndrome X, 96
    in unstable angina pectoris, 85
Psychological function
    after bypass surgery, 161, 162
    in coronary artery disease, 63-64
    heart rate and, 78
    in myocardial infarction, 209
    in myocardial ischemia, 92-93
Psychosocial factors, 187-188

Psyllium mucilloid in hyperlipidemia, 28-29
Pulmonary arteriovenous malformation, 412
Pulmonary artery
    stenosis of
        Fontan procedure in, 402
        stenting in, 398
    in tetralogy of Fallot, 374-375
Pulmonary disease, obstructive, 151-152
Pulmonary embolism, 459-460
Pulmonary hypertension, 474-475
Pulmonary transplantation, 445-457.
    See also Cardiac transplantation
Pulmonary venous connection, anomalous, 389-390
Pulmonic valve
    atresia of, 378-380
    stenosis of, 374-378

QRS morphology in ventricular arrhythmias, 285
QRS prolongation
    in congestive heart failure, 430
    in ventricular arrhythmias, 283
QT interval
    genetics and, 299
    long, 296-298
    in ventricular arrhythmias, 283-284
    in ventricular tachycardia, 395
Quality of care in myocardial infarction, 191-194
Quality of life
    after cardiac transplantation, 447
    after PTCA, 128-129
Quinapril in hypertension, 322
Quinidine in atrial fibrillation, 276
Q-wave infarction, 197
    on Holter monitoring, 205
Q-wave regression, 250

Racial groups
    bypass surgery and, 160-161
    left ventricular hypertrophy and, 49-50
    myocardial infarction and, 181, 208, 209
    PTCA and, 120, 121
    syndrome X and, 95-96
Radiofrequency catheter ablation
    in atrial fibrillation, 278-280
    in ventricular arrhythmias, 288
        with dilated cardiomyopathy, 355-356
Ramipril in hypertension, 322
Raynaud's disease, 475
Recombinant staphylokinase, 247

Recombinant urokinase type plasminogen activator, 247
Reentrant tachycardia, 393
Regionalization of bypass surgery, 150
Regurgitant orifice area, 337
Regurgitant stroke volume, 337
Regurgitation
    aortic, 340
    mitral, 337-338
        after cardiac transplantation, 452
    tricuspid, 452
Rehabilitation
    after bypass surgery, 160-161
    in myocardial infarction, 258-261
Reinnervation after cardiac transplantation, 451, 452
Rejection of cardiac transplantation, 445, 450
Renal function in hypertension, 325-326
Renal replacement therapy, 411
Reoperations in valve replacement, 351
Reperfusion
    biochemical markers of, 249-250
    tissue, 250-251
Resistant atrial fibrillation, 280
Respiratory muscle training, 440
Rest angina pectoris, 119-120
Restenosis
    after directional coronary atherectomy, 138
    in PTCA, 131-136
    stent implantation in, 146
Restenotomy for bleeding, 162
Restrictive cardiomyopathy, 365
Resuscitation, cardiopulmonary, 289-290
Reteplase in thrombolysis, 244-246
Revascularization after myocardial infarction, 186, 187
Rhabdomyoma, 414-415
Right ventricle
    in congenital heart disease, 411-412
    in congestive heart failure, 428
    dysplasia of, 364-365
    after myocardial infarction, 213-214
Risk factors
    in atherosclerosis, 1-5
        lipids in, 5-9
        in men, 50-55
    in atrial fibrillation, 269-270
    in bypass surgery, 159
    in coronary artery disease, 61
    in stable angina pectoris, 89, 90
    in unstable angina pectoris, 79-80
Running, lipid levels and, 17-18
Ruptured plaque, 140

St. Jude medical prosthesis, 342, 343
Saphenous vein graft
  angioplasty of, 146
  narrowing of, 120
Saruplase in thrombolysis, 247
Saturated fat, 19-21
Sclerosis, tuberous, 414-415
Septal aneurysm, 471-473
Septal defect
  atrial, 369-370
  atrioventricular, 370-372
  ventricular, 372-374
Septal myectomy, 361-362
Serum C3 levels, 190-191
Serum lipids, 324-325
Sex. *See* Gender
Shift work, 52-53
Shock, cardiogenic, 215
Shoveling, 473
Shunts
  in congenital heart disease, 409-410
  in hypoplastic anomalies, 385-386
Signal-averaged electrocardiography
  in congestive heart failure, 430
  in myocardial infarction, 210-211
Silent myocardial ischemia, 92-95
Simvastatin
  in hyperlipidemia, 24-27
  in myocardial ischemia, 110, 111
Single-photon emission computed to-
  mography
  after bypass surgery, 164
  in coronary artery disease, 67-68
Sixty-millimeter balloon, 121
Skeletal muscle oxygenation, 428-429
Sleep-disordered breathing, 427
Smoking
  atherosclerosis and, 36-41
  bypass surgery and, 159
  cardiac arrest and, 291
  myocardial infarction and, 188-190,
    193-195
  thrombolysis and, 238
Snow shoveling, 473
Society of Thoracic Surgeons National
  Cardiac Database, 148, 149
Sotalol
  in supraventricular tachycardia, 282
  in tachyarrhythmias, 395
  in ventricular arrhythmias, 288
Soy protein, 18
Spasm, coronary
  in syndrome X, 96
  ultrasonography of, 74
Spastic angina, 95-98
Spironolactone in hypertension, 323
Stable angina pectoris, 88-92
  nitroglycerin patch in, 98-99

Staphylokinase, recombinant, 247
Stenosis
  aortic valve, 339-340, 384-385
  carotid artery, 466-469
  mitral valve, 335-337
  pulmonary artery, 402
  pulmonic valve, 374-378
Stenting
  bypass surgery after, 153-154
  in congenital heart disease, 397-399
  in coronary plaques, 140
  in directional coronary atherectomy,
    141-148
Strecker stent, 141
Streptokinase in thrombolysis, 233,
  243-247
Stress, mental, 78
Stress testing
  in coronary artery disease
    computed tomography in, 67-68
    diagnosis of, 67-68
    echocardiography in, 72
    pharmacologic agents in, 71-72
    prognosis for, 77-78
  in myocardial infarction, 206-207
  after PTCA, 132
  silent myocardial ischemia with, 93-
    94
Stroke
  in atherosclerosis, 109
  carotid endarterectomy in, 155
  in hypertension, 316
  lipids in, 15
Stroke volume, 337
ST segment
  in myocardial infarction, 205-206
  in thrombolysis, 249
Sudden death, 89, 90
Suicide, 15
Superior vena caval flow, 416
Supraventricular aortic stenosis, 385
Supraventricular tachyarrhythmia, 395
Supraventricular tachycardia, 281-282,
  394
Survival. *See* Mortality
Sympathetic reinnervation, 452
Syncope, 293-296
Syndrome X, 95-98
Systemic hypertension, 315-334
  atrial natriuretic peptide in, 318
  drugs, poisons, and foods in, 315
  endothelial function in, 318-319
  late-life cognition and, 317
  mortality in, 316-317
  nonsteroidal anti-inflammatory drugs
    and, 315-316
  small reductions in, 316
  treatment of, 319-332

captopril in, 332
change of, 321-324
dexamethasone in, 332
enalapril in, 326-329
exercise in, 319
losartan in, 329, 331, 332
myocardial infarction in, 320-321
renal function in, 325-326
serum lipids in, 324-325
thiazides in, 326-328
trends in, 319-320, 322-323
Systolic blood pressure, 202

Tachyarrhythmia
supraventricular, 395
ventricular, 395
Tachycardia
atrial, 393-394
supraventricular, 394
Tacrolimus in hypertrophic cardiomyopathy, 362
Tamponade, cardiac, 457-459
Tasks, household, 67, 68
Tea in atherosclerosis, 55
Terazosin in hypertension, 323
Tetralogy of Fallot, 374-378
β-thalassemia major, 364
Thallium imaging
after bypass surgery, 164
in stress testing, 72
Theophylline in myocardial infarction, 223
Thiamine in congestive heart failure, 439-440
Thiazide in hypertension, 323, 326-328
Thoracoscopic surgery, 410-411
Thromboembolism. See Thrombosis
Thrombolysis, 231-255
alteplase in, 246-247
angina effects on, 238-239
anistreplase in, 244
heparin in, 246-247
hirulog in, 246-247
infarction after, 251-252
ischemia after, 251-252
in menstruating women, 237-238
in men vs. women, 235-237
mortality in, 252-255
in myocardial infarction, 192, 194
nitroglycerin in, 248-249
patency after, 247-248
Q-wave regression after, 251
reperfusion in, 249-250
reteplase in, 244-246
in smokers vs. nonsmokers, 238
staphylokinase in, 247
streptokinase in, 243-247
ST segment elevation in, 249

tissue plasminogen activator in, 239-244
tissue reperfusion in, 250-251
urokinase type plasminogen activator in, 247
use of, 232, 236
Thrombosis
in atherosclerosis, 109
atrial, 471
in atrial fibrillation, 273, 277, 280-281
after bypass surgery, 159-160
with complex lesions, 140
mechanical valve, 349
in prosthetic valve replacement, 344-345
stent, 143
in unstable angina pectoris, 84
venous, 459-460
Thyroid hormone treatment, 162-163
Tilt testing in syncope, 293-295
Tissue plasminogen activator in thrombolysis, 239-244
Tissue reperfusion after thrombolysis, 250-251
Tomography
computed
in coronary artery disease, 67-68
coronary calcium by, 69-71
graft patency by, 164-165
positron emission, 67-68
Torsade de Pointes, 298
Training
in coronary artery disease, 34
in dilated cardiomyopathy, 356-357
in hypertension, 319
lipid levels and, 17-18
in myocardial infarction, 212-213
respiratory muscle, 440
in stable angina pectoris, 92
syncope during, 295
Trandolapril in myocardial infarction, 228-229
Transdermal nicotine therapy, 37-38
Transdermal nitroglycerin patch, 98-101
Transesophageal echocardiography, 72-73
Transhepatic cardiac catheterization, 396-397
Transplantation, heart, 445-457
in congenital heart disease, 445-446
in congestive heart failure, 426
coronary artery disease after, 452-457
ejection fraction after, 451-452
in end-stage heart failure, 445
HLA matching in, 449-450
hypercholesterolemia after, 448-449

Transplantation, heart *(Continued)*
immunosuppression after, 451
ketoconazole in, 447-448
mitral regurgitation after, 452
mortality after, 446-447
quality of life after, 447
reinnervation after, 451, 452
rejection of, 445, 450
tricuspid regurgitation after, 452
troponin T in, 451-452
Transposition of great arteries
complete, 380-383
corrected, 383-384
Transradial approach to PTCA, 119
Trauma, lipids in, 15
Triamterene in hypertension, 323
Tricuspid regurgitation, 452
Tricuspid valve replacement, 345-346
Triglycerides
in atherosclerosis, 7
myocardial infarction and, 195
after PTCA, 133
Triiodothyronine after bypass surgery,
162-163
Troponin T
in cardiac transplantation, 451-452
in myocardial infarction, 196-199
Truncus arteriosus, 384
Tuberous sclerosis, 414-415
Tumor necrosis factor soluble receptors,
431-432
Type A personality, 187-188

Ulcer, atherosclerotic plaque, 463
Ultrafast computed tomography, 69-71
Ultrasonography
in congenital heart disease, 413
in coronary aneurysms, 66-67
in coronary artery disease, 73-75
after PTCA, 125
in unstable angina pectoris, 83-84
Univentricular heart, 407-408
Unrecognized myocardial infarction,
191-195
Unstable angina pectoris, 79-88
angiography in, 80-83
angioscopy in, 83-84
aspirin in, 86
atherectomy in, 136-137
diltiazem in, 86, 87
glyceryl trinitrate in, 86, 87
heparin in, 86
hirulog in, 88
ischemic threshold in, 84-85
management of, 79
P-selectin in, 85
risk stratification in, 79-80
thrombotic reactant markers in, 84

ultrasonography in, 83-84
Urokinase in thrombolysis, 247

Valvular heart disease, 335-353
aortic
atresia in, 385-387
regurgitation in, 340
stenosis in, 339-340, 384-385
infective endocarditis in, 340-342
mitral, 392-393
prolapse in, 338-339
regurgitation in, 337-338
stenosis in, 335-337
prosthetic replacement in, 342-351.
See also Prosthetic heart valves
pulmonic
atresia in, 378-380
stenosis in, 374-378
Valvuloplasty, balloon, 335-337
Variant angina, 95-98
Vascular disease, 466-471
bypass surgery after, 154-155
of carotid arteries, 466-469
in hypercholesterolemia, 46
of leg arteries, 470-471
Vasodilation
cigarette smoking and, 38-39
in diabetes mellitus, 41
in hypertension, 318-319
lipid levels and, 324-325
Vasopressor syncope, 295
Vasospasm, coronary, 74
Vena caval flow, 416
Venous graft angioplasty, 165
Venous thrombosis, 459-460
after bypass surgery, 159-160
Ventricular arrhythmias, 282-288
amiodarone in, 286-288
bretylium in, 287-288
coronary narrowing in, 286
origin of, 285
procainamide in, 288
prognostic predictors in, 282-285
radiofrequency catheter ablation in,
288
sotalol in, 288
Ventricular assist device, 441-442
Ventricular dysplasia, 364-365
Ventricular fibrillation, 359
Ventricular function
abdominal aortic aneurysmal surgery
and, 156-157
in aortic regurgitation, 340
in aortic stenosis, 339
after bypass surgery, 158
after cardiac transplantation, 451-452
carvedilol and, 437
in congenital heart disease, 411-412

in congestive heart failure, 428, 433-
434
  carvedilol and, 437
  digoxin and, 20, 435
  losartan and, 434
  thiamine and, 439-440
in HIV, 362
in hypertrophic cardiomyopathy, 358
losartan and, 434
in mitral regurgitation, 338
in myocardial infarction
  gender and, 208, 210
  on Holter monitoring, 205
  quality care and, 193
in myocarditis, 365
in β-thalassemia major, 364
in ventricular arrhythmias, 283-284
Ventricular hypertrophy, 49-50
Ventricular infarction, 213-214
Ventricular septal defect, 372-374
  Fontan procedure in, 405-406
Ventricular tachyarrhythmia, 395
Ventricular tachycardia
  in dilated cardiomyopathy, 355-356
  in hypertrophic cardiomyopathy, 359
  in myocardial infarction, 211
Verapamil

in hypertension, 315-316, 322
  in myocardial ischemia, 103-104
Vitality, after bypass surgery, 161
Vitamins in hyperlipidemia, 29-30

Waist circumference in weight measurement, 32
Warfarin
  in atrial fibrillation, 273, 275-276
  in valve replacement, 348-350
Weight
  in atherosclerosis, 31-34
  with smoking cessation, 38
Wiktor stent, 148
Work, atherosclerosis and, 52-53
Wrinkling in myocardial infarction,
188-189

Xanthelasma, 12

Young adults, myocardial infarction in,
205

Zatebradine in myocardial ischemia,
112-113
Zofenopril in myocardial infarction,
229-230